OPERATING THEATRE TECHNIQUE

*To My Wife Anne
and Son Nigel*

OPERATING THEATRE TECHNIQUE

A Textbook for Nurses, Operating Department Assistants, Medical Students, Junior Medical Staff and Operating Theatre Designers

RAYMOND J. BRIGDEN PhD SRN

Formerly Nursing Officer,
Department of Health and Social Security,
London

FIFTH EDITION

CHURCHILL LIVINGSTONE
EDINBURGH LONDON MELBOURNE AND NEW YORK 1988

CHURCHILL LIVINGSTONE
Medical Division of Longman Group UK Limited

Distributed in the United States of America by Churchill
Livingstone Inc., 1560 Broadway, New York, N.Y. 10036,
and by associated companies, branches and representatives
throughout the world.
© E. & S. Livingstone 1962, 1969
© Longman Group Limited 1974, 1980
© Longman Group UK Limited 1988

First edition 1962
Second edition 1969
Third edition 1974
Fourth edition 1980
Fifth edition 1988

ISBN 0 443 03364 1

British Library Cataloguing in Publication Data
Brigden, Raymond J. (Raymond John), *1931–*
    Operating theatre technique.—5th ed.
    1. Medicine. Surgery. Operations — Manuals
    I. title
    617'.91

Produced by Longman Group (FE) Ltd
Printed in Hong Kong

PREFACE TO THE FIFTH EDITION

This new edition has been thoroughly revised to take account of the advances which have taken place in most surgical specialties during the past six years. These have resulted in corresponding developments in operating theatre technique and instrumentation, particularly in the fields of microsurgery and endoscopy. The first section of the new edition has an additional chapter and the glossary of technical terms is now displayed as an appendix.

There has been increased delegation of capital planning to individual health authorities following the Griffiths management enquiry in 1983 on the United Kingdom National Health Service. Previously, the majority of major capital schemes were managed by regional or area health authorities. These provided appropriate nurse and medical planning expertise to supplement the user input to project teams. In many instances this is no longer possible and nurse managers and medical staff are likely to find themselves very much involved in providing the only user input to a project; the operating department is no exception. For this reason Chapter 1 has been extensively revised and extended to give general planning advice on the preparation of the user input to an operating department design brief. This takes into account the latest advice on operating department design, an example of which is that there is no microbiological basis for the traditional clean and dirty zones. Aspects of operating department management form the content of Chapter 2.

The remaining 11 chapters in the first section follow a similar arrangement as previously adopted, except that Chapter 3 is now devoted entirely to electromedical equipment, and is extended to include surgical lasers, cryoprobes, ultrasonic aspirator and infusion pumps. Chapter 11 Anaesthesia and the anaesthesia room takes account of the developments in anaesthesia systems with electro-mechanical integration. Chapter 12 Operating microscopes and Chapter 13 Fibre-optic endoscopy have been rewritten and represent the latest developments in this field.

The chapters on operative procedures have always aimed to present an overview of surgical procedures, encouraging the reader to seek more detailed information from other specialist textbooks. Within the space available it is difficult to include a description of all those operations which are in common use and also others which may be of more general interest. It is hoped readers will find that an equitable balance has been achieved.

As with previous editions, emphasis has been placed on a fully comprehensive index with extensive cross-referencing. The references included in various chapters have been selected on the basis that they provide detailed information of practical value to the reader.

During the past 26 years I have received help from many individuals in the preparation of Operating Theatre Technique; this edition is no exception. I have received a good deal of cooperation in the provision of material for inclusion in the fifth edition, and this applies particularly to the many manufacturers whose instruments and equipment are illustrated throughout the book. These are acknowledged as appropriate.

Once again space does not permit the inclusion by name of everyone who has helped in this work, but nevertheless grateful thanks are due to the Royal Berkshire Hospital, Reading, which provided facilities for preparing some of the illustrations. In particular, the author would like to thank Sister R. Clarke and Miss G. Griffiths. Thanks are due also to the following who provided material or arranged a critical appraisal of various chapters:

Anaesthesia — Dr Tony Davenport, Northwick Park Hospital, Harrow;

Colour views through endoscopes — Dr J. Leung, Prince of Wales Hospital, Hongkong; Dr D. L. Carr-Locke, University of Leicester Medical School;

Colour views through operating microscope — Professor Gruss and Dr C. Naumann, Wurzburg Neurosurgical Clinic;

Dr W. Werber, Munich; Dr Cognac, Lyon; Dr H. Schobel, St Polton;

Ulm University Eye Clinic; Frieiburg University Eye Clinic;

Fibre-optic endoscopy — Stuart Greengrass, KeyMed Ltd, and Mr H. Morishima of Olympus;

Management and Urology — Philip Clarke, Guy's Hospital, London;

Operating Department and Sterilization — Sheila Scott, DHSS;

Operating microscope — Dr Edward Hinton-Clifton, Carl Zeiss (Oberkochen) Ltd;

Ophthalmic — Philippe Arent; *Ear, Nose & Throat* — Mr T. Hayworth, Royal Berkshire Hospital, Reading;

Orthopaedics — Josephine Fox, Princess Alexandra Hospital, Harlow;

Plastic — Mary Spacy, Royal Orthopaedic Hospital, Birmingham;

Thoracic and cardiovascular — Linda Hurley, John Radcliffe Hospital, Oxford.

The work associated with this revision has been very detailed and prolonged and I am appreciative of the patience and encouragement of my wife and family at all times. As usual, the staff of Churchill Livingstone have been more than helpful in allowing for the idiosyncrasies of the author: the last 26 years have developed into a very satisfactory partnership.

It must be understood that the contents of this book and the opinions expressed by the author do not necessarily reflect the policy of the Department of Health.

Reading 1988   R.J.B.

PREFACE TO THE FIRST EDITION

For some time now the author has felt there is a need for a comprehensive textbook on theatre technique to which nurses, technicians and medical students can refer and supplement their practical experience.

This book is written primarily for personnel who intend to specialise in theatre duties, but it is hoped that house surgeons and others who may be associated with this work may derive some benefit also.

Theatre technique is now a very complex subject, and it would be impossible to include all the operations and procedures associated with the various specialities without producing a rather unwieldy volume. The author appreciates that techniques vary considerably and wishes to impress upon the reader that this book must be regarded as a basis for practical experience and study in individual units. It is hoped that advantage will be taken of the various references which have been listed if a more detailed study of a particular subject is required.

The chapters on electricity and static electricity have been included because it is felt that these subjects are of increasing importance to theatre staff. A better understanding of electrical apparatus and lighting will ensure a sensible approach to the use of such equipment in a modern operating theatre.

Emphasis has been placed upon a packet system of sterilization and the use of heat rather than chemicals whenever possible. Although nylon has been described as a wrapping material, it is accepted that many units are using paper or linen for this purpose. This is, of course, a matter of individual preference.

The chapter on ligature and suture materials has been made comprehensive in order that it may be used for reference. The sizes and technical data quoted are in accordance with BP standards.

'Assisting the surgeon and draping the operation area' is intended to help the reader to understand how this is done, combined, of course, with practical instruction from the surgeon, theatre superintendent or charge nurse. Again, methods of draping the operation area must be adapted to individual needs, but those described, if carried out correctly, will ensure the drapes remain in position during the course of operation.

The instruments described for various operations are those in common use and are arranged in sets. Substitution of instruments may be necessary according to a surgeon's individual preferences, but those shown should be adequate for the particular procedure. The outline of procedure for each operation is not intended to replace the many excellent textbooks on operative procedure, but rather to act as a general guide and handy source of reference. The reader is referred to the appropriate surgery textbook if further details are required.

The Appendix of instruments is an extraction of those in common use from the multitude illustrated in the surgical instrument catalogues. An opportunity has been taken to list technical data of orthopaedic implants as this information is not easily available from other sources at present.

Coventry 1962   R.J.B.

ACKNOWLEDGEMENTS

Acknowledgement is given to the following authors and publishers who have kindly provided illustrations for this edition:

Adams, J. Crawford (1972) *Standard Orthopaedic Operations*. Edinburgh: Churchill Livingstone.

Ballantyne, J. (1986) *Operative Surgery — The Ear, Nose and Throat*. London: Butterworths.

Bruce, J., Walmsley, R. & Ross, J. A. (1964) *Manual of Surgical Anatomy*. Edinburgh: Churchill Livingstone.

Cleland, W. P. (1968) *Operative Surgery — Thorax*. London: Butterworths.

Rintoul, R. F. (1986) *Farquharson's Textbook of Operative Surgery*. Edinburgh: Churchill Livingstone.

Garrey, M. M., Govan, A. D. T., Hodge, C. H. & Callander, R. (1972) *Gynaecology Illustrated*. Edinburgh: Churchill Livingstone.

Gillingham, F. G. (1970) *Operative Surgery — Neurosurgery*. London: Butterworths.

Gardner, J. F. & Peel, M. M. (1986) *Introduction to Sterilization and Disinfection*. Edinburgh: Churchill Livingstone.

Hall, I. S. & Coleman, B. H. (1976) *Diseases of the Nose, Throat and Ear*. Edinburgh: Churchill Livingstone.

Hall, R. M. (1972) *Air Instrument Surgery*. New York: Springer Verlag.

Howkins, J. & Bourne, G. (1977) *Shaw's Textbook of Operative Gynaecology*. Edinburgh: Churchill Livingstone.

Illingworth, C. (1973) *A Short Textbook of Surgery*. Edinburgh: Churchill Livingstone.

Irvine, W. T. (1971) *Modern Trends in Surgery*. London: Butterworths.

MacFarlane, D. A. & Thomas, L. P. (1972) *Textbook of Surgery*. Edinburgh: Churchill Livingstone.

McGregor, I. A. (1975) *Fundamental Techniques of Plastic Surgery*. Edinburgh: Churchill Livingstone.

MacLeod, D. & Hawkins, J. (1966) *Bonney's Gynaecological Surgery*. London: Baillière, Tindall & Cassell.

Martin, P. (1963) *Indications and Techniques in Arterial Surgery*. Edinburgh: Churchill Livingstone.

Movair, T. J. (1972) *Hamilton Bailey's Emergency Surgery*. Bristol: Wright.

Narborough, E. & Densley, G. (1984) Smith and Nephew — Handbook of Plaster Techniques. Hull: T. J. Smith & Nephew Ltd.

O'Brien, B. McC. (1977) *Microvascular Reconstructive Surgery*. Edinburgh: Churchill Livingstone.

Rank, B., Wakefield, A. R. & Hueston, J. T. (1973) *Surgery of Repair as Applied to Hand Injuries*. Edinburgh: Churchill Livingstone.

Robb, C. (1976) *Operative Surgery — Vascular Surgery*. London: Butterworths.

Robinson, J. O. (1965) *Surgery*. London: Longman.

Smith, G. & Aitkenhead, A. R. (1985) *Textbook of Anaesthesia*. Edinburgh: Churchill Livingstone.

Stallard, H. B. (1973) *Eye Surgery*. Bristol: Wright.

Stradling, P. (1976) *Diagnostic Bronchoscopy*. Edinburgh: Churchill Livingstone.

Swinney, J. & Hammersley, D. P. (1963) *Handbook of Operative Urology*. Edinburgh: Churchill Livingstone.

Wilson, J. N. (1976) *Watson-Jones Fractures and Joint Injuries*. Edinburgh: Churchill Livingstone.

Acknowledgement to manufacturers who have kindly provided illustrations of supplies or equipment for this edition, is given as appropriate in each chapter.

CONTENTS

1

The operating department

This chapter deals with the briefing and design of operating theatres. The main objectives are to emphasise the importance of preparing a good design brief which clearly identifies user requirements, and to describe current trends in operating theatre design.

To demonstrate the principles of good design, it is appropriate to identify those features which are considered to be ideal. However, despite the construction of many new operating departments since the previous edition of this book, many hospitals still have to utilise facilities which are *not* ideal, despite extensive upgrading schemes. But even new departments cannot be expected to fulfil all theoretical requirements as new ideas are constantly being developed, and by the time they are incorporated into buildings, fresh ones take their place on the drawing board.

The following definitions are used in this chapter:

1. *Operating department*. Comprises a unit of two or more operating suites and support accommodation.

2. *Operating suite*. Comprises the operating theatre or operating room, together with its immediate ancillary accommodation.

3. *Operating theatre*. This is the room in which surgical operations and some diagnostic procedures are carried out.

BRIEFING

If the reader ever has an opportunity to contribute to a brief for the design of an operating department, the importance of clear identification of user requirements in the brief cannot be over-emphasised. Unless this is achieved, there is a likelihood of experiencing the frustrations which may result from apparent misinterpretation of user requirements into bricks and mortar. Those commissioning a new department or working in it for the first time, who have not been involved at the planning stage, may be unaware of the operational policy assumptions on which the design was based. The adoption of policies markedly different from those originally envisaged during planning may result in day-to-day operational shortcomings and inefficient use of facilities.

The importance of preparing an accurate well thought out brief as a basis for the design of an operating department may seem obvious. But the unsatisfactory design solutions of some present operating departments suggest that in the past this was not always the case. Briefing methods and involvement of users appear to have been varied and haphazard. Often inadequate information of the real user requirements given to the designers has created

misunderstandings. Because the planning process is complex, this information gets further jumbled in the protracted period of time required to prepare the brief (Brigden, 1984). But even when full participation of users is possible, individual experience in understanding planning principles may be non-existent. This can often lead to 're-invention of the wheel', or the introduction of ideas which perhaps unbeknown to the individual have been tried in other projects and found unacceptable.

This chapter is not intended as a treatise on planning, but it can alert the reader to sources of guidance, the availability of planning aids, and give some indication of what is involved in planning operating departments. It is recommended that those readers who are asked to participate in the preparation of a design brief, either for new building or upgrading of existing accommodation, should first study this guidance (additional reading material is listed in the bibliography).

The Department of Health (DHSS) publishes a series of documents which contain information on planning for new health buildings and for upgrading existing buildings. In addition there are promotional videotapes on Briefing, Health Building Guidance and Activity Data. This guidance should be available in all National Health Service (NHS) District Health Authorities (DHAs) or may be purchased from Her Majesty's Stationery Office (HMSO), and includes the following:

Health building notes

Health Building Note No 26 — Operating Department (DHSS, 1989). This provides guidance for those planning an operating department suitable for most types of surgery practised in district general and teaching hospitals, except a few specialties such as ophthalmic or cardiac surgery, which may require modification of the common approach and design. The guidance assumes that all operating facilities in the hospital, with the exception of the maternity unit, are concentrated in the operating department, since this has been shown to be the most economic approach.

Health Building Note No 19 — Sterilizing and Disinfecting Unit (SDU) (DHSS, 1989). This covers the provision of sterilizing and disinfecting facilities for the whole hospital including the operating department. It replaces guidance on the Theatre Sterile Supply Unit (TSSU) contained in the previous edition of HBN 26, and Central Sterile Supply Departments HBN 13.

Design briefing system

Each new or revised health building note is accompanied by a companion Design Briefing System (DBS) note book. The DBS offers a disciplined check list approach, identifying the planning decisions which need to be made. A range of appropriate planning options which concentrate on the intended operational policies is printed on the right hand pages of each DBS document (Fig. 1.2), together with extracts of associated health building guidance on the left (Fig. 1.1). There is a simple referencing system which allows cross checking for compatibility of decisions made, and tracing throughout each document the consequences of changing decisions.

DBS documents are structured so that project team members can make their own record of decisions in the document itself, mostly by ticking options or entering additional text in the appropriate place (Fig. 1.3). The brief for the operating department can then be typed directly from the complete Master Document, supplemented where necessary with information from project team minutes.

Planning unit/dept: OD | Page: 10 | Design Briefing System

OPERATING DEPARTMENT

Guidance

4. ORGANISATION OF SERVICE 4.2 PATIENT MOVEMENT

Patient Transport

The several ways of transporting the patient from the ward to the operation table and then back to the ward are characterised by the points in the process at which the patient is transferred from one means of transport to another.

A transport system should be judged by the following criteria: disturbance of the patient and interference with the conduct of clinical procedures should be minimal; and excessive physical strength should not be required of staff. A satisfactory method, so far as is possible, reconciles these criteria.

Three transport systems are illustrated in Figure 1.8. System A is traditional; its form is a consequence of a belief in the value of the definition of clean and dirty zones, and of the associated transfer procedures and devices. Systems B and C have the following advantages: the number of transfers is small; patients on regaining consciousness are reassured to find themselves in their own bed; and it is convenient for anaesthetists and nursing staff. However, the methods require for successful realisation the manoeuvrability of a variable height bed, and, indeed, corridors which will permit the passage of the bed. It is also essential to ensure that laundering standards conform with HTM 71/49, revised 1987, and that the patient's bedding is changed shortly before leaving the ward.

The commonest means of transferring the patient to theatre trolley or operation table are lateral transfer using a roller system or by canvas and poles. The former consists of a roller frame and rubber/canvas belt or cushioned sleeve covered with a non-friction fabric. Other methods such as detachable table tops, and moveable, rolling trolley systems which permit lateral or longitudinal transfer of patients are available.

Space is required for parking beds and trolleys while the patients are in the theatre. The use of corridors for this purpose is unacceptable.

Planning unit/dept: OD | Page: 10 | Design Briefing System

OPERATING DEPARTMENT

Decisions

4. ORGANISATION OF SERVICE 4.2 PATIENT MOVEMENT

Earlier decision	Ref	
	A	Patients called to the department in advance of their operation will wait in: (a) a holding area at the reception/transfer point (✓) (b) an anaesthesia room ( ) (c)
4B	B	Patients will be brought to the department on: (a) their own beds (✓) (b) ward trolleys having trendelberg tilt mechanism ( ) (c) and will proceed direct to the anaesthesia room (✓) (d) and will be transferred to an operating department trolley before proceeding to the anaesthesia room ( )
	C	Transfer to an operating department trolley will take place in: (a) the reception/transfer area ( ) (b) the anaesthesia room ( ) (d)
	D	Patients will be transferred to the operation table in: (a) the anaesthesia room (✓) (b) the operating theatre ( ) (c)
	E	Before proceeding to the post anaesthesia recovery room, patients will be transferred from the operation table to: (a) their own bed (✓) (b) an operating department trolley ( ) (c) in the operating theatre ( ) (d) in the exit bay (✓) (e)
	F	Patients will be transferred from an operating department trolley to: (a) their own bed ( ) (b) a ward trolley ( ) (c) in the post anaesthesia room ( ) (d) in the reception/transfer area ( ) (e)
	G	The system of transfer preferred is: (a) lateral transfer roller/fabric sleeve system (✓) (b) lateral transfer using canvas and poles ( ) (c)

Fig. 1.1 Design Briefing System — Operating Department; left hand 'guidance' page example. (DHSS Crown Copyright, reproduced by permission.)
Fig. 1.2 Design Briefing System — Operating Department; right hand 'decisions' page example. (DHSS Crown Copyright, reproduced by permission.)

Operating Department extract from brief (example 1)

ORGANISATION OF SERVICE, PATIENT MOVEMENT

Patients called to the department in advance of their operation will wait in:

(a)   a holding area at the reception/transfer point

Patients will be brought to the department on:

(a)   their own beds

(c)   and will proceed direct to the anaesthesia room

Patients will be transferred to the operation table in:

(a)   their own bed

The system of transfer preferred is:

(a)   lateral transfer roller/fabric sleeve system

Operating Department extract from brief (example 2)

ORGANISATION OF SERVICE, PATIENT MOVEMENT

Patients called to the department in advance of their operation will wait in a holding area at the reception/transfer point.

Patients will be brought to the department on their own beds and will proceed direct to the anaesthesia room where they will be transferred to the operation table.

Before proceeding to the post anaesthesia recovery room patients will be transferred from the operation table to their own bed in the exit bay.

The system of transfer preferred is lateral transfer roller/fabric sleeve.

Fig. 1.3   Design Briefing System — Operating Department; example of options selected from Figure 1.2 to form part of a brief.

The DBS leads the user to a selection of the rooms or activity spaces required in the department. Its use enables user requirements to be stated clearly and concisely by the project team, not only in respect of accommodation, but also how that accommodation is to be used. Furthermore, during refinement of the brief as the design work proceeds, use of DBS enables a check to be made on the implications of modifications suggested by the designer which may affect earlier decisions made by the project team. In other words it provides a systematic data chain which can be referred to if at some subsequent stage it is necessary to trace back the decisions made.

Activity data

This comprises a detailed library of *Activity Data Sheets (A and B sheets)*, each of which sets out the functional design requirements (activities which are to take place) in a space or room and technical information such as environmental data (Fig. 1.4). A set of these is available for the operating department. These *A sheets* lead the user to the selection of appropriate *Activity Unit Data Sheets – B sheets* (Fig. 1.5), which display graphically the components and equipment required. Used with *ergonomic data sheets*, this information forms part of the briefing information given to the designer.

The brief

The design brief is prepared by a project team (planning team) acting on behalf of the client/potential user (Curry, 1982a; Dunstan, 1982). The multiprofessional project team which includes users' representatives, health administrator, architect, engineer, quantity surveyor, has to ensure that the design of new buildings or the upgrading of existing buildings is functional and yet remains within the financial limits imposed. To achieve this, it is vital that the designer understands fully the intentions of the project team. This is not only in respect of the accommodation required, but how that accommodation is to be used; in other words the operational policies. The ultimate design solution inevitably will involve some compromise, and unless the designer interprets correctly the requirements of the user, misunderstandings are bound to occur.

For these reasons it is quite wrong to start with a preconceived sketch plan, and then attempt to fit in the operational intentions. This can result in under- or over-provision of activity spaces/rooms, poor space relationships in the department and unacceptable circulation patterns.

Mention has already been made of the DBS which helps project teams to formulate detailed departmental operational policies in a logical systematic manner. Whether DBS or other methods are adopted, the information required in the brief is of the same order. It is an opportunity for users to consider how current developments might be incorporated in the new design, rather than perpetuate present practices. Such changes, however, will need to take into account the existing whole hospital policies; for example, the possible introduction of a different method of patient transport to that generally in use within the hospital — beds rather than trolleys.

The content of a design brief should proceed from the general to the particular. Many of the initial statements in the brief will be predetermined by the service strategy for the health district or organisation. Taking these planning statements into account, the project team will then need to consider every aspect of the operational policies (Curry, 1982b). The

A D B — activity space data sheet — N101 — DATE FEB 1987

ORIGIN DHSS

DEPARTMENT OPERATING DEPARTMENT
ACTIVITY SPACE NAME THEATRE

ACTIVITY
UNIT
SELECTION

See Continuation Sheet

FUNCTIONAL DESIGN REQUIREMENTS
FACILITIES needed for the following activities

(i)   Positioning patient on operating table.
(ii)   Connecting patient to anaesthetic machine.
(iii) Space for parking and subsequent preparation of instrument trolleys.
(iv)   Assembling and connecting mobile equipment.
(v)   Performance of operative procedures.
(vi)   Viewing X-ray film and medical records.
(vii) Checking, weighing and recording of used swabs.
(viii) Display of operating list.
(ix)   Recording of patients case notes.
(x)   Transfer of patient from operating table to trolley or bed.

PERSONNEL
An average of 7 staff

ADDITIONAL EQUIPMENT OR ENGINEERING TERMINALS not associated with a specific activity unit

6 No. socket outlet, 13A, switched, double

PLANNING RELATIONSHIP
Direct access to preparation room, anaesthesia room, scrub-up, exit area, and utility

---

Continuation Sheet

A D B — activity space data sheet — N101 — DATE FEB 1987

ORIGIN DHSS

DEPARTMENT OPERATING DEPARTMENT
ACTIVITY SPACE NAME THEATRE

		Code
ACTIVITY	2	OPERATIVE PROCEDURES: Surgeon's platform	A33 AF
	1	OPERATIVE PROCEDURES: parking diathermy	
	1	OPERATIVE PROCEDURES: suction unit, mobile	
	1*	OPERATIVE PROCEDURES: control panel,	A33 CC
		theatres, front access	
	1	OPERATIVE PROCEDURES: operating area,	A33 AL
		general theatre, mobile table and services	
	1	OPERATIVE PROCEDURES: recording, swab count	A33 N111
		board, rack mobile	
UNIT	1	ANAESTHESIA, anaesthetic ventilator cabinet,	A38 AN
		mobile	B31 AR
	1	PARKING, infusion stand, twin hook, mobile	B31 CO
	2	PARKING, portable suction jars, pipeline	B31 CP
	2	PARKING, bowl stand, single	B31 CQ
	1	PARKING, bowl stand, double	B31 CR
	2	PARKING, kickabout	C04 HB
SELECTION	1	CHAIR, anaesthetist, adjustable height	C27 DA
	2	STOOL, surgical, adjustable	C31 CJ
	1**	TROLLEY, instrument	C31 KD
	1	TROLLEY, instrument tray	C31 CH
	2**	TROLLEY, dressing/instrument, 750 x 450 mm	C31 CI
	1	TROLLEY, dressing/instrument, 450 x 450 mm	

*   Front or rear access is a project option
** Size subject to local decision

B

THIS SHEET MAY NEED MODIFICATION TO MEET PROJECT REQUIREMENTS		
A D B	ACTIVITY UNIT DATA SHEET	A33AL

ORIGIN		DATE FEB 1987	PROJECT CODE

ACTIVITY UNIT TITLE OPERATIVE PROCEDURES. Operating area general theatres mobile table and services.

Activities: Preparation of anaesthetised patient, carrying out operative procedures by a surgical team. Ceiling services retractable column type.

scale 1:50

Group	Item	Qty	Size	Ref. No.
1	Shadowless lamp, operating, with satellite	1		
	Services pendant containing:			
	13A double, switched, socket outlet	2		
	Oxygen outlet	1		
	Nitrous oxide outlet	1		
	Suction outlet	1		
	Medical compressed air outlet low pressure (4 bar)	1		
	Scavenging outlet	1		
	Services pendant containing:			
	13A double, switched, socket outlet	2		
	Suction outlet	1		
	Medical compressed air outlet high pressure (7 bar)	1		
3	Table, operating	1		
	* Project option, alternate position of service pendants.			

Fig. 1.5 Activity Data Base — example of component data 'B' sheet. (DHSS Crown Copyright, reproduced by permission.)

A

TECHNICAL DESIGN DATA					
			SPACE LOCATION		NOTES
SPACE REQUIREMENTS		PERIPHERAL	INTERNAL		

AIR CONDITIONING	Air temperature	Winter		20/22°C MECH	
	Air changes	Natural or mechanical			
	Air changes	Rate if mechanical			
★ SPECIAL CRITERIA	Air temperature	Summer		18/24°C	
	Air humidity	Summer		40% minimum minimum efficiency of 95 when tested by the sodium flame method	
	Air humidity	Winter			
	Air filtration				
	Air pressure	(relative to adjoining space)		POSITIVE	

LIGHTING	Lighting intensity	General			T EMERGENCY
	Lighting intensity	Night			BATTERY SUPPLY
	Lighting intensity	Local			H
	Lighting intensity	Emergency			
SAFETY	Glare index				
	Colour rendering		COLOUR CORRECTED		

★	Maximum accessible hot surface temperature				
	Maximum domestic hot water supply temperature				
NOISE	Acceptable level of noise from outside				
	Total acceptable sound level within space		40 dBA at L10		
	Description of noise which cannot be tolerated within space				
	% of time acceptable sound levels can be exceeded				

NOTE ★ Absolute control of these conditions cannot be attained except by the use of costly and complex engineering systems. Values should only be put against these conditions where they are essential to room function at defined in and in accordance with Departmental Guidance.

DESIGN CHARACTER				
INTERNAL FINISHES		WALLS	FLOOR	CEILING
GRADE		1	1	1
SURFACE REFLECTIVITY				
DOORS		To Exit Bay; Patient/trolley access, through vision single swing, self closing.		
IRONMONGERY		See seperate schedule		
WINDOWS		Clear glass		
INTERNAL GLAZING AND METHOD OF OBSCURING	N/A			
HATCH		N/A		

C

Fig. 1.4(A–C) Activity Data Base — example of activity data 'A' sheet. (DHSS Crown Copyright, reproduced by permission.)

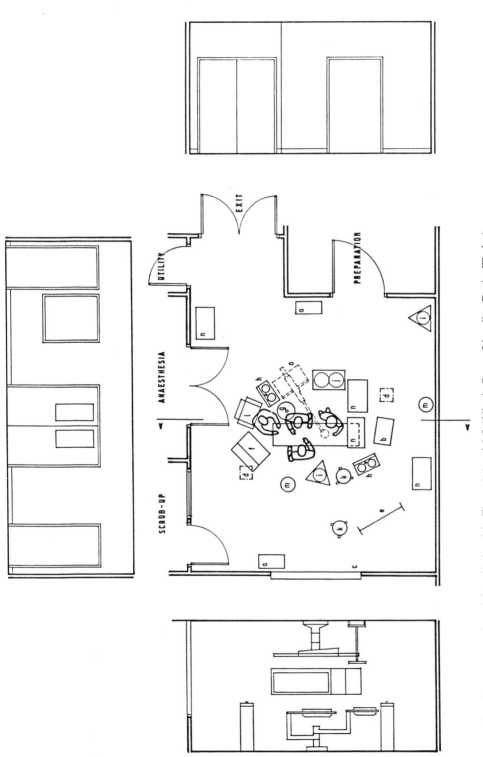

Fig. 1.6 Graphic representation of data displayed in Figure 1.4 and 1.5 (Alistair Green; Llewellyn-Davis, Weeks.)

Top. View towards scrub-up, anaesthesia room and utility.

Right. View towards exit and preparation room.

Left. Cross-section through centre, showing operation table, operating luminaire simple service pendants, and wall control panel in background.

Key to plan view (see also Fig. 1.4 continuation sheet).

a. Surgeons' platform
b. Diathermy machine
c. Control panel, switches, X-ray viewing screen etc.
d. Services pendants (Figs. 1.23 and 1.24)
e. Swab count rack

f. Anaesthesia apparatus
g. Infusion stand
h. Pipeline medical vacuum apparatus
i. Single hand rinse bowl stand
j. Double hand rinse bowl stand

k. Soiled swabs runabout
l. Anaesthetists' chair
m. Surgeons' stool
n. Instrument trolley
o. Mobile X-ray apparatus.

following list, though not exhaustive, gives examples of aspects which should be included in the brief for an operating department:

Scope of service to be provided and estimated workload

Specialities to be excluded

Functional content, e.g. number of theatres

Preferred locational relationships with other hospital departments

Operational policies, e.g.
— access zones
— staff facilities including changing
— patient transportation, reception, documentation, transfer and movement within the operating department and post-anaesthesia recovery
— preparation, recycling, and sterilization of instrument sets, holloware, gowns, etc.
— supplies system and storage
— disposal of used dressings and other waste material
— administration, secretarial support
— teaching
— cleaning
— catering
— communications e.g. telephones, intercom

General design requirements

Statutory regulations.

Functional content, size and location: Guidance on calculating the appropriate size of an operating department is given in HBN 26 Operating Department (DHSS, 1988). A study of hospitals throughout England and a study by the Oxford Regional Health Authority revealed a considerable under-utilisation of operating theatres (MARU, 1981; Oxford RHA, 1982). It was concluded that by more efficient programming and use of operating sessions, the ratio of operating theatres to procedures/beds required in a district hospital could be reduced. Another factor is the development of fibreoptic technology which has revolutionised endoscopy. Whereas most complex endoscopy investigations formerly were carried out in the operating department, these may now be more efficiently and economically undertaken in an adult day care unit treatment suite, thereby reducing the number of operating theatres required. Whilst the HBN gives general guidelines on this matter, it is for individual health authorities and project teams to determine an economical level of provision to match need.

Factors which need to be taken into account when determining the facilities which are to be provided include: the catchment, planning and cross-boundary population; estimated workload; specialities being served (general surgery, ENT, urology etc); and specific exclusions (specialities/type of surgery *not* being undertaken).

The location of the department in relation to the total hospital development is of particular importance. The department must be easily accessible from the inpatient wards, intensive therapy unit — ideally on the same floor level — and with the shortest possible route to the accident and emergency department.

Access zones: Previous editions of this book described the segregation of clean and dirty streams of traffic, and the accepted practice of enforcing rigid restrictions on the entry of personnel to the operating department. Microbiological research does not support these traditional views (Williams, 1966; Ayliffe *et al.*, 1969; Berry and Khon, 1972; Lidwell, 1982; Royal Col. Surg., 1984; DHSS, 1989). The assumption that rigid staff disciplines and rituals can enforce a gradient of decreasing bacterial load is not justified by evidence. However, aseptic discipline is an important aspect of operating theatre technique, and it is common

sense not to permit unrestricted access to all parts of the department. But the use of the traditional terms 'clean', 'sterile' and 'dirty' zones which have long established architectural connotations are no longer appropriate. HBN 26 suggests a definition of four access 'zones' (Fig. 1.7):

1. *general access zone*: through which any authorised person entering the department is admitted; it includes the entrance, reception, patient transfer area, porter's base, staff changing, department store, disposal hold, and some offices.

2. *limited access zone*: comprises the general circulation areas between the department entrance and operating suites, includes post-anaesthesia recovery, staff base, staff rest rooms, some offices, seminar room/teaching facilities where appropriate, equipment parking and special storage, and the exit bays to each operating suite.

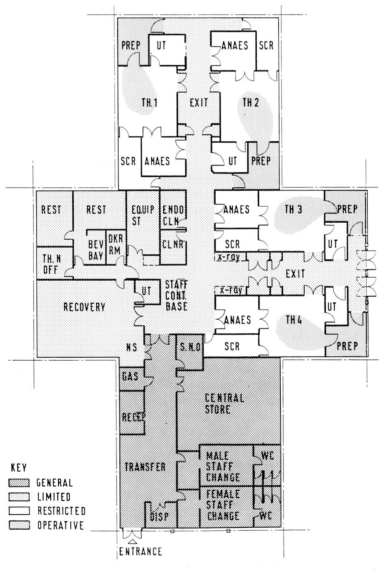

Fig. 1.7 Access zones related to a first phase 4-theatre operating department which can be extended to 6 or 8 theatres. (Nucleus, DHSS Crown Copyright, reproduced by permission.)

3. *restricted access zone*: which is limited to those persons, appropriately attired, whose presence is related to activities in the *operating suite*; comprises the operating theatre, anaesthesia room, scrub up and gowning, preparation/supply, and utility.

4. *operating zone*: defined as the zone which encompasses the operating area, and the preparation room. A decreased bacterial load can be achieved by reducing the number of persons in the operating zone to the minimum, and ensuring sufficient directed ventilatory air flow to the other access zones.

The project team need to determine the policy regarding access to the department. Should it be decided to perpetuate a 'red line' policy*, then the design implications of this must be taken into account, for example, the location of staff changing rooms. An acceptance of recent microbiological research would suggest that it is unnecessary to position changing rooms specifically to ensure that staff and visitors are fully changed before entering the limited access zone.

Patient transport: The method adopted for the transportation of patients from ward to operating department and vice versa has considerable special implications for the design of the operating department; for example, whether beds or trolleys are wheeled to the operating suite for transfer of the patient to the operation table, and the space required for parking of beds during an operating procedure. Account should be taken of the safety and comfort of patients, the need to reduce the number of transfers, manoeuvrability of the bed through hospital corridors, and the locational relationship of wards to the operating department. Where possible, use of the patient's bed throughout is becoming the system of choice, providing the minimum number of transfers and reassurance for the patient who, on regaining consciousness, finds himself in his own bed (Fig. 1.8).

Supplies: The operational policies for supplies must be clearly identified, as these will have a bearing on the design solution. The project team will need to identify the various items involved, such as sterile supplies, pharmaceutical, catering, clean linen and office supplies. Of special importance is the provision of sterile instrument sets; for example, whether all instruments are to be processed and sterilized in the Sterilizing and Disinfecting Unit (SDU), or some such as endoscopes sterilized within the operating department. The methods of delivery and subsequent collection of used instrument sets for recycling should be determined. For example, an SDU distribution trolley will transport sterile instrument sets from the department sterile store to individual theatre suites, and following operation the same trolley will be used for returning sets to the SDU.

Decisions will have to be made on whether all supplies should enter through a single main entrance, or alternatively via a separate entrance to the main departmental store. The amount and distribution of storage space required in the department will need to be considered, together with frequency and estimated time of receipt of supplies and onward distribution to stores at point of use.

Policies for the requisition, storage and care of pharmaceuticals are factors which form part of the brief.

Disposal: The method adopted for the identification and disposal of used items for destruction or recycling, and the need to provide a disposal hold at a convenient point in the department must relate to the 'whole hospital' disposal policy.

Administration and teaching: The policy for nursing and medical administrative facilities required in the department should be considered; e.g. provision for the senior nurse in

---

* This is when a distinctive line of demarcation is adopted between the entrance to the department and inner zones, where patients may be transferred from a bed/ward trolley to theatre trolley, and vice versa. Staff entering by this route and visitors are obliged to change into appropriate protective clothing before crossing the 'red line'.

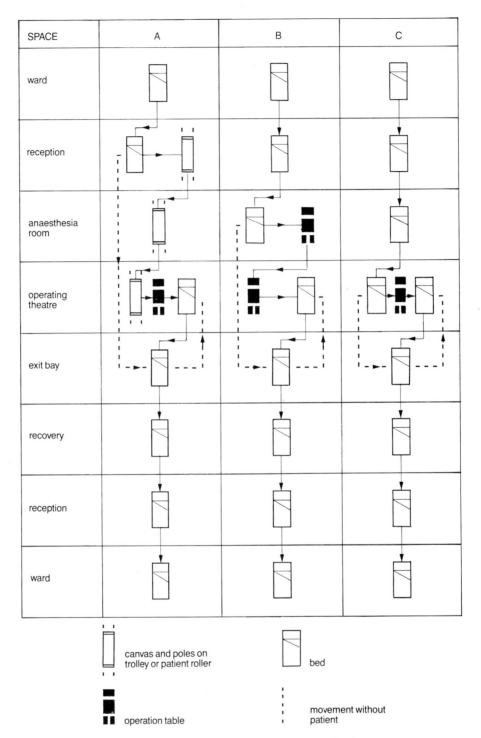

Fig. 1.8 Example of three patient transport systems. In each instance the bed is used for transport to and from the operating department, and for recovery of the patient. Transfer takes place:
(A) From bed to theatre trolley at reception, from trolley to operation table in the operating theatre, and finally from operation table to bed;
(B) From bed to operation table in the anaesthesia room, and finally from operation table to bed in the operating theatre;
(C) From bed to operation table in the operating theatre and finally from operation table to bed.
(DHSS HBN 26 Crown Copyright, reproduced by permission.)

charge, theatre sisters, anaesthetic sisters, nurse tutors, and for medical staff who wish to write up patients' notes or hold confidential discussions.

Account should be taken of the educational needs of nurse learners, post-registration, courses, and medical students, and whether part of these requirements can be met in the hospital education centre.

Catering: A number of options can be considered. The most commonly accepted practice is a basic service for the preparation of beverages and limited snacks, which may include the use of vending machines. This may be augmented by the provision of hot and cold meals from the main hospital kitchen. Each of these options has different design implications.

Cleaning: The brief must specify that the internal construction materials and finishes selected should minimise maintenance and cleaning costs. The designer requires information on the anticipated cleaning policies which can be taken into account when locating facilities for the storage of cleaning materials and equipment, and provision of utilities for cleaning staff.

Communications: Various options need to be considered to ensure an effective communications system within the operating department. These include the use of intercom between critical areas such as preparation rooms, department store, reception and post-anaesthesia recovery; telephones with internal and external facilities in convenient locations; the use of paging receivers (bleeps); and various emergency alarms such as staff to staff in post-anaesthesia recovery, failure of medical gases, blood refrigerator, and those from drug cupboards, with repeater signals in reception and at the staff control base.

General design requirements: These specify general standards of provision, and matters such as the potential sharing of activity spaces for more than one function.

Completion of the narrative brief describing the operational policies will lead to an initial selection of the activity spaces/rooms required. It is the responsibility of the project team to identify clearly the functional requirements for each activity space and provide this information to the designer. Use of the DHSS activity data sheets simplifies this, and later during the design stage facilitates scrutiny of the sketch plans. A good brief forms the basis of documentation for commissioning, and subsequently provides a reference point at the evaluation stage when the building has been in use for a period (Rait, 1982; Williams, 1982).

Statutory regulations

The design will need to comply with mandatory legislation including:
   Building Regulations (or Building Byelaws in inner London)
   Chronically Sick and Disabled Persons Act
   Health and Safety at Work Act
   Fire Precautions Act
   Town and Country Planning Act

These cover a range of building standards which must be achieved and deal with such matters as siting of the building, external appearance, finishes in relation to existing buildings, materials used in the building, health and safety, changing and sanitary accommodation, means of escape in case of fire and access for the fire services.

One of the most important of these which influences the planning of operating departments are the fire regulations. Planners must take fire safety into account and agree with the local fire authority measures to be adopted, e.g. means of escape, fire compartmentation and protection from spread of smoke. HTM81 Fire Safety in Health Buildings (1987) provides a detailed description of the requirements for fire safety in new health buildings including operating departments.

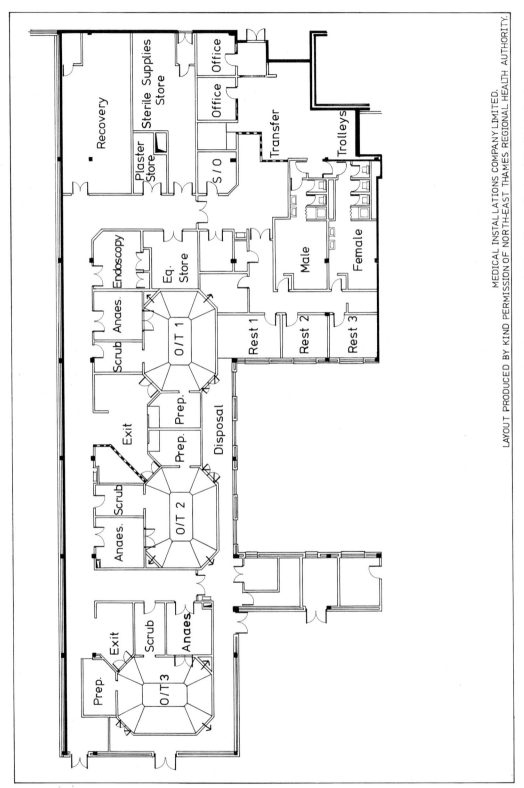

Fig. 1.9 Plan of a three theatre, modular construction operating department. (Harold Wood Hospital, North East Thames Regional Health Authority. Medical Installations Co. Ltd.)

DESIGN

Operating facilities should be centralised in the operating department rather than dispersed in the hospital, since this has been shown to be the most economic approach in terms of engineering services, the use of equipment and deployment of personnel.

Present trends in hospital design favour the low-rise building solution limited to two or three storeys high. This enables maximum advantage to be taken of natural light and ventilation where appropriate, for example by the provision of internal courtyards. The operating department should be constructed so that it is separate from general traffic and air movement in the rest of the hospital (DHSS, 1968). If the department is located on an upper floor, care will need to be taken to eliminate noise transmission from ventilation plants which may be sited on the roof above.

Movement of patients is made easier if there are good planning relationships between the operating department surgical wards and intensive therapy unit (ITU), with easy access to the accident and emergency (AED), and radiodiagnostic (X-RAY) departments. Convenient access is required also to the sterilizing and disinfecting unit (SDU), and laboratory facilities.

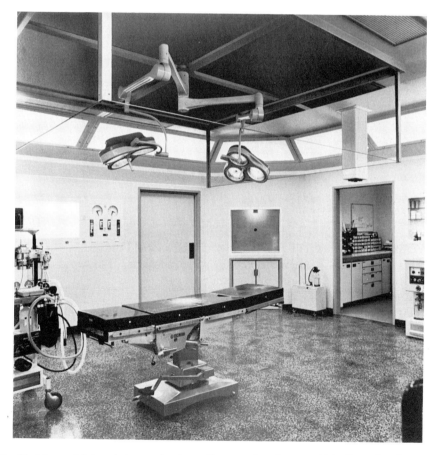

Fig. 1.10 Modular prefabricated theatre showing wall-mounted equipment which allows clear floor space for the surgical team. (Harold Wood Hospital Essex Medical Installations Co. Ltd.)

Examples have been given already of the accommodation which needs to be provided in the four access zones of the operating department (page 10). The design solution should permit the traffic and workflow patterns envisaged by the operational policies to be adopted. Good relationships between the operating suites and support accommodation will simplfy management of the department. The limited access zone should include adequate 'forward' storage for equipment and ready-to-use supplies; an x-ray darkroom may be required.

The processing and sterilization of drape and instrument trays/packs should be centralised, ideally in the SDU which serves the whole hospital. This may not be possible where a Theatre Sterile Supply Unit (TSSU) is already built adjacent to an operating department which is being upgraded. However, such provision is less economical in space and service terms.

Ventilation should be on the principle that the direction of air-flow is from the operating suites towards the department entrance. There should be no interchange air movement between one operating suite and another. Heating and ventilation should allow comfortable climatic conditions for the patient, and staff.

The construction must be such that a high standard of cleanliness may be obtained and maintained (Houghton and Hudd, 1967). All surfaces should be washable and all joins between walls, ceilings and floors curved to facilitate cleaning. Open radiators or pipes for heating the operating suite are totally unacceptable; they are dust traps.

Well established in Europe and the Middle East is the prefabricated modular operating suite. This is constructed from factory-prefabricated sections consisting of a framework of interlocking members which support a variety of wall panels having a hygienic finish. The unit, which may be hexagonal or square, can be erected relatively quickly either within existing buildings or a simple building shell.

The modular operating suite is designed to take the maximum advantage of available space. Several variations in layout can be achieved, ranging from a single operating theatre to a complete department. The system can be incorporated in conventional design solutions and provision can be made for future extensions (Figs. 1.9 and 1.10).

Types of operating departments

The preceding paragraphs have highlighted the policy considerations applicable to the design of new operating departments. These principles can be adopted for theatres designed as part of a new hospital complex, as an extension to existing buildings, or for upgrading. However, readers may find they are working in operating theatres which can be classed in one of three main categories:

1. The single theatre suite containing operating theatre, scrub-up and gowning, anaesthesia room, trolley preparation, utility, and exit bay, plus staff change and limited ancillary accommodation.

2. The twin theatre suite with facilities similar to No. 1, but with duplicated ancillary accommodation immediate to each operating theatre, sharing ancillary accommodation which sometimes includes a small post anaesthesia recovery area.

3. Operating departments consisting of three or more operating suites. Ancillary accommodation will include post-anaesthesia recovery, reception, porter's base, sterile store, and staff change. Examples of operating departments with four and eight operating suites are illustrated in Figures 1.11 and 1.12.

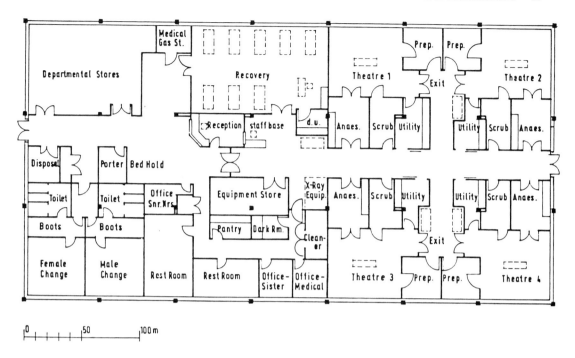

Fig. 1.11 Plan of a four theatre operating department with single circulation corridor. (Alistair Green; Llewellyn-Davis, Weeks.)

Construction

Walls and ceilings. All rooms in the operating suite should have impervious wall and ceiling finishes able to withstand wet cleaning. Walls should withstand damage by trolleys and mobile equipment; additional protection buffers should be placed at especially vunerable points. Suitable finishes include sprayed plastic skin, an epoxy resin type of paint, and plastic sheet with welded joints for walls. Where movement of the structural wall is anticipated, then plastic laminate, steel or glass sheets which can be supported independently of the wall should be used. The joints between these sheets must be sealed to prevent penetration of moisture during cleaning. Although ceramic tiles are durable provided the structural walls remain uncracked, they are not ideal because new building movement may cause crevices which can eventually form at the joints.

A semi-matt wall surface reflects less light than a highly gloss finish and is less tiring to the eyes of the theatre team. With this in mind the colour is important also, and walls, ceilings and floors should be light in colour. Pale green or blue is acceptable as strong colours will distort the colour rendering of light sources and should be avoided.

Floors. These must be able to withstand the rolling loads of heavy operating tables and mobile x-ray machines. The surface should be slip resistant under wet conditions and impervious to frequent cleaning with scrubbing machines. There will be the need to remove stains with cleaning agents. Cleaning policies should take into account recommendations made by the manufacturer of the floor finish material selected.

Terrazo tiles or a cement based poured-in-place finish are suitable where the floor structure is not liable to movement or deflection. An alternative is to use flexible thermoplastic

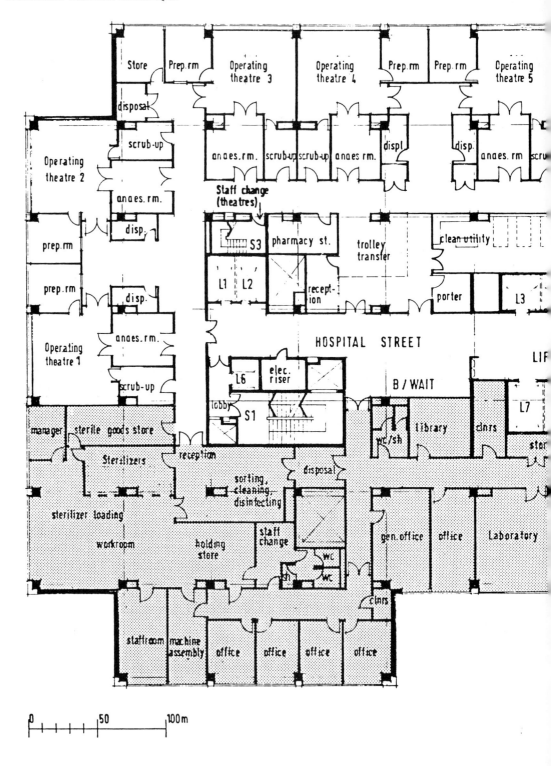

Fig. 1.12 Plan of an eight theatre operating department. (St Mary's Hospital, Paddington, London. Alistair Green; Llewellyn-Davis, Weeks.)

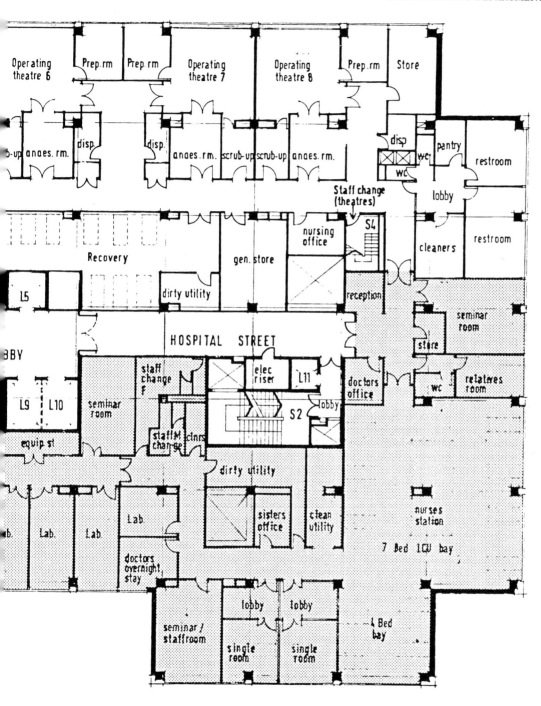

sheet or tiles with welded joints, but these should not run across the theatre floor. Such finishes are more tolerant to small movements in the structural floor, provided the underlying floor screed is perfectly smooth. The adhesives used must be powerful enough to prevent 'waves' in the floor finish which can occur with the movement of heavy wheeled equipment. The surface should be slip resistant under wet conditions.

Antistatic floors. The need for antistatic flooring has diminished now that flammable anaesthetic gases and volatile agents are less commonly used. Regular testing and systematic maintenance are required to ensure that the electrical resistance of such floors remains effective (see Chapter 4). Taking these factors into account, and particularly as antistatic floors can be more costly, a project team with the approval of the Health Authority may decide to omit this specification. In such circumstances, notices must be displayed to warn staff that the use of explosive anaesthetic gases and agents is forbidden. Examples of warning notices are included in HTM65 'Health Signs' (DHSS, 1985). If antistatic floors are installed the requirements are set out in HTM2 (DHSS, 1977).

Lighting

Some natural daylight is preferred by staff. Where possible, high level windows which give a visual appreciation of the 'outside world' should be provided in the operating theatre. Alternatively this can be achieved by means of borrowed light from windows across corridors (Figs. 1.44–1.45).

If external windows are fitted, solar gain or loss which may affect control of environmental conditions must be taken into account. It may be necessary to provide triple glazing, and provision must be made for the windows to be blacked out completely.

Colour-corrected general artificial lighting which permits true colour rendition of patients' skin tones is required, together with a ceiling mounted operating theatre table luminaire (Lovett *et al.*, 1983; Lovett, 1984). If the mains or fuses fail there must be a 'no-break' emergency supply which provides adequate lighting and power to complete the operation and in an emergency commence others. During an emergency, the supply must be switched off as soon as practicable and the use of unnecessary lights in ancillary rooms carefully avoided. This will help to reduce the generator load or battery 'drain'; batteries are usually designed to give one to three hours emergency illumination. The emergency system must be fully automatic and tested frequently.

Sometimes mobile emergency luminaires are in use. The apparatus generally incorporates a trickle charger which should be connected to an electric socket outlet; this keeps the batteries continually charged and the luminaire ready for immediate use. The batteries should be fully sealed, and battery and charger should be kept away from the operating zone as far as is practicable.

General lighting. This should be provided by colour-corrected fluorescent lamps, recessed or surface ceiling mounted and arranged to produce even illumination of at least 500 Lux at working height with minimal glare. There should be means of dimming or switching as procedures such as endoscopy often require dark surroundings, and some surgeons prefer to work in a field that is 'spotlighted'.

Operation (task) area illumination. Choice of operating luminaire will have to take into account such factors as the colour emitted, light intensity and pattern, shadow reduction, the elmination of heat and manoeuvrability (Barlett, 1978). Part of a British Standard BS 4533 (1986) specifies the requirements of operating theatre table luminaires and examination luminaires.

Colour. Mention has been made of the requirement for colour corrected general lighting. The surgeon needs to differentiate between normal and diseased tissue and perform tasks with materials having little colour contrast, for example using blood soaked sutures. The colour quality of light most generally acceptable for this purpose is in the region of 4000 Kelvin (4000K). Operating luminaires are available working at colour temperatures between 3600K and 5000K which should meet most personal preferences.

Intensity/pattern. The density of light achieved in the task area at operation table level is directly dependent on the intensity of light directed upon it. With the luminaire at approximately 1000 mm (40 in) from the task area, the light pattern should be at least 200 mm (8 in) in diameter, with a brightness at the pattern centre of between 50,000 and 100,000 Lux, and at least 15,000 Lux at the periphery. This is very high compared with a normal general intensity of 500 Lux for a working area. The main reason for such large levels of brightness is because of the high light absorption and low degree of reflectivity of the tissues; a large proportion of the light is simply absorbed and thus contributes little to visibility.

Shadow reduction. Operating luminaires are designed to produce beams of light from a variety of angles, so that when the light source is partially obscured by the surgical team's heads or hands, the task area is still illuminated. Total shadow reduction is undesirable, for if all shadows are eliminated there will be no 'modelling' of contours and three-dimensional perception for the surgeon is lost (Bartlett, 1978).

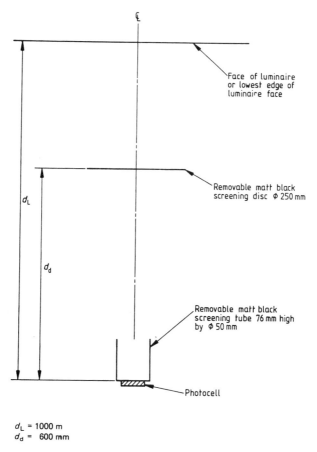

$d_L = 1000$ m
$d_d = 600$ mm

Fig. 1.13   Test rig for operating luminaires; diagram of illuminance test rig for single-head luminaires.

Beck (1980) suggests a 'tunnel test' for testing the shadow-reducing ability of an operating luminaire. In the test specified in the British Standard (1986), the luminaire should provide 40 per cent of the normal (unshadowed) light level inside, and at the bottom of, a tube of 5 cm (2 in) in diameter and 7.6 cm (3 in) long, finished matt black inside, placed at a distance of 110 cm (42 in) from the light source, and when the light beam is obstructed by an opaque disc 25 cm (10 in) in diameter placed 60 cm (23 in) from the surface on which the tube is standing (Fig. 1.13).

Elimination of heat. It is important that the heat from the beams of light is kept as low as possible to prevent 'drying out' or burning of delicate tissue. Most modern operating luminaires reduce this heat by means of dichroic reflectors (cold mirrors) combined with heat-absorbing reflectors or filters. Dichroic filters reflect visible radiation as a light beam but transmit the heat-producing infra red energy backwards for dissipation by the luminaire housing.

The radiant heat emitted by a luminaire light beam providing an illuminance of 100,000 lux will produce a temperature rise in the operating field of approximately 12°C above the ambient temperature. Similarly a temperature rise of approximately 6°C will be produced with an illuminance of 50,000 lux. The BS 4533 (1986) stipulates that this temperature should not exceed 22°C with an illuminance of 100,000 lux (Fig. 1.14).

Manoeuvrability. The ceiling-mounted operating luminaire should be suspended and counterbalanced in such a way that it is easy to move, allows a multiplicity of positions, horizontal and vertical, and does not vibrate or drift once it has been positioned. Some form of removable, sterilizable handle should be provided which enables the surgical team to make minor adjustments if required.

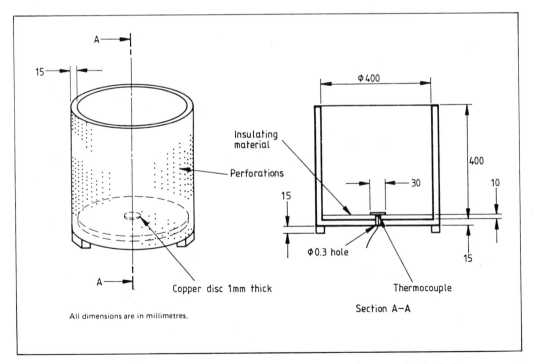

Fig. 1.14 Diagram of test rig for measuring radiant heat from the beam of an operating luminaire.

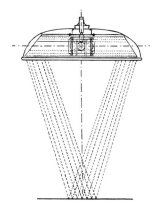

Fig. 1.15 Schematic diagram of the optical system in a scialytic operating luminaire. (Technical Lights and Equipment Co. Ltd.)

Types of operating luminaires*

Luminaires in common use comprise either single light sources using multi-reflectors, or several sources in the form of projectors or spotlights.

Multi-reflector luminaires

Scialytic. This contains an optical lens, similar to a lighthouse lantern, and Chance glass heat filter surrounding a single 24 volt tungsten/tungsten halogen lamp of 150/200 watts (Fig. 1.15). Light rays from the lens are projected on to a circle of mirrors set at 45 degrees to an imaginary perpendicular line running through the centre of the lens, and which surround the inner circumference of the luminaire. These rays are then projected on to the task (operation) area (Fig. 1.16). Focussing is accomplished by movement of the lamp up or down within the lantern lens. Modern versions of this luminaire additionally incorporate multi-light projectors.

Metallic reflector. This is basically the same as the scialytic luminaire in respect of performance, but instead of mirrors the reflector consists of a concave, highly polished metallic surface, either plain or made up of facets. The 24 volt lamp is situated at the central focal point of the reflector and is adjustable in a similar manner to the scialytic type.

A modern development of this concept is the AMSCO Polaris luminaire, incorporating a continuous reflector, folded optical path system and a single 26–34 volt, 235 watt tungsten halogen lamp source, which results in good depth of focus throughout the range of use (Fig. 1.17).

The luminaire produces light intensity variable between 3000–100,000 Lux, at a colour temperature of 4400K. The task area light pattern is adjustable in three stages 170 mm (6.4 in), 208 mm (8.3 in) and 245 mm (9.4 in), preserving 70 per cent of the available visible light energy. Dichroic filtration reduces the heat output of the light beam to 13,000 microwatts per cm^2.

---

* The following terminology is used when describing lighting equipment:
Lamp. Refers to the filament lamp.
Luminaire. Refers to the operation theatre table light fitting suspended from the ceiling; also to mobile equipment, and is then described as a mobile luminaire
Task area. This is the area, usually circular, illuminated by the luminaire.

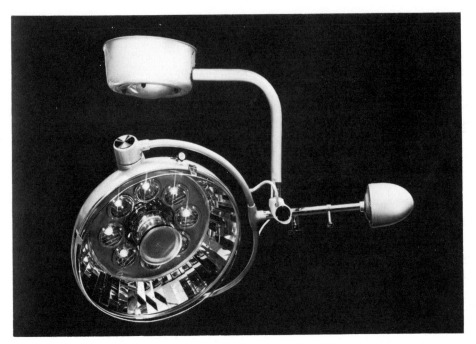

Fig. 1.16   Scialytic operating luminaire fitted with additional multi-lamp projectors. (Technical Lights and Equipment Ltd.)

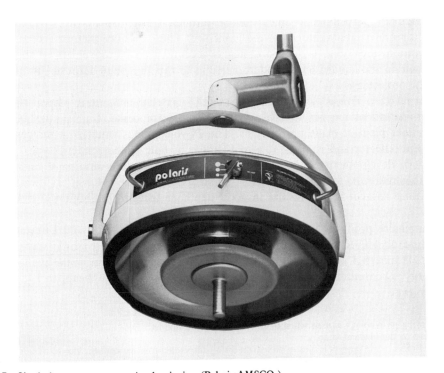

Fig. 1.17   Single lamp source operating luminaire. (Polaris-AMSCO.)

Multi-lamp luminaires

These usually comprise six to nine separate spotlights fitted in a single housing (cupola) or mounted as pods on manoeuvreable arms. The size of the task area can generally be adjusted by manipulating a single knob or switch fitted to the exterior of the luminaire, which adjusts the focus of all the lamps simultaneously.

Although each of the lamps used is of a lower intensity (40 watt) compared with that in the single lamp source luminaire, the cumulative effect of the six to nine lamps is very efficient. There is an advantage in that should one lamp fail during operation, the intensity of the light is only marginally reduced.

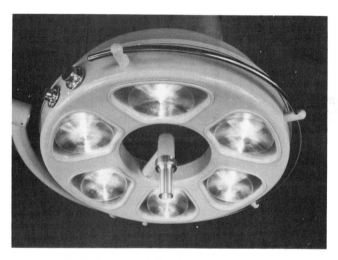

Fig. 1.18   Multi-lamp operating luminaire in cupola housing. (Hanaulux Amsterdam — Siemens.)

Cupola housing. A modern version of this type is the Hanaulux Amsterdam (Fig. 1.18) which comprises six projector lamps plus a central spotlight (combined with a sterilizable handle), which produce a light intensity of up to 115,000 Lux at a distance of 100 cm (40 in) from the front surface of the luminaire. Normally the luminaire provides a light colour temperature of 4300K, although versions are available with colour temperatures of 3500K or 5200K. The size of illuminated task area is infinitely variable between 20–30 cm (8–12 in), and the light intensity can be adjusted for superficial work. The luminaire provides an even field of illumination in a depth of field range of 30 cm (12 in) (Fig. 1.19). This avoids the need for further adjustment of the luminaire during surgery. The illustration also shows on Oslo satellite comprising three lamps, which provide supplementary illumination of 55,000 Lux.

The Castle 2800 series luminaires comprise four lamps mounted in a square housing, plus an optional two lamp satellite. The task area pattern of illumination can be adjusted to three sizes at the prime focus of 106.7 cm (42 in) from the cover glasses.

Pod-mounted lamps: One version of this concept is the Brandon Galaxy which is aerodynamically styled for ultra clean airflow systems to assist uninterrupted airflow without turbulance. The twin five plus four lamp luminaire illustrated in Figure 1.20 produces a task area of 20–30 cm (8–12 in), with a total light intensity of 107,000 Lux, colour temperature 4000K at 100 cm (40 in) from the lamps. The light intensity and diameter of the task area are variable.

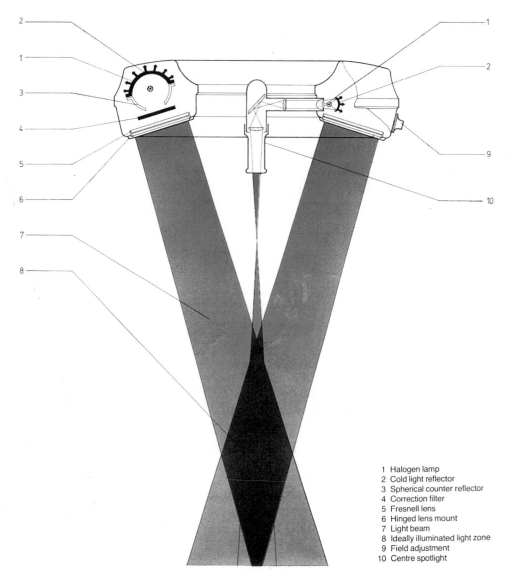

1 Halogen lamp
2 Cold light reflector
3 Spherical counter reflector
4 Correction filter
5 Fresnell lens
6 Hinged lens mount
7 Light beam
8 Ideally illuminated light zone
9 Field adjustment
10 Centre spotlight

Fig. 1.19   Schematic optical system diagram of the operating luminaire illustrated in Figure 1.18. (Hanaulux Amsterdam — Siemens.)

The infra red energy filtration system produces a light beam of low heat characteristics. The surface temperature of the lamp heads is not greater than 29°C, assuming an ambient temperature of 21°C. This low heat generation contributes significantly to the effectiveness of downflow air ventilation by reducing adverse convection currents to a minimum. A schematic diagram of the optical system is shown in Figure 1.21.

Provision can be made to mount a television camera in the luminaire or on an additional arm.

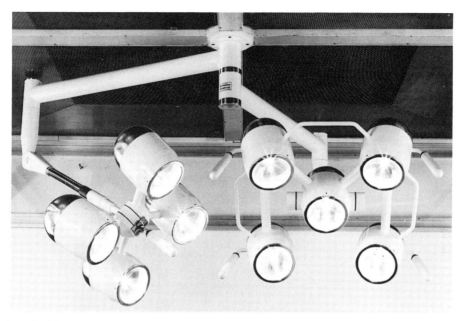

Fig. 1.20 Multi-lamp operating luminaire, pod mounted. (Brandon Galaxy — Brandon Medical Equipment Co.)

Pendant services

Pipeline services in the operating theatre are best provided in two ceiling pendants to minimise the hazard of trailing leads: one for the surgical team and the other for the anaesthetist. These pendants may be rigid, although retractable versions provide adjustment in height and simplify connection of hoses and electric cables. Ideally the anaesthetic pendant should be retractable and have limited lateral movement and provide a shelf for monitoring equipment (Figs. 1.23 and 1.24).

The surgical pendant should contain oxygen, 10-bar medical compressed air and medical vacuum outlets, and at least four electric socket outlets. The anaesthetic pendant requires oxygen, nitrous oxide, 4-bar medical compressed air, medical vacuum, and gas scavenging terminal outlets, and at least four electric socket outlets.

Ventilation

The ventilation system provided in the operating department has three main functions:
1. to control the temperature and humidity of the operating suite.
2. to dilute contamination by airborne micro-organisms and expired anaesthetic gases.
3. to provide an acceptable air movement within the operating suite such that the transfer of airborne micro-organisms from less clean to cleaner areas is minimised.

This is achieved by the supply of heated or cooled, humidified, clean air to the operating suite. Aerobic cultures using a non-selective media should indicate that not more than 35 micro-organism-carrying particles are present in 1 cubic metre (m^3) of the supply air. During surgical operations and preparation of sterile trolleys, the concentration of airborne particles contaminated by micro-organisms in the operating theatre averaged over a five-minute period should not exceed 180 per m^3.

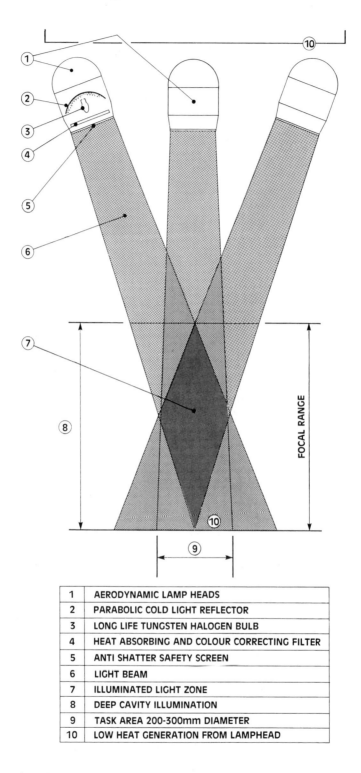

1	AERODYNAMIC LAMP HEADS
2	PARABOLIC COLD LIGHT REFLECTOR
3	LONG LIFE TUNGSTEN HALOGEN BULB
4	HEAT ABSORBING AND COLOUR CORRECTING FILTER
5	ANTI SHATTER SAFETY SCREEN
6	LIGHT BEAM
7	ILLUMINATED LIGHT ZONE
8	DEEP CAVITY ILLUMINATION
9	TASK AREA 200-300mm DIAMETER
10	LOW HEAT GENERATION FROM LAMPHEAD

Fig. 1.21 Schematic optical system diagram of the operating luminaire illustrated in Figure 1.20. (Brandon Medical Equipment Co.)

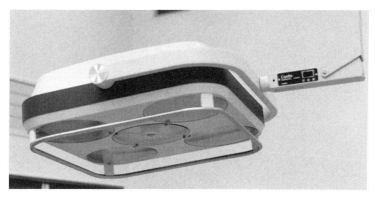

Fig. 1.22 Multi-lamp operating luminaire in a square housing. (Castle Lamp — Peacocks Surgical and Medical Equipment Ltd.)

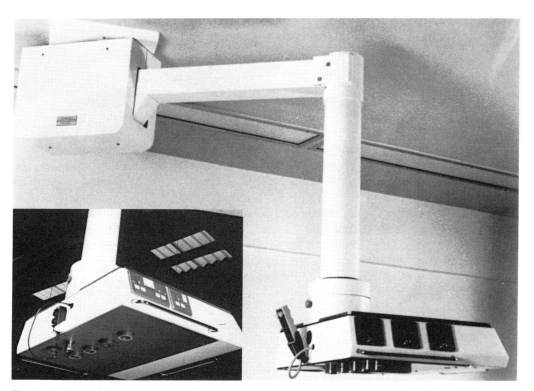

Fig. 1.23 Retractable services pendant, i.e. moveable in both a vertical and horizontal direction. (MGI Manufacturing Ltd.)

The optimum environmental conditions for various operating department staff and patients can be in conflict. Amongst staff, the subjective response to temperature and humidity will depend on factors such as the mode of dress, activity and proximity to direct radiant heat from the operating luminaire. Patients are susceptible to hypothermia during an operation under anaesthesia; this is due to disruption of their heat balance mechanism

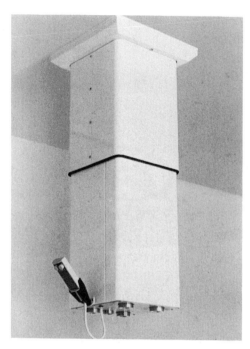

Fig. 1.24 Mobile services pendant, i.e. moveable in a vertical direction. (MGI Manufacturing Ltd.)

resulting from a lowering of metabolic levels, inhibition of muscular activity, and dilatation of peripheral blood vessels. There is a loss of body heat by evaporation which can be increased by the administration of dry anaesthetic gases, and the exposure of moist tissue surfaces.

In 1968, a survey of operating theatre staff (Wyon *et al.*, 1968) indicated that anaesthetists generally preferred temperatures 2.5°C warmer than their surgical colleagues. It would appear that thermal comfort is affected by humidity and air velocity as well as temperature; a 10 per cent fall in humidity or an increase in air velocity of 0.1 m³ per second is equivalent to a lowering of 0.5°C in the ambient air temperature. Similarly, an increase of 1.5°C of radiant heat, for example from the operating luminaire, can be counteracted by lowering the ambient temperature by 0.5°C.

There have been studies also which identify the relationship between ambient temperature and patient hypothermia. A study of patients undergoing abdominal surgery was conducted in America in 1970 and 1971 (Morris, 1971; Morris and Wilkey, 1970). This showed that patients almost invariably became hypothermic in operating theatres having an ambient temperature of less than 21°C. There was a 30 per cent incidence of hypothermia in ambient temperatures between 21°C and 24°C, but no patients became hypothermic in rooms with temperatures between 24°C and 26°C. Some operations are performed under hypothermia anaesthesia and in these situations the theatre temperature may be maintained at below 21°C.

The DHSS Design Guide *Ventilation of Operating Departments* (DHSS, 1983) concludes that the comfort requirements of the operating theatre staff conflict with each other and with the heat balance needs of the anaesthetised patient. It suggests that a compromise is necessary, the requirements of the surgeon usually being accepted, with other staff dressing accordingly. Various methods are being adopted to help maintain the patient's temperature, including warmed infusion fluids, heated mattress table tops, etc. The Design Guide

recommends that:

1. The air conditioning system should be capable of maintaining internal temperatures of 20°C in the summer and 22°C in winter in all but the most extreme outside conditions.

2. In order to ensure optimum selection of conditions, the controls for adjustment of temperature between 15°C and 25°C should be in the operating theatre.

3. The relative humidity should be allowed to vary within the range 40 to 60 per cent under normal working conditions, but be capable of being set to a minimum of 50 per cent saturation when flammable anaesthetics are being administered. The air velocity should be maintained in the range 0.13 to 0.25 m^3 per second.

4. The air distribution equipment in the anaesthesia room, post-anaesthesia recovery and operating theatre should prevent the patient from being exposed to unnecessary 'draughts'.

Most ventilation systems installed in operating departments provide a plenum airflow (Lancet, 1956, 1958; Medical Research Council, 1962; Male, 1978). In the last decade there has been development of high and medium velocity laminar or linear flow ventilation systems, the high-input/high-exhaust enclosures (Charnley, 1964, 1970; Mullick, 1978; Howorth, 1980, 1985; Lidwell et al., 1982; Whyte et al., 1983; Arrowsmith, 1985) and the surgical plastic isolator (McLauchlan, 1974, 1976).

Plenum turbulent air flow system. A medium velocity system of this type is most commonly employed, and if maintained and balanced correctly, is reasonably efficient. Air at roof level is drawn by means of fans through a series of filters, is humidified, cooled or heated, and forced through ducts into the operating suite through high-level diffusers fitted into the walls or ceiling.

The air pressure in the operating suite should always be greater than that in the rest of the department (Medical Research Council et al., 1972). Figure 1.25 illustrates the nominal air pressures, supply and extraction flow rates which are required to minimise the movement of contaminated air from dirtier to cleaner areas (DHSS, 1983). The highest pressure of air should always be in the preparation room when used for the preparation of sterile trolleys (35 Pa), followed by the operating theatre (25 Pa), scrub-up and anaesthesia room (14 Pa), exit bay (3 Pa), and utility/disposal (−5 or 0 Pa). Four examples of air movement control schemes for single and two corridor operating departments are given in Figure 1.26.

Extraction of air from the preparation room and operating theatre is not mechanically aided. Air from the operating theatre flows through the small gaps around closed doors and also spills via balanced pressure relief flap valves set in the walls or lower part of doors. These flaps are hinged and weighted so that the air is allowed to pass in one direction only — any tendency for a back-flow of air from less clean areas will cause them to close. Approximately 10 per cent of the operating theatre air supply is provided by air flowing from the preparation room.

It is relatively easy to maintain an outward flow of air through the gaps around closed doors. Difficulties arise when turbulence is created by a person passing through a doorway, or when the door is left open which allows the transfer of air between the two areas separated by the doorway. Given that the temperature difference between rooms is within 1°C, an open doorway of 2.05 × 1.4 m may allow the transfer of 0.19 m^3 per second in each direction. If the temperature difference increases to say 2°C, the volume of air transferred could be in the order of 0.24 m^3 per second. In normal circumstances the flow rates indicated in Figure 1.24 should protect the operating theatre from the ingress of contaminated air when only one door is open at a time. *If several doors to an operating theatre remain open during operations, this may seriously interfere with the outward airflow pattern.* The total air flow supply to an average operating theatre should be between 0.75 and 1.0 m^3 per second, providing 20 to 30 changes of air at a velocity of between 0.05 and 0.2 m per second.

Class	Room	Nominal pressure Pa (A)	Air flow rate for bacterial contaminant dilution	
			Flow in or supply m³/s	Flow out or extract m³/s
Sterile	Preparation Room			
	(a) lay up	35	0.20	—
	(b) sterile pack store	25 ± 5	0.1	—
	Operating Room	25	0.65	—
	Scrub.			
	(a) open bay	25	0	0 (B)
	(b) semi-open bay	25	0	0.10
Clean	Central Sterile Pack Store.	14	0.10	—
	Anaesthetic Room	14	0.15	0.15
	Scrub Room	14	—	0.10
Transitional	Recovery Room	3	15AC/hr(C)	15AC/hr(C)
	Clean Corridor	3	(D)	7AC/hr
	General Access Corridor	3	(D)	7AC/hr
	Changing Rooms	3	7AC/hr	7AC/hr
	Plaster Room	3	7AC/hr	7AC/hr
Dirty	Disposal Corridor	0	—	(E)
	Disposal Room	–5 or 0	—	0.10

Notes: A. Nominal room pressures are given to facilitate setting up of pressure relief dampers, the calculation process, and the sizing of transfer devices. They are **not** an essential feature of the solution.

B. The open bay is considered to be part of the operating room and provided air movement is satisfactory, no specific extract is required.

C. 15 AC/HR is considered necessary for the control of anaesthetic gas pollution.

D. Supply flow rate necessary to make up 7AC/hr after taking into account secondary air from cleaner areas.

E. No dilution requirement. Temperature control requirements only.

Fig. 1.25   Hierarchy of cleanliness and recommended air supply and extract flow rates for dilution of airborne bacterial contaminants. (*Ventilation of Operating Departments — a Design Guide* — DHSS Crown Copyright, reproduced by permission.)

It was thought at one time that extraction of air at floor level helped to dissipate anaesthetic gases thereby avoiding an accumulation of flammable gases which could ignite under favourable circumstances. However, the zone of such risk associated with flammable anaesthetics is limited to an area extending for 25 cm around any part of the anaesthesia circuit or gas paths of an anaesthesia apparatus; flammable gas mixtures now less frequently used, escaping from anaesthesia breathing circuits, rapidly dilute to a non-flammable level within a few centimetres of the point of escape (DHSS, 1971).

Research has identified potential hazards to staff because of pollution of the theatre atmosphere by anaesthetic gases. In particular there is evidence which points to a risk of spontaneous abortion amongst operating department staff. It is therefore recognised that no staff member should be exposed to anaesthetic gases for at least the first three months of

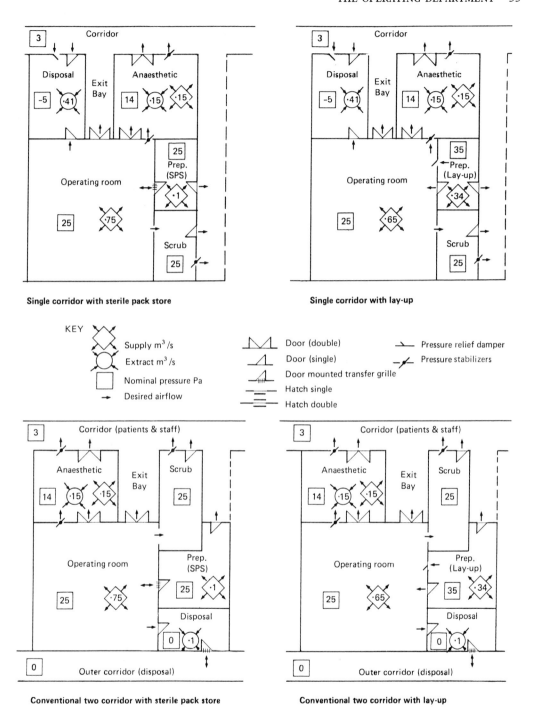

Fig. 1.26 Four examples of air movement control schemes (*Ventilation of Operating Departments — a Design Guide* — DHSS Crown Copyright, reproduced by permission.)

pregnancy. There may be other harmful effects from atmospheric pollution, although at present there is no direct evidence to substantiate this. However, it is a sound principle of health and safety practice to take steps which reduce atmospheric pollution to the lowest practical level.

Good, well-maintained ventilation systems will to a great extent dilute atmospheric pollution. In addition there should be a 'scavenging system' which can remove expired anaesthetic gases (DHSS, 1976, 1983). The active type of system is preferred in which a powered extract device is provided connected to a terminal unit fitted to the services pendant or wall in the operating theatre and anaesthesia room. This can be connected to the expiratory port of the anaesthesia breathing system.

A small positive pressure of air is required in the limited access and general access zones, i.e. the entrance, staff change and circulation areas. There should be 15 air changes per hour in the post-anaesthesia recovery (3 Pa pressure) and 7 air changes per hour in the sterile pack store (14 Pa pressure).

The efficiency of the operating department ventilation system must be checked periodically. Filters must be checked regularly. Some installations incorporate a system of continuous-feed filters which move on automatically as they become clogged. Micro-organisms such as *Pseudomonas sp.* and *Bac. Legionalles* can multiply on cooling coils, eliminator plates and in water reservoirs of humidifying apparatus, and may contaminate the air. The addition of bacteriocides to water reservoirs does not necessarily discourage the growth of bacteria, although periodic flushing with chlorine is recommended. Humidification should preferably be by the injection of clean, dry steam either from the hospital boiler plant or a dedicated supply. Alternatively, spinning disc humidifiers utilising mains water may be considered.

In addition to bacteriological sampling, either by slit samplers or exposure of culture plates, the pressure differentials can be checked visually by the effect on air flows using a smoke test.

One method is to use glacial acetic acid and cyclohexyamine, holding the bottles in rubber gloved hands, close together and with the tops removed. As the fumes rise from the bottles they mix and produce a smoke, enabling the flow of air currents to be detected. Alternatively an applicator, covered lightly at one end with cotton wool, is dipped first into one bottle and then the other to create a flow of smoke. Any solution splashed on the skin should be washed off immediately. Smoke-generating tubes are available also and these are used in a similar manner.

Air currents should be checked at tops and bottoms of doors — both open and closed. If there is any backflow or air currents seem to flow from the less clean to the clean areas, this may indicate either a mechanical fault, or that the filters are blocked and insufficient air is being supplied to the operating suite.

Ultra clean ventilation systems. These originate from developments in the construction of 'clean rooms' for the assembly of electronic components in the electronics and aerospace industries.

Advances in surgical techniques during the past two decades have permitted the development of complex procedures such as joint replacement, high-risk vascular surgery and the transplantation of organs. Such patients are exposed to an increased risk of infection and contamination by particulate matter, especially if they are receiving immunosuppressive drugs. In these circumstances ultra clean ventilation (UCV) by means of unidirectional or laminar air flow systems may be adopted (Charnley, 1964, 1970, 1973; Voda and Withers, 1966; Whitcomb and Clapper, 1966; U.S. Department of Health, Education and Welfare, 1967; Scott, 1970; Scott *et al.*, 1971; Nelson, 1978; Howorth, 1980; Whyte *et al.*, 1983).

The Medical Research Council has conducted a randomised trial into the benefits of UCV in orthopaedic surgery compared with conventional plenum systems (Lidwell *et al.*, 1982). The findings of the MRC study were complex, and in addition to UCV included the relative merits of prophylactic antibiotic cover, and the use of body exhaust suits which will be described shortly. The study showed that the provision of UCV is an effective method of reducing post-operative infection to 0.6 per cent. To what extent this reduction can be achieved exclusively by UCV, rather than using either of the other two measures, singly or in combination, is not entirely resolved. However, a further study by Lidwell (1984) has shown that where at least 100 joint replacement operations are done each year, the cost of installation and maintenance of UCV is more than offset by the financial savings through prevention of infection, even when prophylactic antibiotics are used (Selwyn, 1986).

The term 'laminar or unidirectional flow' refers to the passage of air through an efficient filter to remove inherent contamination, then moving it at a velocity such that it travels in a unidirectional form without eddies or turbulence. The flow of air in vertical UCV systems is directed towards the operation site from a large ceiling diffuser (Fig. 1.27). Horizontal flow UCV systems direct the airflow through a filter bank which consists of an entire wall (Figs. 1.28 and 1.29).

Vertical flow systems are preferred because of their superior performance. In an existing operating theatre, however, horizontal systems, although less effctive, may be the only solution. Their performance may be optimised by the use of special clothing and strict operating theatre discipline to ensure that members of the surgical team do not work between the filter bank and the wound site.

The volume of air passing through the filter bank and ceiling diffusers moves initially at a velocity in the region of 0.35 to 0.55 m per second, making only a single transit over a given area. This reduces to about 0.3 m per second at the periphery of the operating area (Whyte *et al.*, 1973, 1974; Nuegart, 1975; Arrowsmith, 1985). The volume and movement of air is sufficient to give 500–600 air changes per hour in the operating site area. When a solid object is encountered, the air flows round the object, interrupting the unidirectional airflow only momentarily. Surgery is carried out in a uniform flow of clean air and contaminants are flushed away as they are released.

The system incorporates filters which have a minimum efficiency of 90 per cent when tested by the sodium flame method, which is more than adequate to stop bacteria-carrying particles. Some systems do have filters of higher efficiency, but this is usually to assist in maintaining a uniform air flow. Because of the large air volume required for ultra clean ventilation systems, a significant proportion of air is recirculated, usually by means of return air grilles located at high level. However, there is still a need to supply fresh air, and the fresh air supply volume is normally designed to take account of the air conditioning loads of the operating theatre. This is usually half the volume supplied for a conventionally ventilated operating theatre. The excess air volume is allowed to escape through balanced pressure relief valves and door gaps to the peripheral rooms in the operating suite, similar to conventionally ventilated operating theatres (Arrowsmith, 1985).

It has been suggested that a disadvantage of some UCV systems may be the noise created by the fans and constant high velocity flow of air which may prove distracting to the operating team. However, unpleasant odours are quickly dissipated, the drying effect of the air stream reduces perspiration, and the risk of contamination of the operating site is reduced to a minimum. Regarding noise, it is claimed that for one unit — the GEL-OT — the noise level is between 54–55 dBA, and that users quite quickly become accustomed to the background hum (Boulton, 1976). Systems can, however, be installed with remotely sited fans,

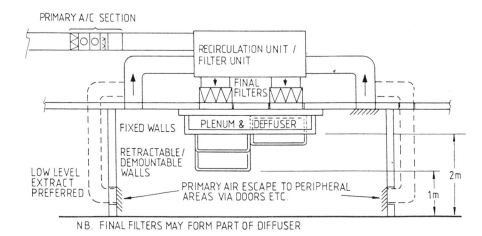

Fig. 1.27 Typical integrated Ultra Clean Ventilation system. (Arrowsmith.)

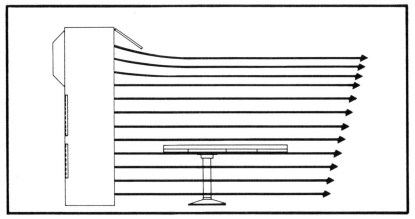

AIR STREAM PATTERN CAUSED BY AIRFOIL

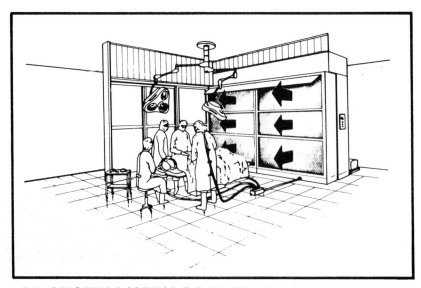

LAF SYSTEM WITH BREATH EXHAUST IN USE

Figs. 1.28 and **1.29** Horizontal laminar air flow unit showing air stream flowing in a horizontal direction across the operation site. (Gelman Hawksley Ltd.)

particularly in new operating theatres; noise levels will be little different from conventional ventilation systems.

Microbiological sampling has shown that virtually no micro-organisms settle in the ultra clean operating area created by the UCV system. This compares with settle counts taken in an operating theatre with conventional ventilation, which have grown from 9 to 19 colonies per culture plate after only one hour's exposure.

High input/high exhaust enclosure. This was first developed by Sir John Charnley in 1962. Further improvements resulted in the Howorth Surgicair enclosure (Charnley, 1973), and the latest Howorth exponential flow system which it is claimed does not require side walls. There have been significant developments, and a number of manufacturers offer similar UCV systems (Figs. 1.30–1.32).

The basic operating principle of a UCV system is to provide an operating zone approximately 2.8 m square in which surgical procedures are performed. Air is discharged vertically from an air diffuser or filter which has fixed high-level partial side walls terminating about 2 m above the floor. The air flows with a uniform velocity of about 0.38 m/sec, this velocity being necessary to avoid buoyancy effects. The Howorth system employs a velocity profile, decreasing from the centre to the perimeter, but has an equivalent air volume of a uniform velocity system. There is, however, considerable debate on the air flow pattern achieved by UCV systems.

Air discharged by any diffuser device is likely to create some degree of entrainment as the discharged air acts upon the surrounding air. The Howorth Exflow system attempts to create an 'expotential' airflow to prevent entrainment at the perimeter of the enclosure. An opposing view is that to do so allows air to short-circuit, perhaps not reaching the extremities of the operating field, and that it is preferable to ensure that all discharged air has sufficient velocity to reach the level of the operating table.

All systems, however, have an outward air flow at some stage, since the air has no alternative escape route; thus they all provide an 'expotential' air flow to some extent. In a working environment other forces are at play (not the least of which is the movement of staff), such

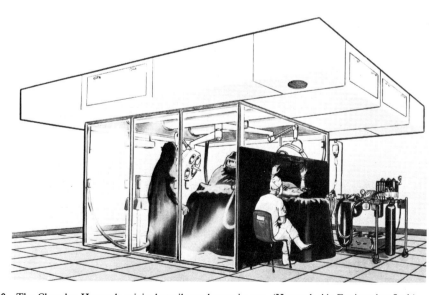

Fig. 1.30 The Charnley-Howorth original sterile enclosure in use. (Howorth Air Engineering Ltd.)

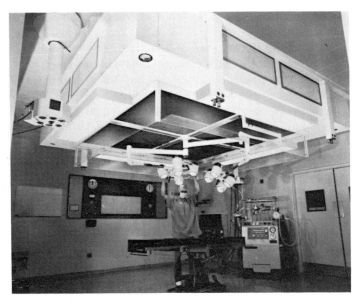

Fig. 1.31   The Howorth EXFLOW Ultra Clean Ventilation system. (Howorth Air Engineering Ltd.)

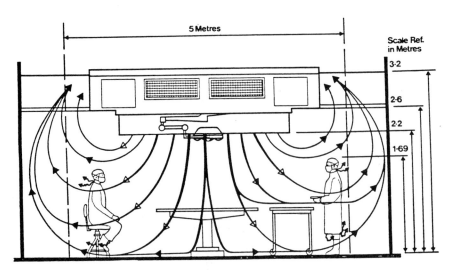

Fig. 1.32   Air flow pattern diagram of the EXFLOW system illustrated in Figure 1.30. (Howorth Air Engineering Ltd.)

that subtle variations in air flow patterns between different systems are unlikely to be significant (Arrowsmith, 1986).

There can be little doubt that the use of side wall extension panels (which attach to the fixed panels and extend down to 1 m above the floor) will assist in optimising the performance of all systems but at some loss of convenience. Nevertheless, the use of enclosing drapes at the anesthetising end should not be discounted, nor should the use of side walls during periods of high occupancy, e.g. during staff training (Whyte *et al.*, 1975; Arrowsmith, 1985).

When planned as part of a new operating theatre, a UCV system can be fully integrated with the general ventilation system. General lighting can be incorporated and full use made of the fixed panels for electrical and gas service outlets.

In association with the original system the *Charnley Body Exhaust System* (BES) was developed to remove body convection currents and the exhaled breath of the operating team, a major source of contamination. A surgical gown is worn, made of Ventile/Scotchguard or non-woven fabric, to reduce the dispersion of bacteria-carrying skin particles which are being shed continually by the operating team (see Ch. 6). This is supplemented by the BES which enables the air under the gown to be extracted constantly at 0.025 m^3 per second, taking away skin particles in addition to cooling the wearer. Perspiration is inhibited and fatigue reduced by improved personal comfort. The original version of the BES consisted of a transparent plastic visor connected to a corrugated extract tube and worn with a hooded gown (Fig. 1.33). This arrangement has been found to be inconvenient in many forms of surgery, particularly when a microscope is used. An alternative is the 'Mandarin' loop which is hung around the neck under a suitable gown with a secure neck band. In this instance it is important to ensure that the hair is completely covered and the conventional mask fits snugly: a simple hood can be worn (Fig. 1.34).

As in the case of the original high performance enclosure, there have been developments in the application of clean room style clothing for use in a UCV system. Unlike body exhaust suits, they do not provide for ventilation of the wearer and may not be considered by some to be as comfortable. However, they do not necessitate the incumbance of an umbilical cord exhaust tube (Whyte *et al.*, 1976).

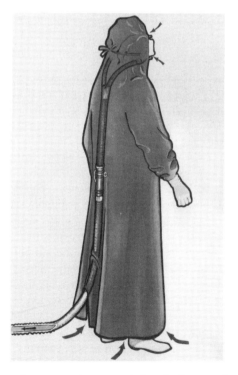

Fig. 1.33 Charnley Body Exhaust System to reduce transmission of micro-organism-carrying skin particles. (Howorth Air Engineering Ltd.)

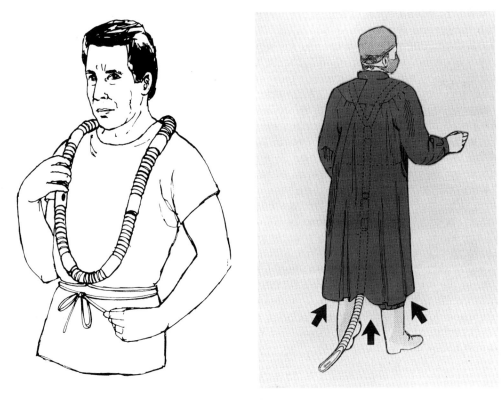

Fig. 1.34   Mandarin Body Exhaust Gown. (Howorth Air Engineering Ltd.)

INDIVIDUAL SPACE REQUIREMENTS

GENERAL ACCESS ZONE

Entrance and transfer

The design of this area will be influenced by the views of the project team on such matters as 'access zones', security, and the movement of patients, staff, supplies and items for disposal.

The provision of a single main entrance to the department through which all traffic passes will simplify security. Entrances to staff changing, the supplies store, and disposal hold, should be easily visible from reception. Alternatively, access to staff changing can be controlled with electronic door locks operated by a personal plastic identity card. The patient transfer area must be under direct observation from reception.

The implications for design of the transfer area have been discussed already (page 11). For example, a policy of patient transportation may be adopted whereby patients are first transferred from their beds to theatre trolleys at the entrance, and their beds are subsequently used after surgery for transport between the operating suite and post-anaesthesia recovery. In this instance space must be provided for handling supplies of clean and soiled linen and materials for damp dusting the bed. Other factors influencing design would

include the adoption of a 'red line' policy, and whether the entrance is to be used as a preoperative 'holding' area for patients on beds or trolleys.

A space should be provided in this area for a porter's base.

Reception

This office may be combined with facilities for general administrative and secretarial activities, but must be planned and sited so as to make possible easy surveillance of the entrance and the reception of visitors.

During normal operating sessions the reception is the control and communication centre for the operating department and the point at which specimens and samples are held for transmission to the laboratory. Account should be taken of communication technology and development of automated data processing, and space should be provided for a micro computer or computer terminal for use by operating department staff.

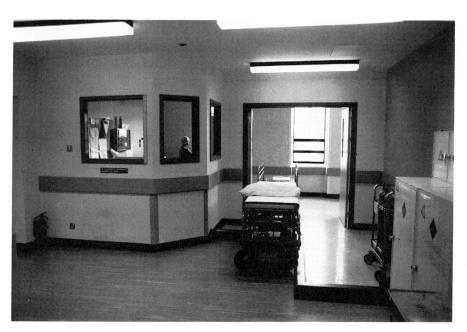

Fig. 1.35   Reception/transfer area at entrance to operating department. (Moriston Hospital, Swansea, Glamorgan.)

Staff changing

Male and female changing rooms and sanitary facilities are required at the entrance where staff can change from uniform or outdoor clothes into theatre protective clothing and footwear before moving into the department, and vice versa.

In addition to personal lockers for indoor clothing and shoes there should be secure racks for outdoor coats and motor cycle crash helmets, and a few lockers suitable for items such as shopping baskets and small cases.

Theatre protective clothing in various sizes can be stored on open shelving. Theatre footwear, whether clean or dirty, should be held on shelving near to a mechanical ventilation

exhaust grille. Washing of theatre footwear can take place in the cleaner's room which should be provided with sufficient space and equipment for this purpose.

The HBN (DHSS, 1989) recommends sanitary facilities for staff as being: 'One wash basin and one WC should be provided for 8–10 persons; the number of showers is a matter for local decision. The inclusion of toilet facilities in the changing rooms is not acceptable; these facilities should be located in an adjacent space.'

Disposal hold

There should be a disposal hold at the entrance for the temporary holding of soiled dressings, linen and general rubbish securely sealed in clearly identifiable bags. All material for disposal associated with a particular operation should be labelled with the operation and theatre number, and released only after the used instrument tray sent direct from the theatre utility has been checked in the Sterilizing and Disinfecting Unit (SDU).

There is no standard formula for deciding the capacity of the disposal hold. Project teams will need to take into account such factors as frequency of collection, whether all items for disposal will be routed through this hold, or whether a proportion will be taken direct from the point of use for disposal outside the department.

LIMITED ACCESS ZONE

Staff control base

This is the control point for the co-ordination of theatre staff activities and the movement of patients within the limited access zone; it should be located centrally in a good relationship to the operating suites. It is the point for temporary storage of blood for transfusion,

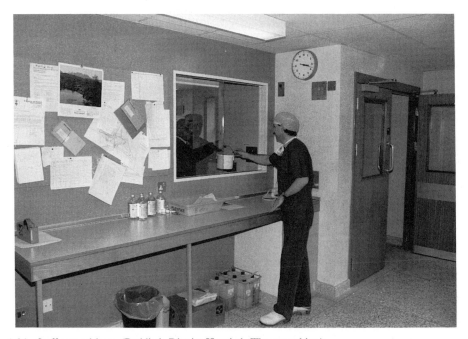

Fig. 1.36   Staff control base. (Redditch District Hospital, Worcestershire.)

routing of pathology samples and specimens via reception for onward transmission to the laboratory, and the storage of drugs including the main controlled drugs cupboard and a lockable drugs refrigerator.

At night, when the reception is unmanned, it may be designated as the communication centre for the department. Fire and other alarms are duplicated in both locations.

Post anaesthesia recovery

This space accommodates patients who, following operative procedures, are recovering from anaesthetics and require the attention of anaesthetists and other trained staff before returning to the ward. The post-anaesthesia recovery should be close to the reception/transfer area, but not remote from the operating suites as it needs to be easily accessible to the anaesthetists.

The HBN (DHSS, 1989) suggests, when planning recovery facilities, a ratio of two beds for each operating suite should be considered, but account will need to be taken of the number of cases per session, average time spent in the recovery room and the arrangements selected for transportation of patients.

Bed spaces should be of a size which permits the bed to be pulled away from the wall to enable an anaesthetist to work at the head end in an emergency, whilst still leaving room for the passage of a bed or trolley at the other end. Each bed space requires wall-mounted piped oxygen, 4-bar medical compressed air and medical vacuum terminal outlets and electric socket outlets. Up to two bed spaces may be provided with piped nitrous oxide for continuing anaesthesia.

The HBN (DHSS, 1989) states that the recovery room is only a secondary source of expired anaesthetic gas pollution and 'provided that exhaust grilles are near the heads of the beds, and the non-circulating ventilation exchange rate in the room does not fall below 15 changes per hour, no additional installation should be necessary'. If piped nitrous oxide

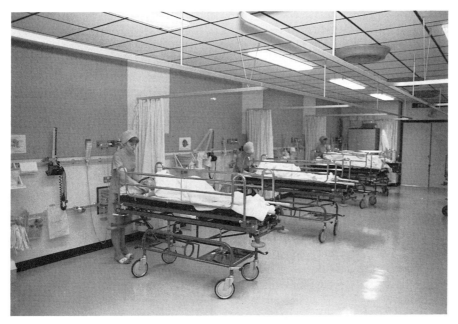

Fig. 1.37   Post-anaesthesia recovery. (Grimsby District Hospital, Lincolnshire.)

outlets have been provided, then these bed spaces should have anaesthetic gas scavenging system terminals also.

Equipment rails at the bed head are a convenient means of mounting equipment such as small work surfaces, oxygen flowmeters, monitors and suction apparatus. The general level of lighting should be suitable for most clinical procedures; supplementary lighting can be provided by means of a mobile spotlight.

Although staff will be mainly engaged at the bedside, there is the need for a staff base in a position from which the whole of the recovery area can be observed. This staff base should be combined with facilities for the storage of clean and sterile commodities, and, subject to local operational policy, drugs. There should be easy access to a utility room and facilities for disposal including suctioned liquids and the contents of vomit bowls. Space is required for parking mobile equipment such as trolleys, a ventilator and resuscitation apparatus.

The decor should be pleasant, walls can be covered with washable paper and the ceiling finished with sound absorbent material. If possible, windows with a pleasant outlook should be provided.

Rest rooms

Pleasant, quiet rest accommodation for staff is required. It is a matter of opinion whether one large rest room should be provided for all grades of staff to sit together. Those who favour this solution argue that this arrangement contributes to a better atmosphere in which teamwork will flourish. Conversely, others consider that there are advantages in providing separate rooms in which various groups of staff can sit and discuss matters privately.

Cost constraints limit the amount of space which can be provided for staff rest accommodation. It is a matter for local decision as to how this space should be allocated. Some projects may opt for the common sitting room, others will prefer separate rooms which may be allocated either on a grade basis, or perhaps for smokers and non-smokers. Whichever solution is adopted, account must be taken of the special needs of medical staff who require facilities for dictation and confidential discussions (Utting, 1984). One solution is to provide a medical staff office adjacent to the rest rooms, for administrative work, confidential discussions and the dictation of case notes (DHSS, 1988).

Rest rooms should have windows with a pleasant outlook, and if these are openable, then an entrance lobby to control ventilation in the limited access zone may be required. The rooms should be pleasantly furnished with comfortable chairs, occasional tables, a bookcase and perhaps a small writing table. The furnishing will to some extent be influenced by the catering policy adopted.

Pantry

In the majority of operating departments a pantry should suffice for the preparation of beverages and snacks, the storage and washing up of a limited amount of crockery and cutlery, and the storage of dry provisions and milk.

Exceptionally this service may be extended to the provision of meals from the hospital kitchen. In this instance consideration will need to be given to the spacial implications in the staff rest rooms, space for washing dishes or holding them for transportation to central wash-up, keeping meals hot or re-heating (i.e. microwave ovens) (DHSS, 1988).

The pantry should be located immediately adjacent to the staff rest rooms.

Offices/seminar

Senior nurse. The operating department manager/senior nurse requires an administrative base near to the transfer/reception area. This office will be used for administrative work and confidential discussions between medical and nursing staff, interviewing visitors and counselling staff. Space may be required for a micro-computer or computer terminal.

Theatre nursing staff. An administrative office for the use of department nursing staff should be provided in the limited access zone. In addition to the storage of documents and records and general administrative work by theatre sisters and senior nurses, this office can be used for discussions, interviews and counselling of staff. This office may be used also by a nurse tutor, although when the workload associated with post-registration courses is great, it may be necessary to provide a separate office for this purpose.

Medical staff. The option for an administrative office for medical staff has already been mentioned in the previous section.

Seminar. Because the demands of hygiene and the specialist nature of theatre work mean that staff cannot easily leave the department, the inclusion of a seminar room in the operating department has many advantages and will save staff time. The room can be used for intra-departmental meetings and case conferences, teaching sessions for staff, and private study. The amount of audio-visual equipment provided will depend on local policy, but provision should be made for secure storage. This room could be used as a base for the clinical nurse teacher.

Storage

Main supplies store. This should provide storage both for sterile packs in protective outer wraps and bulk clean supplies. For convenience of deliveries the store should be located near the entrance/transfer area, but accessible to the limited access zone and operating suites.

The shelving and racking for the sterile supplies section should be appropriate to take various sizes of trays and packs. There should be sufficient space for loading trolleys with large sterile pre-set instrument trays (Fig. 1.38).

Clean supplies will include some pharmacy items such as bulk supplies of lotions, but controlled drugs will not be stored here.

An administrative area including desk, filing system and space for micro-computer or computer terminal may be required.

Equipment store. A centrally positioned store is required for bulky mobile equipment not in daily use such as operating microscopes, lasers, and operation table traction apparatus. The store should be zoned to protect equipment, some of which is delicate and costly. Mobile x-ray equipment and an image intensifier should be parked in a separate space, with easy access to a mains power socket for recharging the batteries.

Gas cylinder store. Storage of a limited quantity of ready-to-use cylinders of oxygen and nitrous oxide for anaesthesia machines and anaesthesia ventilators is required. The store may also contain equipment to supply high pressure, 10-bar medical compressed air to the theatres for driving surgical tools. This may be in the form of an air cylinder manifold, or equipment which boosts air supplied from the 4-bar medical air pipeline system. A code of practice on Safety and Care in the storage, handling and use of medical gas cylinders is contained in Health Equipment Information No 163 (DHSS, 1987).

Cleaner. This room should have sufficient space for the convenient storage of cleaning equipment and materials for exclusive use in the operating department. Facilities are

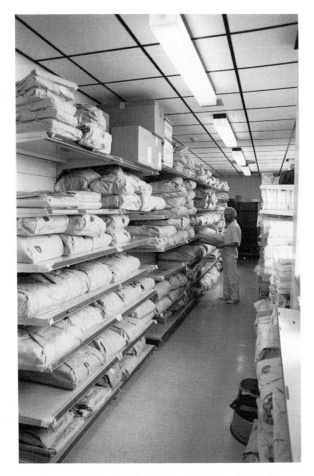

Fig. 1.38   Departmental sterile store. (Grimsby District Hospital, Lincolnshire.)

required for cleaning theatre footwear, and space should be provided for parking floor scrubbing machines, the storage of bulk cleaning supplies and accommodation for cleaning staff.

Endoscope cleaning

Proper cleansing and processing of endoscopes is ideally carried out by skilled staff in the SDU (Chapter 7). However, some endoscopes will require cleansing and sterilization within the operating department; a special room should be provided for this purpose. These endoscopes are most likely to be flexible instruments, e.g. gastroscopes, as rigid endoscopes which can withstand heat sterilization can be processed in the SDU. Equipment may include an automatic washing, rinsing and sterilizing machine. Ventilation to remove obnoxious vapours will be required. The SDU should normally undertake terminal processing and sterilization at the end of an operating session.

RESTRICTED ACCESS ZONE

Anaesthesia room

The anaesthesia room should be of the same hygienic finish as the operating theatre.

Quietness is essential and planning should take into account the need for privacy and sound attenuation to permit the maintenance of an undisturbed environment. The general lighting levels should be adequate for most procedures, although a small mobile spotlight is useful on occasions.

Patient care. The patient will arrive on a bed, conventional theatre trolley, or transfer trolley. Ward staff may escort patients to the anaesthesia room, particularly children who may be accompanied by a parent or member of the paediatric nursing team. The patient may then be transferred to the operation table or top (where this is not incorporated in a trolley transfer system) and safely positioned for surgery either before or after anaesthesia is induced. Procedures may be carried out, such as setting up intravenous infusions, connecting monitoring equipment and the positioning of diathermy electrodes.

Size/layout. All anaesthesia rooms in an operating department should be identical in layout, not handed*, having a work top with writing surface and storage units placed to the left hand side of the patient, and piped services and mobile equipment to the right. There should be a clock with sweep second hand located above the entrance of the door to the operating theatre, and a time elapse clock within easy reach. Equipment should always be kept in the same place and not be interchanged between rooms. To avoid this it is important to ensure that adequate replacements are available.

Depending on the shape of the room, the floor area should be in the region of 15.12 m², with a minimum width of 3.6 m assuming that fitted equipment is confined to one side of the room only.

Storage should include adjustable shelves or modular storage units and cupboards (Figs. 1.39, 1.40). Equipment is arranged neatly on shelves or racks, labelled and in order. All items must be clearly visible and *always* kept in the same place. Equipment such as laryngoscopes should be duplicated as they are known to fail at crucial moments. The cupboards and storage units should not be used as a store for general replacements. Various sizes of endotracheal tubes complete with connectors, and anaesthesia face masks, etc., may be kept separate by storing them in individual disposable bags. In this way equipment can be arranged ready for immediate use, and the preparation of special trolleys simplified.

A dispenser should be provided containing a selection of sterile disposable syringes in sizes ranging from 2 ml to 20 ml, hypodermic and intravenous needles.

A separate lockable cupboard is required in each anaesthesia room for the temporary storage of controlled drugs issued to an anaesthetist for a specific operating session. This is when one main controlled drugs cupboard is provided in the operating department, ideally sited at a central supervised point such as the staff control base. However, local policy may dictate that each anaesthesia room be equipped with a complete controlled drugs cupboard. The drug cupboard in the anaesthesia room may also contain the register used for recording controlled drugs administered. It is the legal obligation of the anaesthetist to enter all use made of controlled drugs, the name of the patient and quantity used. Drugs for immediate use may be stored in a locked drawer fitted to the anaesthesia machine. Provision should be made to secure the anaesthesia machine to a wall when left unattended.

Equipment. An efficient suction machine or pipeline suction device must be available, together with tubing and a selection of suction nozzles and catheters with connectors of appropriate size. Unless being used by the anaesthetist in theatre, this is always kept ready in the anaesthesia room, as timely use of suction can be life-saving on occasions. Unless pipeline gases are available, the use of a suction device working off oxygen supplied from cylinders on an anaesthesia machine is to be deplored. There is the danger that the oxygen

---

* Where the layout of the room is a mirror image of identical rooms elsewhere in the department.

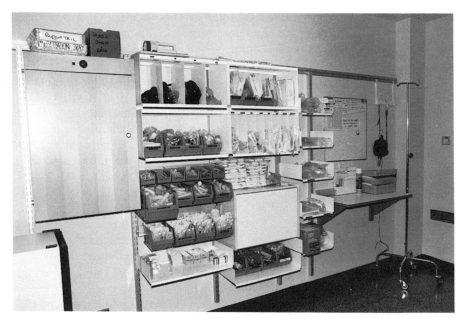

Fig. 1.39 Anaesthesia room demountable storage system. (Moriston Hospital, Swansea, Glamorgan — TopRail, Simple Systems Ltd.)

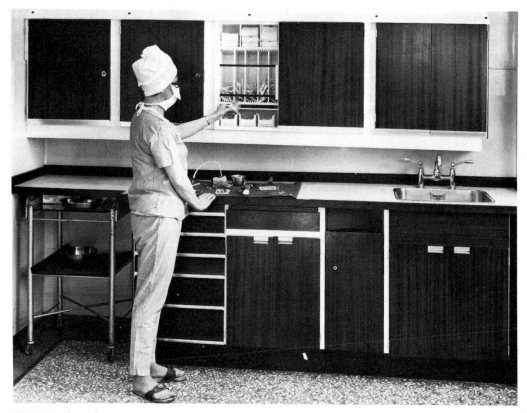

Fig. 1.40 Anaesthesia room storage units at the Royal National Orthopaedic Hospital, London. (Cuxson Gerrard Ltd.)

from a cylinder may be used up very quickly and result in anoxia from lack of oxygen in inspired gases.

Two trolleys about 450 mm (18 in) square are required for the exclusive use of the anaesthetist for transfusions and local anaesthesia procedures. At least two transfusion stands should be available; an infusion pump to enable rapid transfusion of blood should be fitted to one, or ideally to each of the stands, to supplement the pumping device of the plastic recipient sets.

Other items easily accessible and ready for use should include: a sphygmomanometer, stethoscopes, recipient infusion sets, monitoring and resuscitation equipment, e.g. monitors, ventilator, defibrillator, tracheostomy set.

A wash hand-basin with elbow-operated mixing taps and requisites for 'scrubbing up' should be provided in the anaesthesia room. This basin should be located away from areas in which sterile trolleys are being used.

The operating theatre

Size/shape. Mention has been made already of the 'operating zone' which is defined as the operating site and the preparation room (page 9). During an operation, the patient, scrub team, anaesthetist and much of the equipment being used occupy a relatively central area of the operating theatre. The remaining space in the theatre will contain some equipment, and is used by circulating staff and observers. During specialist surgery, the team may be clustered at the head or foot of the table, but there may be trolleys and other equipment at the sides as well. The HBN (DHSS, 1989) recommends that the theatre should be approximately square, with an area of 38 m^2 which is sufficient for most types of surgery.

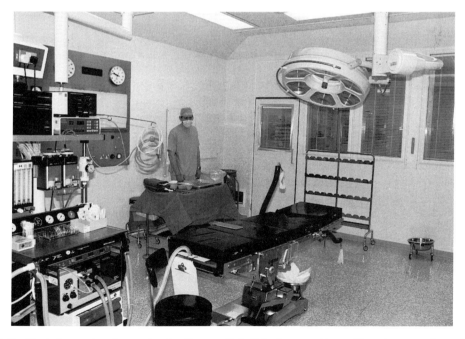

Fig. 1.41 Typical operating theatre showing 'borrowed' daylight from outside corridor, via preparation and scrub rooms. (Milton Keynes District Hospital, Buckinghamshire.)

Services. Electric socket outlets, piped medical gases and anaesthetic gas scavenging terminal outlets (page 27) should be conveniently sited. A single wall mounted control panel can incorporate lighting and temperature controls, clock (including time elapse facility), x-ray viewing screens, and a swab count record board. In addition, a writing surface in the form of a wall desk 45 cm by 61 cm fitted under the x-ray viewing screens, will be found useful for writing up notes and swab registers, etc.

Doors. There must be adequate, wide connecting doors between the theatre and ancillary rooms of the operating suite. Doorways to the anaesthesia room and exit bay must permit the easy passage of a bed with attachments; the doorway to the preparation room should be wide enough to wheel through trolleys with sterile drapes without touching the sides. All doors must be fitted with a mechanism which permits the door to be held in a 90° stand open position. Vision panels are required with an obscurable facility fitted in those to the anaesthesia room and exit bay.

Equipment. All theatre furniture must be of hygienic finish; stainless steel or aluminium are ideal materials for trolleys, lotion bowl stands, etc. (Fig. 1.41).

Exit bay

There must be an exit route from the operating theatre for the patient other than through the anaesthesia room. The main function of this bay is to provide space for the transfer of a patient between operating table and bed or trolley before he is moved to the post-anaesthesia recovery. The bay is not used for recovery and therefore piped services are not required.

Scrub-up and gowning

Scrubbing and gowning should take place in a space or room immediately adjacent to the theatre. This room must be sufficiently large to allow gowning and gloving simultaneously in separate zones.

Scrub-up zone. The most important consideration is the provision of a trough or wash basins of adequate depth and at the optimum height, to avoid splashing the scrub clothes of those using it. Taps should be of the elbow-operated type, mixing hot and cold water into a single faucet, and preferably controlled by a thermostatic mixing valve. The position of the taps should be calculated to minimise 'drumming' noise from the flow of water on the metallic surface of the trough. In the past an angled glass sheet has been used which channelled water into a gulley, but this is now unacceptable as the use of floor gullies in the operating suite is regarded as microbiologically unsound.

There should be a clock or other timing device visible from the scrub-up position. Scrub-up solution, e.g. Hibscrub, Betadine, PHisoHex., is dispensed from foot or elbow-operated dispensers. Individual clean nail brushes are supplied from a suitable dispenser which can be refilled afterwards for terminal disinfection of the used brushes by autoclaving. Alternatively, disposable foam plastic pads impregnated with a scrub-up germicide are available as dispenser packs.

Gowning/gloving area. This should be located as far away from the scrub-up trough as possible. Gown packs can be opened either on a suitable trolley or a cantilever shelf fitted to the wall and having a 15 cm (6 in) space at the rear to facilitate opening out the wrappings. Adjustable shelving is required for storing ready-to-use packs of sterile gowns and

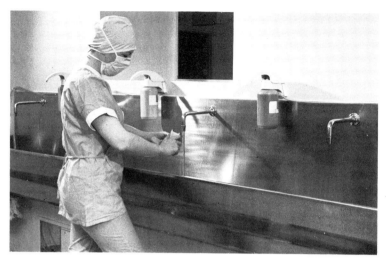

Fig. 1.42 Three-position 'scrubbing up' trough with foot-operated taps and skin disinfectant dispenser. (Northwick Park Hospital, Harrow, Middlesex.)

gloves for at least one session. The main supply of packets should be held in the department's main supply store.

Large bin sack holders are required for the temporary holding of used hand towels and wrappers.

Preparation room

Ideally the use of pre-set tray pack systems for instruments and drapes enables trolleys to be prepared in the operating theatre immediately before an operation starts. However, during a list or series of operations, or when a good deal of pre-operative activity occurs (for example, positioning of the patient for a complex procedure), to avoid delay and possible contamination, the sterile packets should be opened in an adjacent preparation room.

Preparation of trolleys. This space should be sufficient to accommodate two members of staff and sterile trolleys prepared for the next case. The sizes of trolleys envisaged must be taken into account during formulation of the design brief during planning. The nurse preparing the trolley should first scrub up in the scrub room and then gown and glove in the preparation room. Care must be taken to avoid the dissipation of glove powder; ideally powder-free gloves should be used.

Mention has been made previously that the doorway to the theatre must be wide enough to permit the passage of prepared trolleys without contamination of sterile drapes.

Sterile supplies. The provision of a pre-set tray system of sterile instruments and drapes supplied from a Sterilizing and Disinfecting Unit (SDU) is assumed (Chapter 7). Generally, these supplies are first delivered to the main departmental store where the bulk are held until required. Some special instruments may be taken directly to specific preparation rooms for storage. With the possible exception of the disinfection of complex endoscopes with suitable equipment, and sterilizing a 'dropped' instrument in a small portable autoclave, sterilizers are not normally required in the operating department. Similarly, sterile topical fluids are supplied in sealed flasks prepared by the pharmacy or obtained commercially rather than from locally based running water presses or multi-supply tanks (Fig 1.43).

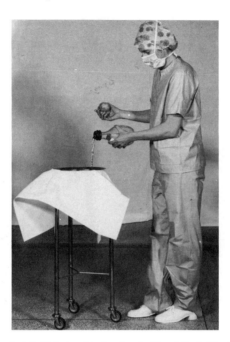

Fig. 1.43 Dispensing sterile topical fluid in hand lotion bowl. (Royal Berkshire Hospital, Reading, Berkshire.)

Storage. Sufficient storage space with adjustable shelving or modular storage units should be provided to contain all the sterile items required for an operating session (Figs. 1.44–1.45). These will include sterile instrument trays, supplementary packs and other items such as suture materials, sterile fluids and lotions. Access to a heated lotion cabinet is required.

The arrangement of storage should be identical in each preparation room as staff, sometimes under pressure, need to easily and swiftly locate a required item. An area of storage may be reserved for those items peculiar to the theatre it serves.

Utility

The use of this space, which should have direct access to the theatre, depends on the extent of service provided by an SDU. After the safe disposal of used 'sharps' in rigid containers, soiled swabs, dressings and linen are sealed in identifiable bags labelled with the operation and theatre numbers for temporary holding and disposal. The used trays of instruments having been over-wrapped with trolley drapes in the theatre, are labelled with the operation and theatre numbers before return to the SDU for processing. Used suction bottles may be sealed and returned to the SDU for emptying, washing and terminal disinfection. This is an alternative to emptying in a slop hopper in the utility which may result in aerosol dissemination of micro-organisms.

Cleaning materials. Cleaning materials for use in theatre between cases are kept in this room which may also be used by surgeons wishing to examine a specimen. Shelves are required for the storage of disposable bags and specimen containers, and hook clips for the vertical storage of mop handles and heads. A slop hopper sink and drainer is required for filling and emptying buckets, suction bottles and other fluids. Space may be needed for parking an SDU collection trolley, either within or adjacent to the utility room.

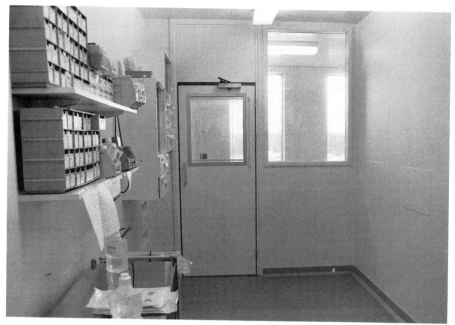

Fig. 1.44

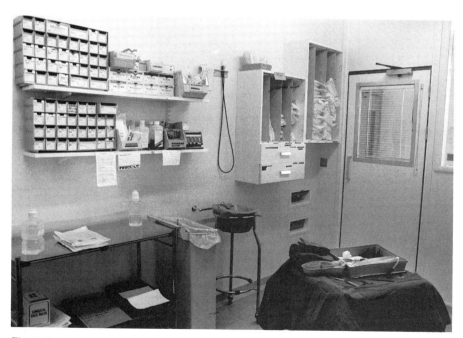

Fig. 1.45

Figs. 1.44 and **1.45** Preparation room showing 'borrowed' daylight from outside corridor. (Milton Keynes District Hospital, Buckinghamshire.)

REFERENCES

ARROWSMITH, L. W. M. (1985) Ultra-clean ventilation systems for operating rooms. *Health Services Estate*, No. 55, February, 65–68.

ARROWSMITH, L. W. M. (1986) Design aspects of ultra clean ventilation systems for operating rooms. *Journal of Sterile Service Management*, 17–18, October.

AYLIFFE, S. A., BABB, J. R., COLLINS, B. J. and LOWBURY, E. J. L. (1969) *Journal of Hygiene (Camb)*, 67, 417–25.

BARTLETT, D. (1978) Operating theatre lighting. *NATNews*, November, 24.

BERRY, E. C. and KHON, L. (1972) *Introduction to Operating Room Techniques*, 4th edn. New York: A Bleninston Publication, McGraw-Hill Book Co.

BECK, W. (1980) Choosing surgical illumination, *American Journal of Surgery*, 2, 327–331.

BRITISH STANDARDS INSTITUTION (1986) BS 4533: Section 103.2. London: BSI.

CHARNLEY, J. (1964) *British Journal of Surgery*, 51, 195.

CHARNLEY, J. (1970) *Lancet*, i, 1053.

CHARNLEY, J. (1973) *Cleveland Clinic Quarterly*, 40, 99.

CURRY, I. (1982a) Planning operating departments, the nursing role. *NATNews*, May, 9–12.

CURRY, I. (1982b) Planning operating departments, operational policies. *NATNews*, August, 14–16.

DEPARTMENT OF HEALTH AND SOCIAL SECURITY (1968) Article on operating departments. *Hospital Management*. September.

DEPARTMENT OF HEALTH AND SOCIAL SECURITY (1971) Anti-static precautions, rubber, plastics and fabrics. *Hospital Technical Memorandum No. 1*. London: HMSO.

DEPARTMENT OF HEALTH AND SOCIAL SECURITY (1976) Pollution of operating departments by anaesthetic gases, *H.C.76(38)*.

DEPARTMENT OF HEALTH AND SOCIAL SECURITY (1977) Anti-static precautions, flooring in anaesthetic areas. *Health Technical Memorandum No. 2*. London: HMSO.

DEPARTMENT OF HEALTH AND SOCIAL SECURITY (1983) Ventilation of operating departments. *A Design Guide*.

DEPARTMENT OF HEALTH AND SOCIAL SECURITY (1985) Signs: a design manual for hospitals and other health buildings, new and old. *Hospital Technical Memorandum No. 65*. London: HMSO.

DEPARTMENT OF HEALTH AND SOCIAL SECURITY (1987) Safety and care in the storage, handling and use of medical gas cylinders — a code of practice. London: DHSS.

DEPARTMENT OF HEALTH AND SOCIAL SECURITY (1989) Sterilizing and disinfecting unit. *Health Building Note No. 19*. London: HMSO.

DEPARTMENT OF HEALTH AND SOCIAL SECURITY (1989) Operating department. *Health Building Note No. 26*. London: HMSO.

DUNSTAN, M. E. (1982) Planning operating departments, Reading Architectural Drawings. *NATNEWS*, June, 13–15.

HOUGHTON, M. AND HUDD, J. (1967) *Aids to Theatre Technique*, 4th edn, Chap 1. London: Bailliere.

HOWORTH, F. H. (1980) Air flow patterns in the operating theatre, *Journal of the Environmental Engineers*, June, 29.

HOWORTH, F. H. (1984) The air in the operating theatre. *The design and use of operating theatres*, edited by I. D. A. Johnston and A. R. Hunter. London: Arnold.

JOURNAL OF BONE AND JOINT SURGERY (1983) Annotation — ultra-clean air, 65, No. 4, August.

LANCET (1956) Leading article — ventilation of operating theatres, ii, 1197.

LANCET (1958) Annotation — air contamination and layout of theatre suites, i, 203.

LIDWELL, O. M., LOWBURY, E. J. L., WHYTE, W., BLOWERS, R., STANLEY, S. J. AND LOWE, D. (1982) Effect of ultraclean air in operating rooms on deep sepsis in the joint after total hip or knee replacement: a randomised study. *British Medical Journal*, 1, 285.

LIDWELL, O. M. (1984) Bacteriological considerations. *The Design and Use of Operating Theatres*, edited by I. D. A. Johnston and A. R. Hunter. London: Arnold.

LOVETT, P. A., HALSTEAD, M. B., HILL, A. R., PALMER, D. A., RYAN, T. J. AND SONNEX, T. S. (1983) Colour rendering of fluorescent lamps for use in hospitals. *Proc. CIE, 20th Session*, 1, E 28/1–2.

LOVETT, P. A. AND HALSTEAD, M. B. (1986) Measurement of the skin colour of babies in hospitals. *Proc. CIBSE National Lighting Conference*, 140–154.

MALE, C. G. (1978) Theatre ventilation. *British Journal of Anaesthesia*, 50, 1257.

MCLAUGHLAN, J., PILCHER, M. F., TREXLER, P. C. AND WHALLEY, R. (1974) *British Medical Journal*, 1, 322.

MEDICAL RESEARCH COUNCIL (1982) Operating theatre hygiene sub committee. *Lancet*, ii, 945.

MEDICAL RESEARCH COUNCIL, DHSS AND REGIONAL ENGINEERS ASSOCIATION (1972) Joint Working Party. *Operating Theatre Requirements*. London: MRC/DHSS.

MORRIS, R. H. (1971) Influence of ambient temperature on patient temperature during intra abdominal surgery. *Annals of Surgery*, 173, 230–3, February.

MORRIS, R. H. (1971) Operating room temperature and the anaesthetized, paralyzed patient. *Archives of Surgery*, 102, 95–7, February.

MORRIS AND WILKEY (1970) The effects of ambient temperature on patient temperature during surgery not involving body cavities. *Anaesthesiology*, **37**, 102–7.

MULLICK, A. (1978) Control of airborne infection using a mobile horizontal laminar air-flow system. *NATNews*, July, 10–12.

NELSON, J. P. (1978) Clinical use of facilities with special air handling equipment. *Hospital Topics*, September/October, 32–35.

NUEGART, H. (1975) *Sulzer Technical Review No. 1.*

OXFORD REGIONAL HEALTH AUTHORITY (1982) *Use of operating theatres, Report.* Oxford: RHA.

RAIT, A. (1982) Planning operating departments, the principles of Commissioning. *NATNews*, October, 11–14.

RAWLINSON, C., KELLY, J. AND COALSLEY, A (1982) An evaluation of the provision and utilisation of operating suites. Medical Architecture Research Unit, Polytechnic of North London. London: DHSS.

SCOTT, C. C. (1970) *Lancet*, **i**, 989.

SCOTT, C. C., ANDERSON, J. T. AND GUTHRIE, T. D. (1971) *Lancet*, **i**, 1288.

SELWYN, S. (1986) Airing operating theatres. *British Medical Journal*, **292**, 1544.

SILVESTER, J. C. (1978) *Nursing Times*, August 24, 1411.

U.S. DEPARTMENT OF HEALTH AND EDUCATION AND WELFARE (1967) *Circular*, May.

VODA, A. M. AND WITHERS, J. E. (1966) *American Journal of Nursing*, **66**, 2454.

WEEKS, J. (1982) Planning operating departments, the planning of operating theatre suites, *NATNews*, July 9–12.

WHITCOMBE, J. G. AND CLAPPER, W. E. (1966) *American Journal of Surgery*, **112**, 681–685.

WHYTE, W., SHAW, B. H. AND BARNES, R. (1973) *Journal of Hygiene (Camb)*, **73**, 559.

WHYTE, W., SHAW, B. H. AND FREEMAN, M. A. (1974) *Journal of Hygiene (Camb)*, **73**, 61.

WHYTE, W., LIDWELL, O. M., LOWBURY, E. J. L. AND BLOWERS, R. (1983) Suggested bacteriological standards for air in ultraclean operating rooms, *Journal of Hospital Infection*, **4**, 133.

WILLIAMS, R. E. O., BLOWERS, R., GARROD, L. P. AND SHOOTER, R. A. (1966) *Hospital Infection — Causes and Prevention, 2nd edn.* London: Lloyd Luke.

WILLIAMS, M. (1983) Planning operating departments, commissioning theatres. *NATNews*, April, 15–18.

WYON, D. P., LIDWELL, O. M. AND WILLIAMS, R. E. O. (1968) Thermal comfort during surgical operations. *Journal of Hygiene*, **66**, No. 2, 229–248, London

2

Organisation and management

An introductory paragraph in the book *The Design and Utilisation of Operating Theatres* states: 'Organisation is necessary in the operating department in order to integrate a complexity of skills, expertise and technology in the interests of patients requiring surgery. It must be planned round a central point which in the operating theatre should be the patient undergoing surgery . . . . . The patient is unaware of the implications of standards of design and care in theatre and has placed his trust temporarily in people, many of whom he will never see. This imposes a great responsibility on those who plan and those who work in the theatre, not because they will be unrecognised but because the patient has given them complete trust' (Clarke *et al.*, 1984). In simple terms, this is what good management of the operating department is all about.

Care of the patient in the operating department is shared by surgeon, anaesthetist and nurse. Each has a specific field of responsibility as part of a team, although some tasks such as checking instruments, swabs and packs are shared. The surgeon decides if and when to operate and the procedure to perform; the anaesthetist is responsible for the patient's safety and survival during the operation and immediate post-operative period; the nurse provides the staff, instruments and equipment, and co-ordinates technical services for the team (Bevan, 1984).

PERSONNEL

Operating department manager

The senior nurse responsible for operating department services influences to a great extent how working relationships develop between members of the medical, nursing and technical team (Douglas, 1962; Clarke *et al.*, 1984). This person should be a good leader, experienced in all aspects of theatre technique, having managerial skills and qualifications of kindness, tolerance and total commitment.

The capacity to plan ahead with good judgement, and the ability to accept constructive criticism is very important. There should always be a willingness to adapt to new developments in surgery and theatre technique. The need for loyalty to the patient and other members of the team is obvious. The importance of good communication between the operating department manager and members of the team cannot be over emphasised. He*

---

* Refers equally to the feminine gender

should tackle problems and contentious issues as soon as possible; they should not be shelved, otherwise morale can suffer as a result of resentment or misunderstandings. In short, he should be a good 'manager', but essentially a leader of a nursing and technical team.

The previous edition suggested that the visible signs of good leadership can be summed up in seven observable qualities; this remains relevant (McKenzie, 1971).

1. A leader should be able and willing to assist his team and individual members of the team to carry out their roles, and in so doing think out clearly what are the roles and functions of all members of the team and then facilitate their carrying out of these functions.

2. He is capable of thinking out and bringing about *desirable* changes, for not all changes result in progress.

3. Since changes may be resisted, the leader will know the most acceptable and effective method of introducing them.

4. He will be seen and known to assist the team and members of the team to overcome difficulties and hardships.

5. The leader will observe and develop the initiative and potentialities of members of his team.

6. He will preserve and transmit those appropriate features of the team pattern which are desirable.

7. Finally, the leader will encourage and help the members of his team to express, whether in words or actions, their hopes, desires, apprehensions and wishes.

The operating department manager should endeavour to establish a harmonious but disciplined working atmosphere, so as to secure the safety and welfare of patients and staff. He must be certain that there is a clear understanding by all members of the team as to whom they are directly responsible. He should review operational policies from time to time so as to improve efficiency. These policies and procedures must be planned in detail, discussed, and when agreed be accepted by the whole team (AORN, 1982; NATN, 1983; Clarke *et al.*, 1984; Bevan, 1984).

In order to maintain a continuing high standard of care for patients undergoing surgery, the manager must ensure that all staff are adequately trained and experienced for the tasks they undertake. He should set up well-planned orientation and training programmes for all grades of staff including nurse learners. Nurses in training must have the opportunity of working in the operating department to enable them to appreciate specific pre- and post-operative anaesthesia care of patients, as well as acquiring some understanding of operating theatre technique and the nature of the surgical procedures carried out.

When nurse learners are in the department for only a period of observation, the manager must regard them as supernumerary to the establishment. Even when they are allocated for longer periods, it is essential to maintain a practical ratio between trained and untrained staff.

Whether or not the nurse will continue to co-ordinate the services of the operating department will depend on a number of factors. One of these is the ability of nurses to develop expertise both in clinical matters and management techniques including the control of financial budgets. Another factor is a dependency on sufficient numbers being prepared to pursue a nursing career in this specialty. This is why it is important that nurse learners obtain an understanding of work carried out in the operating department, to encourage them to undertake a 'theatre' career when their training is completed (Cain, 1985; Mazza, 1986).

Staff

Operating department personnel must aim to achieve the highest possible standards in their

work. Strict asepsis would perhaps not be achieved during tonsillectomy operations as compared with a bone graft, but the same amount of care must be taken during the preparation for each. Commitment to the work requires high personal standards to set an example to others; dexterity, accuracy and efficiency are vital. The ability of nurses to be part of an operating team and contribute towards a happy professional atmosphere helps toward the attainment and maintenance of the high standards required.

The last two decades following the Lewin Report (1970) have seen the introduction of the operating department assistant (ODA) into the theatre team. The National Association of Theatre Nurses (NATN) recommends that there should be a basic non-medical team of five people for an operating session (NATN, 1980). The NATN assumes that the team leader will be a trained nurse qualified in operating theatre techniques. In addition to nurses and specialist technical staff, the team may include ODAs, the overall nurse/assistant ratio within the department being not more than one ODA to two nurses (NATN, 1980).

The introduction of the ODA has resulted in a person who can provide skilled assistance in the operating department. Although having a largely technical role, he has become a valuable member of an integrated team, sharing in its responsibility for patient care. Unfortunately, there is still controversy in some quarters regarding the extent and nature of the ODA's role, and this can effect working relationships in the team (Fox, 1985; Thompson and Newall, 1986). This need not occur, for an objective appraisal of the nurse's and ODA's roles can result in some interchangeability of tasks, and better deployment of trained nurses in areas where it is considered their skills are essential. For example, one member of the team should be working with the anaesthetist at least during the induction of anaesthesia and positioning of the patient prior to surgery: this could be a trained ODA or nurse. The ODA could be assigned as scrub nurse with the trained nurse circulating and providing supervision. Nurses will be required in the post-anaesthesia recovery area and at the point where patients for surgery are received and checked for identity.

Just as the ODA is becoming increasingly a full member of the theatre team, there are in addition other highly trained personnel who provide special services such as the operation of radiological or cardiopulmonary bypass equipment. These paramedical staff are from departments normally outside the jurisdiction of the operating department manager, but provide a service to the team as required.

Whenever possible, duties not requiring the skills either of trained nurses or ODAs should be delegated to clerical and ancillary staff (Lewin Report, 1970; Clarke et al., 1984). Some clerical assistance for the operating department manager is essential; where there are four or more operating suites it may be necessary to employ a full-time receptionist in addition to a clerk/typist.

The development of central sterile supply departments (CSSD), theatre sterile supply units (TSSU), and more recently sterilizing and disinfecting units (SDU), has improved the efficiency of cleaning and processing surgical instruments. This has meant that theatre staff have been relieved of these tasks which can be carried out by suitably trained ancillary staff, their work being overseen by skilled supervisors. These units are likely to be under the jurisdiction of the CSSD manager in close co-operation with the operating department manager.

Preparation of the operating theatre between cases and operating sessions will be the responsibility of non-medical members of the team. The policy for cleaning and standards required should be agreed between the operating department manager and domestic manager. This will include major cleaning, such as walls, ceilings and general 24-hour cleaning of the operating department. Domestic staff should be employed to care for staff changing rooms, rest rooms and offices, and for serving beverages and light refreshments

to staff in accordance with a policy agreed with the catering manager. 'Care' in this context includes duties such as general tidiness, the disposal of non-surgical rubbish and the replenishment of supplies items such as linen. These are not duties for which skilled operating department staff should be employed.

Tasks undertaken by operating department porters vary considerably from hospital to hospital. In some cases their duties will be restricted to transfer of patients between the wards and operating department; in others their work many extend to movement of patients within the limited access zone. However, it is preferable that these porters are part of the operating department establishment, rather than being provided on an ad hoc basis from the general portering pool.

MANAGEMENT

A multiplicity of textbooks devoted to management techniques exists, many of which are equally applicable to the operating department and hospital management in general. A list of useful books is included in the bibliography on page 65 and readers may seek specialised information from these. However, the organisation and management of operating departments do include aspects which are not readily available from these sources, and it is appropriate to highlight some of these.

It is important to stress that operating departments cannot be managed in isolation from work in the rest of the hospital. An obvious example is that the provision of surgical facilities should take account of surgical bed throughput and theatre requirements from diagnostic departments in the hospital (Lewin Report, 1970; Rawlinson et al., 1982; Dundas and Meechan, 1986).

The organisation of the department must relate to the overall hospital policies, and for this reason there should be close liaison between the operating department manager and administration, and nursing, medical and paramedical colleagues responsible for other areas of the hospital. The administrative link in the NHS, since the introduction of a revised management structure following the Griffiths management enquiry (DHSS, 1983), will probably be with the unit administrator accountable for overall management of the hospital. The formation of a multidisciplinary 'operating department committee' will help foster liasion with surgeons, anaesthetists and others who are directly concerned with day-to-day matters.

Operating department committee

Although the operating department manager has overall accountability for the service provided, including management of a financial budget, there is need for a multidisciplinary committee to advise on the overall management of the department.

The function of this committee will vary according to local circumstances. Essentially it is advisory to the unit general manager but may have an executive function also; some of the medical members may be responsible for their own financial budgets which could affect management decisions relating to the operating department. Examples of executive function may include the development and monitoring of the management budget including ensuring the most effective use of facilities and staff; keeping under review the incidence of postoperative infection; recommending the purchase of new instruments and equipment within financial constraints and a general monitoring of the standards of care and skill in the

department (AORN, 1982). In their advisory role the committee could, for example, make proposals for changes in the organisation of the department which may effect other departments in the hospital or health district, or advise on staffing patterns and training programmes.

The chairman of this committee should be nominated by the unit general manager. A small group is more efficient and therefore it is suggested that the remaining members would normally be restricted to the operating department manager, representatives of the surgical and anaesthetic consultants, and the unit general manager or his deputy. Other members can be co-opted as required, for example the SDU manager, ward nursing representatives, microbiologist, pharmacist, radiologist, domestic manager or supervisor and the hospital works officer. It is important that these specialists are invited to attend when matters of their particular concern are being considered. Similarly they should also have access to the committee at any time to resolve any matters which require discussion. The committee should meet regularly, ideally monthly; minutes should be kept and circulated to interested parties.

Policies

In conjunction with the operating department committee, the manager should prepare procedure manuals based on agreed policies and standards. The National Association of Theatre Nurses have produced Codes of Practice which give guidelines for the preparation of such manuals (NATN, 1983). Similar guidelines were formulated by the AORN (1982); there have also been published papers which deal with hazards and safety (Hull and English, 1984; Baxter, 1984). Procedures which should be covered include:
1. Accidents to staff, major accident/incident procedures
2. Arrangements for catering in the department
3. Complaints, grievance and disciplinary procedures
4. Supplies and disposal including linen
5. Fire safety, health and safety at work and other safety matters including procedures for safeguards against wrong operations and checking swabs and instruments, safety practices to avoid hazards, for example, relating to the use of x-ray apparatus, radio-isotopes and lasers
6. Handling of laboratory specimens, infection control
7. Patient care including documentation, transport, lifting, organ transplantation
8. Works department including arrangements for repairs and maintenance

Pattern of work

The pattern of work in an operating department should be organised so as to provide cost effective utilisation of accommodation, operating time and manpower consistent with the best interests of patients and staff. This will be simplified if the manager establishes a management information system from which standards can be monitored, and from which accurate costings can be derived without additional effort. Such a system has been developed by the Financial Information Project (1985), which was first set up in 1979 and funded partially by a research grant from the DHSS and partly by the West Midlands Regional Health Authority.

The system is patient-based and is oriented around a form which records the patient's progress through the operating department, identifying key staff who provide the care, procedures carried out and the use of consumables (Fig. 2.1). The system enables a range

```
┌─────────────────────────────────────────────────────────────┐
│ (TPP) Theatre Patient Profile                                │
│                                                              │
│ Theatre number ( )   Operation date (    )   Private Y/N ( ) │
│                                                              │
│ Number (        ) Sex ( ) D.o.B (        ) Adm Type ( ) Op Type ( ) │
│                                                              │
│                 Pre-op    Anaes start   Theatre   Recovery   Out │
│ Times           ( : )     ( : )         ( : )     ( : )     ( : ) │
│                                                              │
│ Consultant ( ) Surg.1 ( ) Surg.2 (    ) Anaes.1 ( ) Anaes.2 (   ) │
│                                                              │
│            CO  SR/R O/S  AN  NT  ODA NU/UO ODA/NA             │
│ Essential ( )( )( )( )( )( )( )( )  ( )( )( )( )              │
│ Other     ( )( )( )( )( )( )( )( ) No.( )( )( )( )            │
│                                                              │
│ Implants  (     )(     )    Anaesthetic Dis. ( )( )( )       │
│ CSSD  ( )x( )  ( )x( )   ( )x( )   ( )x( )                    │
│                                                              │
│ Operation Codes ( )( )( )( )  Research ( )( )                │
│ Operation Descr. (                                    )      │
│ Outcome ( )    Destination ( )                               │
└─────────────────────────────────────────────────────────────┘
```

Fig. 2.1 Computer input screen display for Management Information System – operating theatres. (Reproduced by permission of the Financial Information Project, Alpha Tower, Suffolk Street, Queensway, Birmingham B1 2JP.)

of data to be collected for operating department management purposes, including data for management planning, costing, manpower deployment, monitoring of standards, and statistical returns. The data output includes costs by surgical specialty, by individual clinicians, by patient and by procedure; new sessions, additional consultants, utilisation of theatres and sessions, change in procedures, scheduling of operating sessions etc. (Fig. 2.2).

The operating department management system will supplement other management procedures, for example, patient records or the requisitioning of supplies and stock control (Jones and Stephen, 1986; Przasnyski, 1986).

Operation lists/schedules

Preparation of operation lists by medical staff in collaboration with the operating department manager and ward sisters should ensure that typed copies are available for distribution to all departments concerned not later than the afternoon previous to the morning on which operations are due to take place. The schedule drawn up should be realistic and one which can be reasonably expected to be completed by the surgeons within a defined period. Clarke *et al.* (1984) point out that 'many theatre staff have domestic responsibilities and are often unwilling, or unable, to work beyond their allotted time. Surgical staff can assist greatly the task of nurse managers by ensuring a prompt start, by limiting the length of operating lists to numbers capable of completion in a session, and by early notification of unavoidable alterations to the list'. The Lewin Committee (1970) considered that the average length of an elective operating session should be between three and a half and four hours, with the afternoon session starting at a time which allows it to finish by 17.00 hours.

Utilisation of theatres
1. Booked session time and actual session lengths
2. Individual patient pre-operative waiting period, anaesthesia time, operating time and recovery time
3. Patient throughput data
4. Number of emergency or elective patients per session categorised by time: 0–30 min; 31–120 min; 120 min +
5. Number of cases 'out of hours' (list and emergency)
6. Percentage use of 'available' session time per session, specialty and theatre

Management data
1. Patient average pre-operative waiting period
2. Patient average recovery period
3. Average time taken for specific types and clusters of operation by consultant
4. Number of day patients, Accident and Emergency cases etc.
5. Transfer to location (e.g. wards)
6. Number of cancelled sessions and the reasons for cancellation
7. Names of key medical staff who performed/attended operation sessions

Nurse manpower data
1. Staff duty rotas and actual hours worked
2. Individual nurse records; leave, hours worked, on call, etc.
3. Analysis of above: (a) for manpower purposes (b) returns to finance
4. Average number of staff present at types of operations; analysis related to standards of staffing which should be achieved
5. Nurse used as clinical assistant

Clinical data
1. Types of operations carried out and their time periods, for specialty, firm, surgeon, anaesthetists
2. Evaluation of different procedures
3. Individual patient data related to potential infection
4. Type of implant used per patient; differences between consultants per operation
5. Estimating session lengths (i.e. scheduling theatre)
6. Theatre operating list.

Cost data
1. Individual patient cost
2. Varying costs for patients, e.g. in different age groups, sex, type of operation, consultant
3. Session cost, analysed in subcategories, e.g. total costs including staff time, consumables, overheads
4. Cost by specialty, firm, consultant
5. Cost by individual clinician
6. Cost of emergency procedure
7. Cost of CSSD items per patient
8. Cost of anaesthesia disposables
9. Cost of implants used per patient
10. Cost of used session time
11. Cost of overrunning sessions

Fig. 2.2 Example of data output from Management Information System for operating theatres. (Reproduced by permission of the Financial Information Project. Alpha Tower, Suffolk Street, Queensway, Birmingham B1 2JP.)

Abbreviations should never be used on an operation list which may be generated as a hard copy using computer data, or typed. The following information should be included:

Patient's surname and first name(s)

Age

Sex

Registered hospital or unit number

Nature, site and side of operation

Theatre where the operation took place

Ward or unit

Date and time of operation

Name of surgeon

Name of anaesthetist

Note if there are special requirements.

Self-adhesive labels incorporating identity information, and suitable for attachment to request and other forms, are now in general use. These can be utilised for preparing operation lists to cover the information listed under items 1 to 4. They are an additional safeguard in avoiding errors of transcription.

Last minute changes to operation lists cause concern and possible risk of error. A firm policy should be laid down by the Operating Department Committee for the procedure to be adopted for any changes to the operation list, in order that all relevant personnel are informed (MDU/RCN, 1977). Procedures for checking the identity of patients undergoing surgery are described in Chapter 11.

Records

It is vital that accurate records are kept of operations performed and the personnel involved, nursing care, and any accident or incident which occurs.

Operation records. Information should be entered either in a bound book or on a specially designed sheet which can be filed in a loose leaf folder. Pages should be numbered, and the space allocated for each entry should be reprinted with the serial number of the operation. The design of this record book or sheet will vary according to local policy, but specific sections should be provided for the following information:

Date
Patient's surname and first names
Age
Sex
Registered hospital or identification number
Ward or unit
Operation performed
Time operation commenced and finished
Anaesthetic — local or general
Signatures of surgeons, surgeon's assistant, anaesthetist, anaesthesia nurse/ODA
Signatures of scrub nurse and person who checked the final swab, instrument and needle
    count
Specimens taken
Time tourniquet applied and removed
General additional comments or remarks.

Nursing care records. It is important that the patient's medical and nursing records should accompany him at all times. Following surgery, the medical staff will enter details on the case records including operation performed, anaesthetic given, and drains and packs in position. Instructions for immediate post-operative care will be entered on the nursing record.

Accident record. Where an accident or incident involving a patient or member of staff has occurred, full details must be entered in the official accident book on the designated form.

Operation and swab checking procedures are discussed further in Chapter 6.

REFERENCES

Association of Operating Room Nurses Inc (1982) Standards of Administrative Nursing Practice: OR
    AORN Standards and Recommended Practices for Perioperative Nursing, Denver: AORN.
Bevan, P. G. (1984) Efficiency in the operating suite. In *The design and use of operating theatres*, edited by
    I. D. A. Johnston and A. R. Hunter. London: Arnold.

BAXTER, B. (1984) Hazards in the theatre, *Nursing Times*, **32**, July 18.

CAIN, A. (1985) Constructive criticism – theatre allocation for nurse learners, Theatre nurses supplement, *Nursing Mirror*, **161**, 18.

CLARKE, P. E., DIXON, E., FREEMAN, D AND WHITAKER, M (1984) Nurse staffing and training in the operating suite. *The design and use of operating theatres*, edited by I. D. A. Johnston and A. R. Hunter. London: Arnold.

DEPARTMENT OF HEALTH AND SOCIAL SECURITY (1983) DHSS Management Enquiry. Chairman: Roy Griffiths. London: DHSS.

DEPARTMENT OF HEALTH AND SOCIAL SECURITY (1970) *The organisation and Staffing of Operating Departments* – Lewin Report. London: HMSO.

DOUGLAS, D. M. (1962) *Lancet*, **ii**, 245.

F.I.P. (1986) *Theatre Information System*. Financial Information Project, 12th Floor, Alpha Tower, Suffolk Street, Queensway, Birmingham B1 2JP.

HULL, C. J. AND ENGLISH, M. J. M. (1984) Safety in the operating area. *The Design and Utilisation of Operating Theatres*, edited by I. V. Johnston and A. H. Hunter. London: Arnold.

JONES, H. S. AND STEPHEN, L. E. (1986) Watch the pennies and the pounds will look after themselves – a study of stock control in the operating theatre. *NATNews*, **11**, May.

MAZZA, J. (1986) Student nurse training in theatre. Teaching and Training – Specialty Supplement. *NATNews*, *The British Journal of Theatre Nursing*, **2**, June.

MCKENZIE, N. (1971) *The Professional Ethic and the Hospital Service*, p. 5.

MEDICAL DEFENCE UNION/ROYAL COLLEGE OF NURSING (1977) Safeguards against wrong operations. *Joint Memorandum*. London: MDU/RCN.

NATIONAL ASSOCIATION OF THEATRE NURSES (1980) *Operating Departments Staffing Establishment*, p. 4, paras 8 and 9. Harrogate: NATN.

NATIONAL ASSOCIATION OF THEATRE NURSES (1983) Guidelines – operational policy. *Codes of Practice*, Harrogate: NATN.

PRZASNYSKI, Z. H. (1986) Operating room scheduling – a literature review. *Association of Operating Room Nurses Journal*. Denver: AORN.

3

Electricity and electromedical equipment

The mains voltage in the United Kingdom is supplied at 240 V, 50 Hz; emergency lighting and power for the operating department is provided by an emergency generator at the standard mains voltage, from batteries at 12–24 V, or a combination of both. It is likely that the generator will supply the emergency electrical needs of the operating department through the normal wiring and socket outlets. Alternatively, only a proportion of the electric socket outlets may be connected to the generator. The engineering design must take into account that the emergency generator output should be sufficient to supply the demand likely to be required. However, it is prudent during failure of mains supply to limit the use of lights and equipment to that which is essential.

Upon mains failure, there could be a delay of up to 20 seconds before a generator comes into action. An automatic changeover switch ensures a temporary uninterrupted supply from batteries to the main operating luminaire until the generator takes over (DHSS, 1974). Some electromedical equipment such as infusion pumps may incorporate a battery standby supply.

Unless designated as 'Class II' (double insulated), the outer casing of electrical equipment, including mobile operating luminaires and electromedical equipment, must have a protective earth connection directly through the earth pin of the plug mechanism. The electric flex to such equipment contains three insulated wires: the brown wire is always connected to the live terminal, the blue wire to the neutral terminal, and the green/yellow wire to the longer earth pin at the plug top and the outer casing of the equipment at the other. If a fault to earth occurs, the electric current then generally has a safe passage to earth and not through some unfortunate person who may inadvertently touch the equipment.

It is essential that the earth connections of all non'earth-free' mains powered equipment are checked regularly for integrity. Whether this basic checking is carried out by clinical or technical staff will depend on local policy. However, anything requiring the use of tools to gain access to interior parts, or use of special test equipment, should generally be the responsibility of technical staff. In a well-ordered hospital there will be a system of planned maintenance and safety checking probably operated by the physics or works department. The operating department manager or clinical staff responsible for specific items of electromedical equipment should ensure that the equipment they use does not escape the safety check net.

Another safety protection is an earth-free electricity supply for the operating department, using 'isolating' transformers. Figure 3.1 illustrates the technical aspects of this provision. In this situation, rather than the normal *direct* connection to the mains supply, the electric current is routed through an isolating transformer to socket outlets. With this arrangement, even if faulty equipment allows a direct connection from patient or user to one side the electricity supply, the current that can flow through them to earth is limited to a very low value determined by the characteristics of the 'isolating' transformer. Although this arrange-

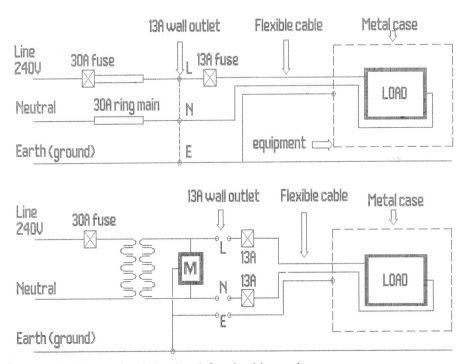

Fig. 3.1 Simplified diagram of earthed and earth-free electricity supply systems.

Top. Earthed mains supply system: electrical equipment obtains supply through 13 amp socket in ring main. Only one supply conductor (L) is 'live'; single pole switches can be used to interrupt current in 'live' conductor.

Bottom. Earth-free mains supply system: electrical equipment obtains supply through 13 amp socket fed from isolating transformer. Both supply conductors (L + N) must be considered 'live'; double pole switches required to interrupt current in both conductors.

ment is provided for operating theatres in the USA, Canada, South Africa and Japan, and recommended in Australia, the present UK view is that isolating transformers do not provide protection commensurate with their cost and complexity (Dobbie, 1972; Hill and English, 1984). Instead, reliance is placed on correct construction and maintenance of the equipment itself.

Further safety measures which may be adopted include the installation of earth leakage or 'residual current' circuit breakers as part of the electricity distribution system. These are devices which detect current faults before they leak to earth, and disconnect the supply automatically. They do provide some protection against electrocution for staff, but are of limited value in patient safety. However, readers may find these in operation, particularly in some Australian theatres where they form part of a comprehensive safety package.

Standard 13 amp electric sockets are now provided in most UK operating departments and these enable any mains-operated equipment to be used on the supply. This applies also to mobile X-ray apparatus; utilising standard 13 amp sockets in 30 amp ring circuits, a special *unfused* plug connected to X-ray apparatus will only take high power from the circuit during a fraction of a second's exposure. This plug is designed to accommodate the larger flexible cable connected to the X-ray apparatus.

No moisture must be allowed to collect on the plug pins. If this should occur, the moisture must be dried off thoroughly before the plug is inserted. Apparatus should be disconnected from the socket by grasping the plug top and not the flex. The use of adaptors for

interchanging plugs of different sizes is not safe and must not be used.

Operating department staff should not disconnect or reconnect any wiring, as this is the responsibility of physicists, an engineer and/or technicians. If any electrical connection or wire is obviously faulty, the equipment must not be used until throughly checked.

Electromedical equipment used in the operating theatre has become increasingly sophisticated. Provided the equipment complies with BS5724 (IEC Publication 601) and is used correctly, it should be safe. But some equipment may deliver potentially dangerous electrical ouputs and must be treated with special care. Theatre staff must be familiar with the manufacturers' operating instructions, be aware of steps which should be taken should equipment malfunction, and have an understanding of safety precautions which need to be adopted.

Care must be taken with the use of electro-medical equipment in the vicinity of anaesthesia apparatus if flammable anaesthetic agents are likely to be used. There is potential risk of sparks originating from switches or motors igniting flammable anaesthetic gases which may leak from anaesthesia breathing circuits. This danger exists within a zone extending to 25 cm from the points where leakage might occur; gases quickly dilute to a non-flammable level beyond this. Electromedical equipment not marked as Type AP should not be allowed to come within the 25 cm zone when a flammable agent is in use.

Extra low-voltage equipment

A considerable amount of electric equipment in the operating department uses an extra low-voltage current. To mention just a few, these include laryngoscopes, bronchoscopes, cystoscopes and head lamps (Smith, 1958). To a great extent extra low-voltage illumination is being superseded by fibre optics (page 387).

It would seem that no other type of apparatus can cause so many problems as the extra low-voltage equipment. It could be argued that the standard of construction should be comparable with that of mains voltage equipment. But as any theatre nurse will confirm, it often seems to go out of action just when needed, and unless considerable care is taken during simple maintenance, with a step-by-step check, much time can be wasted in critical situations. The efficiency of such apparatus depends to a great extent on regular checking of batteries, lamps and electrical contacts, which should generally be the responsibilty of an engineer or trained technician. However, this may not always be possible and an understanding of simple *extra low-voltage* circuit testing, to trace faults can contribute to better care of such apparatus.

Generally, an extra low-voltage circuit used in apparatus for use in theatre may range from 1.5 V for endoscopes to 10 V for a surgeon's headlamp. The electric current may be supplied from batteries or a transformer which reduces the mains voltage to the required level. A transformer may be a separate item of equipment or may be an additional facility in equipment such as diathermy machines (high frequency electrosurgical units). Fibre light sources are discussed in Chapter 13.

In the case of batteries, two or more may be joined together either to give an increased voltage (series circuit) or prolong the period of supply (parallel circuit).

It is quite possible that when batteries or a transformer are working at full-power output the voltage given may be higher than that required for a particular lamp in an apparatus, and using a higher than necessary voltage may burn the lamp out immediately or reduce its life. It is usual in this case to introduce a rheostat into the circuit, which enables the voltage to be varied at will. The batteries or transformer may then be used for a variety of apparatus operating on different voltages.

A rheostat is an electrical resistance operated by turning a knob which when set at the required voltage reduces the slightly higher current to the required level. The rheostat should always be set at zero before switching on and connecting the apparatus.

Care of apparatus

In order that an extra low-voltage circuit may operate satisfactorily all connections must be kept clean, dry and free from corrosion. After sterilization, heat processed apparatus must be well dried before storing away. Good contact of the connections must be maintained and loose soldered contacts repaired immediately by the electrician when they are detected. Lamps must be securely screwed in position and the current source should, if possible, remain fairly constant. With batteries this means a careful watch for battery exhaustion.

Batteries left too long in a metal case tend to sweat, especially in humid atmospheres, causing corrosion and the discharge of power. All batteries not in actual use should be stored under dry conditions.

When a rheostat is connected in the power circuit it is preferable to switch on the full current slowly by commencing at nil volts and raising the current to the required level. This warms up the lamp filament before it receives the full current and increases its life considerably — a very important point as specialised lamps are often expensive and have a comparatively short life.

Checking a suspected faulty low-voltage circuit

This is a simple process if taken stage by stage, if a simple test meter or test lamp and battery are available. The test lamp set consists essentially of a 1.5 V battery to which are connected two insulated wires, having rigid metal points at each of the two free ends, and a small low-voltage lampholder and lamp to which are also connected similar insulated wires. (A diagram of the circuit is shown in the Appendix.)

The battery is used for testing circuits and lamps, the lamp for testing faulty batteries. It is a simple matter for a carpenter to arrange these two items together in a box or on a portable board.

Irrespective of the type of apparatus tested (if, after connecting the apparatus correctly and switching on, as in the case of a laryngoscope, etc., it is found to be out of order) it is usually possible to check the faults as follows:

1. In the case of a transformer especially ensure that it is connected to the wall socket and is switched on correctly.

2. Check that the lamp is firmly screwed into position.

3. Check that all electrical connections appear to be in good contact and are not obviously broken. Where the apparatus has batteries in the handle, ensure that the inside of the case is free from any corrosion. Should there be corrosion, slight scraping of the contacts or tightening of loosened screws will usually suffice.

4. In the absence of a test battery try one or more new lamps in the lampholder or carrier. Small lamps can sometimes vary in size and length of the screw part. Should this be so, the centre contact at the base of the lamp may not reach the contact in the lamp-holder and it will appear that the lamp is out of order. These lamps should not be discarded as faulty until they have been tried with the test battery or in another lampholder or carrier.

Sometimes the centre contact of the lamp is made of a compressed coil of wire. Should the lamp not function in the apparatus but appear satisfactory on test with the testing unit, it may be advantageous to lengthen the contact by pulling out this coil of wire a fraction

of an inch. When re-inserting the lamp be careful that the amount of lengthening is minimal, for if too much this contact may be pushed out of centre during screwing into position. This will then cause the wire to short-circuit across the inside of the lampholder, allowing the current to flow straight back to the battery or transformer and the lamp will still not light or may flicker.

5. If the lamp appears in order, check the batteries by connecting them with another apparatus known to be in working order, or use the test lamp, connecting it directly to the batteries. If the test lamp will not illuminate it is most probable that the batteries are exhausted.

6. Should the lamp still not function it is possible that the wires leading from the batteries or transformer to the lampholder or carrier may be broken somewhere within the insulation. These wires may be checked by connecting to other light carriers or lamps which are known to be in working order, or by using the test apparatus. The test is made by connecting the suspected faulty wires between the test battery and the two wires joined to the test lampholder.

ELECTROMEDICAL EQUIPMENT

The importance of earthing the outer case of non 'earth-free' equipment and possible provision of earth-free supplies or earth leakage contact breakers has already been emphasised (page 68). This protects staff from shocks should an internal fault occur involving heavy electrical leakage or a direct 'line' to case (positive) connection. Unfortunately, earthing does not always give absolute protection to the patient, for if he is connected to 'earthed' electromedical apparatus it is possible under certain fault conditions for a micro-electric shock to occur due to leakage current from another source or another instrument which has an undetected failure in its protective earth connection. This is particularly so where there is a direct intracardiac connection by means of a catheter (either liquid-filled or containing electrode wires, e.g. to an external pacemaker). The order of current which can cause disturbance to the pumping action of the heart, ventricular fibrillation and death, is discussed in papers by Green, Raftery and Gregory. The permissible leakage currents currently quoted from HTM 8 (i.e. less than 100uA) is classified much more completely in the draft IEC Document 62A (Secretariat) 10, ranging from 10 micro amperes to much higher values for permanently installed equipment. *Leakage is the term used in connection with a stray current present to some degree in every engineered electrical system originating from parts connected to the 'live' mains or other electrical energy source* (Hull, 1978).

The principal risk is when the earth connection to the apparatus is accidentally broken; the leakage current may find its way to earth (ground) through other equipment connected to the patient or through some earthed object which the patient may be touching. Another path to earth could be through an attending nurse or doctor, who touches the patient and allows the leakage current to flow through both patient and nurse or doctor.

Another risk associated with the previous one is when the patient is connected to two or more pieces of 'earthed' apparatus, *i.e. utilising separate electrical sockets*. Each instrument will possess a protective device such as a fuse in the electrical circuit or it may have a dedicated ELCB, but if a fault occurs whereby the live cable comes into contact with some part of the earth system, either the metal framework of the instrument or elsewhere in the building, the patient could momentarily be at risk. This is because the fuse or circuit breaker

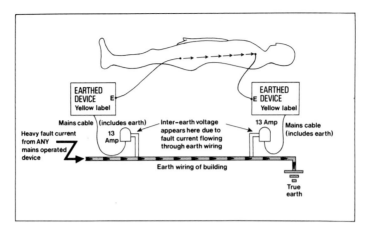

Fig. 3.2   Current through patient. Due to inter-earth resistance, momentary fault current and use of several earthed devices. (Figures 3.2–3.7 reproduced with permission from the Electrical Equipment booklet — Patient Safety M097-72, Northwick Park Hospital, Harrow.)

does not interrupt the supply quickly enough to prevent electric currents flowing momentarily along the earth system and through the patient. An inter-earth current flows due to the voltage existing momentarily between two or more separate electrical sockets, via the earth wires, and the patient for the duration of the fault (Fig. 3.2).

Earth-free patient circuits

Although the above mentioned risks are rare they can be reduced further by various means including that of using equipment having 'earth-free' patient circuits. The electrical design of the inside of 'earth-free' equipment allows connections to the patient to be separated from earth. Consequently, the patient is on a 'floating electrical circuit and *not* connected directly to the earth (Figs 3.3 and 3.4). As a further explanation we can say that the inside of each apparatus is split into two halves — one half going to the patient and the other half obtaining electrical power and being connected to the hospital electrical supply. The equipment is so designed that an electrical failure would not be injurious to the patient. Completely 'earth-free' equipment is therefore safe for connection to the patient, both internally and externally. The patient and all attachments to equipment, are 'separated' from earth (Fig. 3.5).

It is possible that both 'earth-free' and 'earthed' equipment may have to be used on a patient at the same time. Although such a combination is not as safe as exclusively 'earth-free' equipment, the partial use of 'earth-free' equipment will still minimise danger of electric shock (Fig. 3.6).

Earthed patient circuits

If more than one piece of 'earthed' apparatus is connected to the same patient, e.g. 'earthed' diathermy machine and 'earthed' ECG machine, it is possible for an inter-earth current to occur. To avoid this, external earth terminals should be fitted to each apparatus and when in use linked together with an approved safety earth wire which must be kept as short as possible (Fig. 3.7): this connects the patient to a common earth.

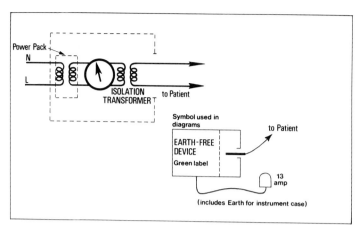

Fig. 3.3   Basic earth-free equipment.

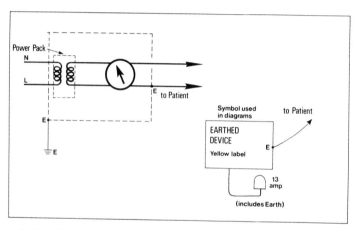

Fig. 3.4   Basic earthed equipment.

It is worth noting that when the expression 'earth-free' is applied to a diathermy machine it is relative; in a fault condition there is no danger of electrocution by external contact, but there is insufficient protection when intracardiac catheters are in place with intraventricular contact. A safety earth should be connected if other 'earthed' equipment is in use. In the more critical situation, therefore, diathermy machines should *not* really be regarded as 'earth-free'.

Safety precautions

Guidance and care are necessary to minimise the risk of injury to patients and staff when using electromedical equipment. Much of the preceding information follows the work of a Safety Committee at Northwick Park Hospital and Clinical Research Centre, Harrow, England. This multidisciplinary group consisted of doctors, biomedical and hospital engineers and nurses who meet to discuss developments in electromedical equipment and all aspects of electrical safety. The group formulated a safety guidance document (Northwick

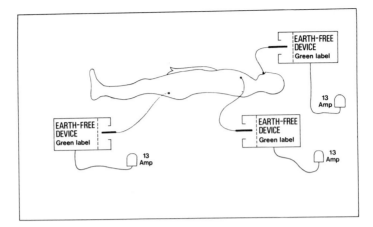

Fig. 3.5 All earth-free devices. The patient is completely protected against current flow through body.

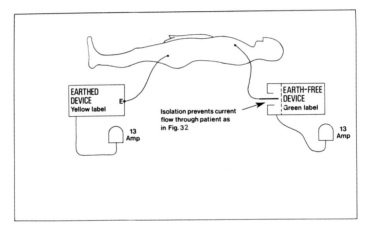

Fig. 3.6 Singled earthed instrument with other earth-free devices. (Generally a satisfactory intermediate standard but shock from a live object is possible because of one direct earth.

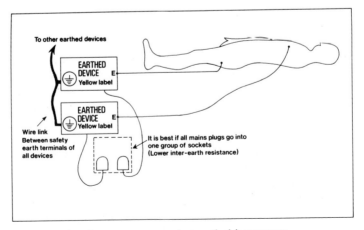

Fig. 3.7 Use of safety earth lines for two or more patient earthed instruments.

Park Hospital and Clinical Research Centre, 1972) which is still relevant and it is useful to reproduce the main points below:

Take care and think!

1. Do not place wet cloths, bottles of fluid or cups etc., on electrical equipment. Liquid seeping into the equipment could not only cause damage but also dangerous short circuits.

2. Never touch exposed pacemaker terminals, intracardiac catheters, or guide wires with one hand while making instrument adjustments or contacting electrically operated devices with the other hand. Wear rubber gloves when touching catheter connected metal fittings (except possibly in emergency).

3. Remove dried out saline solutions or jellies and always reapply the recommended amount of conducting material before placing electrodes on a patient.

4. Ensure that your hands are dry before touching the patient or electrical equipment; moisture allows more current to flow.

5. Disconnect from the patient any electrical equipment which is faulty.

6. Do not touch the patient and any kind of electrical equipment at the same time. You will provide the electrical link between the two, and there could be a fault.

7. Follow the manufacturer's instructions at all times.

8. Ensure that electrical equipment is securely mounted so that it cannot be dislodged by the patient. Unexpected movement could cause breakage of wires, physical injury to the patient or even electrocution if the equipment is damaged.

9. Check all connections to the patient and equipment. Look for:
— loose plugs
— kinks in wires
— worn or frayed wires
— electric cables touching hot surfaces.

Do not use mains extension cables and if in doubt call immediate attention to a suspected fault.

10. Take especial care with 'high power' apparatus, e.g. defibrillators, ECT and diathermy machines. If misused, these can cause serious shock or burns to both patient and staff. *Never test* a defibrillator by power discharge when a synchroniser lead is connected to the patient — use an e.c.g. simulator for test purposes.

11. Use surgical diathermy 'indifferent electrodes' exactly as instructed by the manufacturers. The dry type of plate must make effective contact over a large flat surface of skin; separate small areas of contact could result in high-frequency electrical burns.

Monitoring equipment

Observation and recording a cardiac and respiratory function is called monitoring. A wide range of equipment and systems is available to monitor data such as electrocardiograph wave form, arterial pressures, venous pressures and heart rate, to mention just a few. It is beyond the scope of this book to describe these in detail and the reader who seeks this information will find a number of recommended books listed on page 106. However, the theatre nurse may be concerned in the use of some portable equipment; the safety precautions already enumerated in previous paragraphs are equally as applicable in the operating theatre as in the intensive care situation.

It is common now to manufacture modular equipment which allows maximum flexibility in deciding the range of the measurements to be undertaken. Various items of equipment are designed so that they can be interconnected and plug-in units allow the simple replacement of defective parts. The type of apparatus which the theatre nurse is most likely to meet

is the cardiac monitor, single and multichannel with facilities for ECG pressure wave forms and other cardiac parameters.

The cardiac monitor or electrocardiograph. This is an apparatus which records the electrical currents which are associated inseparably with cardiac contractions. As an electric current is conducted readily through the body (for tissue fluids contain electrolytes, mainly chlorides of sodium and potassium in fairly high concentrations), the electrical currents generated by the heart are carried to the peripheral parts of the body. These can be conducted to the cardiac monitor or electrocardiograph via wires or leads connected to electrodes placed in contact with the skin; thus an electrical circuit is completed. The electrical currents are led from certain paired parts of the body surface, and any pair of electrodes (or rather parts of the body to which they are attached), with their connecting wires are referred to as a 'lead'. Up to 12 pairs of leads may be used in diagnostic electrocardiography, but for monitoring purposes there are generally not more than 3 or 5 pairs.

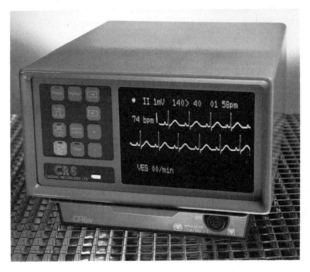

Fig. 3.8 Multiparameter monitor which displays ECG, blood pressure or peripheral pulse, two temperature channels, plus one Delta temperature display. (Cardian III — Cardiac Recorders Ltd.)

Fundamentally the cardiac monitor of cardioscope consists of an electronic amplifier which amplifies the electrical currents of the heart and displays them, either as a trace on an oscilloscope or a continuous band of paper in a writing device (Fig. 3.9).

The basic characteristics of a cardiac monitor are:

1. Power supply; either from the electrical mains or batteries which may be rechargeable or replaceable.

2. Patient monitor cable dividing into three or five different coloured leads with terminals for connecting to the patient electrodes.

3. The oscilloscope screen (which may be green or covered with an orange filter) on which the ECG trace or traces are displayed and may have an overlay grid scale.

4. A selector switch allowing the use of a number of channels (usually up to six) to select the most suitable trace.

5. Control knobs for height of trace (gain), brightness, focus, position and speed of trace (usually 12.5 mm, 25 mm and 50 mm per second).

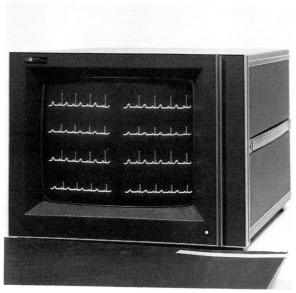

Fig. 3.9 Eight channel non-fade display monitor that presents either moving traces, which simulate a recorder presentation, or fixed traces for ease of wave form comparison and diagnosis. (Hewlett Packard.)

6. Adjustable high/low alarm system which emits visual or audible signals if the heart rate exceeds above or below a pre-set range, e.g. 50 to 110 beats per minute.

7. A recording device or pen writer which records the ECG trace on a continuous band of paper, either at predetermined intervals, e.g. every 15 minutes, when the alarm system actuates or when a button is pressed. This device may be part of the monitor or added as an accessory when required.

The monitor requires some adjustment to achieve optimum viewing conditions. The theatre nurse should first seek a demonstration of the various controls and then adjust them one at a time until the action of each is fully understood. The brightness and focus control in particular may require adjustment; if the trace is surrounded by a ring as it travels across the screen it is too bright, the minimum amount of brightness acceptable should always be selected to avoid burning the screen of the oscilloscope. According to how long each configuration of the wave or complex is required on the screen, so the speed of the trace traverse is adjusted. Generally four to six configurations should be present on the screen as the trace travels across.

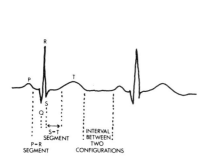

Fig. 3.10 Normal ECG.

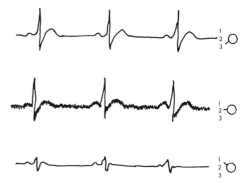

Fig. 3.11 Selecting the most suitable channel.

The channel should be selected so that the trace appears as a thin line rather than a fuzzy one which may obscure smaller waves. If necessary, the size of the waves may be increased by adjusting the gain control. So long as the waves are clearly identifiable, it is not generally important whether they are upright or inverted on the screen. Monitor observation is described further in Chapter 11.

Limb electrodes. These may be oblong brass plates 4 cm by 2 cm, slightly curved, plated with nickel or chrome. A screw socket is incorporated on the top side to which the lead is attached. The electrode is held in place by a band of rubber passing round the limb; one electrode is placed on each limb usually above the wrist or ankle. The leg electrode is positioned on the lateral aspect of the limb to avoid scratching the opposite leg with the screw (Fig. 3.12). Self-adhesive electrodes for limbs are available also.

Chest electrodes. These consist of small circular metal discs about 1 cm in diameter, mounted on a polythene disc and secured to the chest wall with non-irritant adhesive or adhesive tape such as Micropore (3M) or Dermacel (Johnson & Johnson). Usually three or four electrodes are used and positioned over the heart; the exact position of these is not critical and to some extent will be determined by the presence of surgical incisions and the best type of trace produced on the oscilloscope. Suitable sites are on or at either side of the sternum, below the nipples or below the clavicles (Figs 3.13 and 3.14).

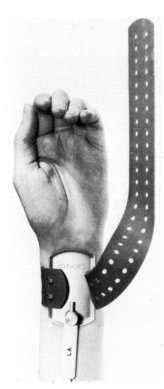

Fig. 3.12

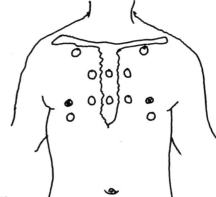

Fig. 3.13

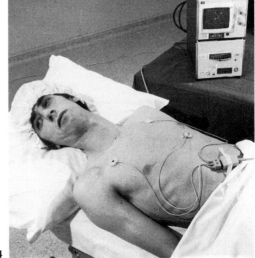

Fig. 3.14

Fig. 3.12   Limb electrode.

Fig. 3.13   Sites for chest electrodes.

Fig. 3.14   Chest electrodes positioned.

Care must be taken in the correct application of electrodes to the skin.

1. It is no use applying chest electrodes over hairy areas, this will prevent a good electrical contact; shave if necessary.

2. The skin must be cleaned thoroughly with ether meths or other solvent to remove traces of perspiration and grease.

3. Be certain that the surface of each electrode is perfectly clean and free from green corrosion; dirty electrodes should be cleaned with ether meths or methylated spirits.

4. A small quantity of a proprietory non-irritant jelly such as Cambridge (blue tube) should be applied to the contact surface of the electrode. With chest electrodes it is particularly important not to smother the electrode with jelly otherwise it may ooze on to the adhesive or fixing tape and prevent secure attachment to the chest with loss of good electrical contact. (Note: The electrically conductive pastes with a high salt content used for routine diagnostic electrocardiography are not suitable for long periods of monitoring. These pastes tend to produce skin reactions and excoriation over extended periods.) Alternatively, pre-jelled disposable electrodes may be used.

5. After attachment to the limbs or chest the electrodes are connected to the leads and thence to the monitor. It is important to ensure that the leads of the monitor cable are secured to the limb, or chest with a suitable non-irritant tap, to avoid pulling the electrodes.

6. In the ward or intensive care situation, the electrodes are checked daily for correct position, security, cleanliness and irritation. If these are all satisfactory, and provided that the trace displayed on the screen is acceptable, the electrodes will be left undisturbed, although generally it will be found necessary to renew them after a period of five to seven days. An interference or absence of a trace may not be due to a faulty electrode. Assuming that the patient's condition is otherwise satisfactory, artifacts may occur with movement of the patient and it is better to check all connections and leads thoroughly before removing a suspect electrode. An artifact appears on the trace as irregularly interrupting spikes of varying height.

Peripheral pulsometers. These consist essentially of a photoelectric plethysmograph (which is a device for measuring peripheral blood flow in the earlobe or fingertip) a receiver and an amplifier. The plethysmograph is clamped to the ear lobe or held in contact with the tip of the finger by means of a Velcro strap. Signals are conveyed by a lead to the receiver/amplifier which may be mains or battery operated. The pulse rate per minute is displayed on a scale or meter and may be monitored also by a bleep from a built-in loud-speaker or buzzer.

Very careful positioning of the electrode is important, the plethysmograph is delicate and sensitive to movement artifacts. Care must be taken to secure the leads and avoid strain on the connections.

Cardiac pacing

The pacemaker is an apparatus which produces a series of electrical shock impulses to stimulate the heart ventricles to contract. Cardiac pacing is generally used for complete heart block although less commonly in the emergency situation it may be used for cardiac asystole applying the shock across the chest wall to cause contraction of the ventricles. In this situation, during surgery if the chest is open, the electrodes may also be applied directly to the heart. External pacing requires an apparatus capable of producing in excess of 20 V as compared to up to 9 V with internal pacemaking.

The apparatus is powered by replaceable mercury batteries or a rechargeable nickel

cadium battery. It has a series of controls allowing adjustment of:

1. Pulse rate per minute, generally 30–160 although models are available with a range of 80–120 per minute.

2. Voltage 0–9 V.

3. Pulse width, i.e. duration, 1–2 milliseconds.

4. Selection of continuous or on demand impulses; continuous pacing impulses to stimulate the ventricles are supplied at a fixed or constant rate; the demand setting only supplies pacing impulses as they are needed, for example, if the heart beat is too slow. If the time interval between two QRS configurations is too long then the apparatus supplies a pacing impulse to cause ventricular contraction thereby increasing the heart rate. When the heart rate is faster than the selected rate on the pacemaker then no pacing impulses are produced.

5. Battery level indicator.

6. Terminals for the active and indifferent electrode leads.

7. A pulse output indicator in the form of a neon lamp and/or buzzer.

An insulated wire or endocardial catheter electrode is passed under local anaesthesia into a suitable vein in the arm or neck and from there, under X-ray control, through the right atrium to the right ventricle where the tip is wedged against the wall of the cavity. This forms the active electrode; the indifferent electrode consists of a wire loop buried subcutaneously near the skin incision. The two wires can then be connected to the terminals of the pacemaker apparatus.

With the epicardial technique, the electrodes are sewn onto the epicardial or outer surface of the heart exposed at thoracotomy. The wires are brought out through the chest wall for connection to the pacemaker.

Alternatively, the wires can be passed subcutaneously to the axilla and connected to a small battery-powered pacemaker buried beneath the skin. When the batteries become exhausted, the patient requires a further operation under general anaesthesia to replace the complete pacemaker; this however, does not need to be done very often; there are batteries having a life of up to 10 years. Developments have taken place in the production of nuclear powered pacemakers for implanation, which provide power almost indefinitely.

The impulses of a heart being paced if viewed on a cardiac monitor show that each QRS-T configuration, instead of being preceded by a P wave is now preceded by a pacing impulse (Fig. 3.15). The pacing impulse may appear as a narrow, bright vertical line immediately before each QRS-T configuration which is often wide and large but constant in shape. Points to note are whether the pacing impulse is present or absent; that the QRS-T shape is constant and immediately preceded by the pacing impulse; that the heart rate is correct and regular; whether any extra pacing impulses or QRS-T configurations are present.

Finally, it is important that theatre staff familiarise themselves with the type of pacemaker in use, particularly whether the power supply is from batteries or rechargeable cells, the method of adjusting controls and the method of attaching electrode leads, especially in the emergency situation.

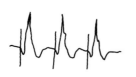

Fig. 3.15   Pacing configurations.

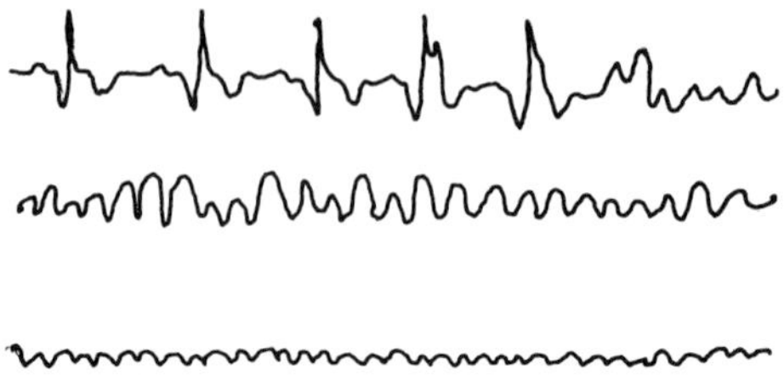

Fig. 3.16   Ventricular fibrillation.

Defibrillator

This apparatus enables an electric shock to be applied to the heart to correct ventricular or atrial fibrillation. The apparatus may be mains or battery operated with a facility to discharge the shock through the chest wall or via electrodes placed directly in contact with the walls of the heart.

When switched on, the defibrillator charges a condenser to a maximum energy of 320 J external application, and 100 J using internal electrodes. The level of stored energy output can be continuously varied between 5 and 320 J and this is released in a pulse having a duration of about 3 milliseconds. In the case of atrial fibrillation the defibrillator is coupled with an electrocardiograph so that the defibrillation discharge is delivered in synchronisation, normally 40 milliseconds delay after the peak of the R wave of the patient's ECG.

Although different makes of defibrillator vary slightly in the method of operation, basically the same technique is used. The following is a description of the method of using a Cardiac Recorders defibrillator in an emergency; instructions are printed on the side of the lid.

Emergency external defibrillation for adults. The defibrillator is equipped with paddle electrodes which can quickly be withdrawn from the lid for emergency use. The main controls, ECG monitor and chart recorder are mounted on a panel which is clearly visible when the lid is opened; the carrying handle acts as a stand which inclines the control panel towards the user.

1. *Set the O–I switch to I to turn unit on.* This sets the defibrillator to deliver a non-synchronised external shock. (A trace will be seen on the monitor screen within 10 seconds; if either battery low lamp is lit the battery must be changed or the unit operated from a mains charger.)

2. *Grip* **paddle electrode** *handles located in lid and pull firmly to remove.*

3. *Apply contact jelly to electrodes and patient's chest.*

4. *Apply both* **paddle electrodes** *to chest as shown* (diagram printed on side of lid indicates position of *sternum* and *apex* electrodes).

5. *Observe ECG on monitor screen.*

6. *Use the rocker* **charge** *+/− switch on the* **apex** *paddle (or the* **Joules** *buttons on the control panel) to achieve the required energy level. This is shown on the monitor screen.* (Output for an adult should generally start at 200 J up to a maximum of 320 J).

7. *Press both electrodes firmly on patient's chest.*

8. **All personnel stand clear of the patient.**

9. *Press both* **defibrillate** *buttons to deliver the countershock.*

10. *Observe ECG on screen which is monitored through the paddles* (Operations 6–9 are repeated if necessary.)

Emergency external defibrillation for a child follows a similar procedure, except for the type of electrodes and power of charge delivered.

Step 2 above consists of substituting child electrodes for the adult paddle electrodes; these are plugged into the same *Apex* and *sternum* sockets on the front control panel. The red light by the *internal defib* button will flash indicating that the shock (approx 50 J to 100 J maximum) can only be delivered by pressing this button.

Steps 3 and 4 are the same. In step 5 displayed above the ECG trace is the heart rate, a heart emblem flashing at each QRS cycle, MON mode, and when appropriate a pacer pulse.

In Step 6 the power of charge to be delivered in *Joules* is indicated above the ECG trace and to the left of the monitor screen. In Step 9 the charge is delivered by pressing the *internal defib* button on the control panel.

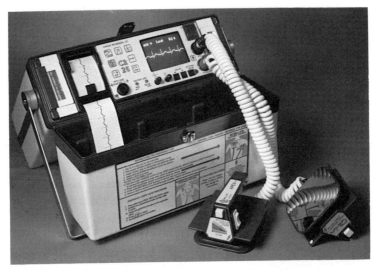

Fig. 3.17   Combined defibrillator, cardioscope and recorder. (Cardiac Recorders Ltd.)

External synchronised cardioversion for adults. The ECG monitoring is via a 5-way chest/limbs patient lead connected to the patient socket on the control panel; the shock is administered with the standard paddle electrodes. The following gives an outline of the steps involved.

1. *The **lead** selector button is pressed* until the desired configuration of leads and paddles being used is displayed above the ECG trace on the monitor screen.

2. *The **gain** button is pressed repeatedly* until the desired height of ECG displayed is obtained.

3. *The **monitor/diagnostic** setting is selected.* (The baseline shifts and muscle potentials are filtered out with the setting at monitor.)

4. *The **sync** button is pressed.* This displays an S on the monitor screen, above the ECG, and the defibrillator firing points will be shown by downward pointing markers superimposed on the ECG. (No changes in gain, leads or filter setting can be made unless the sync button is pressed again. If this is done steps 1–3 are repeated).

5. *Contact jelly is applied to the defibrillator electrodes and the patient's chest.*

6. *The **charge+** switch on the **apex** paddle or the **Joules up** switch on the control panel is pressed.* This creates the desired charge in Joules which is displayed on the monitor screen above the ECG trace. (If necessary the *charge−* switch on the *apex* paddle or the *Joules down* button on the control panel can be used to reduce the charge.)

7. *The paddles are applied to the patient's chest and both **defibrillate** buttons are pressed.* This delivers a shock which occurs on the second QRS wave after the buttons are pressed.

If a charge is unused within 30 seconds, a continuous warning tone is heard. If unused after a further 10 seconds, the charge is 'dumped' and the *charge* procedure must be repeated. Any unused charge may be 'dumped' safely by holding the separated paddles in the air and pressing both *defibrillate* buttons. After use the unit is switched off and connected to the charger.

Again, a final point of importance; although defibrillation apparatus is designed for safe operation it is important that regular checks are made to ensure that it is in working order. Special testing devices are available to check the level of discharge between the two elec-

trodes. A defibrillator is *not* a piece of apparatus to be stored away in some obscure cupboard and forgotten, because every second may count when it is needed during cardiac resuscitation. Its whereabouts must be known to *all* who work in theatre, and *all* must familiarise themselves with the correct method of operation of the particular apparatus in use.

INFUSION CONTROL

There are two distinct types of equipment used for the control of infusion.

Infusion controllers

Infusion controllers rely solely on gravity to provide the infusion pressure, the container of liquid being positioned at an appropriate height above the infusion site. A drip sensor is attached to the drip chamber of the administration set, and this monitors the drip rate which is controlled automatically by a mechanical clamp acting on the delivery tube. The degree of control achieved will depend to some extent on the conditions at the infusion site. Under-infusion can occur as a result of increased resistance, but because of the low delivery pressure control against over infusion is good, and the risk of extra-vascular infusion is reduced. Controllers have alarm systems which operate when there is any significant departure from the set drip-rate, or other malfunctions occur.

Controllers are more suitable for use in the ward situation, involving non-critical infusions where there are advantages in low delivery pressure, rapid alarm, and no likelihood that air will be pumped into the infusion line.

Infusion pumps

Infusion pumps have the ability to overcome resistance to flow in the infusion line by generating increased delivery pressure. However, if an intravenous cannula becomes occluded or blocked there is a risk of extra-vascular infusion, or a 'bolus' delivery of excess liquid into the infusion line following correction of the occlusion or blockage. Pumps permit the rapid infusion in emergency of blood and other intravenous fluids; there are three types:

Syringe pumps are designed to deliver a limited volume of fluid from a given size of syringe. Although high volumetric accuracy is possible with these pumps, they are not generally used in the operating department and are more suited to other applications, e.g. injection of intravenous contrast media for radiodiagnostic procedures.

Drip-rate pumps use sensors attached to the administration set which count the frequency of drops in order to control the infusion rate. The fluid in the infusion line is pressurised by the rotary peristaltic action of rollers, or linear peristaltic action of mechanical fingers on the tubing of the administration set. Some rotary pumps require special administration sets which incorporate an insert of softer tubing. Air-infusion line detectors are not usually provided, and very high pressures can result from an occlusion. The occlusion line may be slow to operate at low delivery rates.

Volumetric pumps are designed to overcome variations in drop size and enable the infusion rate to be set in ml/hour rather than drops/min. They have features which are appropriate to critical areas such as the operating theatre and post-anaesthesia recovery, where the initial high equipment cost and running costs can be justified.

There are two types of volumetric pumps:

1. Those using an administration set which incorporates a special cassette to meter the fluid being infused by the mechanical action of a tiny pump or syringe-like mechanism.

2. Those which apply a peristaltic pumping action to an accurately formed section of an administration set, which generally is suitable for use only with that particular pump. The cost of this is likely to be higher than that of a conventional gravity drip set.

These pumps provide a number of features:

Automatic alarm and shut down if air enters the infusion system.

Pre-set control of total volume to be infused with a digital display of the volume infused.

Automatic setting of a 'keep vein open' rate at the end of the comprehensive alarm systems to detect faults/failure.

Automatic changeover to battery standby in the event of mains supply.

Some pumps provide additional features such as computer interface detector.

There is a large range of drip rate and volumetric rate infusion pumps available. It is important to fully understand the manufacturers' operating instructions, especially regarding the type of administration set which must be used with a particular pump.

HEI No. 135 (1985) gives useful information regarding drip-rate infusion pumps and makes a number of recommendations.

Administration sets for solutions. Provided that an administration set is 'primed' correctly and joints are sound, there will be no problem of air being introduced into the infusion line until the fluid supply is almost exhausted. However, blood sets should not be used with drip-rate infusion pumps for solution delivery; this is because:

Blood sets may deliver air to the patient if the infusion is not stopped before the fluid in the container reaches a low level.

The drop-forming orifice of a blood set is designed to give the correct nominal drop volume when using blood, and the drop volume with solutions will differ.

The tubing of a blood set generally is too large in diameter and too stiff for satisfactory operation in a pump or controller.

The main difference between a blood set and a solution set is the filter chamber which comprises a small semi-rigid container above the drip chamber. It is this chamber, containing liquid, which gives rise to the increased risk of air delivery from a blood set when using a pump. The risk is minimal when a 'vented' liquid container such as a rigid glass bottle is used. However, the majority of intravenous fluids are now supplied in unvented collapsible plastic bags or semi-rigid plastic containers which may or may not be vented.

When an unvented container becomes almost empty, the flow of fluid diminishes and the pump attempts to maintain the set drip rate by working harder. The air pressure is lowered both in the fluid container and administration set, and, as a result, what air remains in the system (container, filter chamber and drip chamber) expands considerably. As the pressure reduces and the air expands, the liquid level in the drip chamber falls, but provided the pump can extract drops from the filter chamber or folds in the fluid container the pump will not alarm. When the drip chamber eventually empties, air interspersed with drops of fluid may enter the infusion line and reach the patient before the alarm is raised.

With vented infusion systems air enters the container as the fluid level falls, and when the container is empty the supply of drops ceases abruptly giving an alarm, and no lowering of air pressure occurs. Similarly, the use of solution sets eliminates the source of continued drops after the container is empty; there is a rapid cessation of drops and the alarm is raised. The use of solution sets with drip-rate pumps does not guarantee that air will not enter an infusion line, but the risk is less than using blood sets.

General precautions which should be observed when using infusion pumps (HEI No 135, 1985) are:

Do — use solution sets for administering solutions, especially if a drip-rate infusion pump is to be used.

Do — prime the drip chamber to at least one third full.

Do — squeeze the bottom of the drip chamber when priming solution sets which incorporate a filter-sack.

Do — hang the drip chamber vertically.

Do — check that the air inlet of a vented infusion is open.

Do — carefully position drop sensors on the drip chamber as recommended by the manufacturer.

Do not — leave a pump or controller unattended until sure that the desired drip-rate has been established.

Do not — allow the drip chamber or container to empty during an infusion.

Do not — rely upon the pump alarm system as a detector of an empty container/or air-in-line hazard.

Do not — remove the air from a non-vented container during the priming operation.

Do not — allow air inlet filters to be contaminated with solution. If a filter does become affected it should be replaced immediately.

If air does enter the infusion line, before opening the door of the equipment:

Do — switch off the equipment.

Do — clamp the delivery line close to the infusion site.

Do — disconnect the set from the patient.

The risk of air being introduced into the infusion line with volumetric pumps is virtually eliminated as this type of pump generally is incapable of pumping air. Care must be taken when priming, particularly those pumps which utilise cassettes incorporating small pumping chambers, as even a tiny bubble of air can significantly reduce the efficiency of the flow-rate.

Figure 3.18 shows a volumetric infusion pump of the linear peristaltic type which permits user fully variable alarm pressure settings, and incorporates a facility for the measurement of central venous pressures (CVP) during infusion. This is achieved by a pressure sensing disc in the disposable special administration set connected to a very accurate pressure transducer. The measurement and read-out of infusion pressure is constant; CVP is measured using the same infusion line, the infusion being stopped momentarily whilst static pressure measurements are taken. The information is displayed as red alpha-numeric which shows the units of measurement, alarm condition status, pump running, and start-up prompting messages. The pump can be operated from the mains electricity supply or a standby battery supply.

The logic of the sealed membrane type tactile controls is easy to follow. Flow-rate in increments of 1 ml/hr, within the range 1–999 ml/hr, is selected by three up and down touch buttons. Volume to be infused is similarly selected with same touch push buttons, which also set the maximum pressure 0–499 mmHg in 1 mmHg increments. As a safeguard there are three touch buttons marked *set volume limit*, *set max. pressure* and *set rate*, the appropriate one of which must be pressed first before changing any one of these functions. A further two touch buttons activate the display of *pressure* and *volume infused*, the latter being cleared by a third touch button marked *clear volume infused*. There are also separate *stop/start* and power *on/off* touch buttons and indicators to show operation from mains or battery.

The alarm system is comprehensive; alarms are generally audible and visible; the audible alarms can be muted for a maximum of two minutes.

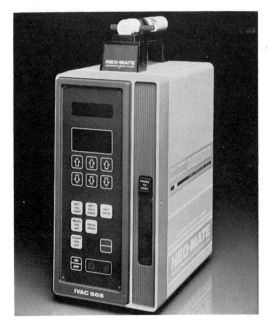

Fig. 3.18   Volumetric infusion pump, paediatric version. (Model 565, Ivac.)

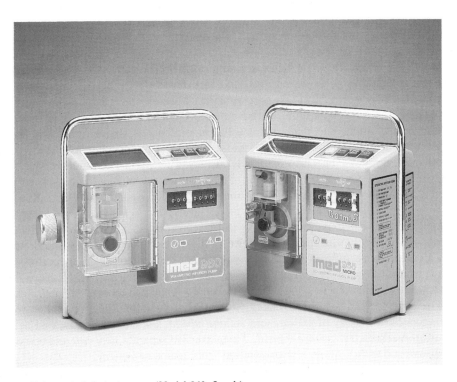

Fig. 3.19   Volumetric infusion pump. (Model 960, Imed.)

Zero-rate set — immediate alarm, display = *rate 000*.

Door opened when pump running — pump stops, immediate alarm. Display = *door*.

Drip chamber displacement — Detector gradually moved towards liquid level. Gross displacement is tolerated until detector centre line is very close to liquid level, then pump alarms and stops. Display = *flow sensor*.

Gross tilting of drip chamber is tolerated up to 45° from vertical when pump alarms and stops. Display *flow sensor* or *bottle clamp*.

Transportation — moderate and intermittent shaking tolerated as pump travels well. Severe shaking gives alarm and pump stops. Display = *flow sensor*.

Clamp or supply/empty container — Alarm given, pump stops after delay ranging from 4 seconds at 500 ml/hr, through 12 seconds at 125 ml/hr, 53 seconds at 30 ml/hr, $6\frac{1}{2}$ minutes at 4 ml/hr, to 22 minutes at 1 ml/hr. Display = *bottle clamp*.

Infusion complete — pump automatically switches over to 'keep vein open' (KVO) rate of 5 ml/hr, or the flow rate setting if less than 5 ml/hr. Display = *infusion complete, KVO xml/hr*.

Occlusion — operates according to the pressure set by the user over the range 0–499 mmHg, pump alarms and stops. Display = *occluded*.

Air-in-line — air bubble of approximately 0.01 ml detected; detector can be placed anywhere on the patient line, pump alarms and stops. Display = *air-in-line*.

Infusion set removed or mispositioned — immediate alarm, pump will not run. Display = *set out*.

Pump hold — if pump is left on 'hold' for more than two minutes, alarm is actuated and pump will not run. Display = *time out*.

Malfunction — if internal malfunction occurs, pump alarm will activate. Display = *fix me*.

Pressure transducer out of calibration — alarm activated. Display = *cal reqd*.

Low battery — the pump will run at 125 ml/hr for 8 hours before alarm is activated. Display = *low batt*.

Another type of volumetric infusion pump is illustrated in Figure 3.19. This has similar features to that in Figure 3.18 except measurement of CVP.

Surgical diathermy

Surgical diathermy is a high frequency electric current. When this current is passed through the patient's body between two electrodes, the effect is to produce a concentration of current at the electrode being used by the surgeon. As the surgeon applies his 'live' (small) electrode to the tissues, the current passes through the adjacent tissue cells and owing to their electrical resistance, heat is generated at this point. The effect is localised because with monopolar output the current from the 'live' (small) electrode spreads out in the patient's body and travels to the 'indifferent' electrode which is a large electrode placed in contact with the patient's body (Fig. 3.20). A high density of current occurs only immediately beneath the live electrode because further away (except under fault conditions) the current density is too small to have any heating effect. With bipolar output the surgeon's instrument, usually in the form of forceps, combines both electrodes so that current flows only through the tissue gripped between the tips of the forceps, thereby eliminating the need for an indifferent electrode (Fig. 3.21).

When electro-section or cutting current is selected and used with a needle electrode, an arc is struck between the point of this electrode and the underlying tissues. The arc is very hot (in excess of 1,000°C) and causes tissue cells to disintegrate instantly in front of the electrode which may be moved with a cutting effect.

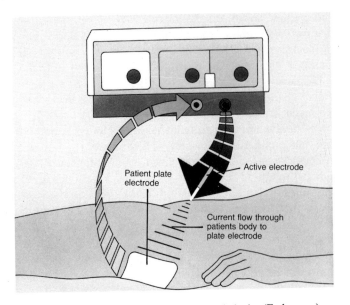

Fig. 3.20   Monopolar passage of diathermy current through patient's body. (Eschmann.)

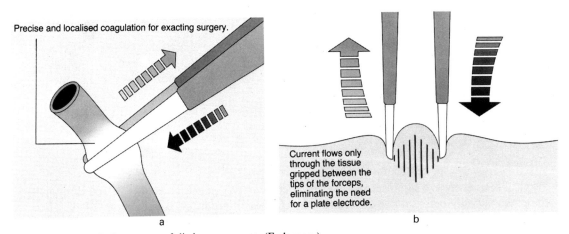

Fig. 3.21   Bipolar passage of diathermy current. (Eschmann.)

Blood vessels which are cut may continue to bleed and it is necessary to apply the diathermy current specifically to the vessel to effect coagulation. The vessel is gripped with artery forceps and an electro-coagulation current is applied via the artery forceps until sufficient heat is generated to cause coagulation of the blood and arrest further bleeding.

Electricity direct from the mains could achieve coagulation of blood, but the current needed to do this at 50 Hz (the mains frequency) would cause intense activation of muscle, thereby preventing the surgeon from working. Also, such a current is likely to cause ventricular fibrillation (page 80) and probable death of the patient. A diathermy current operates at high frequencies and equivalent to 1 amp may be used, the current can pass through the tissues without activating muscles.

Diathermy machines or high frequency electrosurgical units generate currents within the

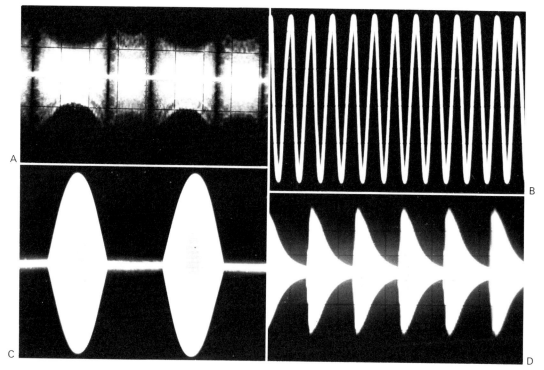

Fig. 3.22   Oscilloscope traces of diathermy (electrosurgical) output: (A) Spark-generated diathermy, 100 bursts per second at about 400 Hz; (B & C) Valve-generated diathermy, 50 bursts per second at between 1.6 and 3 MHz. (D) Valve-generated diathermy, modulated at 20,000 to 60,000 bursts per second at 1.75 MHz. (A. K. Dobbie.)

range of 400 kHz (400,000 cycles per second) to 3 MHz (3,000,000 cycles per second). In one type of machine, the energy for diathermy is created by an electrical discharge across a spark gap. The spark generator produces 100 blocks of energy per second, the oscillating current being at about 400 KHz, but has a high harmonic content extending over a wide band of frequencies. (Fig. 3.22).

The valve generator unit usually produces bursts of energy 50 times per second, each burst oscillating at between 1.6 and 3 MHz per second (Fig. 3.22B and C). Usually the lower frequencies are suitable for coagulation and the higher frequencies more suitable for cutting of tissue. Such factors as the composition of the oscillating wave affect its working characteristics and are beyond the scope of this book.

These two systems may cause severe interference with certain electromedical recording apparatus. This is caused by the fact that both machines release their energy in pulses at 50 or 100 times per second which is broadcast through electric wiring and through the air. This frequency lies within the frequency reception band for such apparatus as ECG and EEG. This means that even with efficient radio suppression, e.g. mains electrical filters, the pulse repetition of the diathermy energy will be detected, amplified by the electromedical recording apparatus and will obliterate any physiological data.

A type of high frequency electrosurgical unit is available which releases its energy at a frequency of 500 KHz in a square waveform (Fig. 3.23), which is outside the frequency band for physiological instruments. This unit provides two modes of use, monopolar and bipolar, with outputs between 15 and 400 watts (Fig. 3.24).

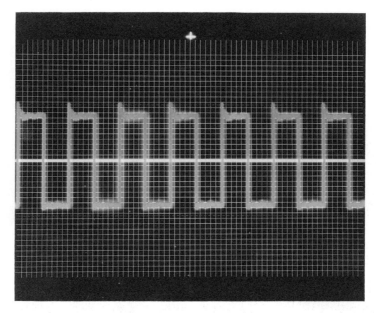

Fig. 3.23 Diathermy square wave form which produces more energy from a given amplitude than from the wave forms illustrated in Figure 3.22. (Eschmann.)

Monopolar cutting/coagulation requires the use of two separate electrodes connected by heavy insulated cable to the terminals on the unit. There are controls for coagulation and cutting, and for blending the output to provide between 150 watts pure coagulation and 400 watts pure cutting. There is a spark-free footswitch which has separate sections to select either coagulation or cutting output.

The *live electrode* which is used in the operating site is sterilized before connecting to the live terminal on the unit. There is a variety of different shaped electrodes ranging from a slender needle to a disc or ball-type point. These are connected to an insulated handle which is then coupled to the wire. Changing of these electrodes is made simply by the provision of a socket on the operating end of the wire.

The purpose of the indifferent electrode is to provide a surface of sufficient area to avoid any physiological effects at the site of application. This is because the indifferent electrode is in contact with hundreds or even thousands more cells than the live electrode which results in a correspondingly lower density of current in each cell. If the electrode is applied correctly, negligible heat is generated in this area.

The commonest types of indifferent electrodes are flexible metal plates. The thin flexible metal plate electrode can either be placed under the patient's body or carefully bandaged round the thigh to ensure even contact with the skin. It is unnecessary to use electrode jelly, though if a hairy site is chosen for application, shaving beforehand is advisable — the hair acts as an electrical resistance. If the patient's skin is dry, moistening with water or saline can be done with advantage before applying the plate. Care must be taken to renew a plate electrode which becomes buckled otherwise areas of irregular contact with the skin result which could allow points of high current density and risk of burns. The electrode is connected to the high frequency electrosurgical unit indifferent or earth terminal by a heavy insulated wire.

Another satisfactory type of indifferent electrode consists of aluminium foil half a thousandth of an inch thick backed with paper. A sheet of foil about 45.5 cm (18 in) square

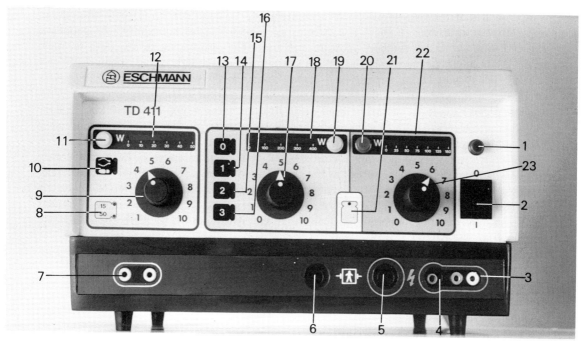

Fig. 3.24 Multi-output electrosurgical unit. (TD411 — Eschmann.)

1. Mains pilot lamp (green).
2. Mains on/off switch.
3. Active sockets for three-pin hand switching instruments.
4. Active socket for 4 mm single-pin footswitch-operated instruments.
5. Active socket for 8 mm single-pin footswitch-operated instruments (Bovie-type).
6. Plate socket for 6 mm jack indifferent plate electrode.
7. Bipolar forceps sockets.
8. Bipolar 15 watt or 50 watt power range selector buttons and indicators (amber).
9. Bipolar power output control.
10. Forceps switching or footswitch selector touch button and indicators (amber).
11. Bipolar pilot lamp (white).
12. Bipolar power display (Red).
13. Pure cutting current 0 touch button.
14. Blend cutting/coagulation current 1 touch button.
15. Blend cutting/coagulation current 2 touch button.
16. Blend cutting/coagulation current 3 touch button. (*Haemostasis increases with blend number*)
17. Cutting current power output control.
18. Cutting current power display (red).
19. Cutting current pilot lamp (yellow).
20. Coagulating current pilot lamp (blue).
21. Monopolar selector touch button and indicator (amber).
22. Coagulation current power display (red).
23. Coagulation current power output control.

is placed under the patient's body and connected to the insulated wire with stainless steel clips. It has the advantages that it is cheap, can be autoclaved and is transparent to X-rays. The foil electrode is particularly suitable for use with infants.

It is important that electrodes are connected correctly to the terminals on the electrosurgical unit. The connections being reversed will almost certainly result in diathermy burns to the patient; modern electrosurgical units incorporate non-interchangeable connections to avoid this danger.

Bipolar coagulation is achieved by two electrodes which are combined into one instrument. This permits greater accuracy and safety in delicate procedures such as neurosurgery, ophthalmic, plastic and microsurgery. There is a control which selects either 15 or 50 watt output, each of which can be finely adjusted within this range by means of a rheostat. The unit illustrated in Figure 3.24 permits on/off switching directly from the forceps as an alternative to the footswitch.

It is vital that the indifferent electrode remains in electrical continuity with the patient and electrosurgical unit. If there is a defect and a break in this continuity, the patient is exposed to grave risk of diathermy burns. Failure of the return path to the earth terminal of the diathermy machine causes the patient's body to rise to a high voltage when diathermy is used. If any part of the patient then makes contact with earthed metal or a large mass of metal, e.g. the operation table, then a burn is likely to occur at the point of contact. This is why special ECG leads should be used in theatre; i.e. those which have a 10 kHz resistor moulded into the extremity of each lead which ensures that a diathermy burn cannot occur with any type of electrode.

Patient plate continuity monitor. Electrosurgical units should incorporate a monitoring device which detects a possible break in the continuity of the indifferent electrode. Generally this is achieved with two separate insulated wires within the indifferent electrode cable. A low voltage electric current is passed out to the plate electrode via one wire, and returns to the unit by the other, thereby ensuring that the 'earth' return path for the diathermy current from the patient is intact. Failure of one wire activates an alarm.

In addition to the above, the unit in Figure 3.24 has two additional safety features (Fig. 3.25).

Patient earth monitor. This protects the patient from the dangers of accidental connection or current leakage to earth via any conductive object which may touch the patient, for example, a transfusion stand or anaesthetic screen.

Patient voltage monitor. The circuitry of the patient voltage monitor activates an alarm in the presence of a dangerous diathermy voltage on the patient's body that is likely to cause a burn. An example would be if an active electrode touches an earthed conductor, or if contact is lost between the patient and the indifferent electrode. This patented circuit prevents the voltage on the patient's body reaching a level at which burns may be produced.

As an additional precaution the patient should be protected by a **thick** layer of insulating material such as rubber sheeting if there is a danger of his coming into contact with metal parts of the table.

Diathermy machine not working

If a diathermy machine will not work when connected the following should be checked:

1. *After switching off at the wall socket*, check the wire leading from the plug top to ensure that there are no loose wires.

2. Ensure that the *on off* switch on the machine is correctly positioned; check with another socket.

If the machine will still not work consult an electrician. However, if an audible hum is made by the machine as it is switched on, but the current does not flow between the electrodes, the diathermy circuit should be checked:

1. *After switching off at the wall socket*, check that the electrode wires are connected correctly and securely to the machine.

2. Check that the insulated wires are still firmly attached to both of the terminal connections in addition to the electrode handle and the plate connection. If a plate monitoring device is fitted, a broken indifferent electrode wire will be detected under 2 above.

3. Check that the metal connections are not corroded.

4. Check that the indifferent electrode is in good contact with the patient's skin.

Any further checks on the machine circuit are beyond the scope of theatre staff, and the electrician should be consulted.

The strength of current required depends upon the purpose for which diathermy is being

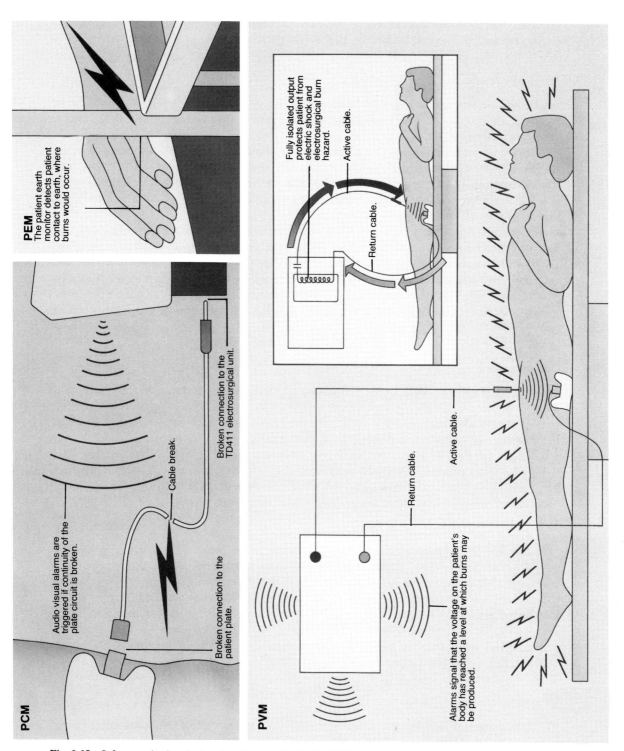

PEM
The patient earth monitor detects patient contact to earth, where burns would occur.

PCM

Audio visual alarms are triggered if continuity of the plate circuit is broken.

Cable break.

Broken connection to the TD411 electrosurgical unit.

Broken connection to the patient plate.

Fully isolated output protects patient from electric shock and electrosurgical burn hazard.

Active cable.

Return cable.

PVM

Return cable.

Active cable.

Alarms signal that the voltage on the patient's body has reached a level at which burns may be produced.

Fig. 3.25 Safety monitoring devices for electrosurgical unit. PCM — Patient Plate Continuity Monitor. PEM — Patient Earth Monitor. PVM — Patient Voltage Monitor. (TD411 — Eschmann.)

used and on the type of machine. As a general rule maximum output is not needed, and for most cases one-third to a half of the maximum will often be sufficient. This current setting must of course be checked by the 'scrub nurse' assisting at the operation.

Surgical cautery

An electric cautery consists of a platinum wire loop or point which is raised to red heat by means of an electric current. This heated cautery point is then applied to the tissue area to cause coagulation.

The current may be produced by a low-voltage battery or transformer, although the transformer is preferable, as the output is more constant than that of a battery. The transformer has a rheostat knob which may be adjusted to alter the voltage applied to the platinum point. The cautery must not be used any hotter than at red heat, as too high a current will cause rapid burning out of the cautery point.

The cautery points, of which there is a varied selection, are mounted in a heat-resisting handle to which are connected two wires. These wires are then connected to the transformer *which must be switched off at the wall socket*. Sometimes a transformer has two sets of low-voltage output terminals, one set being marked *Lights*, the other set being marked *Cautery*. The cautery must not be connected to the lights terminals as this may overload the transformer and cause it to burn out. After connecting the wires the transformer may then be switched on.

Cautery apparatus not working

If the cautery will not work check the circuit in the following order, *after switching off at the wall socket*:

1. Inspect the cautery points to see if they are broken, the most usual points of breakage being where the platinum wire joins the thicker mount.

2. Check through all of the electrical connections — cautery point to handle, handle to wire, wire to transformer terminals — to see if they are clean and not corroded. Corrosion may cause poor electrical contact and failure of the current to flow to the cautery point. Cleaning of the points on these low-voltage connections with a small piece of emery cloth is often all that is necessary.

3. Check that the cautery *on off* switch is correctly positioned.

4. See that the cable leading from the transformer to the plug socket has not been pulled away from its connections. This may be done by manipulating the cable a little to see if any wires are loose at the points of connection to the transformer and plug top.

5. Re-connect the transformer and switch on. If it still does not operate, the plug socket may be tested by connecting another item of apparatus, such as a portable light fitting which is known to be in working order.

Should this reveal that the socket is operating correctly, it is advisable to have the apparatus checked by an electrician.

Lasers

The development of surgical lasers during the last decade has made a significant contribution to microsurgery. Used in conjunction with operating microscopes and fibrescopes (Chapters 13 and 14), a wide range of microsurgical procedures have now become possible, for example, sutureless microvascular anastomosis (Jain and Gorisch, 1979; Jain, 1980), excision

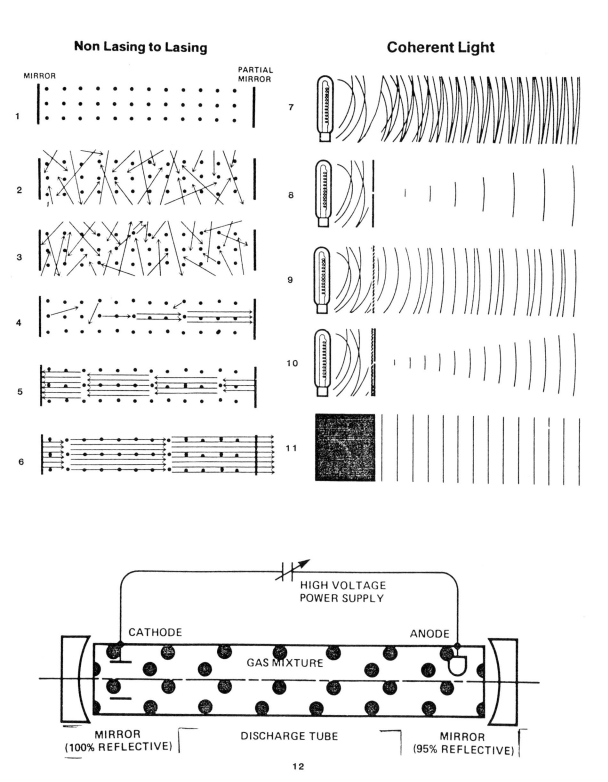

Fig. 3.26 Principles of a carbon dioxide surgical laser. (Coherent (UK) Ltd.)

of the posterior capsule through the tranparent cornea (Cochrane, 1984), coagulation of bleeding peptic ulcers using a flexible gastroscope (Swain et al., 1981).

A laser is an apparatus which produces a fine parallel beam of high intensity light which can be focused on a very small spot. In laser surgery, the light beam heats the target tissue and causes thermal tissue destruction, first with local oedema, then denaturation of protein, contraction of tissue due to alteration of fibrous tissue protein, and finally boiling of cell water and vaporisation. Generally, low energy exposure results in coagulation of blood vessels; higher energy exposure produces a precise incision by vaporisation of the tissue at the focal point.

Laser is an acronym for Light Amplification by the Simulated Emission of Radiation. The laser is produced when light is fed into a 'lasing medium' which causes electrons to jump to a higher level of energy. When a photon strikes an electron in this situation, the electron decays to a lower level of energy and emits another photon which has the same wavelength as the first; both waves are also in phase with each other. The light is bounced back and forth through the lasing medium by mirrors at each end; this releases more and more photons and increases the energy of the light (Cochrane, 1985). One of the mirrors has a central hole or semi-reflective area permitting a beam of highly concentrated light to emerge through the laser aperture which is collimated (parallel), coherent (waves all in phase) and monochromatic (of a single wavelength) (Fig. 3.26). This beam of light can be channelled along flexible optic fibres or reflected by an optical mirror system, to a surgical handpiece or operating microscope.

Present surgical lasers use various materials as the lasing medium. Three types of lasers are in general use:

Carbon dioxide laser. This produces an infra-red beam which is highly absorbed by water and therefore very suitable for vaporising tissue. It enables precise incisions to be made with minimal damage to adjacent tissue, and can seal blood vessels up to about 0.5 mm diameter. This type of laser incorporates a red aiming beam as the infra-red beam is invisible. Carbon dioxide lasers use mirrors to transmit the beams, although suitable flexible fibres are presently under development.

Figure 3.27 illustrates a CO_2 laser attached to an operating microscope. This provides a continuously adjustable laser power of 2–30 watts, with a laser wavelength of 10.6 μ (far infra-red), aiming beam wavelength of 632.8 nm (red), target spot sizes between 0.2 and 1 mm, and exposure times of 0.05, 0.1, 0.2, 0.5 seconds and continuous, with 1 to 4 pulses per second at a variable time interval. The CO_2 gas cylinder provides 25–40 hours use, and the gas pressure is controlled electronically. The laser, which is suitable for a wide range of surgical specialties, can also be used freehand with a special handpiece.

Argon laser. This produces a blue-green light of a wavelength between 448–514 nm well absorbed by melolin and blood. The beam can be transmitted by flexible optic fibres and is very suitable for haemostasis in gastro-endoscopy, ophthalmic and dermatological procedures. The laser power is variable between 0 and 5 watts.

Neodymium-yttrium-aluminium-garnet laser (Nd-YAG). The wavelength of 1064 nm, and energy emission of up to 70 watts, gives deep penetration into tissue and effective haemostasis of blood vessels up to about 1 mm diameter. The beam will pass along optic fibres and can be used in conjunction with flexible endoscopes.

Hazards. Great care is needed in the use of lasers which are potentially dangerous to patients, surgeons or observers. The Department of Health (1980) has issued guidance on safety codes which should be observed, based on BS4803: Part 3 (1980). The National Association of Nurses (NATN) set out safety guidelines on the use of laser beams in their Codes of Practice (1983); other references include the Association of Operating Nurses

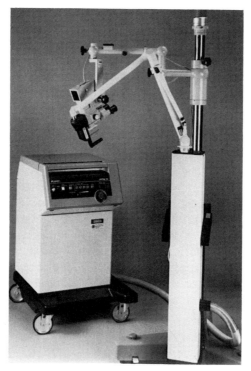

Fig. 3.27 Carbon dioxide surgical laser fitted to an operating microscope. (Coherent (UK) Ltd.)

(AORN, 1985) and McKenzie (1980).

The following safety precautions, which take into account the NATN codes of practice are recommended.

1. When not in use laser equipment must be protected against unauthorised use by the removal of a master control key.

2. The theatre in which the laser is to be used should be designated a laser controlled area.

3. Entry into this area should be limited to personnel whose presence is essential.

All personnel participating in a procedure must wear approved protective eyewear. When the laser is being used in the presence of the patient's face *or* when laser light can reach the patient's eyes, eye protection for the patient is recommended. Specification of suitable protective eyewear should take into account:

The laser wavelength(s)

Irradiance or radiant exposure

Maximum possible exposure

Optical density of eyewear at laser output wavelength

Visible light transmission requirements

Irradiance/radiant exposure at which damage to eyewear may occur

Requirement for prescription lenses for wearer

Comfort and ventilation

Degradation of absorbing media

Resistance of material to shock

Requirements for peripheral vision

Relevant statutory requirements.

The protective eyewear must be clearly labelled with the optical density value and wave-length(s) for which protection is afforded.

While there is no hazard to skin from diffuse reflection of the laser beam off matt surfaces, specular, mirror-type reflection and direct intra-beam exposure may exceed the maximum permissible exposure for skin. Although complete protection of skin is impracticable, beam stops or beam attenuators should be maintained and used whenever possible. It is the responsibility of the surgeon to ensure that the laser is fired only when it has been aimed correctly at the target tissue.

The laser should be activated only by the surgeon who is responsible at that time for the safe custody of the master control key to the system.

Care is needed with the direction of both the aiming and therapeutic beam of the laser.

Care must be taken to avoid directing the laser beam at metallic instruments and specularly reflecting surfaces such as a patient's ring, glass and plastic objects, and walls.

Plastic or rubber anaesthesia tubes may be pierced by a laser beam and constitute a potential explosion hazard. In the case of patients under general anaesthesia, therefore, particular care should be exercised to avoid directing the beam close to such tubing.

The safety circuits of the laser apparatus should be tested at regular intervals; care should be taken during testing to ensure that the beam is directed at non-flammable material sufficient to absorb all energy emitted from the laser aperture, e.g. a special asbestos block or moist gauze pad.

Cryosurgical systems

Cryotherapy, the application of extreme cold, is a useful technique for the destruction of tissues and is characterised by minimal bleeding or pain in the post-operative phase. Cryosurgical systems are well established in many surgical specialties including general surgery, gynaecology, dermatology, neurology, and urology.

The first practical apparatus for the control and maintenance of extreme low temperature in surgery was realised in 1962 (Cooper *et al*). The apparatus was very sophisticated and used liquid nitrogen to achieve a minimum temperature in the region of $-196°C$. This very low temperature was subsequently found to exceed requirements, and Amoils (1967) developed a more simple apparatus which used nitrous oxide or carbon dioxide to achieve temperatures in the region of $-70°C$. The design principles established by Amoils are still used in modern cryosurgical equipment which employs high-pressure, non-syphon cylinders of N_2O and CO_2.

Cryosurgical systems consist of flexible tubing connecting the gas flow control unit to a cryoprobe or working tip which comprises two concentric tubes. The inner tube delivers nitrous oxide or carbon dioxide at pressures between 4,000 kPa and 6,000 kPa to a narrow orifice in the end. The sudden expansion of this gas through the 'Joule Thompson Orifice' (Fig. 3.28a), produces a rapid drop in temperature of the probe surface forming an ice ball (Fig. 3.28b). The expanded gas is then returned at atmospheric pressure along the outer tube. Some extension of cooling along the shaft of the probe occurs and can be a disadvantage, for example in neurosurgery. To overcome this, Spembley manufacture a probe which employs a reversed gas flow (Evans, 1981). This design enables the incoming gas to be carried to the probe tip via the outer of the two concentric tubes; it is allowed to expand through an annular orifice, being finally released through the central tube (Fig. 3.28c). The incoming gas acts as an insulating barrier and effectively confines freezing to the probe tip.

Cryoprobes incorporate a thermocouple in the tip to enable control of the operating temperature. Defrosting is achieved swiftly by supplying a controlled build up of high

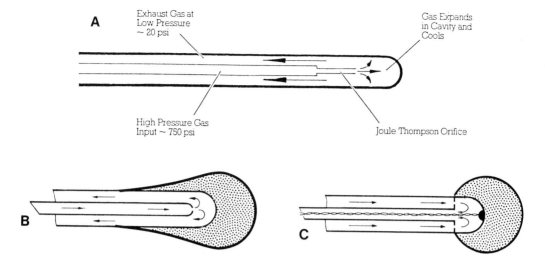

Fig. 3.28 Principles of a cryoprobe. (Spembley Medical Ltd.) (A) the Joule Thompson effect. (B) Flow in a typical Amoils cryoprobe. (C) Reverse flow principles.

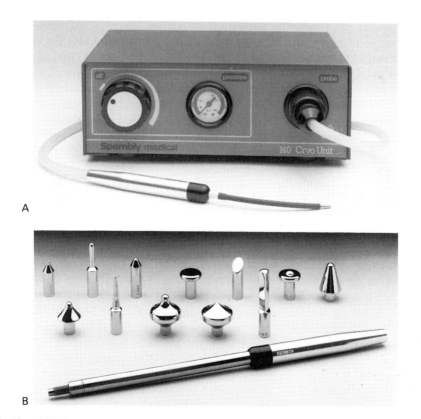

Fig. 3.29 (A and B) Cryosurgical system — utilising nitrous oxide or carbon dioxide. (Model 140, Spembley Medical Ltd.)

pressure gas in the probe tip. This gas condenses on the cold inner surface of the probe and rewarms the probe tip rapidly as the latent heat of condensation is given up. The cryosurgical system illustrated in Figure 3.29 employs a range of detachable handles and probe tips.

When the cryoprobe probe tip is applied to living tissue, heat is extracted and a rapid temperature drop occurs. By the formation of intra-cellular and extra-cellular ice in the tissues adjacent to the probe tip, biological systems are disturbed and cells destroyed (Barnard, 1977). The adherence of tissue to the freezing probe tip can be used to advantage, for example, to extract the ocular lens in cataract operations.

Ultrasonic equipment

Ultrasonic techniques are well established in neurosurgery for rapid, efficient removal of intracranial and spinal cord tumours. Their use in resection and dissection applications for liver, kidney, spleen, pancreas and urology surgery is gaining momentum.

Ultrasonic surgery is carried out with the aid of a magneto-strictive instrument known as the CUSA™ — Cavitron™ Ultrasonic Surgical Aspirator. This is an acoustic vibrator which consists of three distinct components:

1. *Transducer* — a magneto-strictive device which converts electromagnetic energy into mechanical vibrations. The transducer is composed of a stack of nickel alloy laminations. A magnetic field is produced by a coil placed around the laminations and causes mechanical motion of approximately 300 microns.

2. *Connecting body* — mechanically couples the motion of the transducer to the surgical tip; it also amplifies the vibrational motion of the transducer.

3. *Surgical tip* — completes the motion amplification and also contacts the tissue. The tip, relatively long with respect to its diameter, is machined to exacting tolerances to provide proper motion amplification.

The electric coil which is permanently fitted in the hand piece, surrounds the transducer. This coil receives 23,000 cycles per second (hertz) alternating electric current from the console and activates the transducer. The handpiece is connected to the console by a cable which includes the tubing for circulating fluid between the cooling water canister in the console and the handpiece.

Since the electric coil has a current flowing through it and the transducer laminations are moving back and forth 23,000 times per second, heat is generated and absorbed by the water circulating within the handpiece. This keeps the handpiece at a comfortable temperature for the surgeon, whilst preserving the mechanical properties of the acoustic vibrator.

The irrigating solution and medical vacuum are routed from the console to the hand piece. The irrigation and vacuum tubes are sealed side by side to form a single unit called the 'manifold' which is attached to the handpiece cable. The end of the irrigation tube is attached to a port on the nosecone of the handpiece; irrigating fluid is directed co-axially between the surgical tip and a protective flue. The end of the vacuum tube is attached to the proximal port of the surgical tip; suction is then available at the end of the tip.

The CUSA™ utilises a hollow vibrating titanium tip to dissect or fragment tissue. The vibration of the tip of 23,000 hertz is above the audible range and therefore called ultrasonic. No light beams or sound waves are emitted; the CUSA tip must make contact with the tissue in order to fragment it. As tissue is fragmented, a co-axial flow of irrigation fluid suspends the particles. Simultaneously, aspiration or suction removes debris from the operation field. This unique three-fold system of fragmentation, irrigation and aspiration greatly improves visibility during surgery.

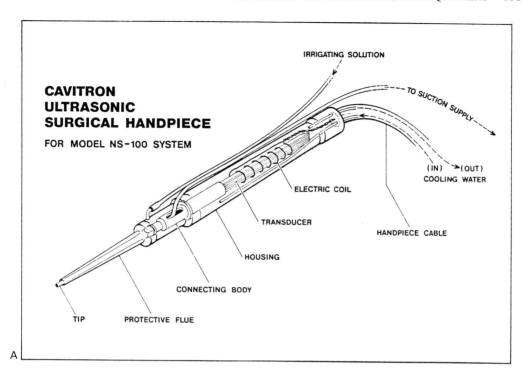

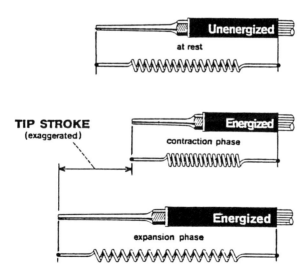

Principle of an Acoustic Vibrator

B   The Acoustic Vibrator changes shape at each moment in time

Fig. 3.30 Principles of the ultrasonic surgical aspirator system. (CUSA — Cavitron Surgical Systems, Division of Cooper Laser Sonics Inc.)

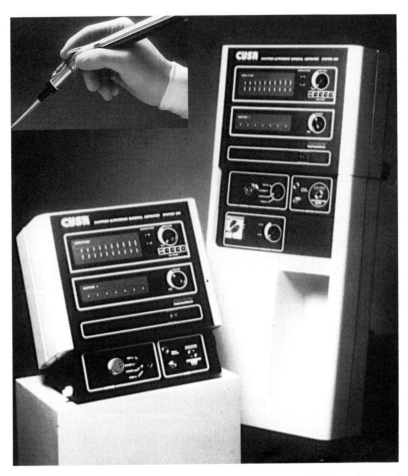

Fig. 3.31 Ultrasonic surgical aspirator. (CUSA — Cavitron Surgical Systems, Division of Cooper Laser Sonics Inc.)

The CUSA™ tip oscillates longitudinally. The amplitude of this movement can be adjusted to allow for selective tissue removal and to provide a high degree of tactile feedback providing controlled tissue fragmentation, a distinct advantage when debulking large tumours. The instrument selectively fragments tissue with high water content, whilst sparing elastic and collagen-rich tissue such as intracapsular walls and blood vessels, as well as reducing trauma to surrounding neural structures.

Electric and pipeline suction units

These are a vital part of the theatre equipment for aspirating fluid, e.g. from the abdominal cavity or nasopharynx, etc.

The suction may be obtained with a mobile machine or a larger central pump unit, connected by a pipe line system to wards and operating suites (Burns, 1958). With the pipe system coupling sockets are placed conveniently in the operating theatre, anaesthesia and recovery rooms, etc., for connection to a mobile suction bottle unit in which aspirated fluids are collected (Fig. 3.32) (DHSS, 1972).

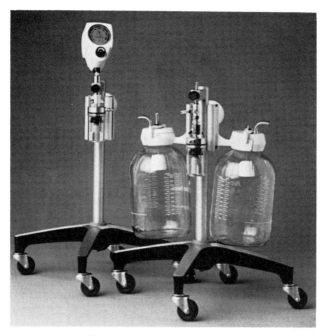

Fig. 3.32 Pipeline suction apparatus. (Ohmeda.)

Mobile suction machines are mainly of two types: (1) the high-vacuum rotary compressor pump, and (2) the reciprocating pump. The first type is most suitable for use in theatre and recovery room as it has the advantage of producing a good vacuum at a high rate of free air displacement, that is, rapid suction of large quantities of fluid. The second type is more suitable for ward use, for although the vacuum produced is reasonably high the displacement of free air is much less, and the speed of suction is correspondingly reduced.

Any mobile suction machines used in the operating theatre must have a spark-free switching mechanism and a flame-proof motor. All the well-known makes of rotary compressor or reciprocating pumps fulfil these requirements, and as the former are the most suitable for use in operating theatres they will be dealt with in more detail.

Although the various machines differ somewhat in design, they are basically similar in the method of fluid collection. The pump creates a vacuum in the glass suction bottle, into which the aspirated fluid is collected. This jar, which should be of 1.5 litre capacity for use in theatre, is provided with some method of quick release from its sealing cap. In some cases this will be a quick-release removable cap, and in others a method of securing the jar against a fixed metal cap which has a rubber washer or liner.

Incorporated in this cap are internal connections to the pump unit, and one or two external connections for suction tubing. Where two external connections are fitted, it is usual to have a selective tap to enable two suction tubes to be connected to the machine at once, e.g. one for the anaesthetist and one for the operation area. The tap is then positioned correctly for the suction tube in use at that particular time. Ideally, of course, it is preferable to have two suction machines for this purpose as both the surgeon and anaesthetist may require suction simultaneously.

In addition to the external suction tube connections a negative pressure gauge is fitted to the unit indicating the degree of vacuum, controllable by an adjacent screw valve. The

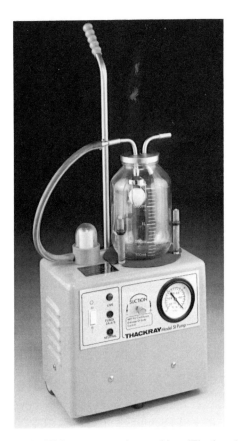

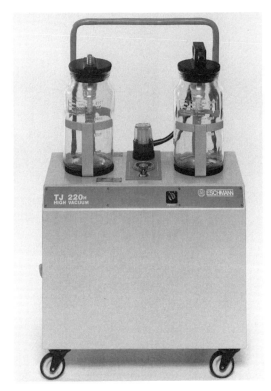

Fig. 3.33 High vacuum suction machine. (Thackray.)

Fig. 3.34 Another type of high-vacuum suction machine. (VP 45, Eschmann.)

degree of vacuum obtainable with the rotary compressor vacuum pump is about 66 cm (26 in) of mercury, which is ideal for the rapid aspiration of large quantities of fluid. However, as in the case of suction required for neurosurgical and other delicate operations, this must be considerably less, about 13 cm (5 in) of mercury, hence the value of the adjustable screw valve.

To avoid the danger of foreign matter entering the pump unit should the bottle become overfilled an automatic cut-out is fitted at some point between the bottle and the pump. This generally consists of a float which rises as the bottle contents approach overflow and seals off the connection to the pump. A space suction bottle is usually provided and some machines incorporate a quick change-over device between the two bottles (Fig. 3.34). The exhaust outlet from the pump should be fitted with a filter to prevent dissipation of contaminated air into the atmosphere. Modern rotary compressor pumps have an exhaust system which safeguards the machine to a certain extent in this respect, but nevertheless unnecessary strain should be avoided whenever possible. A fully disposable closed suction collecting system is available for connection to any suction apparatus. This is of particular value when special cross infection measures are required in Hepatitis B, HIV (Fig. 3.35).

The machine is mounted on strong antistatic castors and is connected with durable electric cable to a plug top.

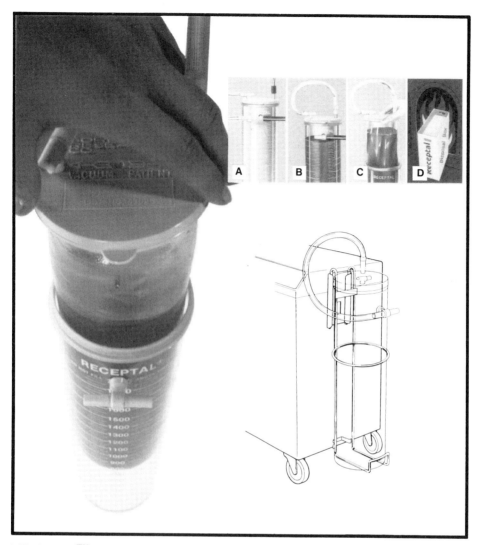

Fig. 3.35 Receptal™ closed disposable suction system. The simple liner/canister (left) allows easy collection of suction waste in a controlled, confined manner. On completion of the operation or procedure, or when the liner is full, it is sealed, removed and disposed of by incineration. The method of use is as follows (top right):
(A) Liner is placed in canister and tubing is connected to suction source
(B) when operation or procedure is completed or the liner shuts off automatically, the lid tubing is reconnected for intact disposal
(C) The full liner is removed . . . .
(D) . . . and disposed of by incineration. Tests have shown that no additional harmful fumes are given off by incineration.
The Receptal™ system can be fitted to any suction machine or stand (bottom right). (Abbott Laboratories Ltd.)

Points to observe when using suction units

1. The suction tubing must be of adequate bore to avoid blockage and collapse. The size will depend upon the tubing connections fitted to the machine and the suction nozzles used, but generally an antistatic tubing of 0.75 cm ($\frac{5}{16}$ in) bore and 0.3 cm ($\frac{1}{8}$ in) wall will suffice.

2. The tubing must be in good condition, without punctures and with a clean lumen.

3. The degree of suction required is regulated initially by compressing the tubing (after switching on the machine) whilst setting the adjustable valve at the necessary position, e.g. to maintain a suction of 25 cm (10 in) of mercury.

4. If the aspirated fluid 'froths up', the froth may be reduced by turning the suction tube connection tap so that the other unused connection is opened to the atmosphere, or alternatively opening fully the suction control valve. If this is not done, the froth may overflow and operate the cut-out mechanism prematurely.

5. The suction bottle must be emptied when the fluid reaches a pre-determined mark. If, by accident, it is overfilled thereby operating the cut-out, the machine is switched off, vacuum broken by opening the suction control valve and the bottle emptied before replacing and recommencing suction. If the cut-out is fitted in a separate chamber adjacent to the suction bottle, it may be necessary to empty this chamber before commencing suction again.

6. Do *not* cause excessive strain to a suction pump by maintaining a constant high vacuum which occurs, for example, when the tubing is accidentally compressed or when the suction nozzle becomes occluded by contact with a towel.

7. After use, the bottle, cap, float and float chamber must be washed with an anti-bacterial agent (Chapter 7) and thoroughly dried. Movable taps, etc. must be lightly oiled at frequent intervals.

8. A final caution — do not leave a residual vacuum in the suction bottle after switching off. Possible cause: kinks in a coil of suction tubing wound round pegs fitted to the machine so that it is ready for emergency use. This may cause a back aspiration of oil from the vacuum pump with 'drying out' of the mechanism and consequent loss of efficiency. It is possible to lose half a pint, or more, of oil in this way.

REFERENCES

AMOILS, S. P. (1967) *Archives of Ophthalmology*, **78**, 201.
ARNOLD, V. F. (1958) In *Medical Electrical Equipment*, p. 177. Edited by R. E. Molloy. London: Newnes.
ASSOCIATION OF OPERATING ROOM NURSES (1985) Recommended Practices — Radiation Safety in the Operating Room (including lasers). *AORN Journal*, **42**, No. 6, 920.
BARNARD, J. D. W. (1977) Cryoanalgesia. *Nursing Times*, June 16.
BRITISH STANDARDS INSTITUTION (1983) British Standard, Radiation Safety of Laser Products and Systems, Part 3 Guidance for Users. B.S. 4803: Part 3. London: BSI.
BURNS, J. T. (1958) In *Medical Electrical Equipment*, p. 229. Edited by R. E. Molloy. London: Newnes.
COCHRANE, J. P. S. (1985) Lasers in Surgical Practice. In *Recent Advances in Surgery-12*. Edited by R. C. G. Russell. Edinburgh: Churchill Livingstone.
COOPER, I. S., GRISSMAN, F. AND JOHNSON R. (1962) *St Barnab. Hospital Medical Bulletin*, **1**, 11–16.
DEPARTMENT OF HEALTH AND SOCIAL SECURITY (1972) *Hospital Technical Memorandum No. 22*. London: HMSO.
DEPARTMENT OF HEALTH AND SOCIAL SECURITY (1974) *Hospital Technical Memorandum No. 11*. London: HMSO.
DEPARTMENT OF HEALTH AND SOCIAL SECURITY (1980) *Guidance on the Safe Use of Lasers in Medical Practice*. London: HMSO.
DEPARTMENT OF HEALTH AND SOCIAL SECURITY (1985) Infusion pumps and controllers. *Health Equipment Information*, No. 135. London: HMSO.
DOBBIE, A. K. (1969) *Biomedical Engineering*, 4, No. 5, pp. 206–216.
DOBBIE, A. K. (1972) *Medical and Biological Engineering*, 7, 2.
EVANS, P. J. D. (1981) Cryoanalgesia. *Anaesthesia*, **36**, 1003–1013.
GREEN, H. L., RAFTERY, E. B. AND GREGORY, I. C. (1972) *Biomedical Engineering*, 7, No. 9, pp. 408–414.
HULL, C. J. (1978) *British Journal of Anaesthesia*, **50**, 647.
HULL, C. J. AND ENGLISH, M. J. M. (1984) Safety in the operating area. *The Design and Use of Operating Theatres*, Edited by I. D. A. Johnstone and A. R. Hunter. London: Arnold.

JAIN, K. K. AND GORISCH, W. (1979) Repair of small blood vessels with the neodymium-YAG laser; a preliminary report. *Surgery*, **85**, 684.

JAIN, K. K. (1980) Sutureless microvascular anastomosis using a neodymium-YAG laser, *Journal of Microsurgery*, May/June, 436.

MCKENZIE, L. A. (1980) Laser safety codes. *Journal of Laryngology and Otology*. XCIV, April

NATIONAL ASSOCIATION OF THEATRE NURSES (1983) Codes of Practice. Harrogate: NATN.

NORTHWICK PARK HOSPITAL AND CLINICAL RESEARCH CENTRE (1972) Electrical Equipment Booklet. *Patient Safety* (M097-72). London: Holborn Press.

SAVAGE, B. (1954) *Preliminary Electricity for the Physiotherapist*. London: Faber.

SMITH, A. C. (1958) In *Medical Electrical Equipment*, p. 156. Edited by R. E. Molloy. London: Newnes.

SMITH, E. A. (1958) In *Medical Electrical Equipment*, p. 30. Edited by R. E. Molloy. London: Newnes.

STEVENS, W. R. (1951) *The Principles of Lighting*. London: Constable.

SWAIN, C. P., BOWEN, S. G., SOTEY, D. W., NORTHFIELD, T. C., KIRKHAM, J. S. AND SALMON, P. R. (1981) Controlled trial of argon laser photocoagulation in bleeding peptic ulcers. *Lancet*, **2**, 1313.

4

Static electricity

From the previous chapter the reader will realise the importance of using spark-free electrical apparatus in the immediate vicinity of anaesthesia apparatus. Even if a great deal of attention is paid to the safety of electrical apparatus and the elimination of naked flames from the operating suite, explosion risks are not entirely obviated, for there remains the danger of a spark caused by static electricity (Vickers, 1970, 1978).

The extent of the risk of electrostatic sparks causing anaesthetic explosions was set out in a report from the Department of Health (1956). The report described an investigation of 36 anaesthetic explosions occurring during a seven year period, 1947 to 1954. Of these 36 accidents, 22 were almost certainly due to an electrostatic spark. The report recommended that antistatic precautions should be taken in all areas where anaesthesia apparatus employing a closed or partially closed breathing circuit is used with flammable anaesthetics. In the light of further experimental evidence, these recommendations were updated (Department of Health, 1977a,b).

What is static electricity, how does it occur and why should it be of so much concern when anaesthetic explosions are relatively infrequent? (Several million anaesthetics are administered each year without an explosion mishap.) The majority of operating department staff complete their careers without being witness to a single anaesthetic explosion. However, this is no excuse for overlooking simple precautions which will result in these small risks in the presence of flammable gases being almost entirely eliminated.

The generation of static electricity

The formation of this condition is a very simple matter and occurs whenever two dissimilar materials are separated. It is not necessary to cause friction, although this will increase the amount of static electricity produced. The surface of one material or object becomes positively charged and the other negatively charged, but to what degree depends not only on the briskness of separation of the surfaces (friction) but also on the ability of the material to absorb moisture readily from the atmosphere and in this way become antistatic for all practical purposes.

These charges of electricity can continue to build up an electric potential or pressure on the surface of the object until earthed or the object comes into contact with another object of a different potential. When this occurs the discharge of static between the two can cause a spark. It is as if the object stores up the static charge like a condenser and when earthed discharges the static as a spark which may be capable of igniting a flammable anaesthetic mixture.

Very high voltages can be created under favourable conditions, especially in a dry atmosphere, e.g., a person walking on a dry floor wearing ordinary rubber-soled shoes is capable

of acquiring or being charged with a potential of 30,000 volts; the act of 'whipping off' a blanket lying on a rubber sorbo pad covering a trolley can produce a similar charge.

These dangers may be very real and steps which should be taken to minimise the formation of dangerous charges of static electricity are:

1. The elimination of materials which predispose towards the formation of static.

2. Allowing the charges to leak away as they are generated and before high potentials are built up.

1. Static forming materials

Some materials are more inclined to form static electricity than others. High on this list are most plastics and some man-made fibres which do not readily absorb moisture, and woollen blankets, which are a grave potential source of sparks.

The following list indicates the materials which may be found in the vicinity of an operating theatre. The order of the list shows that each becomes positively electrified when rubbed with any of the materials following, but negatively when rubbed with any of the materials preceding. The list also indicates that the further apart the materials are on the list the greater the charge produced upon rubbing together.

(a) Nylon
(b) Flannel and wool
(c) Viscose rayon
(d) Glass
(e) Cotton and linen
(f) Dry skin
(g) Wood
(h) Rubber
(i) Various plastics.

Of the materials listed, cotton, linen and viscose rayon are certainly ideal for theatre clothing and towels, blanket covers, etc., unless they have been specially treated to render them water repellent. They have to be quite dry to generate a charge under normal atmospheric conditions, as they readily absorb moisture. It is this property which makes them excellent for theatre use. The only blankets which should be brought into the operating theatre are those of the cotton cellular type, which do not predispose towards the formation of static electricity and are easily sterilized.

2. The dissipation of static charges

If all objects were conductive to electricity and all floors conductive, static electricity would be dissipated as rapidly as it formed; unfortunately this is not so.

All ordinary rubber articles are very highly insulating and many items of theatre equipment are made from rubber, including sorbo trolley mattresses and wheels, macintoshes and tubing, etc. The use of ordinary rubber in the manufacture of these articles will prevent the leakage away to earth of any electrostatic charges which may form on the object. These charges will build up potential and leak away slowly unless they are earthed suddenly and dissipated as a spark.

The answer to this problem has been the discovery that, if during the manufacture of rubber, carbon black is finely dispersed through it, the resultant rubber is electrically conductive to a degree dependent on the quantities of carbon present.

This antistatic rubber has sufficient insulation to ordinary mains electricity, but does allow electrostatic charges to dissipate rapidly as they are formed. Unfortunately antistatic rubber is necessarily black, and in order to distinguish this rubber from other types all antistatic rubber components have a distinctive yellow mark.

The risk of an electrostatic ignition is now considered to be confined to an area extending for 25 cm around the anaesthesia gas circuit or gas paths. Flammable gas mixtures escaping from anaesthesia breathing circuits rapidly dilute to a non-flammable level within a few centimetres of the point of escape. All equipment used in this danger zone must be antistatic and all metal parts must be electrically continuous with the floor, e.g. by fitting antistatic castors or feet. All rubber must be antistatic and have effective contact with metal connections used in the breathing circuit of the patient.

Although plastics are regarded as highly electrostatic, it is not practicable to eliminate them entirely from anaesthesia apparatus. The degree of electrostatic risk depends upon the size of the component and whether, due to its position, an electrostatic charge may be formed by the component being rubbed or brushed against. Rotameters, for example, although consisting of some clear plastic parts, do not constitute a great risk due to their location (DHSS, 1977a). Plastic soda lime canisters, on the other hand, may be located where they can be brushed against with clothing very easily. In order to minimise a charge building-up on the surface of the canister it is prudent to incorporate an electrically conductive mesh, either buried in the plastic or in contact with the inner or outer surface. This mesh must be made electrically continuous with other antistatic components which are in discharge contact with the floor.

Antistatic polish applied to plastic has a limited effect. The polish is liable to get rubbed off and requires reapplication following cleaning or sterilisation.

As endotracheal tubes are moist in use they need not be made from an antistatic material. There is very little electrostatic risk associated with plastic transfusion tubing although the metal supports associated should have a satisfactory antistatic contact with the floor.

Diathermy quivers are intended to insulate a live electrode from possible shorting through towels or with metal/antistatic equipment. They should be made from either ordinary rubber or plastic; the electrostatic risk with these items is negligible.

The efficiency of antistatic rubber is calculated by measuring the electrical resistance in ohms. This ohmic resistance is in effect the degree of insulation to electricity: the higher the ohms figure, the more insulating is the rubber.

A normal high insulation rubber will have a high electrical resistance in excess of 1,000 million ohms (1,000 $M\Omega$), whereas antistatic rubber in service should have a resistance not exceeding 100 $M\Omega$. This ohmic resistance is determined by measuring the amount of electricity which the rubber will pass under test.

Two insulated wire conductors, connected to a 500 V d.c. tester generator (Megger) are placed separately on two moistened areas of approximately 6.25 cm^2 (1 in^2), but 5 cm (2 in) apart, on the surfaces of the rubber being tested. By turning the handle on the tester a voltage of 500 V is generated and the amount of electricity passing between these conductors through the rubber will move a pointer on the tester scale, indicating the resistance in ohms.

There are many ways of testing various rubber objects; the more common tests include the following:

(*a*) Rubber boots and shoes; the resistance is measured between the inside of the sole or heel and the under sole.

(*b*) Rubber tubing, etc.; the resistance is measured between spacings of every 1.5 m (5 ft) if the tubing exceeds this length.

(*c*) Furniture feet; the resistance is measured between the surface at the bottom of the cavity, and that normally in contact with the floor.

(*d*) Castors are tested by placing on a wet metal plate, and measuring the resistance between the plate and the metal framework of the trolley or hub of the wheel. When testing

a castor fitted to a trolley, etc., the other castors should be insulated from the floor during the test.

(*e*) Sorbo pads or mattresses are tested by measuring the resistance between the top and underside, the electrodes being opposite.

(*f*) On thin sheeting the test areas should be on the same surface with approximately 50 mm (2 in) dry spacing between. (Measurements made through the thickness of thin sheeting are unreliable as they may be affected by small areas of conductivity.)

The recommended resistance limits for new equipment are as follows:

Anaesthesia tubing connecting machine to patient, per 1.5 m (5 ft) length: 25,000 Ω minimum, 1 MΩ maximum.

Mattresses or pads: 5,000 Ω minimum, 1 MΩ maximum.

Rubber boots and shoes: 75,000 Ω minimum, 10 MΩ maximum.

Castor tyres and other antistatic items: no lower limit but 10,000 Ω maximum.

The electrical resistance of some antistatic rubber items may increase with use. The maximum permitted electrical resistance of equipment in service is 100 MΩ and equipment exceeding this level should be replaced as having lost its antistatic properties.

All rubber operating theatre equipment, including tubing, sheeting, anaesthesia accessories, operation table mattresses, etc., should be made from an antistatic material and it is important to note that if the surfaces of these are damped, the electrical conductivity will be greater.

Antistatic Floors. If the surface of antistatic rubber is kept clean, the static charges will leak away to earth as they are formed, but the floor must also be antistatic. The efficient dissipation of static does depend a great deal on the provision of a suitable antistatic floor which has a resistance of not more than 2 MΩ new or less than 50,000 Ω in service measured between two separate electrodes placed 60 cm (2 ft) apart, but see also page 20.

One of the most satisfactory materials for theatre floors from the antistatic aspect are *in situ* terrazzo or terrazzo tiles (DHSS, 1977b) laid upon a metal mesh. A direct-to-earth connection for antistatic floors has been found unnecessary. If the floor is laid correctly and has satisfactory antistatic properties, it is capable of equalising any electrostatic charges which are likely to develop on persons or objects which are in electrical contact with the floor.

Wood, linoleum or composition floors are not satisfactory in the theatre suite but antistatic PVC containing granules of carbon may be used. Damp mopping of the floor regularly during an operation list will increase the electrical conductivity considerably. Even if the surface dries rapidly, some moisture will be retained by the floor to a degree dependent on its composition, e.g. a tiled floor will be more absorbent than a PVC one.

3. Humidity

A highly humid atmosphere is a deterrent to the formation of static electricity, but should not be regarded as a guarantee against it. Humidity is much less effective as an antistatic measure with plastics or synthetic fibres which have an inherent tendency to be moisture repellent.

The relative humidity in an operating theatre should be between 50 and 55 per cent, or compatible with comfort.

The humidity should be maintained at a satisfactory level by the ventilation system (Chapter 1, page 31). This can be automatic, being coupled directly to a hygrometer or may be controlled manually in conjunction with direct reading 'gold beater' hygrometers situated in the theatre and anaesthesia room. These hygrometers which indicate the relative

humidity as a direct reading on a scale should be checked periodically against a wet/dry bulb thermometer.

Conclusion

The simple precautions necessary to minimise the possibility of an anaesthetic explosion being initiated by a spark of static electricity do not inconvenience the work of an operating suite.

All rubber components should be of antistatic rubber, tested regularly and renewed when the electrical resistance exceeds 100 MΩ.

Non-antistatic rubber or plastic components such as tubes, airways, etc., should be moistened inside and out before use.

No one should enter the theatre unless wearing antistatic shoes or boots and their clothes covered with a cotton or linen gown. This will reduce the amount of personal static electricity produced by walking.

All theatre outer clothing, etc., should be made of a relatively antistatic material, such as cotton or linen.

Woollen blankets must never be used. Cotton cellular blankets are very suitable from an antistatic as well as a bacteriological aspect. Hot blankets are more likely to generate a static charge than cold or warm ones; in no case must a blanket be 'whipped off' a trolley.

REFERENCES

DEPARTMENT OF HEALTH (1956) *Report of a Working Party on Anaesthetic Explosions.* London: HMSO.
DEPARTMENT OF HEALTH (1977a) *Hospital Technical Memorandum* No. 1. *Antistatic Precautions: Rubber, Plastics and Fabric.* London: HMSO.
DEPARTMENT OF HEALTH (1977b) *Hospital Technical Memorandum* No. 2. *Flooring in Anaesthetic Areas.* London: HMSO.
VICKERS, M. D. (1970) *British Journal of Anaesthesia*, 25, 482.
VICKERS, M. D. (1978) *British Journal of Anaesthesia*, 50, 659.

5

The operation table and positions used for surgery

The modern operation table is a sophisticated piece of apparatus capable of adjustment to give a variety of safe positions for a patient undergoing surgery. Most tables are designed as an all-purpose apparatus suitable for a wide range of general operations, but can be adapted for specialised procedures by the addition of suitable accessories. The operation tables illustrated in this chapter provide raising, lowering, Trendelenberg and lateral tilting mechanisms for the table top; adjustable head and foot ends and a full range of accessories. Each table top is covered with a sectional antistatic sponge rubber mattress which is removable for cleaning.

Figure 5.1 illustrates a versatile four-section general purpose operating table with the Trendelenburg tilt, lateral tilt, 'break back' and chair mechanisms operated by a gear box and control handle at the head of the table. The head and foot table top sections can be interchanged to allow foot end control to be chosen when required. This type of operating table was first introduced in 1955 and is still widely used in operating departments. A similar

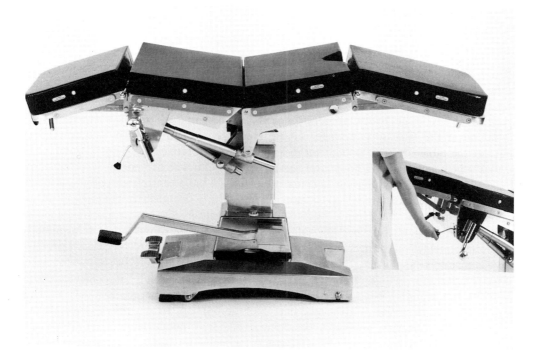

Fig. 5.1   General purpose 4-sections operation table. (Model M, Eschmann.)

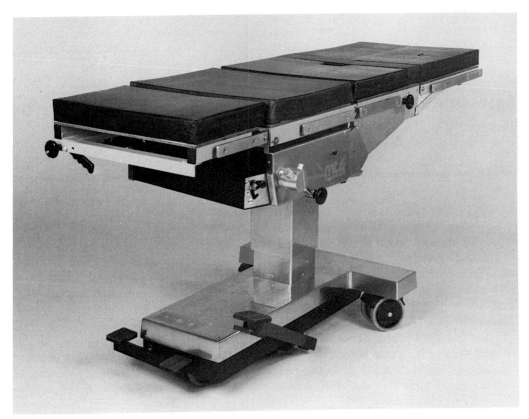

Fig. 5.2   General purpose 4-sections operation table. (Mt4, Thackray.)

manually-operated table with the combined gear box/handle fitted to one side of the table top is illustrated in Figure 5.2.

The introduction of complex operative procedures has been accompanied by the manufacture of more sophisticated operation tables. Early developments in this field included a fixed operation table base in the centre of the theatre on to which was fitted a removable top. The electrical or hydraulic services installed in the base enabled power-operated positioning of the table top. Transfer to and from the operating theatre was achieved by removing the table top with patient on to a mobile trolley frame.

Other schemes provided a floor level services plinth into which a power-operated mobile table could be slotted. In addition to connections for the table controls and electrical outlets this plinth also included medical vacuum outlets which channelled suctioned fluids via tubing embedded in the floor to suction collection bottles sited in a glass-fronted wall cupboard. Although these types are still in use, generally the provision of floor-mounted services and integration of the suction facility in the plinth is considered to present problems of hygiene and maintenance.

An operation table which offers the advantages of power operation, interchangeability of table tops and mobility is illustrated in Figure 5.3. The power source is a self-contained rechargeable battery giving up to several days operation. There are five interchangeable table tops (Fig. 5.4), providing a versatile basic power-operated mobile table. This table can be used in conjunction with a theatre transfer system, whereby a patient is first transferred from his bed to a table top mounted on a transporter (Fig. 5.6). This transporter permits Tren-

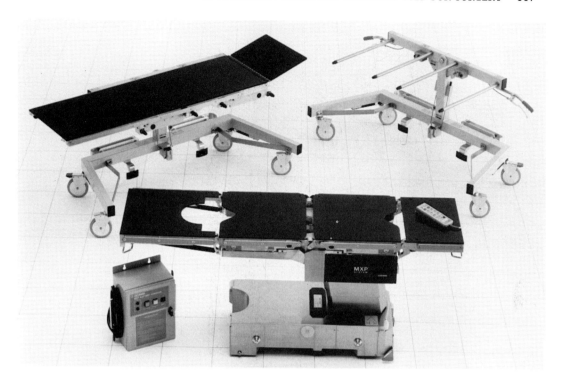

Fig. 5.3   General purpose 2 to 5 sections power-controlled operation table. (MXP System, Eschmann.)

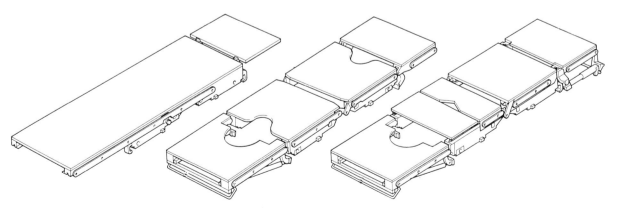

Fig. 5.4   Type of removable tops available for power-controlled operation table. (MXP System, Eschmann.)

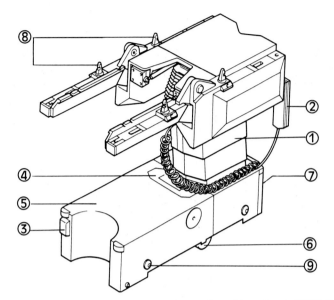

1. Battery-powered pedestal.
2. Handset for remote-control table top positioning.
3. Foot controller socket.
4. Manual override panel.
5. Stainless steel base.
6. Large wheels for easy mobility.
7. Hydraulic brake lever.
8. Table top location latches.
9. Orthotec attachment studs.

Fig. 5.5   Details of power-controlled operation table pedestal. (MXP System, Eschmann.)

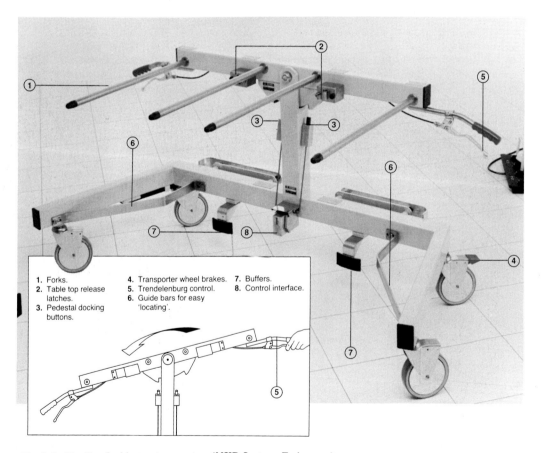

1. Forks.
2. Table top release latches.
3. Pedestal docking buttons.
4. Transporter wheel brakes.
5. Trendelenburg control.
6. Guide bars for easy 'locating'.
7. Buffers.
8. Control interface.

Fig. 5.6   Details of table top transporter. (MXP System, Eschmann.)

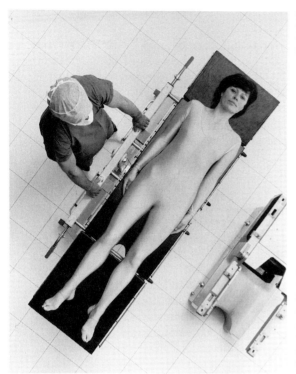

Fig. 5.7 Patient and table top transporter wheeled sideways towards pedestal. (MXP System, Eschmann.)

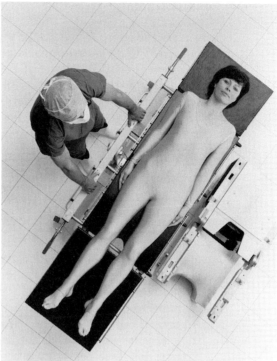

Fig. 5.8 Transporter forks are aligned with location slots on pedestal. (MPX System Eschmann.)

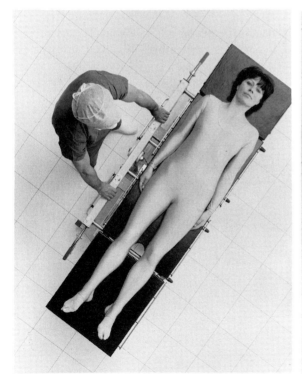

Fig. 5.9 Transporter forks are pushed into location slots on pedestal. (MXP System, Eschmann.)

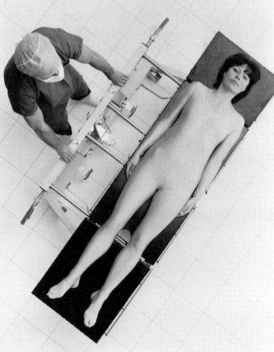

Fig. 5.10 Table top locked on to pedestal, transporter is withdrawn. (MXP System, Eschmann.)

delenburg tilt of the table top and can be used during induction of anaesthesia. The patient is then transferred to the operation table pedestal by docking the forks of the transporter into location slots (Figs. 5.7–5.10). Self-levelling controls position the height of the table top correctly for removal and attachment of the table top to the pedestal.

It is essential that all members of the theatre staff familiarise themselves with the operation table and its accessories which must be easily available and ready for immediate use. The whole apparatus must be maintained in good working order and checked before each operation list.

POSITIONS USED FOR SURGERY

Careful and correct positioning of the patient is very important. It is essential to provide good access for surgery and also to take into account patient safety, anaesthesia technique, monitoring and position of i.v. lines etc. (Smith and Aitken head, 1985) to prevent harm to the patient due to pressure, especially on nerves and bony prominences. These positions which are described can only be learned by repeated practical demonstrations, but the illustrations show essential points to be noted for various operations. The drapes have been omitted in order that these points are easily discernible (Jolly, 1950; Houghton and Hudd, 1967; Pearce, 1967; Ballinger et al., 1972).

Supine or dorsal recumbent position

This and most of the following positions are demonstrated on an Eshmann M general purpose operation table which incorporates the majority of the features described already, plus accessories for orthopaedic procedures.

The position is used for many operations, including those on the eye, ear, face, chest,

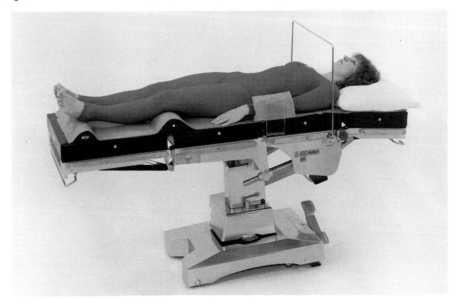

Fig. 5.11 Supine or dorsal recumbent position.

abdomen, legs or feet, and with modifications is suitable for operations on the breast and arms or hands, which may be placed across the chest or extended on an arm table.

Operations on the flexed knee are performed by lowering the foot end of the table with the division between the centre and foot sections situated at the point of knee flexion. Alternatively the foot end of the table can be removed completely.

An anaesthesia screen can be used for this and other positions when it is desirable, for local anaesthesia, or to isolate the anaesthetist from the operative field (Chapter 10, Fig. 10.5).

Important points

1. The arms should be at the sides and secured by L-shaped arm retainers which are slipped under the mattress. This applies unless of course otherwise indicated by surgery or for transfusion. Alternatively the arms may be secured across the chest by pinning the operation gown around them.

2. Pressure points to watch and protect with folded towels or soft pillows are: the heels and the forearms where the arm retainer is in contact with the skin. A soft pillow behind the knees (which should be slightly flexed) will prevent hyperextension of the knee joints which may have painful consequences postoperatively.

Trendelenburg position

This position, a modification of supine, is used for intrapelvic operations, the object being to allow the intestines to displace away from the pelvic cavity by gravity towards the upper abdomen. They may then be packed off readily to leave easier access to the pelvic organs.

Important points

1. The arms are at the sides and secured in the usual manner.
2. The flexion of the knees must be directly over the junction of the foot and central sections of the table.

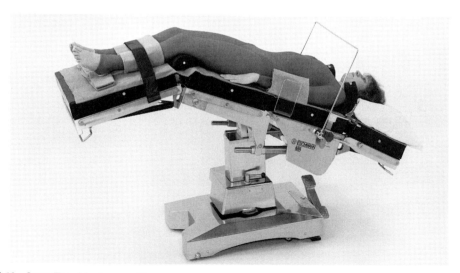

Fig. 5.12   Steep Trendelenburg position.

3. Pressure points to watch and protect are: the heels, leg strap (folded towel between the strap and legs has been omitted from the illustration in order to show the heel pad), behind the knees and the shoulders.

The well-padded shoulder rests must be positioned to the point of the shoulders. On no account must they be placed at the root of the neck, because this would cause pressure upon the brachial plexus and result in paralysis. These rests must prevent the patient from slipping and becoming suspended by flexed knees, which would cause pressure on the lateral popliteal nerve.

Alternatively, well-padded pelvic supports or a Langton Hewer corrugated ribbed mattress (in direct contact with the patient's exposed skin) may be used to retain the patient in position. These avoid the danger of pressure on the brachial plexus.

Gall-bladder and liver position

This is another modified supine position which is used for operations on the gall-bladder or liver. The patient is positioned over the back elevator which is raised to produce extension, and thereby push the gall-bladder towards the anterior abdominal wall. One arm is shown extended on an arm table for transfusion. Alternatively the patient can be positioned over the hinged section of a 'break back' table which when flexed produces a similar effect.

Important points

1. Both arms may be secured in the usual manner, or one extended on an arm table as illustrated, but the abduction must not exceed 90 degrees to the body otherwise the brachial plexus may be stretched.

2. Pressure points to watch and protect are: the heels, behind the knees and at the point where the arm is extended from the table.

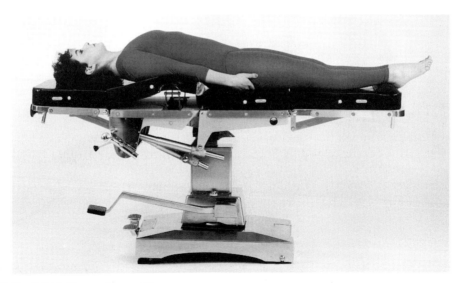

Fig. 5.13 Gall bladder, or liver position.

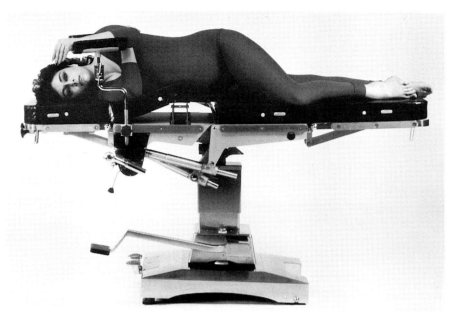

Fig. 5.14   Lateral position of extension for kidney and chest surgery.

Lateral position of extension

This is used for operations on the kidney and chest, but may be modified slightly for operations on the hip. For the former operations the patient is positioned over the kidney elevator which is raised to extend this region. Alternatively if an operation which incorporates a 'break back' is used, extension is achieved by positioning the patient over the division in the centre section before adjusting the angle of the table top.

For hip operations in the lateral position the patient lies on his side in a similar manner to that illustrated, but with no extension.

Important points

1. The upper arm is supported by a Carter Braine's arm support. The lower hand is placed at the side of the face and secured if necessary in the usual manner.
2. The underneath leg is flexed under the upper which is kept straight and secured to the table top with a padded bandage.
3. The patient is supported by pelvic and chest supports, which are well padded, and for additional security a bandage (padded strap or adhesive strapping) may be placed round the thighs and table top.
4. Pressure points to watch and protect are: the heels, between the legs, under the thigh retainer, upper and lower arms.

Lithotomy position

This is used for operations on the external genital organs, perineum and anal region. The buttocks project well over the edge of the table at the junction of the centre and foot section

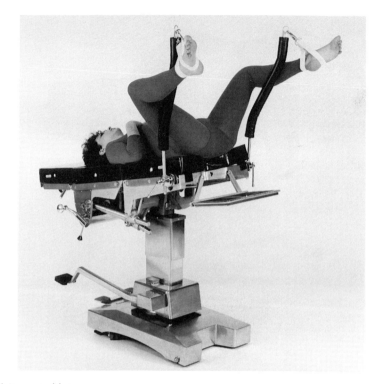

Fig. 5.15   Lithotomy position.

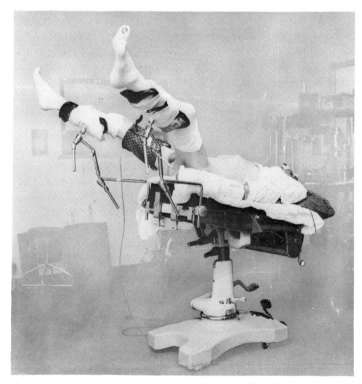

Fig. 5.16   Position for synchronous combined abdomino-perineal excision of the rectum. (Rintoul.)

which is lowered or removed. The legs are flexed at the hips and knees, and raised with the feet supported in webbing slings suspended from the lithotomy poles. A douching funnel may be fitted below the perineal area.

Important points

1. The arms are secured in the usual manner.
2. The patient is first placed supine on the table and is then lifted down until his buttocks are at the edge of the centre section (foot section lowered or removed). *Both* legs are then flexed at the same time, abducted and secured by the webbing slings outside the poles.
3. Pressure points to watch and protect are: the forearms, buttocks and inner aspects of the thighs, which must be protected from pressure by the poles with pads of gamgee or sponge rubber. Note that the lithotomy poles are padded with sponge rubber to minimise still further any pressure on the patient's legs.

Breast and axilla position

This is the position for operations on the breast and axilla. It is a modified supine position, either with both arms extended and secured on arm tables, or one arm secured and the other on the affected side supported by a nurse.

Important points

1. The extended arms must not be abducted more than 90 degrees to the body.
2. Pressure points to watch and protect are: the heels, behind the knees and at the point where the arms are extended from the table.

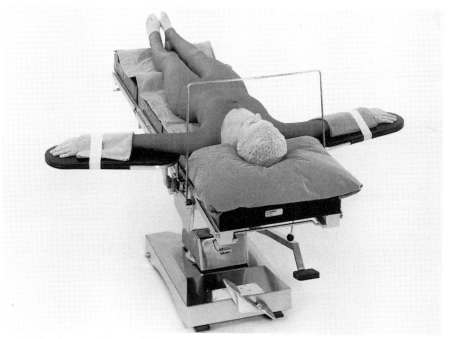

Fig. 5.17   Position for operations on the breast and axilla.

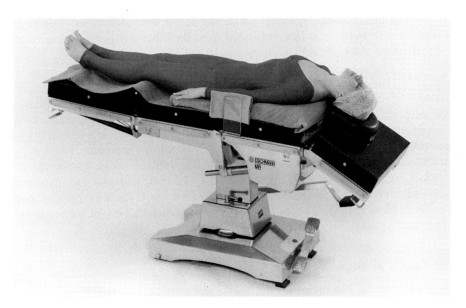

Fig. 5.18   Position for operations on the neck.

Neck position

This position is used for operations on the neck, especially thyroidectomy and tracheostomy. The patient is placed in the supine position with a pillow or sandbag under the shoulder blades, and the head is held by a nurse or assistant with the neck well extended. Alternatively, a padded horse-shoe provides a good support for the head in such operations. If local anaesthesia is being used, e.g., for tracheostomy, further restraint may be required and the patient is held by another assistant who immobilises him by the arms and thighs.

Important points

1. The head must be held exactly in the mid-line with the chin upwards and the neck extended.
2. The arms are secured in the usual manner unless being restrained by an assistant.
3. Pressure points to watch and protect are: the heels, behind the knees, the arms where they are secured, between the shoulder blades, and the occiput if the operating time is lengthy.

Prone cranial position

This position is used for cerebellar operations and high cervical laminectomy. Some reverse Trendelenburg tilt is used and a padded strap placed round the thighs and the table top for additional security. The shoulders and thorax are supported by shoulder supports in conjunction with small pillows.

Important points

1. The degree of flexion or extension of the neck depends upon the surgeon's wishes and the most suitable position for maintenance of a clear airway.

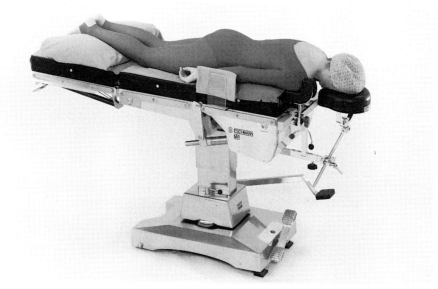

Fig. 5.19 Prone position for cerebellar and high cervical operations.

2. The arms are secured in the usual manner.

3. Pressure points to watch and protect are: the feet (the toes must project either over the foot end of the table or a soft pillow sufficiently large to prevent them being compressed against the table top), under the strap, the arms where they are secured, and the shoulder supports which must be positioned to the points of the shoulders and not pressing on the root of the neck.

Sitting cranial position

This is a position for cerebellar cranial operations and high cervical laminectomy and is an alternative to that described in Figure 5.19. The patient is sitting and stabilised by the cranial support. The hands are placed in the lap and the body immobilised by securing the arms with body supports which are attached to the operation table at each side. These have been omitted in the illustration in order to show the position of the arms.

Important points

1. The weight of the patient must not be entirely supported by the cranial support. Body supports must be used to retain the patient in what would be a fairly comfortable position if he were conscious.

2. The degree of flexion of the neck depends upon the surgeon's wishes and the most suitable position for maintenance of a clear airway.

3. Pressure points to watch and protect are: the heels, behind the knees, the buttocks and the arms (which are protected by small pillows or folded towels).

Supine hip position

This is used mainly for nailing a femoral neck fracture, but is suitable for osteotomy, slipped

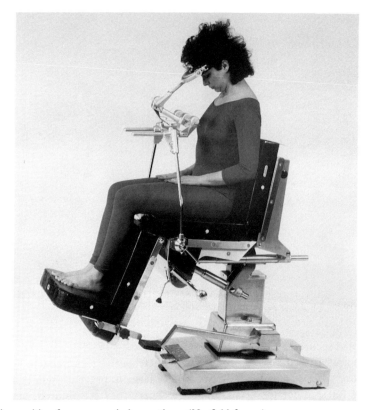

Fig. 5.20   Sitting position for neurosurgical operations. (Mayfield frame.)

femoral epiphysis, etc. The patient is in a supine position, with his pelvis supported by a supplementary table top which is translucent to X-rays and incorporates a slot for introducing anterior position film cassettes under the pelvis. The lower section of the table is removed, the feet are secured to foot pieces and traction applied to both legs. Counter traction is obtained against a perineal post fitted at the pubis. Body supports are needed only when lateral tilting of the table top is necessary in order to obtain greater exposure of the hip being operated on (Fig. 5.22).

Two X-ray machines or an image intensifier is positioned to obtain anterior and lateral position X-rays. The lateral film cassette is fitted into a holder at the side of the patient, corresponding to the hip being operated on. Any lateral tilting would be away from this side.

Important points

1. Both arms are placed across the chest or one is extended on an arm table for transfusion purposes.

2. The degree of abduction of the legs depends on the surgeon's wishes but must be adequate to allow positioning of the lateral X-ray machine. In the case of femoral neck fractures the foot on the affected side is usually internally rotated.

3. Pressure points to watch and protect are: where the feet are secured in the leather boot attachments, the buttocks (supported by a sponge rubber pad), the perineum, the arms and, if lateral tilting is used, at each body support.

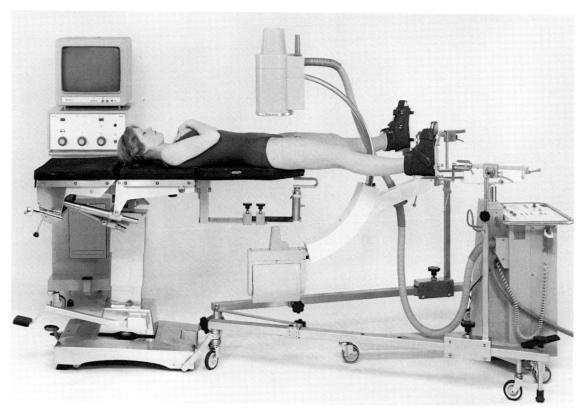

Fig. 5.21 Supine position for femoral intramedullary nailing.

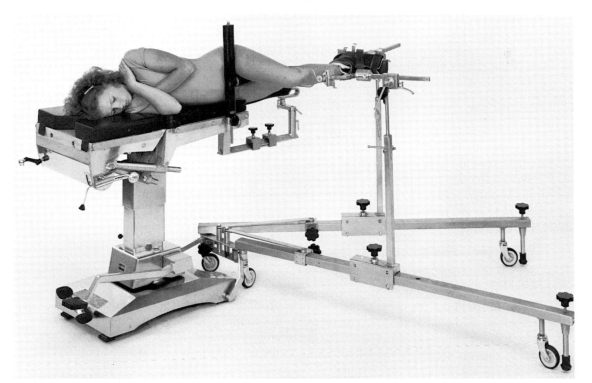

Fig. 5.22 Lateral position for femoral intramedullary nailing.

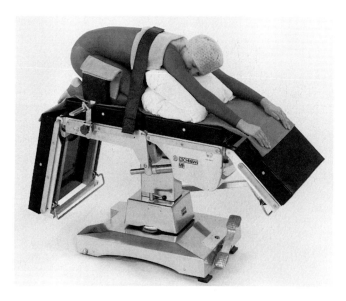

Fig. 5.23   Knee/elbow (rabbit) position for laminectomy.

Knee/elbow (rabbit) position

This is an alternative to lateral position (described under spinal puncture, Chapter 10) for lumbar laminectomy and removal of prolapsed intervertebral disc. The patient kneels with his head and arms supported on a pillow, and his body stabilised with body supports at each side of the table. For additional security a bandage or adhesive strapping may be placed round the thorax and table top.

Important points

1. The pillow under the thorax and the retaining bandage may require adjustment in order that the patient's respiratory excursions are not impeded in any way. It may be necessary to use a pillow under the upper part of the chest and head only, to leave the abdomen free for excursion.

2. The foot section of the table is lowered or removed, and the feet must project slightly beyond to avoid pressure on the toes.

3. Pressure points to watch and protect are: the insteps, between the thighs and the lower legs.

Jack knife position

One of the positions for rectal surgery or occasionally for lumbar laminectomy.

The patient should be placed in prone position with hips directly over the break in the foot section of the table. The arms should be flexed around the head of the patient and the lower part of the legs supported by a foot extension piece. The whole table is tilted into reverse Trendelenburg to the desired position.

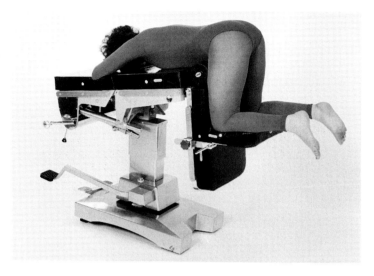

Fig. 5.24 Jack knife position for rectal surgery.

Important points

1. A small pillow should be placed under the symphysis to avoid undue pressure and,
2. The patient's weight should be so balanced as to avoid pressure on the knees.

Endoscopy position

This is a modification of supine position. The head is raised slightly and the endoscope introduced into the pharynx. The head is supported by an assistant and the upper part of the table lowered. The endoscope is introduced with the head held in the degree of flexion or extension required by the surgeon. In the case of an oesophagoscope the head is lowered so that the oesophagus, pharynx and mouth are in a straight line. In the case of a broncho-scope the head is turned to the side opposite to that of the bronchus being examined.

REFERENCES

BALLINGER, W. F., TREYBAL, J. C. AND VOSE, A. B. (1972) *Alexander's Care of the Patient in Surgery.* St Louis: Mosby.
HOUGHTON, M. AND HUDD, J. (1967) *Aids to Theatre Technique*, 4th edn, chap. 4. London: Baillière, Tindall and Cassell.
JOLLY, J. D. (1950) *Operating Room Procedures for Nurses*, 3rd edn, London: Faber.
PEARCE, E. (1967) *Instruments, Appliances and Theatre Technique*, 5th edn. London: Faber.
SMITH, G. AND AITKENHEAD, A. R. (1985) *Textbook of Anaesthesia*, chap. 17, p. 247. Edinburgh Churchill Livingstone.
YEAGER, M. E. (1966) *Operating Room Manual*, 2nd edn, chap. 3. New York: Putnam.

6

Preparation of the operating theatre and sterile supplies

Preparation of personnel

No one should enter the operating suite without first washing his hands and changing into clean protective clothing and footwear such as theatre rubber boots, sandals or clogs. The main purpose for this is to prevent the transfer of pathogenic organisms into the operating department. This rule must apply equally when there are no operations in progress (Medical Research Council, 1968; Ballenger et al., 1972; Lidwell, 1984).

Personnel preparing for operations cover their hair and generally wear masks in addition to wearing suitable clothing and footwear. Visitors and other staff are similarly attired.

Research has demonstrated that personnel should *not* take pre-operative showers. This apparently causes shedding of minute skin particles for several hours afterwards, thereby increasing the risk of dispersion of micro-organisms, particularly staphylococcus (Bethune et al., 1965; Medical Research Council, 1968; Lidwell, 1984). At time of writing, studies are being undertaken into the use of a bland cream for total body application, which inhibits the shedding of skin particles and micro-organisms from theatre personnel.

Surgeons, anaesthetists, other personnel and visitors should wear a scrub suit which obviates the need for an additional gown when not assisting at operation. This applies equally to female staff, for it has been demonstrated that suits minimise the dispersion of micro-organisms compared with the standard dress (Hill et al., 1974; Mitchell and Gamble, 1974; Dankart et al., 1979). Ideally the trousers and sleeves of tops should have stockinette-type cuffs to retain the skin particles shed from the axillae and perineum.

Cotton poplin or polyester cotton (Dankart et al., 1979) are the most commonly used materials for theatre clothing: blue or grey colour for scrub suits, and green colour for operating gowns. But special fabrics such as Ventile and Scotchguard, and non-woven fabrics including Tyvek, Azo44[TM] and Fabric 450[TM], have been found to possess a superior resistance to bacterial permeation (Speers et al., 1965; Blowers and McClusky, 1966; Le Bourdais, 1975; Mitchell et al., 1978; Whyte et al., 1978; Lidwell et al., 1978; Nagai et al., 1986). One of these, Fabric 450[TM], a spun laced fabric, when tested was found to contribute to a reduction in post-operative infection (Molan, 1986), and gave a similar if not equal performance to that of total body exhaust gowns (Whyte et al., 1983). Whyte and Bailey (1984) considered that 'it was better to prevent the dispersion of bacteria from people in theatre rather than allow the bacteria to be dispersed, and then removed by air ventilation. Low airborne dispersion of bacteria from people can be achieved by well designed clothing using fabrics effective in preventing bacterial dispersion.'

The hair should be completely covered with a closely fitting cap manufactured from a non-woven fabric. For the surgical team the most efficient means of controlling bacterial shedding from the head and neck is a hooded helmet exhaust system (page 39). One piece of

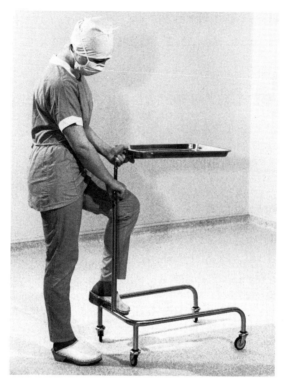

Fig. 6.1 Poplin suit for theatre nurses.

research suggests there is little statistical difference between environment counts when other head coverings are used, e.g. caps or non-exhaust hoods (Ritter *et al.*, 1980).

Masks are probably the greatest potential source of infection. The traditional four to six layers of muslin offer little protection as the mask soon becomes saturated with moisture from the wearer's breath.

The most efficient mask is one made from synthetic fibres or fibre glass (Ford *et al.*, 1967; Furunhasi, 1978; Meffin, 1980). These masks, which should be moulded to fit the facial contour snugly when worn, actually filter the respirations rather than deflect as with the original paper or cellophane insert types. It is claimed that such masks achieve a 98 per cent efficient filtration as compared with only 40 per cent with the muslin masks; however, not all filtration masks are equally efficient (Rogers, 1980).

Examples of these types of masks include Bardic (Bard International), Deseret (Becton Dickinson) and Surgine (Johnson and Johnson).

When removing a mask, care should be taken to avoid touching that part which has acted as a filter, for the hands can easily become contaminated with micro-organisms. Masks should be changed at least every operating session and should *never* be worn 'around the neck'. Mask 'wiggling' is also a potential source of infection (Schweizer, 1976).

Although the use of masks during surgery is generally accepted practice, during quiet talking and breathing there is little or no expulsion of bacteria-laden particles (Shooter *et al.*, 1959). Several papers have been written challenging whether masks are necessary at all (Taylor, 1980; Orr Neil, 1981). Another study has shown that for transurethral prostatectomy, the wearing of face masks had no significant effect on post-operative urinary tract infection (Porter, 1984). The evidence at present does not support the total abandonment

of face masks, but does suggest that for some procedures such as endoscopy they are unnecessary.

Preparation of the operating theatre

Before an operating list, equipment is checked by the senior operating theatre nurse or the scrub nurse who also selects sterile packs, or may prepare instruments and special apparatus for sterilization. Special attention is given to the operation table and accessories to ensure that these are correct and in working order. The operating theatre table luminaire and other mobile luminaires are inspected for illumination and focus. All electromedical apparatus such as the diathermy and suction machines or pipeline suction set are switched on and tested as described in the chapter on electro-medical equipment.

Anaesthesia equipment is checked by the anaesthesia nurse or operating department assistant, under the ultimate supervision of the anaesthetist. Vital inspection includes gas cylinders, soda lime canisters, lamps and batteries of laryngoscopes, etc., and the replenishment of drugs required by the anaesthetist.

All equipment, particularly the operating theatre table luminaire and ledges, etc., within the suite, should be damp dusted followed by cleansing of the floor before sterile trolleys are prepared (Minter, 1952). Supplies of sterile nail brushes, scrub solution, gown packs and supplementary items should be replenished. The required number of bottles or flasks of sterile saline or water for hand-lotion bowls are placed in the warming cupboard until the correct temperature has been reached. Replenishment of bandages, strapping, splints and lotions, etc., should be arranged before the operation list commences.

Preparation of instrument trolleys

Instrument trolleys should be prepared *immediately before* an operation. It is a bad practice to prepare all trolleys required for a list in advance, for even if they are covered carefully, it is impossible to guarantee sterility when required later.

All surfaces of trolleys and tables which are to be used for setting out individual sterile instruments and apparatus should first be covered with a sterile impervious material before the application of sterile drapes. This will prevent contamination of apparatus occurring should the sterile drapes become soiled or wet. Suitable materials are disposable water-repellent paper sheets, proofed non-woven fabrics such as Fabric 450 (Barrier) and Azo44 (Azo drape), and proofed fabrics such as Ventile and Scotchguard.

After the instrument trays have been placed on the trolleys aseptically, the instruments are laid out by a nurse wearing sterile gown and gloves. It is a thoroughly bad practice for an 'unscrubbed' person to complete this arrangement using Cheatle transfer forceps, because of the great risk of contamination occurring when ungloved hands are moved to and fro over the sterile trolley. *There is no place in a modern operating suite for use of sterilized forceps stored half submerged in a container of disinfectant.*

Comprehensive sterile packs containing all the necessary equipment, and incorporating trolley drapes which fall into position as the pack is opened, will shorten the time taken for preparation and minimise bacterial contamination before operation (p. 150).

The scrub nurse

The nurse or operating department assistant (ODA) acting as scrub nurse, scrubs up carefully to disinfect the hands, covers her operating theatre clothing with a sterile gown, and

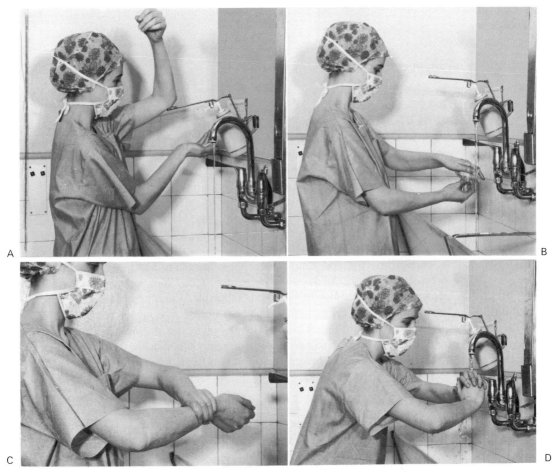

Fig. 6.2 (A) When using ordinary soap the scrub-up or presurgical wash should last five minutes under running water. Less time is required when a detergent solution containing chlorhexidine (Hibitane) or an iodophor (Betadine) is used. With these the forearms and hands are washed for one minute with a small quantity of the solution and then rinsed. (B) Particular attention is then paid to the nails, utilising either a sterilized nail-brush with light friction or orange-stick which is then discarded. (C) The main wash should occupy a further full two minutes and consists of reasonably vigorous massage of the hands and forearms up to elbow level with a mixture of solution and water as shown. Care must be taken to ensure adequate cleansing between the digits and skin folds. (D) Finally the hands and forearms are rinsed thoroughly under running water. The taps are turned off with the elbows and the hands kept in an elevated position to prevent water running down from the elbows. The hands and forearms should then be rinsed or wiped with alcohol (see text, page 140) and dried with a sterile towel before assuming the sterile gown and gloves. (Royal Berkshire Hospital, Reading.)

hands with sterile gloves. When scrubbing up to carry out surgical hand disinfection, care must be taken to ensure that all parts of the hands and forearms are cleansed thoroughly, special attention being given to the nails and between the fingers.

It is important that no person should scrub unless free from upper respiratory infection and skin lesions. Cuts and abrasions or infected pimples can endanger the patient by increasing the possibility of post-operative infection.

Surgical hand disinfection. This is the term used for the pre-operative disinfection of the surgeons, assistants' and scrub nurses' hands. The scrub up procedure should be effective

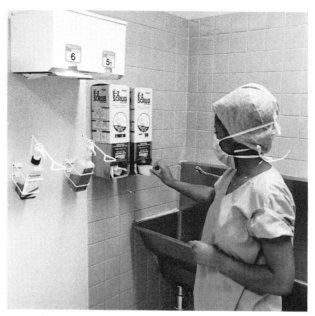

Fig. 6.3   Disposable sponge/nailbrushes Deseret E-2 Scrub (Radcliffe Infirmary Oxford).

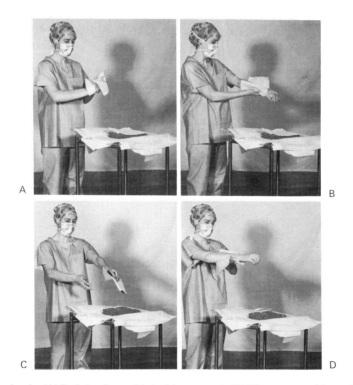

Fig. 6.4   Drying hands. (A) Both hands are dried with one towel. (B) The same towel is used to dry one forearm, taking care to avoid contamination of the hand. (C and D) The second towel is used to dry the other forearm. Nurse is wearing non-woven Fabric 450 disposable suit (Surgikos). (Royal Berkshire Hospital, Reading.)

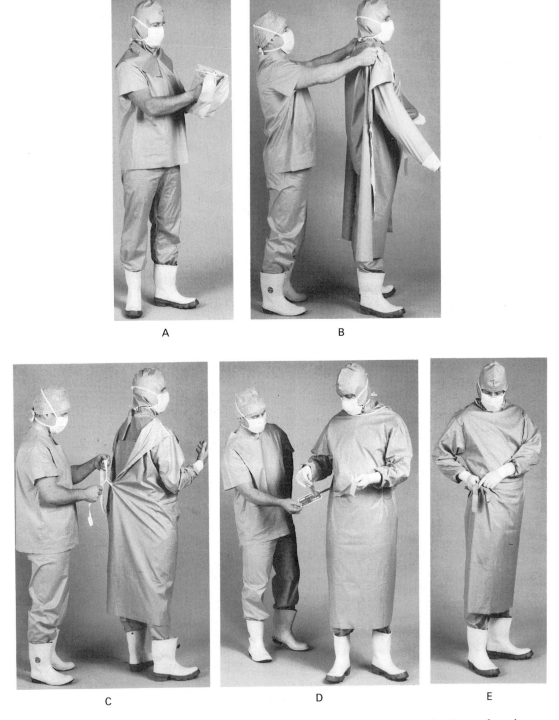

Fig. 6.5 Correct method of putting on a sterile gown. (A and B) The gown is opened well away from the scrub suit. The arms are plunged into the sleeves and the gown is drawn on by an assistant holding only the taped back edges. (C) The tapes of an ordinary gown are secured. (D and E) The back of a wrap-around gown which covers unsterile ties is secured in this fashion. (Surgikos.)

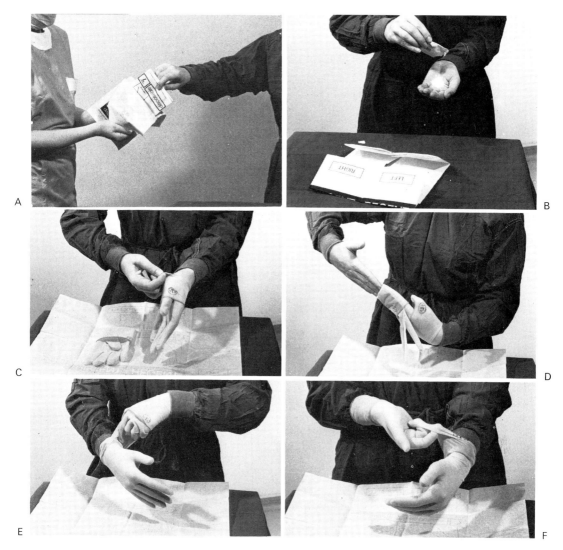

Fig. 6.6 Showing open method of putting on sterile gloves. (A) The pack containing the gloves is first peeled open by the circulating nurse. (B) Powdering the hands — away from the sterile gloves. (C) Inserting first hand, holding by inside of cuff only. (D) Inserting second hand; glove on first hand in contact with *outside* of second glove only. (E) The cuff of the second glove is pulled over the stockinette sleeve. (F) The remaining cuff is pulled over the stockinette sleeve.

against the resident flora as well as transient micro-organisms. Further, it is important that the surgical teams' hands remain as germ free as possible for several hours during the course of lengthy operations. Studies have shown that a large percentage of surgical gloves appear to be perforated at the end of the operation (Devenish and Miles, 1939; Church and Sanderson, 1980). For this reason the method adopted should achieve an immediate antibacterial effect with a sustained activity lasting at least 2–6 hours (Reybrouck, 1986).

Present day opinion generally approves of a surgical scrub or wash which lasts no longer than five minutes. Before the first case of a list, the conventional scrub up technique using a nail brush and a detergent preparation is followed by a rinse containing 1 per cent chlor-

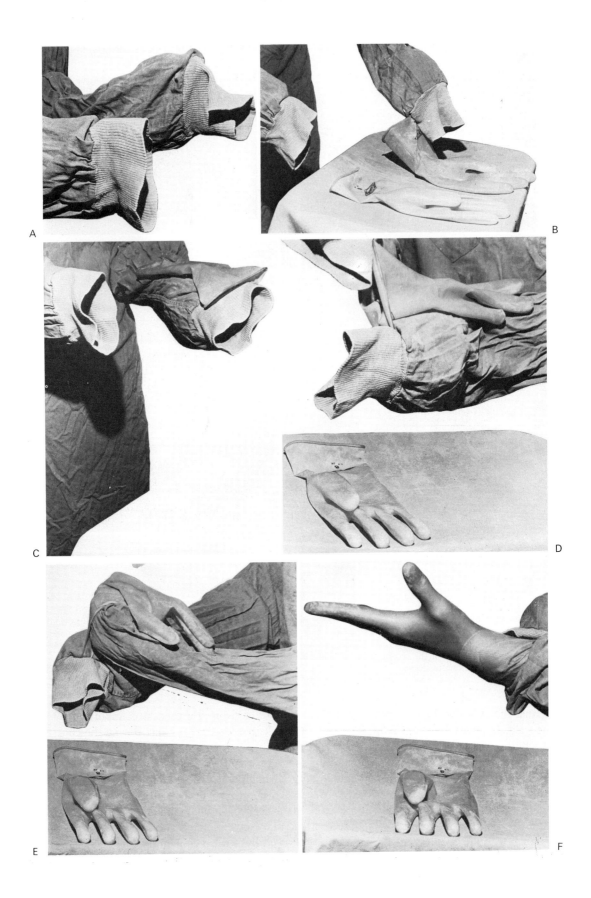

A

B

C

D

E

F

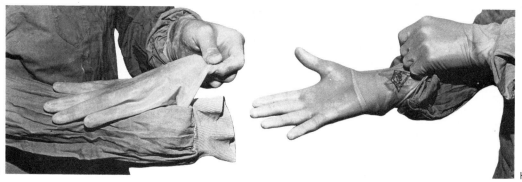

Fig. 6.7 Closed glove technique. (A) The hands are not pushed beyond the stockinette cuffs. (B) The left-hand glove is grasped *through* the left sleeve. (C) The glove is flipped over the wrist and (D) grasped by the second hand (through the gown sleeve). (E) After stretching the cuff the glove is pulled over the sleeve and (F) the hand is forced through the stockinette cuff into the glove. (G) The second glove is put on in a similar manner except that one side of the cuff can be grasped with the already gloved hand and (H) the right hand is forced through the stockinette cuff into the glove. (Figs. 6.7 and 6.8 reproduced by courtesy of the Pioneer Rubber Co. Ltd., U.S.A.)

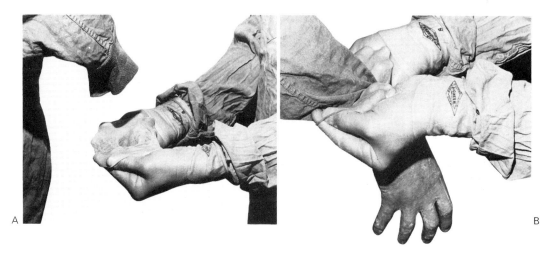

Fig. 6.8 Method of gloving a second person. (A) The cuff is stretched over the fingers of the helper, thumb of glove downwards and (B) the hand is forced through the stockinette cuff and into the glove.

hexidine (Hibitane) in isopropyl alcohol. Prolonged scrubbing can cause excoriations of the skin and predisposes towards post-operative infection. It has been shown that the use of nail brushes can be limited to the nails only, provided an effective detergent preparation containing iodophor (Betadine) or chlorhexidine (Hibscrub) is used as a pre-surgical wash (White and Duncan, 1972; Murie and Macpherson, 1980, Rotter, 1981; Reybrouck, 1986).

If brushes are used for scrubbing up they should be of a good quality soft nylon bristle with grooved plastic backs and of a size which fits the hand easily. These should be terminally sterilized in metal dispensers which fit wall brackets and permit the extraction of single brushes without contaminating the others. Alternatively, a disposable combined sponge/nailbrush is available, impregnated with dehydrated chlorhexidine, iodophor, or wet with alcohol/detergent (Deseret E–Z Scrub) (Fig. 6.3).

Between cases, the hands can be disinfected with a 0.5 per cent solution of chlorhexidine in isopropyl alcohol. This is applied with friction and rubbed to dryness before donning a fresh sterile gown and gloves (Lilley *et al.*, 1979; Reybrouck, 1986).

Gowning and gloving. As it is impossible to render the hands sterile, they must not come into contact with any part of the outside of the gown or gloves. The correct method of putting on gown and gloves in this way is illustrated. Nurses scrubbing up to assist at operations should keep their nails short and endeavour to avoid handling contaminated objects at all times, especially immediately before scrubbing up.

The scrub nurse is responsible for selecting, checking and arranging instruments required on the instrument table. She is responsible also for accounting for all instruments, needles and swabs or sponges at any stage of the operation, especially before any cavity is closed, and must inform the surgeon that these three items are correct, even though he may not ask. It is her duty also to prepare the ligatures and sutures, having them ready immediately when required.

A good scrub nurse will learn to anticipate a surgeon's needs, often having an instrument ready before being asked for it. Sometimes it may be necessary for the instrument nurse to act as surgeon's assistant in the absence of a house surgeon. The most advantageous way of placing the towels in position and assisting the surgeon are dealt with in a later chapter.

The theatre runners or circulating nurses

In addition to the scrub nurse, one or two nurses or ODAs are detailed to act as circulators. One stays in the operating theatre, watching the scrub nurse and ready to bring anything she requires. Dispensing articles from sterile bags or packs, she replenishes sterile gowns and gloves on a sterile trolley or work top reserved for the purpose.

The first circulating nurse also ties up the gowns, being careful to avoid touching any of the gown other than the tapes. She replenishes sterile warm or cold water in the lotion bowls and checks the swabs, displaying them on the counting rack in the required order, or placing them in 5s in a plastic bag before displaying on a count board. (Godfrey, 1983; Shaw, 1984.)

The main duties of the second circulating nurse are to see that the instruments and trolleys are ready for the next case, and she should help in placing the patient on the operation table if a porter or technician is not available. She should also help the scrub nurse if the first circulating nurse has to leave the theatre, for on no account must it be left without one circulator.

It is impossible to define in a textbook the exact duties of circulating nurses. These duties will, of course, depend on the layout and system of particular operating departments.

All notes and X-rays relating to the patient must be available and it is the duty of the operating theatre staff to ensure that these are easily at hand.

The ward staff

Case notes and X-rays should be brought to the operating department by the ward nurse accompanying the patient. She must be able to answer the questions of the theatre nurse or anaesthetist regarding the pre-operative preparation of the patient, especially the premedication, the nature of the drug, the time it was given, whether urine has been passed and the time the patient last ate. After changing into protective clothing, ideally she stays with her patient as the anaesthetic is being administered. This may not always be possible in large operating departments, especially if there is a staff shortage on the ward. In this event, the ward nurse must convey all possible information regarding the patient to a

member of the operating department staff at the point of check and transfer to the limited access zone (MDU *et al.*, 1986).

The patient may be brought to the operating department on a trolley but, where possible, use of the patient's bed throughout is becoming the system of choice. This method provides the minimum number of transfers and reassurance for the patient who, on regaining consciousness, finds himself in his own bed (page 11).

An unconscious patient should remain in the recovery area at least until his reflexes return. If, for some reason, the anaesthetist authorises the return of a patient not fully recovered to the ward, he must be accompanied by a competent nurse. The patient's gown and blankets (preferably cotton) should be ready to cover him when leaving the theatre. Handling the unconscious patient is dealt with in Chapter 11.

Details of the operation, together with any special instructions regarding the patient's post-operative care, are conveyed to the ward sister either by the ward nurse who has stayed in theatre, or by the nurse designated to return with the patient after operation. These instructions should be written down to ensure accuracy.

Swab checking and operation register

It is essential to adopt safeguards against failure to remove swabs etc. from patients (MDU *et al.*; 1986, NATN, 1983). Whatever system of swabs, packs, sponges, needles and instrument checking is in force, it must be the practice to record the check in a register or on a record sheet securely attached to the patient's notes. The system, of course, will vary according to the method of checking, but it is necessary to state the total number of swabs used during an operation and to have the signatures of the scrub nurse and the circulating nurse, one of whom should be a registered nurse. Any mistakes made in this register must be rectified immediately by re-writing the whole entry before recording the next swab check (Fig. 6.9).

All swab checking systems, however efficient, are dependent to a great extent on the human elements, but certain precautions will help to avoid accidental discrepancies in the actual count.

No loose swabs should be allowed in the theatre; those used by the anaesthetist are dyed a distinctive green colour. Those used for application of skin disinfectant should be coloured blue. Swabs needed for dressings must be packed in fixed numbers in a dressings packet and are not introduced into the sterile area until required. Swabs used for operation must be radio-opaque and are made into packets of 5s. These are checked very carefully both before and after they are used.

A nurse should *never* bring a loose swab into the operating theatre for any purpose. For wiping a surgeon's brow a small towel should be used, whereas for the mopping of a small area of bloodstained or soiled floor a clean mop or cloth is preferable. Similarly, a circulating nurse should *never* remove a swab from the theatre without permission of the scrub nurse. It is often the odd swab removed or introduced accidentally which is the cause for concern during a count.

Swab location. This is very important and any swab which is packed into a wound and left in position for any period must have a suitable length of tape or thread attached to one corner, e.g. tonsil swabs 15 cm by 2.5 cm (6 in by 1 in). This tape or thread is clipped with a haemostat and indicates the presence of a swab.

The swabs must be prepared from gauze which contains a continuous strand of barium (Raytec,[TM] Chex,[TM] etc.) and if there is any doubt regarding a missing swab, an X-ray can be taken before the wound is closed. The presence of a swab is indicated by the X-ray

Date	Name	Hosp. No.	AGE	Ward	Operation	Surgeon Assistant	Anaesthetist Assistant	Swab/Instrument Check		TOURNIQUET				Serial Number
								Instrument Nurse/Assistant	Circulating Nurse/Assistant	Time On	Signature	Time Off	Signature	
1.3.88	John Brown	Z3265	22	A2	Laparotomy	Mr Jones Dr Stevens	Dr Green Dr Fells	S/N George ODA Smith	S/N Broad	–	–	–	–	1001
1.3.88	Mavis South	D2323	39	B3	Herniorraphy	Mr Jones Dr Stevens	Dr Fells	ODA Smith	S/N Brown	–	–	–	–	1002
1.3.88	Michael West	B5679	56	A2	Varicose Vein Stripping	Dr Stevens Dr Howe	Dr Fells	S/N George	S/N Broad	–	–	–	–	1003
1.3.88	Jack Dunn	C1212	62	E1	Arthroplasty of Hip	Mr Bones Dr Oseous	Dr Hard Dr Tims	S/N Ward	ODA Smith S/N Evans	–	–	–	–	1004
1.3.88	William White	A2215	20	E1	Menisectomy	Mr Bones Dr Oseous	Dr Hard	S/N Evans	ODA Smith	11.30	ODA Brown	11.50	ODA Brown	1005
														1006
														1007
														1008
														1009
														1010

Fig. 6.9 Sample page from a swab and instrument check register which records application of tourniquets also. (The printed names in columns 7–9 would appear as signatures.)

shadow of a barium strand. This is, of course, an additional safeguard and should not replace an efficient swab-checking system.

Large quantities of swabs may be used during a major procedure and even with the most careful swab count, with numbers reaching three figures, theoretically it is possible to lose a complete packet of swabs.

Most operating departments have a special operation register into which details of the operations are entered each day. This book usually contains information about the patient, operation, surgeon and assistants, anaesthetist, anaesthetic and sometimes the name of the scrub nurse.

The preparation of dressings

At one time preparation of dressings or swabs was usually the duty of the theatre staff. Nowadays manufacturers' pre-prepared dressings are available in sizes to suit all requirements.

Swabs or sponges are prepared from gauze which may be cotton or rayon, both materials having excellent absorbency. The gauze must contain a continuous filament of X-ray opaque barium (Raytec (Johnson & Johnson), Chex (Vernon-Carus), etc.) Available also are X-ray opaque sheets of foam cellulose which have a very high absorbency, and are very useful for abdominal packs and minute ophthalmic mops when cut to a suitable size.

Although the sizes of swabs vary enormously according to the type of operation and individual preference of the surgeon, there are some average types and sizes which are in common use.

Large abdominal packs. These can be made 46 cm (18 in) square, from about 36 layers of gauze. These should be stitched around the edges, and a short length of tape attached to one corner. A pair of haemostats is clipped to this tape which is left protruding when the packs are placed inside the abdomen. Soiled packs should not be washed for re-use. It has been proved that laundered packs predispose towards abdominal adhesions, probably due to detergent or soap residue.

Large swabs or sponges. These may be made as a pad 23 cm by 7.5 cm (9 in by 3 in) containing about 24 layers of gauze when folded, and 23 cm by 46 cm (9 in by 18 in) containing four layers when opened out. These sizes may be varied more or less as required but it is better to standardise to one size of large swab in a particular unit. Alternative sizes range from 15 cm by 10 cm to 23 cm by 23 cm (6 in by 4 in to 9 in by 9 in).

Small swabs. These range from 5 cm square to 7.5 cm by 10 cm (2 in square to 3 in by 4 in), having about 16 layers. The important point is to ensure that there is sufficient difference of size between these and the larger types in use, to avoid any confusion during the swab checking procedure at operation.

Swabs and packs. These should be bundled in fixed numbers (fives) by tying with thread, a narrow bandage, rubber bands or lightly stitching together. These bundles are checked by a second person before packing and are checked again by two persons before the operation commences. Manufacturers such as Chex (Vernon Carus) supply swabs and packs already securely bundled in fives (MDU *et al.*, 1986).

Anaesthesia swabs. These must be made smaller than those in general use and green coloured gauze prepared by the manufacturers is available for this purpose. The size of swabs required will vary according to individual preference but a 2.5 cm (1 in) square swab is usually adequate.

If the dyed gauze is not available it may be made simply by dyeing white gauze with a weak solution of brilliant green, gentian violet, Bonney's blue or proflavine. The gauze is then

dried before making into swabs. Throat packs for the anaesthetist should also be made from green dyed gauze 5 cm (2 in) wide by 3 m to 6 m (3 yd to 6 yd) long, depending on the thickness of gauze.

Rolls of gauze 7.5 cm or 11.5 cm (3 in or $4\frac{1}{2}$ in) wide by 3 m or 4 m (3 yd or 4 yd) long made by folding 23 cm (9 in) wide gauze with a barium filament into three or two respectively are often used for packing off cavities, e.g., during gall-bladder operations or as a pack prior to the secondary suture of a septic wound. These may be used also for bandaging amputation stumps, to obtain even pressure over a skin graft although, for these purposes the gauze should not contain a radio-opaque filament.

Pieces of gamgee. For the application of skin disinfectant, pieces of gamgee about 10 cm (4 in) square, are very useful for they seem to hold the disinfectant better than the conventional gauze swab. If swabs are used for this purpose they must be coloured blue. Although these materials are not generally used in the operation area, they must be accounted for within the swab check.

Alternatively, polyurethane sponge cubes 4 cm ($1\frac{1}{2}$ in) in size are very suitable for applying skin antiseptic and withstand sterilization quite well.

Small dissection swabs, 'bits', 'pledgets' or 'patties'. These are used during general surgery, thoracic surgery, neurosurgery and vascular surgery.

1. Compressed dental cotton-wool rolls 9 mm by 2.5 cm ($\frac{1}{8}$ in by 1 in) securely clamped in the jaws of a haemostat may be used as dissection swabs. These require very careful checking at operation as they conflict with the radio-opaque checking concept.

2. 'Bits' or 'pledgets' are prepared from pieces of Raytec, Chex, etc., gauze folded to form a mop about 1.25 cm ($\frac{1}{2}$ in) square.

3. 'Patties' are made from B.P.C. cotton-wool or lintine. A piece of cotton-wool about 2.5 cm (1 in) square is moistened and stitched with a length of strong black radio-opaque thread. After autoclaving these fluff out into a suitable size.

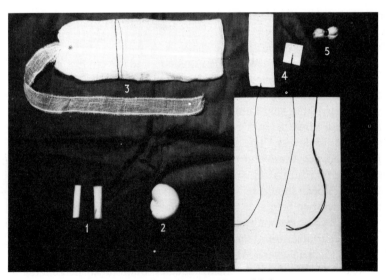

Fig. 6.10 Dissection swabs, wool ball, 'tapped' swab and patties or 'bits'.
1. Compressed cotton dental rolls for dissection swabs.
2. Wool ball covered with tubular gauze.
3. 'Taped' swab with barium strand.
4. Patties made from cottonoid.
5. Pattie or 'bit' made from ribbon gauze rolled into suitable size.

Lintine or 'Cottonoid' is supplied in sheets 31 cm by 7.6 cm (12 in by 3 in), which are cut into suitable sized 'patties'. These are stitched with a length of black thread, care being taken to avoid using actual knots to secure it in position. Knots and rough surfaces will damage delicate nerve tissue, and it is for this reason also that the 'patties' must be moistened slightly at operation. All these small mops are made into bundles of 5 or 10 and are checked carefully before and after operation.

Alternatively, prepared patties are available commercially. One manufacturer (Macarthys) produces patties in packs of 20 (4 × 5 s) or 10 secured on a count card.

Wool rolls. If required sterile these are cut to suitable size and re-rolled loosely before packing into the packets. If a high vacuum/high-pressure autoclave is available they need not be rerolled.

Sterile bandages of all materials, especially crêpe, are frequently required and may be packed into a separate dressings packet or container. A tightly wound bandage cannot be completely sterilized because the steam will not penetrate into the actual centre of the bandage. However the outer layers coming into contact with the dressings are sterile, and are therefore preferable to non-sterile bandages.

ENT and ophthalmic dressings. These are prepared and generally kept in separate packets containing suitable dressings for the eye and ear, including fast-edge bandages, ribbon gauze, and eye pads made from best quality cotton-wool, covered each side with cotton bandage.

Operation linen

Operation towels, sheets and gowns are made from a strong close-weave material such as balloon fabric or repp, or a disposable non-woven fabric such as Fabric 450 or AZO 44, generally green in colour which is restful to the eyes of the operation team.

It is better to minimise the number of towel sizes in an operating suite and generally three or four sizes and types will suffice. The average towel for covering a trolley should measure at least 122 cm (48 in) square, although a trolley measuring 122 cm (48 in) by 61 cm (24 in) will require an oblong towel measuring 183 cm by 152 cm (72 in by 60 in). This enables easier packet preparation by using one towel for the trolley drapes even if the trolley sizes are large.

For draping lower limbs, these larger size towels 183 cm by 152 cm (72 in by 60 in) will be found useful also and will reduce the number of towels required to the minimum.

For abdominal surgery, there may be a preference for a large sheet measuring about 213 cm by 183 cm (84 in by 72 in) and having a longitudinal reinforced slit 31 cm (12 in) by 10 cm (4 in) placed centrally and slightly towards one end. This holed sheet or towel may be utilised also for operations in the lithotomy position, or a lateral thigh operation such as the insertion of a Smith-Peterson nail. The addition of two bag-shaped leg covers stitched to the edges of suitable holes, 30 cm (12 in) from each side of the central slit in a holed towel, obviates the need for extra towels to cover the legs in lithotomy position.

Gowns are made with long sleeves with a stockinette cuff for the operation team. They should be made with an overlap of material at the back which, when tied correctly, covers the unsterile tapes. This is especially useful if the surgeon turns his back to the operation area as may happen during intra-abdominal manipulations.

All linen materials should be kept in a good state of repair and examined for tears, etc., before packing in the packets or containers.

The preparation of packs

Sterile pack systems for operative procedures are now well established. Separate linen or paper packets of sterile materials and instruments are prepared for individual operations, a fresh set of packs always being opened for each operation.

There is no place for the outdated 'drum' system, for the risk of bacterial contamination due to ill-fitting shutters and lids is considerable. In addition, the use of a multi-item container for unwrapped items cannot guarantee sterility indefinitely especially if it remains open for a considerable period of time during an operation list.

Small items may be double wrapped and sterilized in individual packets or paper bags.

Small towels. These are folded or rolled into a convenient size. A 'criss-cross' method of packing facilitates efficient air removal and steam penetration and is preferable to packing the articles in unbroken columns.

Large towels or abdominal sheets. These are packed in a similar manner but it will be found advantageous to fold them in such a way that, when opened at operation, they are conveniently arranged for easy draping.

This is accomplished (see illustrations) by folding the towels lengthways in sections about 23 cm (9 in) wide from each side to the centre. The 23 cm (9 in) wide finished folds are then folded again in 23 cm (9 in) sections equally from each end to the centre, making a folded towel about 23 cm (9 in) square which is a convenient size for packing. Towels folded in this way are less liable to become contaminated, especially in the centre, when opened out by two persons at operation.

Gowns. These are folded inside out in three or four folds, care being taken to contain all

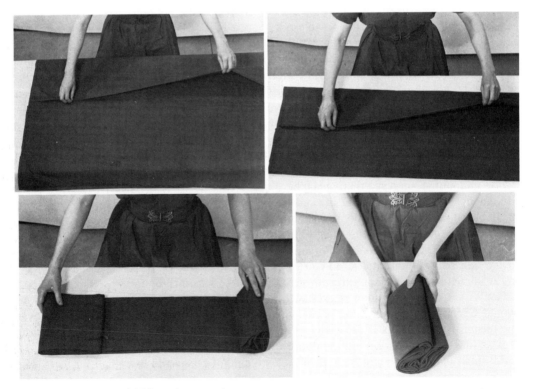

Fig. 6.11 Four stages of folding a large towel.

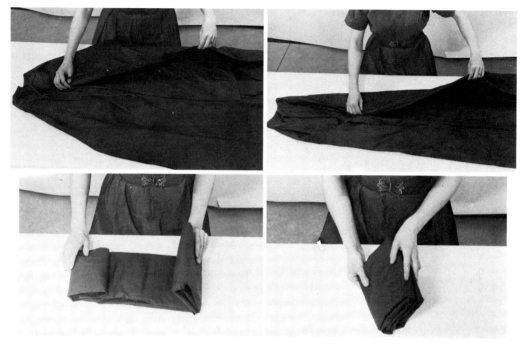

Fig. 6.12   Four stages of folding a gown.

the tapes within the folds. The gowns are then rolled or folded equally from each end to the centre (see illustrations). This will ensure that when the gown is opened at operation, whichever end is grasped the gown will only unroll halfway and avoid touching the floor.

Macintoshes. In the operating theatre these have now been replaced either with a water-repellent disposable non woven fabric such as Azo77 (Vernon-Carus), or fabric such as Ventile and Scotchguard which can be laundered and re-proofed.

These items can be packed and sterilized in a similar manner to fabric towels or drapes.

Gloves. These are supplied presterilized in peel-open packs. Alternatively, if re-processing is unavoidable or special types of gloves are in use they may be put in individual packets which are placed in outer protective paper bags.

Dressings and bandages. These, including materials such as gauze and wool, are packed loosely and sterilized under the same conditions as towels and gowns.

Sterile pack systems

These methods have supplanted the use of drums and caskets. In principle they are quite simple and mean the preparation of sterile supplies either in packs (parcels) or sealed bags, the contents of which are used for one procedure only. Any supplies remaining are discarded for re-sterilization and a fresh pack opened for the next procedure.

There are a number of different methods of packing sterile supplies. Each has its advantages and disadvantages but basically all the items required for an operation are prepared together either in one or several packs, i.e., items required for an abdominal operation could be prepared as a comprehensive single set or divided into the various components as separate packs.

In the latter instance, one would contain the requisite number of gowns and small hand

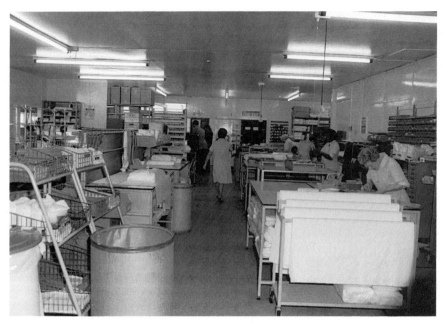

Fig. 6.13   CSSD instrument tray packing area. (District Sterile Supplies Department, Bloomsbury Health Authority, London.)

towels, a second rubber gloves, a third the requisite towels or drapes, swabs and gauze packs, etc., and a fourth the instruments and other steam-sterilizable items.

The packs are covered with a material which enables sterilization to take place, acting also as a barrier to bacteria during the periods of storage before use. Amongst suitable wrapping materials are linen, crêpe paper and non-woven fabrics.

No material is ideal for wrapping all items and although it is desirable to standardise to the most suitable, two or three types may need to be utilised according to requirements. The correct gauge of linen or paper must be selected for wrapping fabrics and instruments. Paper manufacturers in the United Kingdom now conform to a Department of Health specification in respect of sterilizing wrapping papers (Crepe paper — TSS/5/330/005; plain paper — TSS/5/330/007; paper bags — TTS/5/330/004). Items must always be double wrapped to prevent contamination after sterilization or during opening of the packet (Allen, 1965; Speers and Shooter, 1966; Medical Research Council, 1968).

Irrespective of whether the packs are prepared in a Sterilizing and Disinfecting Unit (SDU), Central Sterile Supply Department, or the Operating Department, basic techniques are similar. Space would not permit a description of all methods in use but there are several which are more generally approved, i.e., the comprehensive Edinburgh Pre-Set Tray system prepared in an SDU; modified forms of the Pre-Set Tray system; separate drape and instrument sets and supplementary items in paper or non-woven fabric packs.

The Edinburgh pre-set tray system (in brief)

The most logical and time-saving method is to prepare all the requirements in one comprehensive pack. This is not a new idea for it has been in use for several decades particularly in the United States but there are several problems associated with the method. Some

difficulty may be experienced after sterilization in completely drying out the packet containing a large number of instruments combined with drapes. This is specially so in the High-vacuum/High-pressure autoclave and is due to excessive condensate forming on the instruments during the steam phase.

Secondly, unless the correct packing procedure is carried out, instruments tend to become displaced during handling and transit and this is inconvenient when the packet is opened for use.

Research conducted by the Royal Infirmary at Edinburgh revealed that if instruments and drapes are packed and sterilized on solid aluminium trays of 12 s.w.g. or 14 s.w.g. weight, there is sufficient residual heat left to vaporise this excess condensate during the drying phase.

The trays are made to conform in width and depth to the British Standard High-vacuum/High-pressure rectangular sterilizers, i.e., 66 cm by 66 cm (26 in by 26 in). The sizes of the trays are such as to allow setting out of instruments and drapes in the order of their use. The largest size 61 cm by 61 cm (2 ft by 2 ft) is adequate for a major surgery set, the medium 61 cm by 31 cm (2 ft by 1 ft) for smaller sets and the smallest 31 cm by 31 cm (1 ft by 1 ft) is designed for other supplementary items. Full details of tray specifications are given in the Appendix.

The Edinburgh trays are ideal, particularly when a considerable number of instruments are needed in a surgery set. However, they are not absolutely essential and smaller heavy-gauge aluminium press-out trays about 4 cm ($1\frac{1}{2}$ in) in depth may be utilised as an alternative.

Theatre sterile supplies

These can be supplied by the Sterilizing and Disinfecting Unit (SDU) which is sited to provide a total hospital service, or, exceptionally, built adjacent to the operating department to provide an exclusive service. It is basically the same layout as any CSSD which handles the processing of ward instruments and dressings. It should have a soiled truck unloading area; processing area for soiled instruments and which includes mechanical and ultrasonic washing machines; a tray assembly area; supplementary pack assembly area; soft goods supply storage area; prepared pack and tray holding area; sterilizing area; processed stores area and administrative areas. Linen repair and inspection facilities may be incorporated in the unit or may form part of the hospital laundry services.

Sterile instrument sets are held ready for use in the operating department sterile store for delivery when required to each operating suite. Special instrument sets and supplementary items may be stored in the preparation room of specific theatre suites, e.g. cardiothoracic, orthopaedic. After use, sets are returned immediately to the SDU for processing and rester-ilization. Each operating suite does, of course, maintain a fixed stock of supplementary instrument packs for emergency use and linen packets including sterile gowns, swabs, dressings and other small items.

At the end of the operation, prior to folding over the linen covers of the used trays ready for removal from the operating theatre, the scrub nurse should dispose of any contents of gallipots, separate the used and unused instruments, collect used knife blades, broken glass vials, ligature packets and non-traumatic suture needles in a foil dish or other protective packet before placing in the paper disposal bag or sharps disposal container.

The used trays, salvaged drapes and dressings, empty hand basins and other holloware are returned to the SDU. The disposal bags containing soiled swabs and soiled linen bags are sealed and marked with the operation number. These are held in the operating depart-

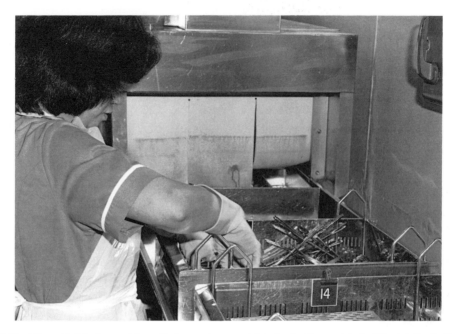

Fig. 6.14   Dismantled instrument trays (instruments are put into basket for washing). (District Sterile Supplies Department, Bloomsbury Health Authority, London.)

ment disposal area until the used trays have been checked and found to be correct. This is to ensure that the bags can be identified later if an instrument is found to be missing. If the loss of an instrument is not detected at the off-loading bench it certainly will be detected while the instruments are being re-set. When the instruments have been re-set and it is clear that the numbers are correct, the laundry bag, disposal and swab bags held in the operating department are disposed of in the appropriate manner (ASSA, 1975).

Salvaged dressings and drapes are returned to the supply storage area and the tray with its linen covers is disassembled. Special instruments such as scissors, skin hooks and amputation knives are separated from the general instruments and washed separately. The remainder of the instruments are loaded into baskets for processing in the washing machine. Unused instruments are generally loaded into a separate basket and the used instruments into as many further baskets as may be required. Jointed instruments should be opened widely and those such as probes and nerve hooks which might drop out of the basket during washing can be clipped or thrust through plastic sponges to keep them within the basket.

There may be several instrument baskets per surgical operation and if the trays arrive at the SDU in rapid succession from different operating theatres, it is important to be able to distinguish instruments used at one operation from those used at another. The Edinburgh Royal Infirmary devised a labelling system to overcome this difficulty.

Above the tray off-loading bench there is a board on which hang groups of four metal discs. The discs are marked with the operating theatre number and the serial number of the particular operation on the list. As each basket is loaded with instruments, an appropriate disc is hooked on to the rim of the basket and is left there till the instruments have been removed from the basket for re-setting at the end of the processing line. The tray checker removes the discs after checking the re-set tray. The discs are then returned to the board for further use.

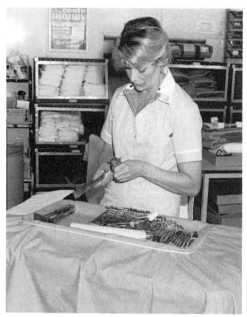

Fig. 6.15

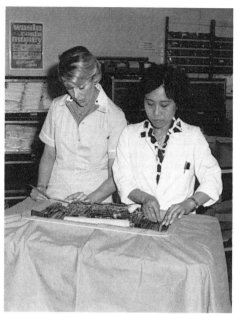

Fig. 6.16

Fig. 6.15 The drapes have been fixed to the tray and the assistant assembles instruments and utensils. (District Sterile Supplies Department, Bloomsbury Health Authority, London.)

Fig. 6.16 Two persons check the instruments against the list. (District Sterile Supplies Department, Bloomsbury Health Authority, London.)

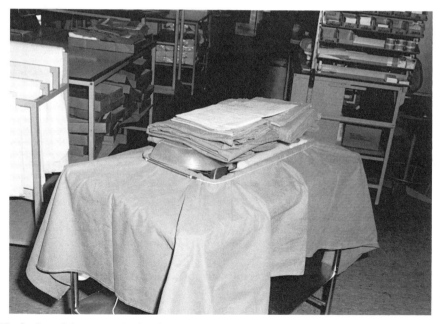

Fig. 6.17 Swabs and drapes are added to the tray. (District Sterile Supplies Department, Bloomsbury Health Authority, London.)

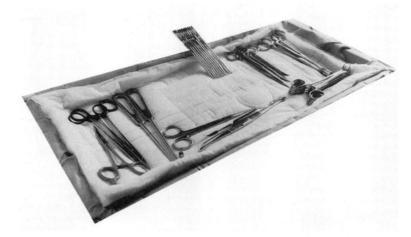

Fig. 6.18   Tray liner made from gamgee to hold instruments in position. (Vernon-Carus.)

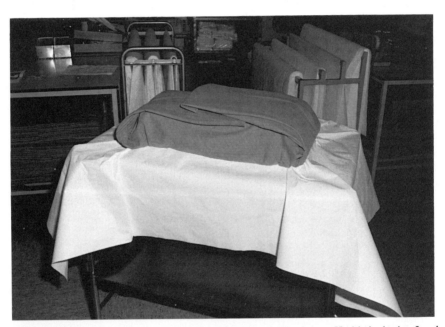

Fig. 6.19   Inner wraps folded. (District Sterile Supplies Department, Bloomsbury Health Authority, London.)

Whilst the instruments are being processed the large trays are cleansed with a suitable solution such as spiritous Hibitane 0.05 per cent and then transferred to the tray assembly area on to a 61 cm by 61 cm (2 ft by 2 ft) trolley. Two layers of fabric covers, one blue and one green are arranged over both the tray and the trolley. (The different colours are to differentiate between the cover handled by the circulating nurse and the cover handled by the scrub nurse wearing sterile gown and gloves.) These covers are pushed down into the tray by a mould of appropriate size for the tray; and a spring-retaining cord is stretched over the covers into the gutter round the upper aspect of the tray.

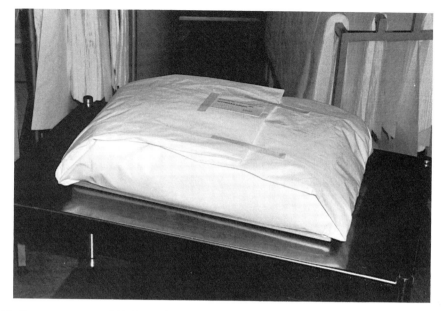

Fig. 6.20 Outer paper wraps folded over the contents and sealed with heat sensitive tape. The set is identified by a printed label (District Sterile Supplies Department, Bloomsbury Health Authority, London.)

After the instruments have been washed, ultrasonically cleansed, dried and inspected they are set out according to the particular arrangement (Fig. 6.15). The instruments are checked by two persons against a list (Fig. 6.16). A set of swabs and fabric drapes are placed over the instruments to retain them in position during transit and sterilization (Fig. 6.17). Alternatively a tray liner made from gamgee-type cotton can be used, one layer beneath the instruments and another above (Fig. 6.18). The covers are folded over as illustrated (Figs. 6.19, 6.20). After sterilization, the trays are held in the processed stores area until required. If prolonged storage is necessary after sterilization an additional plastic dust cover is used.

A modified pre-set tray system

The 61 cm by 61 cm (2 ft by 2 ft) special tray is ideal, particularly when large instrument sets are needed, e.g. major laparotomy. As stated previously, if no SDU is available the system is quite suitable for preparation and sterilization within the operating suite. However, the autoclaves may be too small to take the large size tray and the alternative medium size, i.e., 61 cm by 31 cm (2 ft by 1 ft) may be inadequate for an average general set, or perhaps neither of these trays may be easily available. In these circumstances the Pre-Set Tray system can be introduced utilising any convenient deep aluminium tray, providing it is of sufficient gauge to retain enough residual heat for drying the instrument set during the post-steam cycle. Alternatively, cardboard or polypropylene trays may be used although prolonged drying may be necessary.

Basically the method is similar to the Edinburgh system but as the trays generally do not have the special double gutter to accommodate the spring-retaining cord one layer of fabric cover is placed *outside* the aluminium tray (Fig. 6.25).

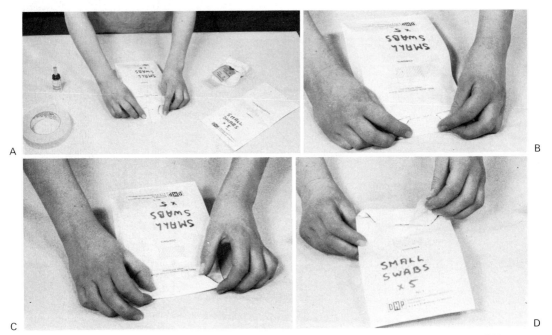

Fig. 6.21 *Supplementary items in Kraft paper bags.* (A) Folded top — first diagonal folds. (B) Second fold. (C) Final fold which is held in position with (D) a piece of 3M autoclave tape.

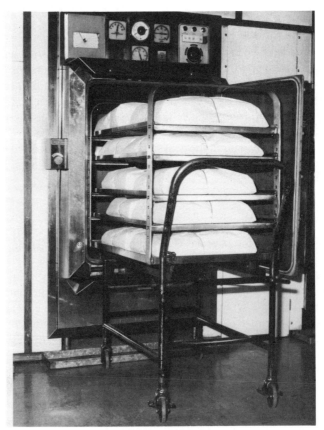

Fig. 6.22 Trolley loaded with theatre trays placed in sterilization chamber. (ASSA Training Handbook for Sterile Supply Assistants.)

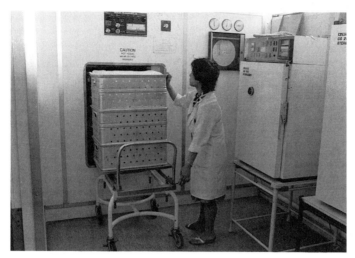

Fig. 6.23 Perforated aluminium baskets used to contain soft packs for sterilization (District Sterile Supplies Department, Bloomsbury Health Authority.)

Separate drape and instrument sets

The Pre-Set Tray system is only suitable when there are sufficient instruments to allow adequate time for processing and sterilization. When this is impossible, the alternative is to sterilize the instruments separately and then add these to a suitable operation packet.

All the swabs, and drapes, are prepared in a linen or paper pack. The method of folding is basically the same as that described under the modified tray system. Pack covers should consist of not less than two layers of fabric which act as a trolley drape also. Suitable materials include Repp, Ventile and Scotchguard (which are water-repellent and can be re-proofed in the hospital laundry (Brigden, 1964), see Appendix), and non woven fabrics (Fabric 450*, Azo44). In addition, there should be a plastic or paper outer wrap if the pack is to be stored for extended periods.

Instrument trays can be wrapped as in Figure 6.25 I to L. This is preferable to open trays, which require the use of Cheatle transfer forceps.

Supplementary items

Single instruments and other supplementary items such as orthopaedic implants, additional packets of swabs, etc., can be packed into small packs or paper bags. Rigid containers can be used for some instruments and for steam sterilization are made from cardboard. Metal containers are generally only suitable for the dry heat process.

Packs are prepared similar to those described previously utilising a diagonal method of folding the two layers.

Paper bags can either be heat-sealed or have a plain folded top. In the former case the Kraft bag incorporates a heat-sensitive adhesive band inside the open end (Thermotop). After the contents have been placed inside, the open end is sealed by squeezing between the heated jaws of a special heat-sealing machine. The bag generally has a small panel of heat-sensitive ink which changes colour after the packet has been sterilized. If this has not been provided a small piece of 3M indicator tape should be affixed to the bag for the same purpose. (3M indicator tape is in the form of dark stripes which appear on the surface of

the tape if it has been through the sterilization process. No 1222 is designed for steam sterilization, No 1226 [Indair] is for dry heat and No 1224 [Indox] is for ethylene oxide.)

Folded top bags are prepared as illustrated (Fig. 6.21) and the folds held in position with a small piece of 3M indicator tape. The cardinal rule with paper bags is that two must always be used. The outer bag acts as a dust cover during storage so that when the inner is opened in the operation area, the possible dissipation of dust is avoided (page 166).

Metal containers are generally made from aluminium in the form of tubes or boxes. They are most suitable for dry heat sterilizable items such as osteotomes, special knives and syringes, etc., and as sterilization is by conduction of heat the container can be sealed before processing.

Sterilization and storage

Sterilization of packs is dealt with at great length in the following chapter. After sterilization a piece of cellulose tape imprinted STERILE may be applied to the pack and stamped with

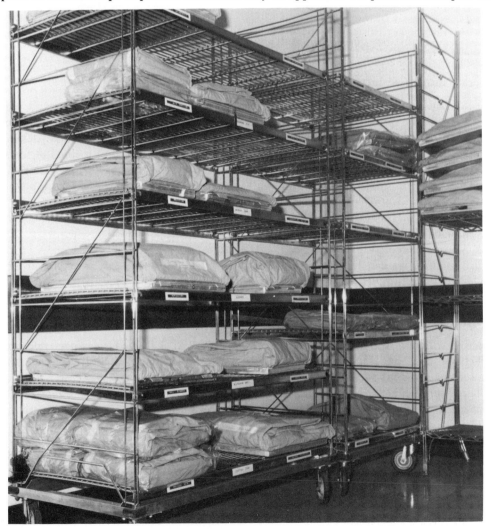

Fig. 6.24 Sterilized sets on 'cooling racks'. (ASSA Training Handbook for Sterile Supply Assistants.)

the date of autoclaving. Alternatively, the date can be marked on the 3M indicator tape used to secure pack folds. This date is a guide to turnover rather than sterility.

The packs should be stored in a clean dry environment until required (Fig. 6.24). If storage is likely to be prolonged for more than a few hours, the packs should have an outer dust cover made from plastic or paper. In a properly air-conditioned operating department normally it should be unnecessary to have dust covers but the packs must be stacked carefully in rotation of sterilization date. This ensures that none are stored for too long a period.

Packs which usually require some form of dust cover within the operating suite are items such as orthopaedic implants or specialised instruments used infrequently. In this case, if the item is small enough, Bri-pac boxes are suitable and enable quite a number to be stored in a small area.

A high standard of cleanliness is necessary in pack storage areas. Shelving or cupboards should be damp-dusted regularly with a suitable anti-bacterial agent (e.g., spiritous Hibitane 0.05 per cent).

Preparation for operation

The outer cover of the pack is opened by hand (Fig. 6.26A), care being taken to avoid contamination of the inner pack which is opened by the scrub nurse as illustrated. With the Pre-Set tray very little additional preparation is needed with the exception of a few supplementary items.

Where separate drape and instrument packs are in use these are opened aseptically and transferred to the main trolley by the scrub nurse. Items in paper bags should, preferably, be removed with sterile forceps by the scrub nurse (Fig. 6.27) although they can be dropped on to a sterile surface with care.

Gown packs should be opened only to the inner layers, which are left folded for opening by the instrument nurse just before gowning up. Gloves are dispensed from individual paper bags as required (Fig. 6.6A, page 139).

Using this type of pack system, even during busy operation lists, the preparation time of trolleys is shortened considerably. Only one trolley should be prepared, the next instrument pack is opened as the next operation is ready to start. This ensures minimal bacterial contamination and reduces the rush or tension which previously tended to be present during preparations in the operating theatre.

The care of instruments and apparatus

After use the instruments should ideally be cleansed in an ultrasonic cleanser or mechanical washing machine combined with a suitable caustic based detergent solution, e.g., Neodian, Lab-brite, Sumazon XL, Helpex No 1 etc. The process should include a cycle of cold water followed by a detergent wash and finally a very hot rinse 85°C containing a neutral rinse aid such as Sumabrite (Fig. 6.28). Alternatively the instruments are soaked in a bactericidal solution such as 1 per cent Titan Sanitizer SU357 or Titan Quatdet SU321 before being cleansed with a stiff brush under running cold water, although this is not as effective as mechanical cleansing. Staff must be adequately protected by wearing aprons and rubber gloves.

If excessive contamination has occurred, e.g. following a septic operation, it is better to autoclave them for four minutes at 134°C before processing. However, during subsequent cleansing the instruments must still be regarded as potentially infected due to the debris adhering.

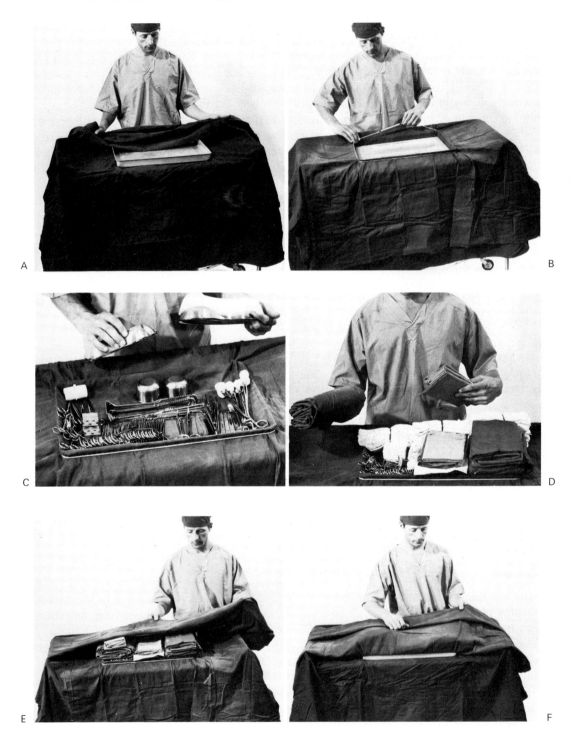

A

B

C

D

E

F

Fig. 6.25 (caption on page 162)

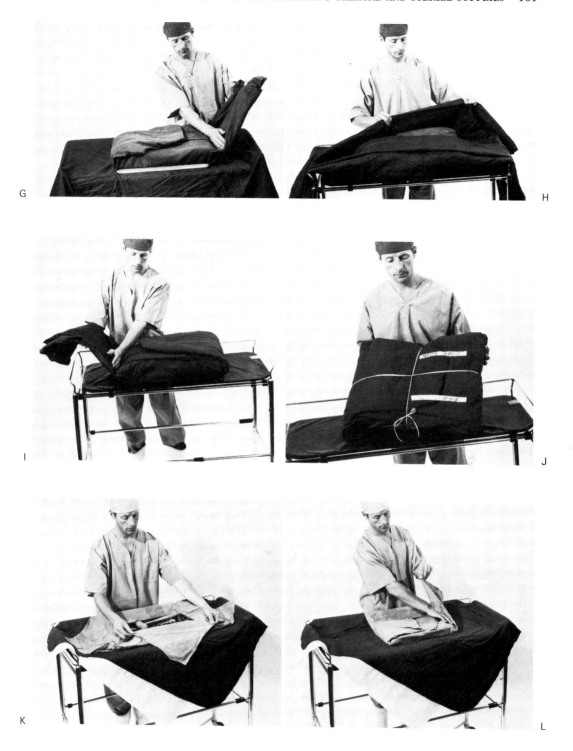

Fig. 6.25 (caption on page 162)

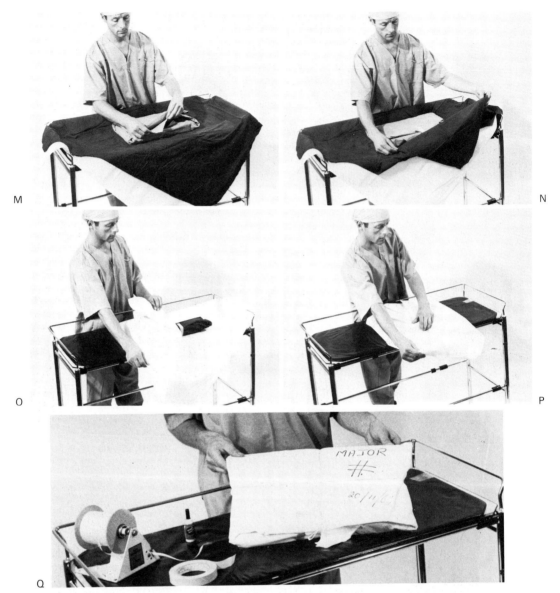

M

N

O

P

Q

Fig. 6.25 *The modified pre-set tray system.* (A) aluminium tray placed on outer piece of blue fabric. (B) Green trolley drape in position over aluminium tray, wooden former pushes drape flat, which is then held in position with a cord and spring. (C) Major basic instruments set out. (D) Swabs and drapes placed over instruments. This helps to retain them in position during sterilization and handling afterwards. (E) Rear part of green trolley drape folded to the front and then turned back on itself. (F) Front part of green trolley drape folded towards the back and then folded back on itself. (G) Second side fold of green trolley drape. (H) The outer blue piece of fabric is folded as previously described. (I) The final side folds of the blue fabric. (J) The completed major basic instrument set ready for sterilization. (The contents, date packed and initials of tray assembler and checker are written on the 3M autoclave tape with felt pen magic marker). (K) *Instruments packed separately to drapes*; a fracture and bone set which is wrapped in three layers, green and blue fabric and crêpe paper. A diagonal method of folding is used with corners turned back for easy aseptic opening at operation. The first front fold, green fabric. (L) The second side fold. (M) Tucking in the final fold, green fabric. (N) The blue fabric layer is folded in a similar manner. (O) The final paper layer folded diagonally as before, first side fold. (P) The front paper fold. (Q) The completed pack ready for sterilization. This paper layer is required only if the packet is being sterilized outside the operating suite. Note the packet is tied with cotton tape and a piece of 3M indicator autoclave tape has been applied.

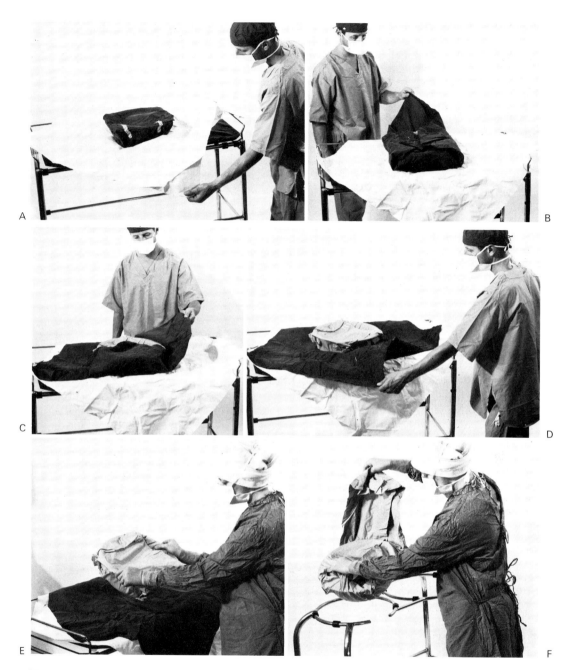

Fig. 6.26 (caption on page 165)

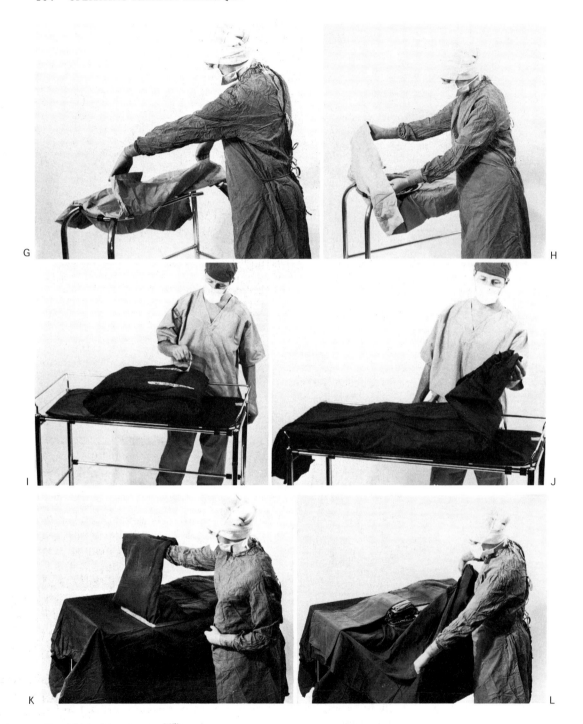

Fig. 6.26 (caption on page 165)

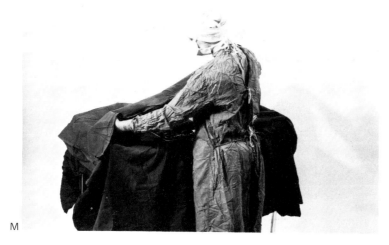

M

Fig. 6.26 *Opening sterile packs at operation.* (A) The outer crêpe paper layers are opened, utilising the turned-back diagonal corners. (B) The inner blue layer is also opened by the circulating nurse, fold one. (C) Opening the second side fold. (D) The final blue fold which exposes the innermost green wrapped pack. (E) The scrub nurse lifts out the inner pack (which contains a hand lotion bowl set complete with bowl stand drape). (F) Grasping the topmost part of the drape, the scrub nurse lowers the bowl and drape into the lotion bowl stand. (G) The drapes are opened to cover the lotion bowl stand, (H) exposing the hand lotion bowl which is then filled with sterile water or saline. (Fig. 1.42, page 51). (I) *Opening the pre-set tray of instruments*; removing the autoclave tape after checking that it is the correct set and has been autoclaved. (J) The blue layers are opened by the circulating nurse. (K) The inner green trolley drape is opened by the scrub nurse, the side folds. (L) The front fold of the trolley drape. (M) The rear fold is opened: note the front fold already opened protects the sterile gown of the scrub nurse as she stretches over the trolley.

Instruments should be dried hot soon after removal from the washing machine, ultrasonic cleaner or a hot detergent solution such as 0.5 per cent cetrimide. After cleaning and drying they should always be examined carefully each time for defects, i.e., loose rivets and screws, cracking of forceps' jaws, lack of apposition between grooves and, in cutting instruments, blunt cutting edges, etc.

Sharp instruments. These should be handled with very great care. The cutting edges of fine cataract knives, scalpels, osteotomes and gouges, etc., must not be damaged. These instruments must be dried thoroughly after use to avoid rusting, as they are often manufactured from carbon steel.

The cutting edges of knives, etc., may be examined by viewing the edge under a strong light. A sharp knife edge will appear black, but if the edge appears as a broken or continuous white line, the knife is blunt and should be discarded for resharpening.

Scissors. These should have even edges and secure rivets. Good quality scissors require only occasional sharpening. In any case the scissors remain semi-closed during sterilization, thereby protecting the edges.

Suture needles. These are generally disposable but, if for reasons of economy, re-use is necessary, they must be washed thoroughly after use, special attention being paid to the needle eye. Rust marks should be removed with fine steel wool and soap, following which the needles are carefully dried. They are sterilized by dry heat or autoclaving (utilising a piece of anti-rust paper) after packing in paper envelopes. Needles having blunt or rough edges should not be kept for further use and must be discarded.

Syringes and hypodermic or serum needles (Non-disposable). These are rinsed thoroughly after use. Care must always be taken to remove blood from the inside of barrels and needles

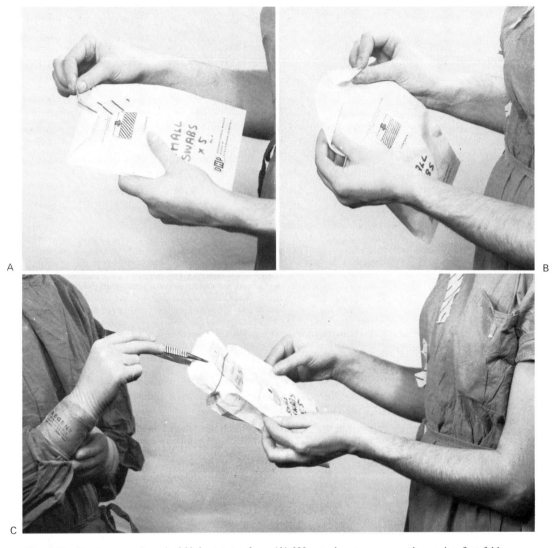

Fig. 6.27 *Supplementary items in folded top paper bags.* (A) 3M autoclave tape removed, opening first folds. (B) Utilising gusset to open remaining folds of bag. (C) Contents removed with sterile forceps.

otherwise it will be impossible to sterilize them. An ultrasonic cleanser or good non-pyrogenic detergent such as Neodian, Lab-brite, Helpex No 1, etc., should be used, and the needles checked for blockage by passing a stilette through.

Glass/metal special syringes are always dismantled before sterilization; the different degrees of expansion between the metal and glass will cause cracking of the barrel. *All glass* syringes are sterilized assembled in the dry-heat oven or infra-red apparatus, and un-assembled in the autoclave, as in the latter case it is possible that sufficient moist heat will not reach the piston of an assembled syringe.

With the exception of syringes having interchangeable barrels and pistons, care must be taken to avoid the exchange of components. Manufacturers generally engrave corresponding

numbers or letters on the pistons and barrels to ensure correct assembly. Incorrect assembly may result in an ill-fitting piston.

If the syringes are to be sterilized by the dry-heat method, after cleaning they should be carefully dried inside and out with acetone or ether before *very lightly* lubricating the piston with sterile liquid paraffin or silicone solution. Silicone solution is preferable if the syringes are sterilized assembled as it obviates the risk of pistons becoming jammed in the barrel. They may then be sterilized in packets, metal containers or glass tubes.

Some special instruments such as cystoscopes, laryngoscopes and other endoscopic apparatus may be sterilized by moist heat, but manufacturers' instructions regarding sterilization should be followed carefully. Endoscopes may be disinfected by 'pasteurisation' or sterilized, or in a chemical solution, e.g., Cidex, Hibitane 0.5 per cent. Sterilization can be achieved by formaldehyde at subatmospheric steam pressure, or ethylene oxide vapour can also be used if suitable apparatus and bacteriological control is available (Medical Research Council, 1968).

After use, endoscopes are cleansed carefully, first under cold running water, and then in a hot detergent solution, special attention being given to the inside tube. A cotton-wool swab on a metal probe or a pipe cleaner can be used for cleaning and drying the inside of a rigid endoscope. After drying, the instruments are lightly lubricated, inspected for general defects, including the lamps and lamp carriers which are tested before putting them away (see Chapter 14).

Non-disposable rubber drainage or suction tubing is washed through with cold water after use. The lumen of suction tubing can easily become blocked with hardened blood and debris caused by inefficient cleansing and repeated sterilization. To avoid this, the tubing should be rolled between the hand and a board, or stretched in sections to dislodge any particles adherent to the lumen wall. The tubing is then flushed by attaching it to a pressure nozzle or tap and forcing cold water through it.

Following this, the tubing is washed with hot detergent solution and hung up to dry partially before sterlization.

In most operating theatres a stock of assorted sterile drainage tubes is kept ready in plastic or paper packs. Special drains, such as Marian's suprapubic tubing for draining the bladder, may be sterilized with the instruments when they are likely to be needed during an operation.

Non-disposable rubber catheters are cleansed as tubing, being rinsed through from the 'eye' end. After detergent washing and drying, the surface of a catheter must be examined for irregularities or deterioration and if found, the catheter should be discarded. A smooth surface is essential to avoid trauma to the delicate urethral mucosa.

Some catheters have an inflatable cuff or obturator bag which should always be tested before and after use.

Non-disposable plastic drainage tubing and catheters. Those made from vinyl resins (vinyl Portex), nylon, polythene, polypropylene, silicones and polycarbonates, are cleansed in a similar manner to rubber.

This type of tubing should be sterilized only when needed or stored dry in sterile packs. Many catheters are now supplied disposable and sterile in a pack.

Reusable solution rubber gloves. These should be washed thoroughly in cold water before removing from the hands. They should be washed again in cold water to ensure complete removal of blood stains.

If the gloves have been used for a septic case they should be discarded. Following a clean case, they are scrubbed inside and out with a detergent solution.

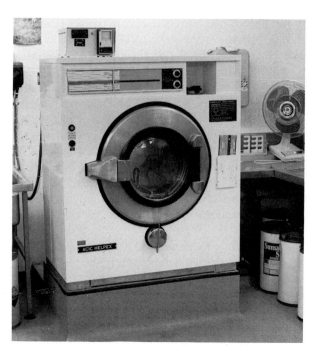

Fig. 6.28 Helpex automatic washing machine for instruments and apparatus. The machine drum rotates in both directions, repeatedly plunging the moving items into a heated washing solution. Rinsing is accomplished by repeated immersion in hot water, cold water and, if desired, distilled water. Drying is accomplished by centrifuging to throw off water droplets, at the same time introducing a blast of hot (or cold) air. The cycle is controlled automatically by a punched card control system shown top left. (Peacocks Surgical and Medical Equipment Ltd.)

The gloves are then dried either by hanging up until the outside is dry, turning, and then repeating the process, or rubbing each side with a towel whilst holding them on a warm surface.

Each glove is then tested for perforations by inflating with a foot pump, twisting the wristband so that the palm and fingers are under air pressure and plunging below the surface of a fluid (Williams *et al.*, 1966). Alternatively a proprietary glove tester is available (Helpex, Peacocks). Following this the sound gloves are finally dried and lightly powdered inside.

Gloves with perforations should be discarded as resistant tetanus spores may remain in the patch of a rubber glove.

Tests have shown that granulomata may form in wounds if a talcum glove powder is used. Talc deposition in the wound may occur if the surfaces of gloves are inadequately wiped before operation, or if a glove should become punctured during use.

Talc-free absorbable powders containing basically either starch or magnesium are less likely to cause this complication, although by 1965 the sixteenth case of starch granuloma had been reported (Bates, 1965). If this type of powder is used (Biosorb, K285, Diastol) the minimum should be applied to the inside of the gloves only (British Medical Journal, (1973).

After powdering, the gloves are grouped in sizes, each cuff being folded over about 6.5 cm (2½ in). They are packed as pairs in separate paper or linen bags having two compartments, one for each glove. A small green or similarly dyed swab should be placed just inside the palm of each glove to ensure adequate penetration of the steam.

A small quantity of powder is required for use with each pair of gloves to lubricate the hands. This may be contained in small cellophane bags which are filled with about one teaspoonful of powder and placed *with the end open* in one compartment of the glove pack. Alternatively it is possible to purchase one brand of glove powder already packed in small sterilizable paper packets (Biosorb).

Most surgeons' rubber gloves used nowadays are disposable (Regent, Velvex, Pioneer, etc.). These are made from a latex rubber and are supplied presterilized together with a suitable glove powder or specially treated powder-free surfaces. They are designed to be used only once for surgery but afterwards following decontamination, may be utilised in the wards and departments for non-sterile procedures.

Gum elastic catheters. These are rarely used as they are easily damaged and require very careful handling. They are cleansed in the usual manner, and after use *may* be submerged vertically in a suitable anti-bacterial agent such as Cidex or Hibitane 0.5 per cent. Ureteric catheters should be syringed through with a fine needle and syringe before resterilizing and the lumen must be filled with the solution by means of a syringe and needle. Alternatively, subatmospheric steam/formaldehyde may be used to sterilize these types of catheters.

Sterilization by heat is always more reliable, and if this is difficult it may be advisable to consider using catheters made of a heat sterilizable material. It is for this reason that the latest forms of plastic are being found very useful for catheters and bougies.

REFERENCES

ALLEN, S. M. *et al.* (1965) *Lancet*, ii, 1343.

BALLINGER, W. F., TREYBAL, J. C. AND VOSE, A. B. (1972) *Alexander's Care of the Patient in Surgery*. St. Louis: Mosby.

BATES, B. (1965) *Annals of Internal Medicine*, **62**, 335.

BRIGDEN, R. J. (1960) *The Nylon Packet System of Sterilisation*. London: Nursing Mirror.

BRIGDEN, R. J. (1964) *Nursing Times*, December 11.

BETHUNE, D. W., BLOWERS, R., PARKER, M. AND PASK, E. A. (1965) *Lancet*, ii, 458.

BRITISH MEDICAL JOURNAL (1973) ii, 502.

CHURCH, J AND SANDERSON, P. J. (1980) Surgical glove punctures. *Journal of Hospital Infection*, 1, 84.

DANKERT, J., ZIJLSTRA, J. B. AND LUBBERDING, H. (1979) A garment for use in the operating theatre: the effect on bacterial shedding. *Journal of Hygiene*, 82, 7.

DEVENISH, E. A. AND MILES, A. A. (1939) Control of *Staphylococcus aureus* in an operating theatre. *Lancet*, i, 1088–1094.

FALK, H. C. (1942) *Operation Room Procedure for Nurses and Internes*, 3rd edn, pp. 24, 83. London: Putnam.

FORD, C. R., PETERSON, D. E. AND MITCHELL, C. R. (1967) *American Journal of Surgery*, **6**, 787.

FURUHASHI, M. (1978) *Bulletin Tokyo Medical Dental University*, **25**, 7.

GODFREY, B. (1983) Checking swabs without using a swab rack, *NATNews*, **21**, September.

HILL, J., HOWELL, A. AND BLOWERS, R. (1974) *Lancet*, ii, 1131.

LE BOURDAS, E. (1975) *Dimensions in Health Services*. 52, (2), 27 (Toronto).

LIDWELL, O. M., MACKINTOSH, C. A. AND TOWERS, A. G. (1978) *Journal of Hygiene, Cambridge*, **81**, 43.

LIDWELL, O. M. (1984) Bacterial considerations in *The Design and Utilisation of Operating Theatres*. Edited by I. D. A. Johnston and A. R. Hunter. London: Edward Arnold.

LILY, H. A., LOWBURY, E. J. L., WILKINS, M. D. AND ZAGGY, A. (1979) Delayed antimicrobial effects of skin disinfection by alcohol. *Journal of Hygiene*, 82, 497–500.

LOWBURY, E. J. L., LILLY, H. A. AND BULL, J. P. (1964) *British Medical Journal*, ii, 531.

MEDICAL RESEARCH COUNCIL (1968) Aseptic methods in the operating suite. *Lancet*, i, 763.

MEDICAL DEFENCE UNION, MEDICAL PROTECTION SOCIETY., MEDICAL AND DEFENCE UNION OF SCOTLAND., NATIONAL ASSOCIATION OF THEATRE NURSES, AND ROYAL COLLEGE OF NURSING OF THE UNITED KINGDOM (1986) *Theatre Safeguards*, MDU, MPS, MDU of S, NATN, RCN.

MEFFEN, K. (1980) The good and the bad. *Nursing Mirror NATN Supplement*, Oct 9,

MINISTRY OF HEALTH (1959) *Report on Subcommittee on Staphylococcal Infection in Hospitals*, p. 35. London: HMSO.

MINTER, S. (1952) *Theatre Technique for Nurses*, pp. 2, 10. London: Nursing Mirror.

MITCHELL, N. J. AND GAMBLE, D. R. (1974) *Lancet*, ii, 1133.

MITCHELL, N. J., EVANS, D. S. AND KERR, ANN. (1978) *Lancet*, **i**, 696.

MOYLON, J. (1986) The importance of gown and drape barriers in the reduction of the incidence of post-operative wound infection. *NATNews*, June.

MURIE, J. A. AND MACPHERSON, S. G. (1980) Chlorhexidine in methanol for the pre-operative cleansing of surgeons' hands: a clinical trial. *Scottish Medical Journal*, **25**, 309–311.

NAGAI, I., KADOTA, M., TAKECHI, M., KUMAMOTO, R., NAKANO, S. AND JITSUKAWA, S. (1986) Studies on the bacterial permeability of non-woven fabrics and cotton fabrics. *Journal of Hospital Infection*, **7**, 261–268.

NATIONAL ASSOCIATION OF THEATRE NURSES (1983) *Guidelines to the total patient care and safe practice in operating theatres. Codes of Practice*, NATN, Harrogate.

ORR NEIL, W. M. (1981) Is a mask necessary in the operating theatre? *Annals of the Royal College of Surgeons of England*, **63**, 390–1.

PORTER, A. (1984) Unmasking the facts. *Nursing Mirror NATN Supplement*, Oct 10.

REYBROUCK, G. (1986) Hand washing and hand disinfection — a review article. *Journal of Hospital Infection*, **8**, 5–23.

RITTER, M. A., EITZEN, H. E., HART, J. B. AND FRENCH, M. L. V. (1980) The surgeon's garb. *Clinical Orthopaedics and Related Research*, **153**, Nov/Dec.

ROTTER, M. L. (1981) Povidone-iodine and chlorhexidine gluconate containing detergents for disinfection of hands. *Journal of Hospital Infection*, **2**, 273–275.

ROGERS, K. B. (1980) An investigation into the efficiency of disposable face masks. *Journal of Clinical Pathology*, **33**, 1086–1091.

SMYLIE, H. G., WEBSTER, C. V. AND BRUCE, M. L. (1959) *British Medical Journal*, **ii**, 606.

SPEERS, R. AND SHOOTER, R. A. (1966) *Lancet*, **ii**, 469.

SCHWEIZER, R. T. (1976) *Lancet*, **ii**, 1129.

SHAW, H. (1984) Checking swabs without using a swab rack, *NATNews*, **22**, February.

TAYLOR, L. J. (1980) Are face masks necessary in operating theatres. *Journal of Hospital Infection*, **1**, 173–4.

WÄLLENBERG, E. AND JÄRNHALL, B. (1956) *Svenska Läkartidningen*. **53**, 2578.

WHITE, J. J. AND DUNCAN, A. (1972) The comparative effectiveness of iodophor and hexachlorophane surgical scrub solutions. *Surgery, Gynaecology and Obstetrics*, **135**, 890–892.

WHYTE, W., HODGSON, R., BAILEY, P. V. AND GRAHAM, J. (1978) *British Journal of Surgery*, **65**, 469.

WHYTE, W., BAILEY, P. V., HAMBLIN, D. L., FISHER, W. D. AND KELLY, I. G. (1983) A bacteriologically occlusive clothing system for use in the operating room. *Journal of Bone and Joint Surgery*, **65-B**, No 4, August.

WHYTE, W. AND BAILEY, P. V. (1984) Reduction of microbial dispersion by clothing. *Journal of Parenteral Science and Technology*, **39**, No 1, Jan/Feb.

WILLIAMS, R. F. O., BLOWERS, R. AND GARRARD, L. P. (1966) *Hospital Infection — Causes and Prevention*.

YEAGER, M. E. (1966) *Operating Room Manual*, 2nd edn, p. 18. London: Putnam.

7

Sterilization

An understanding of the methods adopted for the sterilization of instruments, utensils and materials used in the operating theatre is one of the most important aspects of theatre technique.

The preferred method of sterilization (i.e. the destruction of all micro-organisms *including bacterial spores*) is by heat. However, gamma irradiation is used commercially for the sterilization of ligatures and sutures, implants, catheters and other heat labile products.

Disinfection (i.e. the destruction of all micro-organisms *except bacterial spores*) can be achieved by low temperature steam and chemicals. The addition of measured quantities of formaldehyde to the low temperature steam process will effect sterilization.

A great deal of research and many tests have been made regarding the minimal times and temperatures for sterilization by a particular method. Times and temperatures quoted in this chapter allow a margin of safety.

Bacteria and their destruction

A simple bacterium consists mainly of a cell wall surrounding protoplasm, which is a suspension of proteins in a solution of organic substances and salts.

One of the easiest ways of destroying bacteria is to upset the equilibrium of the protoplasm. The simplest and surest way is to apply heat to cause some irreversible protoplasmic change within the bacterial cell. This coagulation of protein depends to a great extent on the quantity of water contained within the bacteria. Vegetative bacteria contain about 80 per cent water, and as a result their protein coagulates readily at a relatively low temperature, and they are easily destroyed by five minutes exposure to boiling water (Perkins, 1956a; Gardner and Peel, 1986). However, some bacteria contain within their protoplasms, oval or spherical bodies which will survive boiling; these bodies are called spores. During sterilization, the aim must be to destroy all bacteria including their spores.

The effect of moisture on the coagulation temperature of proteins bears a relationship to the temperatures at which bacteria are destroyed. Moist heat rather than dry heat is the preferred sterilization agent, for when moisture is present bacteria are destroyed at much lower temperatures and shorter times than when moisture is absent.

When dry heat is used for sterilization the process is primarily one of oxidation. When bacteria are exposed to dry heat, before the temperature can rise sufficiently to cause death by coagulation, a process of dehydration has taken place. It is for this reason that death by dry heat is regarded as a slow burning-up process or oxidation.

It is inadvisable to refer to the destruction of bacteria at a certain point (thermal death point) (McCulloch, 1945). A more accurate term refers to the combination of temperature and time (thermal death time): the higher the temperature, the shorter the time of exposure

needed. Generally speaking, a temperature of 121°C at 1.05 kg per cm^2 (101 kPa), 15 lb per square inch [p.s.i] of pressure steam for 15 minutes, will kill the most resistant spores. This timing commences only *when the correct temperature of steam has reached* **all** *parts of the materials being sterilized*. It is therefore considered necessary to allow a safety margin of time equivalent usually to about double the thermal death time to ensure adequate penetration of packs. However, *individual tests must be conducted to determine the penetration time with a particular type of sterilizer and pack.*

Sterilization by dry heat requires much higher thermal death times. As bacteria show a marked resistance to dry heat, a temperature of 160°C with an exposure of one hour is necessary to achieve the destruction of micro-organisms. This exposure period of one hour does not, of course, include the period of time necessary for all parts of the load to reach the temperature of 160°C.

Although dry heat is destructive to rubber and fabrics, it can be used for the sterilization of glassware and instruments, such as fine knives, made from carbon steel which may otherwise rust if exposed to moist heat, and where sterilization of surfaces only is required.

The effect of chemicals on bacteria is rather a complex action which varies with the nature of the chemicals used. A chemical reaction occurs between the bacteria and the chemical, being dependent on several factors including temperature, chemical strength, freshness of the chemical, resistance of the organism and, most important, the duration of free contact between the two. The chemical effect can be one of oxidation, halogenation, poisoning of vital enzymes, hydrolysis and coagulation.

METHODS OF STERILIZATION (GENERAL PRINCIPLES)

Heat sterilization

1. Autoclaving (steam under pressure).
2. Dry heat.
3. Low temperature steam/formaldehyde.

Cold sterilization

4. Gamma-irradiation.
5. Ethylene Oxide.
6. Glutaraldehyde.

HEAT STERILIZATION

1. AUTOCLAVING

This is by far the most efficient method of sterilization for materials that will stand up to heat and moisture (Medical Research Council, 1968).

The highest temperature that can be reached by boiling water in an open vessel is 100°C.

With increased pressure, the water can be raised to much higher temperatures before it boils, e.g., at a pressure of 0.35 kg per cm² (34.5 kPa, 5 p.s.i.) the temperature reaches 105.5°C; at 0.7 kg per cm² (69 kPa, 10 p.s.i.). 115°C; and at 1.05 kg per cm² (103 kPa, 15 p.s.i.) the temperature will reach 121°C, etc.

High pressures of steam, however, are not the only consideration for efficient sterilization, as a pressure could result from a mixture of air and steam with a relatively low temperature (Gardner and Peel, 1986). It is the high *temperatures* that really matter but, in addition, the steam should be at a point where it has just changed from water into steam (phase boundary of saturated steam) (Walter, 1948). In this condition the steam not only has an increased temperature in relation to the pressure (sensible heat), but when it condenses on a cold surface (the materials being sterilized) a great deal of extra heat (latent heat) is given up. The latent heat absorbed by the materials being sterilized is more important for the destruction of bacteria than the sensible heat.

The steam heating of fabrics being sterilized by a process of condensation is relatively rapid (McCulloch, 1945), as compared with dry-heat sterilization, which is slow, heat being conducted from one instrument to another and from one container to the next, etc.

The physical process of heating the fabrics to the sterilizing temperature can be described as follows:

In a sterilizer chamber (autoclave) which has been well exhausted of air the steam entering promptly fills the free spaces surrounding the load. As steam contacts the cool outer layers of the fabrics a film of steam condenses, leaving a minute quantity of moisture in the fibres of the fabrics. Air contained in the fabric interstices, being heavier than steam, is displaced by gravity in a downward direction, and the latent heat given off during the process of condensation is absorbed by that layer of the fabrics.

The next film of steam immediately fills the space created when the first film condensed into water, and it does not condense on the outer layer of the fabrics but penetrates into the second layer, condenses and heats it. This process continues until the whole load is heated through, and no further condensation occurs, the temperature within the pack remaining at that of the surrounding steam.

If initial air elimination from the chamber is not good it will be difficult for the steam to displace air from the interstices of the fabrics, due to the small difference in density between the air pockets in the packs or caskets, and the air that has gravitated below the load to the bottom of the chamber. This means that the pocketed air and steam may eventually mix, but it will be impossible to attain a sterilizing temperature which is equivalent to that of the surrounding steam without prolonged exposure. A procedure involving steam pulsing or a multi-vacuum technique helps to extract this air and thoroughly heat the load before sterilization commences (Knox and Pickerill, 1964, 1967). Exceptions to this rule are instruments, which require only one pre-vacuum, as the air displacement from these loads is comparatively rapid if they are packed correctly.

In the high-vacuum/high-pressure sterilizer where an electric pump is used to obtain a vacuum, all air may be extracted in one operation, or there may be a series of pre-vacuums and steam pulsations before the sterilizing cycle. This breaks down any small airpockets and results in a final pressure of air left in the chamber of less than minus 98.8 kPa below atmospheric pressure (2.5 kPa to 0.066 kPa or 20–0.5 mmHg absolute pressure).

It will be observed that the steam used for sterilization of materials must have a certain temperature and pressure in order to be effective. Furthermore, the steam must reach all parts of the load and unless packs are prepared very carefully, adequate penetration cannot be ensured. Materials should be packed with good spacing between the articles, with folds placed vertically to allow steam to pass easily in a downward direction through them, any

Table 7.1 Sterilization by heat

A. Steam sterilizer, gravity or downward displacement type

Materials Being Sterilized	Initial Vacuum (Twice)		Initial Steam Cycle		Sterilizing Steam Cycle			Final Vacuum (Drying)		Total Cycle (Approx.)
	Degree	Holding Time	Pressure	Temp.	Pressure	Temp.	Holding Time	Degree	Holding Time	
Gowns, towels, dressings, etc.; in paper or linen packets	300 mmHg (39.47 kPa) to 250 mmHg (32.8 kPa)	5 min (each time)	1.41 kg per cm² (136 kPa, 20 p.s.i.)	125°C	1.41 kg per cm² (136 kPa, 20 p.s.i.)	125°C	30 min	300 mmHg (39.47 kPa) to 250 mmHg (32.8 kPa)	40 min	90 min
			1.76 kg per cm² (169 kPa, 25 p.s.i.)	130°C	1.76 kg per cm² (169 kPa, 25 p.s.i.)	130°C	25 min		30 min	75 min
Metal instruments unwrapped on open trays, ligatures, etc.	Not needed		Not needed		1.76 kg per cm² (169 kPa, 25 p.s.i.)	130°C	6 min	Not needed		7 min
Metal instruments with minimal wrappings, ligatures, etc.	Not needed		Not needed		1.76 kg per cm² (169 kPa, 25 p.s.i.)	130°C	6 min	450 mmHg (59.2 kPa)	1 to 2 min	9 min
Metal instruments, ligatures, etc., in packets with normal wrappings	300 mmHg (39.47 kPa) to 250 mmHg (32.8 kPa)	5 min (once only)	Not needed		1.76 kg per cm² (169 kPa, 25 p.s.i.)	130°C	15 min	300 mmHg (39.47 kPa) to 250 mmHg (32.8 kPa)	7 to 10 min	27 to 30 min
Rubber gloves. (With gloves in upper part of chamber)	300 mmHg (39.47 kPa) to 250 mmHg (32.8 kPa)	5 min (once only)	1.76 kg per cm² (169 kPa, 25 p.s.i.)	130°C	1.76 kg per cm² (169 kPa, 25 p.s.i.)	130°C	6 min	450 mmHg (59.2 kPa)	5 min	30 min
			2.25 kg per cm² (218 kPa, 32 p.s.i.)	134°C	2.25 kg per cm² (218 kPa, 32 p.s.i.)	134°C	3 min	450 mmHg (59.2 kPa)	3 min	20 min
Topical fluids	Not needed		Not needed		0.7 kg per cm² (69 kPa, 10 p.s.i.)	116°C	60 min	Gradual exhaust of steam from chamber		
					1.05 kg per cm² (101 kPa, 15 p.s.i.)	121°C	45 min			

Table 7.1 Sterilization by heat (*contd.*)
B. Steam sterilizer, High-vacuum/High pressure type

Materials Being Sterilized	Initial Vacuum	Sterilizing Steam Cycle	Final Vacuum (Drying)	Total Cycle
Gowns, towels, dressings, metal instruments etc., in packs	Approximately 0.5 to 1 mmHg (0.066 to 0.132 kPa)	$3\frac{1}{2}$ min 134°C	5 to 10 min	Approximately 25 min

C. Dry-heat steriliser

Articles Being Sterilized	Period
Syringes, compressed air drills, some types of electric drills and saws, powders, osteotomes, etc.	With efficient circulation of hot air these should be exposed for a period of 60 minutes when the temperature has reached 160°C in all parts of the load. This may mean a total cycle of between $1\frac{1}{2}$ and $2\frac{1}{2}$ hours, or more.

D. Pasteurization

Articles Being Sterilized	Period
Endoscopes (cystoscopes, etc.)	Process in low temperature steam/formaldehyde sterilizer at 82°C for 90 minutes, total-cycle approximately $2\frac{1}{2}$ hours. Maintain in a hot-water bath at 75°C for 10 minutes (ensure they are completely covered and allow time for water to regain temperature when cool endoscope is added to the bath).

tendency to force too many items in one pack being avoided. A linen or paper pack should not be wrapped tightly to fit in an inadequate size of cover.

Unless a pre-set tray is used, utilising heavy-gauge aluminium trays (p. 150) it is difficult to dry large quantities of metal instruments with bulky drapes. The unequal rate of condensation between the fabrics and instruments will require an extended drying cycle.

Arrangements for the correct supply of steam and maintenance of the apparatus is not a responsibility of the nurse, but if packs are wet or damaged when removed from the autoclave there is something wrong with the apparatus or its operation and the sterilizer engineer should be consulted before the apparatus is used again.

In the gravity displacement sterilizer after a partial vacuum of about 500 mm (minus 66 kPa) has been created, (an absolute pressure of 250 mmHg, 33 kPa); standard atmospheric pressure being 760 mmHg), steam is admitted to the chamber and applied to the load until the selected temperature/pressure has been reached *in the chamber*. (Very low pressures are generally quoted with reference to the perfect vacuum.) Air from the interstices of the fabrics which has been displaced into the lower part of the chamber, but has not been discharged by the special thermostatic condensate release valve, is extracted by a second vacuum. A second application of steam displaces most of the remaining air pockets and thoroughly heats the load throughout to the surrounding steam temperature.

Sterilization by autoclaving (application of methods)

'Mains steam' (supplied from a boiler house) is used to operate most moist heat sterilizers which are generally of three types, (1) the high-vacuum/high pressure machines, (2) the gravity or downward displacement porous load machines, and (3) the 'flash' instrument sterilizers. Sterilizers are available which generate their own steam by electricity, and these are used in a similar manner to the mains steam models.

The high-vacuum/high pressure sterilizer

This operates at a pressure of between 2.25 and 2.46 kg cm^2 (221 to 241 kPa) (32 to 35 p.s.i), at a temperature of 134°C to 136°C. A high vacuum pump removes air from the chamber down to a final pressure of less than 0.5 mmHg absolute (0.066 kPa). The process is controlled automatically.

Although in earlier models of this apparatus attempts were made to obtain a high vacuum in one stage, it has been found that utilising a vacuum pump only will not achieve a vacuum much lower than minus 98.8 kPa below atmospheric pressure (2.5 kPa or 20 mmHg absolute pressure). This was followed by steam at 134°C for 3 minutes, a post vacuum of varying degree and admission of filtered air to the chamber. This type of cycle did not give consistent results for it often depended upon how the chamber was loaded and the kind of materials being sterilized.

Research has shown that a pre-vacuum/steam pulsation technique will achieve a much better removal of air from the sterilizer chamber before sterilization (Bolton, 1966; Knox and Pickerill, 1967). Basically, steam pulsation technique consists of allowing a charge of steam to enter the chamber after an initial high vacuum has been drawn, then following this by another vacuum draw and repeating the process to give two or more steam pulses. The logic is that any residual air is diluted each time and replaced with water vapour; each steam pulse and vacuum draw resulting in repeated reduction of air content without reducing the total pressure in the chamber. The high-vacuum/high-pressure sterilizer relies upon a pre-

vacuum stage which reduces the air content in the chamber to 0.5 mmHg absolute (0.066 kPa) or less.

With negligible air in the chamber and some pre-heating of the load, penetration of steam into the items being sterilized is very rapid. High temperatures in the region of 134°C are reached very quickly and an exposure to this temperature for 3.5 minutes will ensure sterility. It is important though, as mentioned previously, that all parts of the load must reach this temperature before timing commences. For automatic control of process a simple and accurate means of measuring the partial air pressure (pre-vacuum) and a load simulator which simulates the conditions within the pack are required. This obviates the need for a thermocouple within the load to control the process.

Depending on the size of a load the total cycle in this type of sterilizer is from 25 to 35 minutes. The chamber can be fully loaded with soft packs provided a few centimetres of space is allowed between the load and the chamber wall. An angled condensate plate should be fitted underneath each shelf on which pre-set trays are being sterilized. These slope downwards to one or other side of the chamber in order to prevent drips of condensate from the lower surface of a tray above wetting a tray below (Fig. 6.22).

The cycle of operation

For a high-vacuum/high-pressure sterilizer, this can be summarised as follows.

After loading the chamber and closing the door:

Stage 1. Pre-vacuum — air removal. The air is removed from the chamber by a vacuum pump and controlled steam pulsations. The vacuum achieved should be in the order of 0.5 mmHg absolute (0.066 to 0.132 kPa) (Fig. 7.2).

Stage 2. Sterilization — hold period at operating temperature. Steam is admitted to the chamber and when all parts of the load have reached a temperature of 134°C this is maintained for 3.5 minutes (Fig. 7.3).

Stage 3. Drying. Achieved by an adequate post vacuum, checked periodically by a test pack of towels which when removed from the sterilizer, unfolded and allowed to cool are not damp (Fig. 7.4).

Stage 4. Breaking the vacuum — air replacement. This should be completed within 3 minutes, through a glass fibre or ceramic type filter (Fig. 7.5).

The chamber is unloaded and the packs marked with the batch number of that particular load. Pre-set trays should have a water repellent or plastic dust cover applied if they are to be stored for more than a few hours. This cover should be applied only after the trays have cooled off.

Performance tests for high-vacuum/high-pressure sterilizers

Sterilizers are complex pieces of machinery which incorporate built-in safeguards which should interrupt the sterilization cycle should a fault occur. But this is not always so and the sterilizer may appear to function correctly when in fact it does not.

There are many faults which can occur, for example inadequate extraction of air from the sterilizer chamber during the pre-vacuum stage. This may be due to a faulty pump or to air that is trapped or has leaked back through faulty door seals or valves. This means that steam can penetrate the load only slowly and in an irregular manner, which can result in unsterile packs.

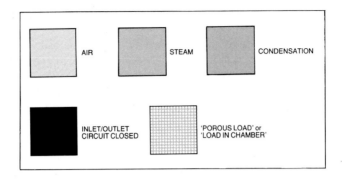

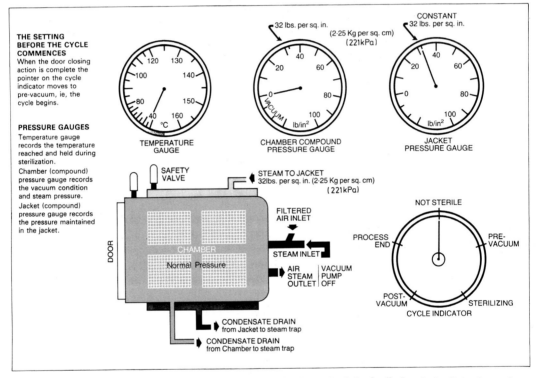

Fig. 7.1   The setting before the cycle commences. (*A Training Handbook for Sterile Supply Staff*, Institute of Sterile Services Management.)

The efficient functioning of a sterilizer depends on regular planned maintenance. This may be undertaken by a hospital engineer trained in sterilizer maintenance, but if the expertise is unavailable locally then it is essential that the sterilizer manufacturer services the machine periodically. This will involve performance tests, some of which should also be carried out on a daily or weekly basis by suitably qualified hospital staff (HTM 10, DHSS).

The performance tests required are:

1. Bowie/Dick test *performed daily.*
2. Vacuum and leak rate test *performed weekly.*
3. Air detector function test *performed weekly.*

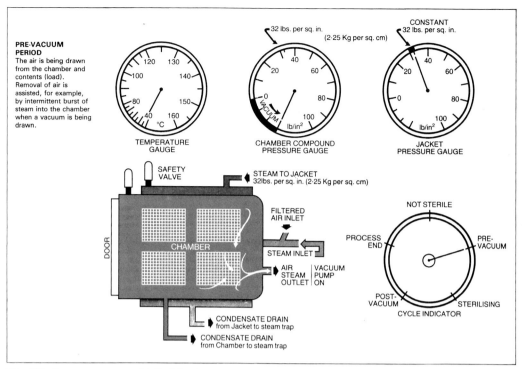

Fig. 7.2 Pre-vacuum stage. (*A Training Handbook for Sterile Supply Staff*, Institute of Sterile Services Management.)

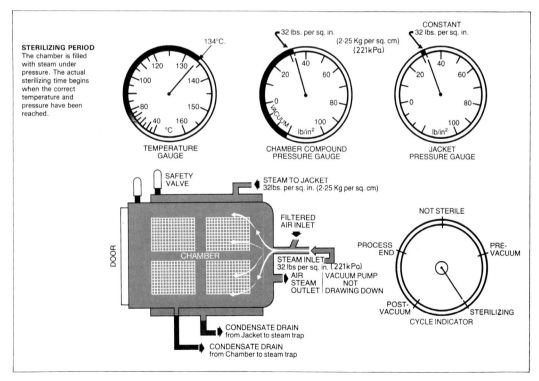

Fig. 7.3 Sterilizing stage. (*A Training Handbook for Sterile Supply Staff*, Institute of Sterile Services Management.)

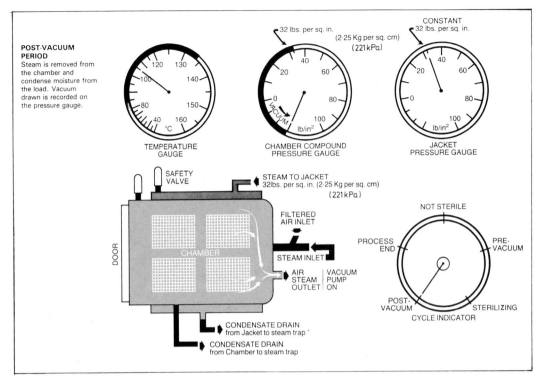

Fig. 7.4 Post-vacuum stage. (*A Training Handbook for Sterile Supply Staff*, Institute of Sterile Services Management.)

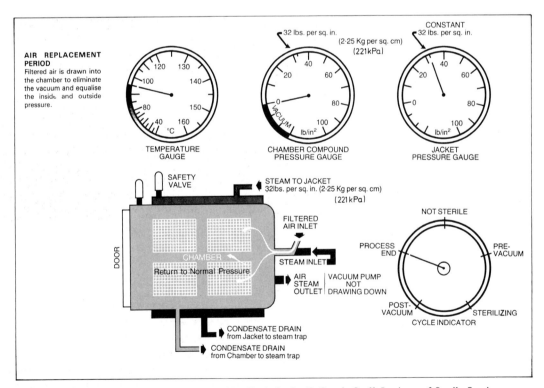

Fig. 7.5 Air-replacement stage. (*A Training Handbook for Sterile Supply Staff*, Institute of Sterile Services Management.)

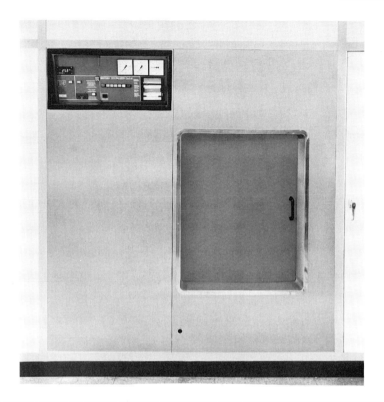

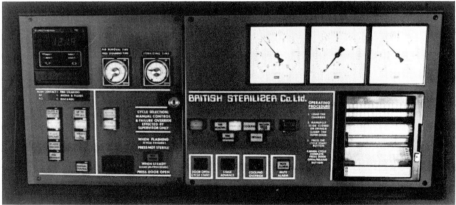

Fig. 7.6   High-vacuum/high pressure autoclave. (British Sterilizer Co. Ltd.)

4. Temperature and automatic control test *performed weekly*.
5. Steam quality test *performed during commissioning/recommissioning*.
6. Air detector performance test (small load) *performed yearly*.
7. Air detector performance test (full load) *performed yearly*.
8. Commissioning and re-commissioning tests *quarterly and yearly*.

Tests may also involve the use of thermocouples (temperature sensors) in addition to those fitted as part of the operating system. These sensors are placed in various positions within a test pack, and are connected to a control panel via wires which are contained in heat

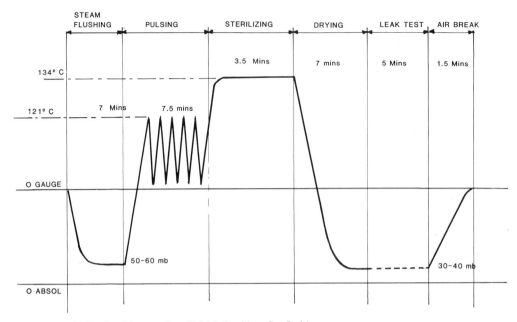

Fig. 7.7 Graph showing hi-vac cycles. (British Sterilizer Co. Ltd.)

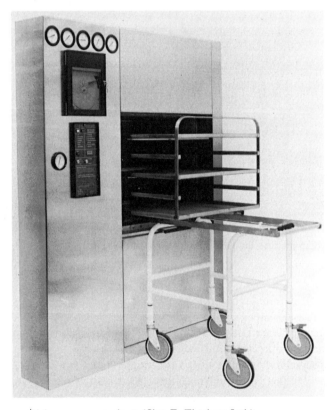

Fig. 7.8 High-vacuum/high pressure autoclave. (Chas.F. Thackray Ltd.)

resistant insulation. The wires of these thermocouples generally enter the chamber through steam-tight glands in the chamber wall. Such thermocouples are also used during tests on dry heat sterilizers and the low temperature steam and formaldehyde sterilizers which will be described later. Thermocouples enable temperatures in the test pack to be checked at any time during the sterilization process, and the rate of temperature rise during heat penetration to various parts of the load is clearly shown.

A very important instrument on the sterilizer is a time chart recording the sterilizing cycles. This chart will indicate the pre-vacuum, temperatures reached, and relative time periods of each stage in the sterilizing process. It is a reliable check for the SDU manager or operating department manager, who is often unable to supervise every sterilizing laod. Once the correct operating procedure has been determined, any variation by the sterilizer operator is easily observed, and the record chart is permanent for future reference. The Department of Health specify that temperature and pressure readings should be taken at least three times during the sterilizing stage (DHSS, 1987).

Two of the physical performance tests will be described in detail: the Bowie/Dick test and the Vacuum and Air leak rate test.

The Bowie/Dick indicator tape test. This test is a means of determining the efficiency of air removal from the sterilizer chamber during the pre-vacuum cycle. It does not indicate directly that sterilization is achieved, but that air removal has been adequate to allow sterilization to take place at 134°C for 3.5 minutes. In practice this is very simple. A standard test pack is made up consisting of 36 towels, 0.6 m^2 (2 ft^2), (complying with B.S.I. 1781.TL.5 and HTM 10) folded and forming a stack 25 to 28 cm (10 to 11 in) high (Bowie, 1961; Bowie *et al.*, 1963, 1975; Morris and Everall, 1975; DHSS, 1986). In the centre is placed a piece of paper 30 cm (12 in) square to which has been fixed a cross of sterilizer indicator tape (or a complete sheet of indicator tape (TSS/S/330/013, DHSS). The towels should be washed initially before using and whenever they become soiled or discoloured. Between tests they are unfolded and hung out to air for at least one hour. Alternatively two cubes of spun bonded polypropylene — the Lantor cube — can be used; the test sheet is placed between the two (Hambleton, 1986).

The test pack is placed in a perforated metal casket (BS1, 1960) or wrapped in fabric or paper. It is now placed by itself in the sterilizer and subjected to a standard sterilizing cycle.

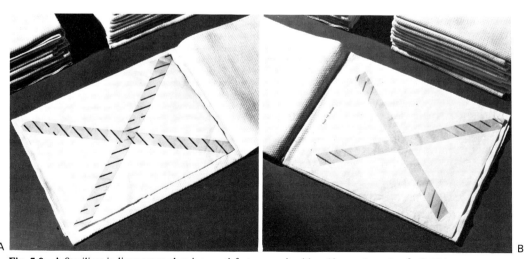

A   B

Fig. 7.9 A Sterilizer indicator tape showing a satisfactory result with uniform colour change. B This is an unsatisfactory result — the colour change is irregular and incomplete in the centre.

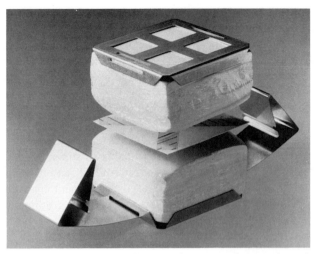

Fig. 7.10 Lantor test cube: a synthetic polypropylene autoclave test pack as an alternative to the Bowie/Dick towel pack. (3M Health Care.)

Care must be taken to ensure that the 'Holding' or 'Sterilizing' time does not exceed 3.5 minutes at 134°C. If the automatic cycle is set for a longer holding time this must be cut short, for the purposes of the test, to 3.5 minutes, by using the manual control. Should there be any doubt about this the technician or engineer responsible for maintenance of the sterilizer should be asked for advice.

When the cycle is finished the pack is removed and the paper with the tape is examined. After a satisfactory run the tape will show a colour change *which is the same at the centre as the edges.* If the tape at the centre is paler than it is at the edges, it means there was a bubble of air there and the sterilizer was not working correctly. If this happens, the sterilizer must be taken out of service immediately until the fault has been rectified.

Unless the test is carried out exactly as described it may not be truly reliable. In particular the following points should be noted.

1. The test should be carried out each day. The first cycle of the sterilizer should be an empty chamber, followed by the second cycle with only the Bowie/Dick test. This is followed by subsequent runs.

2. The more air there is to remove, the more exacting will be the test and that is why the test pack is used by itself in an otherwise empty chamber.

3. The exact colour change shown by the processed tape may depend upon the storage conditions of that tape. The important thing is whether the *same colour change* occurs at the centre and the edges.

4. The contrast in colour change from centre to edge will be reduced to an unreadable level if long 'holding' periods are used. That is why the *'holding' period must not exceed 3.5 minutes at 134°C.* Even an extra minute or two may seriously affect a comparison of results.

5. *Because of this it is very important to realise that if an autoclave fails to pass the Bowie/Dick test as described, it cannot be made safe merely by increasing the 'holding' time until a uniform colour change is produced. Such a sterilizer is in urgent need of skilled attention.*

6. The Bowie/Dick test is relevant only to high-vacuum/high-pressure autoclaves. It is valueless in downward displacement autoclaves.

Vacuum and leak test (instrumentation required). In order to carry out this test the ster-

ilizer requires additional instrumentation fitted, which is capable of measuring small variations in the degree of vacuum attainable within the chamber. Most autoclaves already incorporate the necessary instrumentation as follows:

1. The control camshaft is modified so that a position can be obtained manually directly subsequent to the *pre-vacuum* position, when all valves on the camshaft are closed. This position has a location cam and a significant reference mark on the camshaft position indicator, known as the *leak test* position.

2. A 0 to 100 mmHg (0 to minus 13.17 kPa) absolute pressure gauge (tolerance ± one per cent F.S. reading) is mounted on the front panel, and connected via a manual valve directly beneath it in series with an electrical solenoid valve (normally closed to the chamber by the shortest route in copper pipe of a least 0.6 cm (0.25 in) diameter, in such a way that the pipe will drain into the chamber.

The solenoid is operated by a micro-switch actuated by the control camshaft so that the valve is opened only when the camshaft is in the 'pre-vacuum' and the 'leak test' positions.

3. A toggle switch is mounted on the front panel adjacent to the absolute pressure gauge. This switch is wired in series with the coil of the vacuum pump motor contactor, so that the contactor may be de-energised and the motor stopped.

4. A Smith's or similar 0 to 30 minutes timer is useful mounted on the front panel adjacent to the absolute pressure gauge.

5. An extra outlet may be fitted in parallel with, and adjacent to the absolute pressure gauge, so that the gauge can be calibrated regularly against either a standard gauge or mercury column.

Note: Any other method may be used provided that the chamber is isolated by the valves which are normally used during a process, so that they are tested for leakage. Indeed, the micro processor which controls the sterilizer may be programmed to carry out this test automatically.

The recommended post-vacuum pressure should be less than 50 mmHg (6.6 kPa absolute pressure) and it is possible to modify the camshaft in such a way that the solenoid valve to the leak test gauge can be opened and the post-vacuum pressure checked.

From this rather technical description of the instrumentation required the reader may imagine that the actual test is equally complex. This is not so for the vacuum and leak test can be conducted effectively by any supervisor of an SDU or operating department service unit.

Method of performing the test (autoclave instrumentation as described):

1. Close and lock the door with the chamber empty. The sterilizer must be on manual control.

2. Turn the control cam-shaft to *pre-vacuum* position and open manual valve beneath the absolute pressure gauge.

3. When the pressure indicated on the absolute pressure gauge is less than 20 mmHg (2.6 kPa), turn the control camshaft to *leak test* position, and wait 10 seconds for the vacuum valve to close.

4. Turn the toggle switch to the *off* position and wait until the needle on the absolute pressure gauge starts to return.

5. When the gauge needle starts to return, take a reading, set and start the timer for 10 minutes. When the timer reaches zero take another reading on the absolute pressure gauge.

6. Close the manual valve beneath the absolute pressure gauge and turn the toggle switch to *on*.

7. Rotate the control camshaft to *post-vacuum* position and hold for 4 minutes. Note the reading on the absolute pressure gauge and rotate control camshaft once again to the *break-*

vacuum' or *'off'* position. Finally where applicable, press the automatic *re-set* button and with the control camshaft in the *'off'* position, the door may be opened.

The test can be deemed a failure if the vacuum fails to reach 20 mmHg (2.6 kPa), or the leak at stage 4 is greater than 1 mmHg (0.132 kPa) per minute. If this result is observed, skilled engineering assistance must be obtained and the cause of the fault investigated immediately.

Use of the high-vacuum/high-pressure sterilizer is a very effective method of steam sterilization, providing regular efficiency tests and maintenance are instituted. It may not be possible to perform the vacuum and leak tests due to the appropriate instrumentation being non-existent. However, the Bowie/Dick Test must be carried out daily as described and will provide a reliable means of assessing the efficiency of the sterilizer.

The gravity-displacement sterilizer

Working pressure is 1.05 kg to 2.11 kg per cm² (103 to 207 kPa) 15 p.s.i. to 30 p.s.i., vacuum is 380 to 508 mmHg (minus 50 to minus 67 kPa) via an ejector valve. It consists basically of a circular or rectangular metal chamber, surrounded by a hollow jacket of a similar material, being designed to withstand pressures of steam in excess of those in use. A suitable door, also designed to withstand high pressures of steam, and controlled by a single hand wheel is fitted to one end of the chamber.

Steam reaching the sterilizer from the boiler house is usually at a much higher pressure than required. A reducing valve reduces this pressure from about 5.55 kg per cm² (552 kPa,

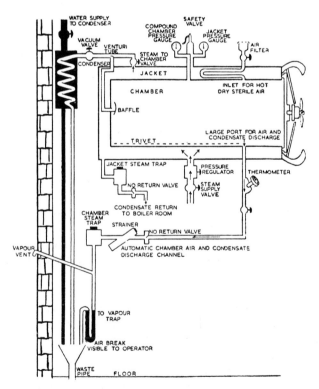

Fig. 7.11 Diagram of a steam-pressure sterilizer of the gravity air displacement type. (The late J. M. Bowie — by kind permission.)

80 p.s.i.) to the level required and prevents any greater pressure of steam entering the sterilizer than the maximum pressure at which it is designed to operate.

To sterilize

1. The inner chamber is loaded with packs which are placed in such a way that free passage of steam through the material is possible. This usually means placing the packs on their sides so that the steam passes through the folded layers. As steam is lighter than the air which is displaced it should enter the chamber at the top, pass through the load, and be discharged at the bottom through the thermostatic release valve.

2. The door is securely closed with the bolts 'well home' and attempts must not be made to open it until the sterilization is complete and the chamber pressure gauge reads zero.

There are two important gauges that are fitted to a steam sterilizer, one recording the jacket pressure and one the chamber pressure. The pressure in the jacket may be kept on all day, but that in the chamber rises only when the appropriate valve is opened. Another essential accessory is the provision of a thermometer or thermocouple in the steam condensate release or discharge line, and when the correct temperature in relation to the pressure used has been reached by this thermometer the sterilization cycle commences.

3. The first stage is an initial vacuum, which is created and held for about 5 minutes, followed by the admittance of steam to the chamber. When the selected temperature/pressure has been reached *in the chamber*, a second vacuum is created and also held for 5 minutes. On the gravity displacement sterilizer there is a limiting factor to the greatest degree of vacuum obtainable. With some types, fitted with a powerful ejector, this may be in the region of 457 to 508 mmHg (minus 60 to 67 kPa), but the average vacuum does not usually exceed 380 mmHg (minus 50 kPa).

4. In the second stage the steam is admitted to the chamber again and raised to the selected temperature/pressure. For dressings, gowns and instruments, etc., in packs a temperature/pressure of 126°C, 1.41 kg per cm^2 (138 kPa, 20 p.s.i.) is maintained for 30 minutes.

During this second steam stage the holding time is correlated to the temperature indicated by the thermometer in the discharge line, which is always the coldest part of the chamber. During the period of sterilization this thermometer must register one of the following temperatures and the holding time from this point must be *not less than the time period stated*:

        134°C for 3 minutes.
        130°C for 4 minutes.
        125°C for 8 minutes.
        121°C for 12 minutes.
        115°C for 18 minutes.

This is the temperature and time relationship at which all parts of the load must be held and *it is advisable to increase the time by 50 per cent of that stated to ensure absolute safety.* The appropriate composite holding times and temperatures listed in Table 7.1 allows a margin of safety.

5. The steam is released from the chamber, and the materials, with the exception of gloves, are dried in a vacuum for 40 minutes to one hour. Gloves need only 6 minutes drying from the time the vacuum reaches 380 mm (minus 50 kPa).

The moisture remaining finely distributed in the dressings, etc., during the period of sterilization is at the same temperature as the surrounding steam. As soon as the pressure is reduced and the steam exhausted, this moisture flashes into vapour by virtue of the residual heat in the fabrics and from the surrounding hot jacket, the temperature of which is above

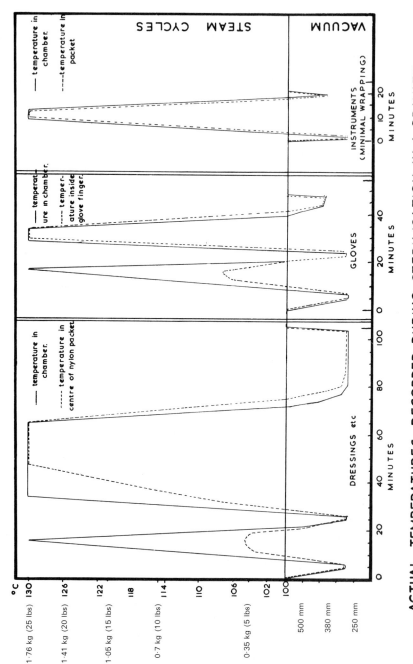

Fig. 7.12 Record of sterilizing temperature showing double-vacuum technique.

boiling point. The real drying process therefore consists of getting rid of this steam vapour as fast as it forms.

This constitutes the final stage of sterilization, and with an efficient sterilizer using steam at phase boundary point it should not be necessary to suck in air, which may be contaminated, except to break the vacuum. The air required for breaking the vacuum must be well-filtered, to avoid recontamination of the load, using a release valve incorporating a high-efficiency filter such as one made from glass fibre or ceramic material. This filter is flushed during the steam cycle by allowing free steam to permeate through it.

6. After the correct period of drying the sterilizer is switched off, the vacuum broken, *and when the chamber pressure gauge reads zero*, the door is opened. The operator should be wearing a clean overall and should wash his hands before unloading the chamber; an identification batch number should be applied to packs as they are unloaded.

Instrument and utensil sterilizers

Ideally all instruments used at operation should be wrapped in a pack for sterilization, but there may be occasions in the operating department when this is not possible. For example, the need to sterilize between operations a special instrument which has no duplicate; or more rarely the 'dropped instrument'.

In these instances the 'flash sterilizer' may be utilised. This is a gravity displacement sterilizer designed specifically for the sterilization of unwrapped instruments and utensils. Because the articles are unwrapped, special care is necessary to avoid contamination when removing from the sterilizer chamber and handling following sterilization.

The sterilizer chamber is non-jacketed, relatively small and generally cylindrical; air is removed during the cycle by gravity displacement. Although mains piped steam may be utilised, most 'flash sterilizers' are free standing bench models which use electricity to

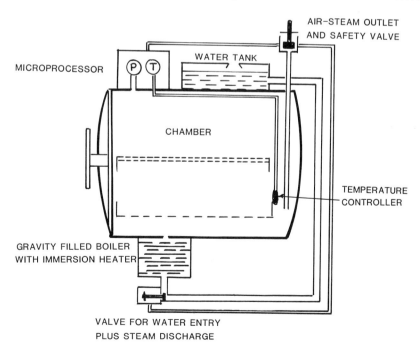

Fig. 7.13 Diagram of portable electrically heated 'flash' sterilizer.

generate their own steam from a self-contained water tank (Fig. 7.13). To avoid deposits of lime on instruments it is preferable to use demineralised or distilled water in the water tank.

Most modern 'flash sterilizers' incorporate microprocessors which control the operation of the machine automatically, taking account of the correct time/temperature relationships (Fig. 7.14). The procedure for operation is generally along the following lines:

1. Time can be saved by switching on the sterilizer in advance of requirement to preheat the water tank and warm the chamber. This will enable a cycle to be completed in about 10 minutes.

2. The perforated tray or basket in the chamber should not be overloaded. Each article must be positioned so as not to impede the flow of air out of the chamber. Bowls are placed on their sides and hinged instruments are sterilized in the open position.

3. The automatic cycle comprises:
   a. Removal of air and heating the chamber to the sterilizing temperature.
   b. Sterilization for 4 minutes at 132°C, or for 3 minutes at 134°C.
   c. Restoration of the chamber to atmospheric pressure by rapid exhaustion of steam.
   d. Venting of the chamber and opening immediately atmospheric pressure has been reached.

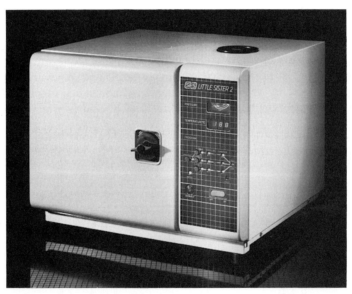

Fig. 7.14   Portable autoclave (Little Sister) which can be operated from a standard 13A power socket outlet. (Surgical Equipment Supplies Ltd.)

2. DRY HEAT (IN THE FORM OF HOT AIR)

This can be used for sterilizing many items, but is destructive to linen and rubber or plastic articles, etc. (Perkins, 1956b).

The articles which can be sterilized include non-disposable syringes, glassware, needles, mechanical power drills (some compressed air types), fine knives and other delicate instruments that will withstand this dry heat but not the wet methods. (The method is also applicable for sterilizing heat stable powders and non-aqueous liquids such as Vaseline, paraffin

oil, paraffin gauze dressings, eye 'ointment bases, oily injections, silicone lubricant and pure glycerol.) Suitable containers for sterilization and storage can be made from aluminium. Larger items can be folded in sheets of aluminium foil, but care must be taken not to compress the pack as puncture of the foil will occur.

Design of sterilizing ovens

The hot air electric oven is designed to achieve a uniform temperature throughout all parts of the load. The non-pressurized sterilizing chamber, insulated against heat loss, is fitted with perforated shelves to separate the packs or containers (Fig. 7.15). The heater bank is contained in a chamber on one side of, and separated from the sterilizing chamber by a perforated diffuser wall. An adjustable external air inlet opens into the heater chamber directly in front of the heater bank and a motor fan. Air is drawn through the air inlet over the heaters and forced into the sterilizer chamber through the perforated diffuser wall. As the warm air circulates and gives off some of its heat to the load, it passes back into the heater chamber, mixes with the incoming fresh air and the cycle is repeated. This forced circulation of air promotes even heating of the load being sterilized. Provision is made for the insertion of twelve thermocouples into the chamber for performance tests.

The most suitable dry heat sterilizers are those with automatic controls. These incorporate a sterilizing timer which returns to zero on power loss, and does not restart automatically; a control which prevents the cycle being started unless the door is locked, and prevents the door being opened until the cycle is finished; and a manually resettable overheat cut-out mechanism. There is an indicating thermometer and a chart recorder connected to heat sensors positioned in the chamber. Indicator lights are provided for power on, sterilizing in progress, and process complete. If a fault develops the door remains closed until the sterilizer is checked by an authorised person. Non-automatic dry heat sterilizers may be used but the door should be locked with a key retained by the person supervising the process.

Packing and loading

Instruments and glass syringes are cleansed and dried as described in Chapter 6 and packed in metal containers or aluminium foil. Glass syringes are sterilized assembled, and forceps are closed. Delicate instruments such as ophthalmic knives should be sterilized in a suitable metal rack to protect against damage during the handling process. Heavy metal instruments require a metal cradle in the sterilizing container to promote the conduction of heat. The chamber must not be overloaded; space should be allowed between instrument containers to permit the circulation of hot air.

Sterilization process

Pre-heating the oven before loading will reduce the time taken for the oven to reach sterilizing temperature. Timing is commenced *when all parts of the load* have attained the required temperature. HTM 10 (DHSS, 1987) recommends a temperature of 160°C held for a minimum of 60 minutes. This can be reduced to 40 minutes at 170°C and 20 minutes at 180°C. However, these higher temperatures may prove detrimental to the materials being sterilized, and 160°C for 60 minutes is the norm. Readers should note that the holding times/temperatures recommended in the United Kingdom conform to the British Pharmocopoeia (1980). In the United States, the US Pharmocopeia quotes a temperature of 160°C held for at least two hours.

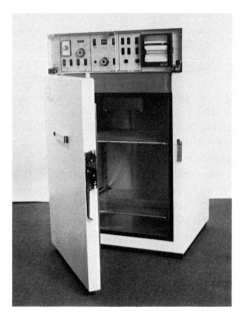

Fig. 7.15   Dry heat sterilizer. (Baird and Tatlock Ltd.)

The period taken for even heating of the load varies considerably with the capacity of the oven, type of load, and the containers in which the articles are packed. The total cycle time can extend to two hours or more, including heating the sterilizing chamber to the selected temperature, sterilizing, and eventually cooling the load.

It is possible to demonstrate the tidal movement of air out of, and subsequently into, metal containers during the sterilization process and cooling period. As the remaining sterile air in the container cools and contracts, a tidal flow of air occurs from the oven into the container. If containers are removed from the oven before adequate cooling occurs, there is a possibility that contaminated room air could be entrained. For this reason it is advisable to keep the oven door shut until the thermometer or recording pen indicates that the chamber temperature has dropped to 50°C. Dry heat sterilizers with automatic controls may prevent the door opening until this occurs.

When a new oven is purchased, and at periodic intervals, the performance of the oven and effectiveness of the sterilization process should be checked. Temperature levels are recorded with twelve thermocouples inserted into various packs or containers in a 'worst case' load. Chemical indicators such as Brownes tubes (page 196) are useful to show that containers have been processed.

3. LOW TEMPERATURE STEAM/FORMALDEHYDE STERILIZATION

Whilst the two previous methods are practical and effective ways of sterilizing most fabrics and instruments, there is still the problem of heat-labile articles such as plastics and optical devices. Three cold methods that can be relied upon to kill spores are: gamma irradiation (impracticable in most hospitals), the use of glutaraldehyde for sterilizing endoscopes, and careful microbiologically controlled ethylene oxide gas. But work by Alder and Gillespie at the Bristol Royal Infirmary in 1966 using steam at 90°C to disinfect blankets led to the

development of a method for the disinfection of heat-labile articles able to withstand temperatures up to 80°C. Subsequently, the method was modified to include exposure to formaldehyde vapour to effect sterilization.

In an appropriately designed sterilizer, steam under sub-atmospheric pressure at temperatures below 90°C will rapidly kill non-sporing organisms after the air in the chamber has been removed by a high-vacuum pump. Most bacterial spores are killed also but a small proportion are very resistant. *If formaldehyde vapour is added to the steam, it can destroy all spores and effect sterilization.* Low-temperature steam, and low-temperature steam/formaldehyde cycles can be incorporated in one and the same sterilizer (Hurrell, 1980; Deverill and Cripps, 1981).

The cycle of operation

The typical characteristics of low-temperature steam formaldehyde sterilization can be summarised as follows:

After loading the chamber and closing the door:

Stage 1. Pre-vacuum — air removal stage. A flush of steam is drawn by the vacuum pump through the surrounding jacket and the chamber whilst the pressure is reduced to approximately 380 mmHg (50 kPa). At this point the jacket pressure is held steady and the pump continues to evacuate the chamber until a pressure of about 50 mmHg (6.56 kPa) is reached. This is maintained for 10 minutes to effect complete air clearance from both the chamber and the load.

Stage 2. Sterilization — hold period at operating temperature. A predetermined quantity of formalin is automatically delivered into the chamber from an externally fitted dispenser or container. The valves of the autoclave are so arranged as to admit in two stages about 40 ml of formalin⋆ (34–38 per cent formalin solution) per m^3 of sterilizer chamber space. The formalin first enters a heated vapouriser where it is converted to steam and gaseous formaldehyde before passing into the chamber. At the same time there is a controlled injection of steam which allows the chamber pressure to rise into equilibrium with that of the jacket at about 380 mmHg (50 kPa). Once this equilibrium pressure is reached (82°C saturated steam temperature), continuous pressure waves of steam, followed by condensation, are applied within the upper and lower absolute pressure limits of 380 mmHg and 330 mmHg (50 kPa and 43.42 kPa). These pressure waves occurring at approximately once every 90 seconds, promote penetration of the formaldehyde vapour into all parts of the load.

In order to maintain the formaldehyde concentration in a sub-atmospheric cycle, the chamber must remain virtually closed. This does produce a problem of the extraction of condensate which is formed during the decompression phase of each pressure wave. The removal of condensate is achieved through an automatic condensate release valve fitted in the chamber drain. Duration of the sterilization stage is normally in the order of 90 minutes and this is determined by bacteriological check of a standard load.

Stage 3. Flushing. The pressure is once more reduced in the chamber by means of the vacuum pump and two continuous flushes of steam are applied. Pumping and steam flushing is carried out at an absolute pressure of about 1 mmHg (0.132 kPa) and this ensures that most of the formaldehyde is removed from the chamber and the materials being sterilized. This stage lasts for approximately 12 minutes.

⋆ Formalin is a synonym for Formaldehyde Solution BP that contains, nominally, 36 per cent w/w Formaldehyde (limits 34–38 per cent w/w)

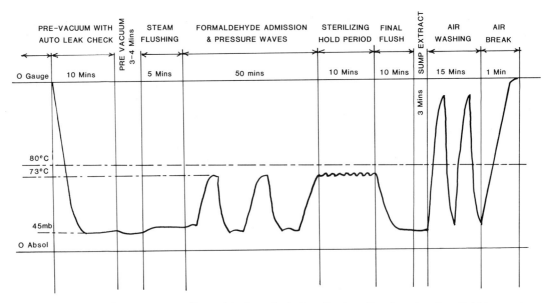

Fig. 7.16 Graph of low temperature/formaldehyde method of sterilization. (Based on data from British Sterilizer Co. Ltd.)

Stage 4. Drying. A final reduction of pressure to 0.5 mmHg (0.066 kPa) or less, achieves drying of materials over a period of approximately eight minutes.

Stage 5. Breaking the vacuum. Filtered air is admitted until atmospheric pressure is reached in the chamber. This generally takes about two minutes.

Performance tests for low temperature steam/formaldehyde sterilizers (LTS and F)

In a similar manner to high-vacuum/high-pressure sterilizers (page 178), LTS & F machines require regular performance efficiency tests to be carried out by a sterilizer engineer as part of a planned maintenance programme. Physical tests and microbiological tests are required for LTS & F machines used for sterilization; the procedure for this is detailed in HTM 10 (DHSS, 1987).

Physical tests. One test using an empty chamber consists of observing and recording the process variables of each stage of a test cycle, i.e. time taken, number of steam pulses, chamber temperatures, pressures and levels of vacuum at significant points in the cycle. Other tests are carried out with small and full chamber loads. These include temperature measurements with electric sensors (thermocouples) in various parts of the chamber and in the centre of a test pack, and a leak monitor test (page 178). The concentration of formaldehyde vapour discharged from the chamber after completion of the LTS and F cycle is also measured.

Microbiological tests. Each production cycle should include a spore test which is used to monitor satisfactory operation of the sterilizer. Provided the physical performance of the machine during a cycle meets the standard, the load can be released for use without waiting for the results of the spore test.

The spore test strip consists of 10^6 to 10^7 recoverable spores of *Bacillus Stearothermophilus* NTCT 10003 prepared in accordance with DHSS specification TSS/S/330/013 (DHSS, 1987). These are placed in the sterilizer chamber and in a number of test packs used to evaluate formaldehyde distribution, penetration and the suitability of the packs.

Lengths of narrow lumen tubing form a suitable vehicle for microbiological test pieces used to determine gas penetration. They are realistic, relatively easy to prepare in the microbiological laboratory, and are readily included with any routine load. One such device is the Line and Pickerill test helix (1973) which consists of stainless-steel tubing 3 mm lumen by 455 mm long with a gas-tight capsule for the spore strip at one end. The capsule is in two parts which fit together against an O-ring seal, and are secured by a knurled ring. The formaldehyde gas must penetrate the tubing lumen to reach the spore test strip. Two of these test pieces are placed in the chamber, one located at the front and the other in the rear. To test the compatibility of packaging, a further two helices are inserted into two layers of paper bags (BS6257, 1982) and placed in the corners of the chamber.

Chemical indicators. Formaldehyde indicator tests are not sufficiently reliable to guarantee that sterilization has taken place, but may be used as a managerial aid to show an item has been processed by LTS and F. The Browne's formaldehyde test consists of a square of white paper, enclosed in a small envelope of thin transparent plastic, which is permeable to steam and formaldehyde vapour. The paper gradually changes from white to coloured as the vapour reaches it. It is recommended that a test-piece is placed on the outside and in the centre of each pack. The outside test indicates that the pack has been exposed to the LTS & F process; the inner test-piece should be examined when the pack is opened, and if found not to have changed colour, the pack should be discarded. Other LTS and F chemical indicators in the form of adhesive paper tape are available.

Safety measures. Formalin is toxic and potentially hazardous. The chemical requires careful handling and secure storage. Exposure to 2–5 p.p.m. in the air causes immediate irritation of the respiratory tract and eyes, with the shedding of tears (Gardner and Peel, 1986). Skin irritation or allergic contact dermatitis may result from contact with formaldehyde solution. It is important that suitable protective clothing is provided for the sterilizer operator, together with adequate washing and eye irrigation facilities which will be needed should spillage occur.

During installation of the machine checks should have been carried out to determine the concentrations of formaldehyde resulting in the environment. Regular checks are necessary to ensure that the statutory levels specified by the Health and Safety Executive (HSE) are not exceeded. Additional ventilation, independent of the normal ventilation should be provided (HTM 10). This consists of an extract system sited on the opening side of the sterilizer door to scavenge formaldehyde vapour discharged from the chamber.

A space or room is required for the storage and 'aeration' of LTS & F sterilized packs before release. Although levels of formaldehyde residues in articles sterilized by LTS & F have not yet been accurately established, it is recommended that the aeration periods are the same as for ethylene oxide (page 198).

The following are some of the items suitable for sterilization by this method: nylon, Terylene, Acrilan and rayon fabrics; polyurethane; teflon tubing; perspex; silicone rubber; anaesthesia equipment such as endotracheal tubes, valves, connectors etc.; cystoscopes and other endoscopic instruments having electrical systems (low-voltage); catheters and tracheostomy tubes, etc.

Chemical indicators

External chemical indicators have already been mentioned in Chapter 6. These take the form of printed stripes on paper tape or patterns printed directly on the outside of sterilizer wrapping materials. Such indicators are intended only to distinguish packs which have been through the sterilizing process from those which have not. They do not confirm that ster-

ilization has taken place. Similarly there are internal chemical indicators which, when placed routinely inside packs, can provide immediate evidence of gross deficiency in the sterilizing process. These indicators should NEVER be used as the sole criterion of sterilization efficiency.

These chemical indicators are available as solutions or solids in sealed tubes, and dye patterns printed on paper or card. The indicators undergo a specified change in colour when exposed over time/temperature to a particular sterilizing agent.

Browne's tubes contain a fluid which changes colour from red, through yellow to green, when the correct conditions for sterilization by steam or dry heat have been reached during the cycle (Gardner and Peel, 1986; Howie and Timbury, 1956; Howie, 1961; Knox, 1961; Kelsey, 1967). It is important to store these tubes at a temperature less than 21°C, and away from sunlight, otherwise there may be a variable degree of premature chemical reaction, resulting in inaccurate readings when used for test purposes.

Browne's tubes are available in three different types, covering the sterilization in high vacuum/high pressure porous load sterilizers, gravity displacement sterilizers, and dry heat ovens. These three types are:

Type Two: Yellow Spot for testing all articles in the high-vacuum/high-pressure sterilizer. Correct exposure to the sterilizing process is indicated after 3.5 minutes at 120°C.

Type One: Black Spot, for testing the sterilization of dressings, gowns and gloves etc., in the gravity displacement sterilizer. Correct exposure to the sterilizing process is indicated after 10 minutes at 125°C or approximately 6 minutes at 130°C.

Type Three: Green Spot, for testing sterilization of syringes, glassware, and instruments by the dry heat process. Correct exposure is indicated after one hour at 160°C.

In all cases the tubes are operative over a range of temperatures and times. A lower temperature must be compensated by a longer exposure, and vice versa.

In some operating departments a separate pack is used into which is placed some of the indicator tubes, and after being processed in the lower part of the sterilizer chamber this is opened immediately. If the tubes have not changed colour correctly, several other packs are opened at random and their tubes examined. If the liquid in the Browne's tubes is amber or red the function of the sterilizer is checked. Subsequently the articles in the faulty load must be repacked and resterilized, fresh indicator tubes being used.

Diack Controls consist of glass tubes containing chemical pellets which fuse and change colour at 121°C. *Vac Controls* are similar and used for temperatures above 130°C. *Steamclox* consists of a card with printed segments which change from pink to green according to time/temperature reached.

Microbiological indicators

It has been emphasised that chemical indicators do not confirm the lethal effect of the sterilizing process. Microbiologists therefore use a biological test packet containing a standardised preparation of bacterial spores. The nature of the spore test pack depends on the type of sterilizing process, but generally it contains spores of the thermophil group such as *Bacillus stearothermophilus* which is extremely resistant to sterilization (Gardner and Peel, 1986; Oxborrow *et al.* 1983).

After exposure to the sterilizing process, the spore pack is returned unopened to the microbiologist for culture and examination. However, microbiological tests are not necessary for routine use provided that regular physical performance checks are carried out on the sterilizer. They should be restricted to use for occasional check on sterilizing efficiency, for the test takes up to three days to complete.

COLD STERILIZATION

4. IONIZING RADIATION

Generally limited to sterilisation on a commercial scale there are two methods in general use, gamma irradiation from a Cobalt 60 source and electron bombardment from a linear accelerator (Mackenzie, 1966; Gardner and Peel, 1986).

The usual dose is in the region of 2.5 Mrad, although this may be increased to 3.2 to 5.0 Mrad depending on the number of contaminants present initially (Gardner and Peel, 1986), and the technique is highly successful for most disposable items which require sterilization only once. Degradation and ageing does occur when sterilizing some materials so care is taken to select those suitable for irradiation.

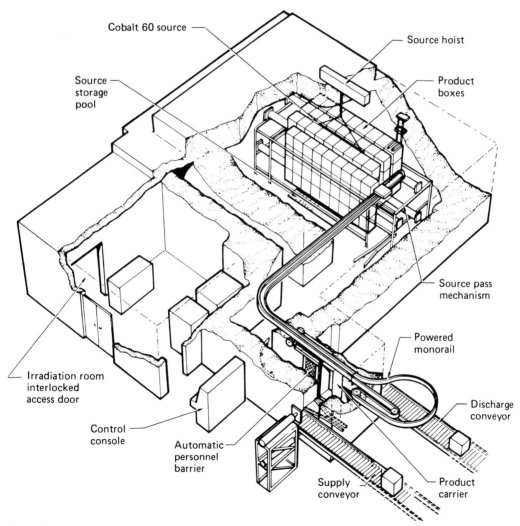

Fig. 7.17 A Cobalt-60 installation for radiation sterilization (built by Atomic Energy of Canada Ltd, reproduced with permission from *An Introduction to Sterilization and Disinfection*, Gardner and Peel)

The Cobalt source is the most economical process if it can be kept running the full 24 hours. It has greater penetrating power than the linear accelerator which is more suitable for thin packets such as catgut, scalpel blades, needles, etc.

An irradiation sterilization service is available commercially to hospitals. Advice on this can be obtained from the Pharmaceutical Technology and Supplies Group, Procurement Directorate, DHSS, Russell Square, London W2. Articles which have been sterilized by gamma irradiation should not subsequently be re-sterilized by ethylene oxide.

5. ETHYLENE OXIDE

Ethylene oxide (EO) is suitable for sterilizing heat labile articles which will withstand temperatures of 50–60°C. It is a method which requires careful control in respect of its explosive characteristics, toxicity, and for monitoring the efficiency of the process.

Ethylene oxide gas has been used as an industrial disinfectant for over fifty years, and was introduced as a clinical sterilizing agent in 1949 by Philip and Kays. The chemical acts by alkylating the proteins of micro-organisms, thereby upsetting their equilibrium. If the process is applied correctly, this reaction is irreversible, and reanimation of the alkylated micro-organism is prevented.

Ethylene oxide boils at a temperature of 10.7°C at ambient temperature and pressure and is liquified at a relatively low pressure in storage cylinders. The gas diffuses rapidly, moving through air pockets and dissolving in plastics, rubber, silicones and oils.

The pure gas which is 1.5 times as heavy as air, is flammable and highly explosive at concentrations above 3.6 per cent by volume in air. The exothermic reaction is violent and has on a number of occasions caused serious accidents. This explosive polymerisation can be avoided by mixing EO with an inert gas such as carbon dioxide or fluorocarbon-12, or employing a sterilization process which extracts most of the air from the chamber before the introduction of EO (Fischer, 1971). Mixtures of 10 per cent by volume of ethylene oxide and 90 per cent carbon dioxode or 12 per cent ethylene oxide and 88 per cent fluorocarbon-12, are non-flammable.

Strict safety precautions must be observed by those involved in the use of ethylene oxide. The inhalation of EO by sterilizer operators or other persons who are in the vicinity of the sterilizer can cause acute toxicity with irritation of the eyes and respiratory tract, headache, dizziness, nausea and vomiting. Any detectable level of EO in the atmosphere should be considered hazardous if it extends throughout working hours (Gardner and Peel, 1986). Care must be taken to minimise the period of time during which staff are exposed to risk. Dermatitis and burns to patients can result from contact with items such as anaesthesia facemasks, endotracheal tubes and catheters etc., which have not been aerated adequately following sterilization by ethylene oxide (Gardner and Peel, 1986).

The ethylene oxide gases from the sterilizer chamber and aeration chamber must be vented directly to the outside atmosphere. Ventilation of the room in which these functions take place should achieve 8 to 10 air changes per hour at the least.

The main risk to staff occurs when the sterilizer door is opened and the load transferred to the aeration cabinet. Unless an extract hood has been fitted over the door, the room in which the sterilizer is situated should be vacated for 15 minutes to allow residual gas to dissipate (Gardner and Peel, 1986). Rubber or fabric gloves should be worn for handling packs which are loaded onto a transfer trolley, which should then be wheeled by the operator moving ahead to avoid exposure to the gas that trails behind (Samuels, 1978).

Policies must be determined for dealing with leaks and spills; these should be clearly documented and understood by all staff working in the SDU or CSSD. Should personnel

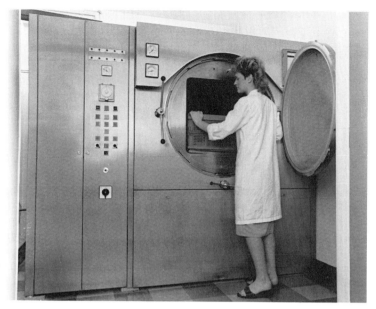

Fig. 7.18 Ethylene oxide sterilizer; positive pressure type. (Sterivit, Atesmo Ltd.)

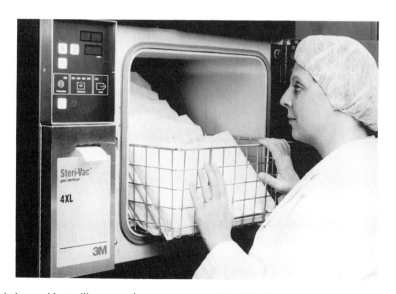

Fig. 7.19 Ethylene oxide sterilizer, negative pressure type. (Steri-Vac Model 4XL, 3M Health Care.)

come into contact with liquid ethylene oxide, then clothing, shoes and any rubber materials must be removed immediately and washed or aerated. Staff may need to shower and flush their eyes with water.

Special consideration must be given to the installation of EO sterilizers, particularly regarding the potential fire hazard and fire escape routes. Large machines are usually installed in the SDU or CSSD in a space separate to that containing steam sterilizers; the space must be bounded by an outside wall. The manifold cylinder in use and standby

cylinders can be housed in external accommodation, and cylinders of ethylene oxide in use should be fitted within 2 to 2.5 metres (6 to 8 feet) of the sterilizer served. If a leak in the pipe system occurs, air may be drawn into the sterilizer chamber to form a highly combustable mixture.

Small machines using an ethylene oxide/inert gas mixture or pure ethylene oxide cartridges do not require separate accommodation, but should not be sited near to steam sterilizers.

Principles of use

Initially care must be taken to thoroughly cleanse instruments and apparatus so that all protein material is removed.

The articles being sterilized must be dry, for if they are wrapped in polythene film while still wet, they will remain wet after sterilization. The most suitable packing material is low-density 300 gauge polyethylene or nylon film, used as one of two layers which are rapidly penetrated by ethylene oxide, moisture and heat under the appropriate controlled conditions.

An essential part of the sterilizing process using EO is the maintenance of adequate humidity (70–80 per cent) with effective moisture distribution throughout the load. Humidification should be achieved automatically by the sterilizer and there must be fail-safe mechanisms to monitor this and any other parameters of the process. Although it is thought that adequate humidity can be achieved by preconditioning the items to be sterilized, holding them in a room at 50–60 per cent humidity for several hours before sterilization, this method is somewhat haphazard as compared to automatic humidification in the sterilizer.

It is essential to aerate packs sterilized by EO in order to remove residual gas. This is done either in the sterilizer chamber, or by placing the packs in an aeration chamber; the recommended period of aeration may be up to twelve hours for PVC. In both instances venting to the atmosphere outside the building is essential. The packs will be held in quarantine for an additional period allowing further dilution of EO gas to an acceptable clinical level, and to await the results of microbiological tests. The store used should have negative pressure ventilation and be entirely separate from the sterile goods store.

There are two types of EO sterilizers used in hospitals:

1. A positive pressure machine using a mixture of ethylene oxide and an inert gas — generally carbon dioxide supplied from a cylinder; this design is used for large machines, although cabinet versions are available for small loads.

2. A machine operating at a negative pressure, using pure ethylene oxide supplied from a single cartridge; these are cabinet machines suitable for small loads (Weymes, 1966).

Positive pressure machines. The Sterivit apparatus (Fig. 7.18) utilises a 15 per cent ethylene oxide, 85 per cent carbon dioxide mixture under pressure and with controlled humidity. Two pressure cycles are available; 5.74 kg per cm^2 (565 kPa, 82 p.s.i.) and 1.75 kg per cm^2 (172 kPa, 25 p.s.i.). There are a range of chamber sizes available between 100 litres and 2,000 litres, although one with a capacity of 100 to 500 litres (0.382 to 0.496 m^3) will be adequate for most requirements of an SDU OR CSSD. The larger chambers are used mainly for sterilizing bulky items of equipment such as complete ventilators or cardiovascular bypass machines. There is microprocessor control of the sterilizing process and safety features such as a continuous ventilation system within the sterilizer cabinet. Briefly the sterilizing process consists of the following stages:

1. The sterilizer is loaded, the door closed and start button activated. An automatic gas tightness test of the high and low pressure systems and the chamber is carried out.

2. The first stage consists of raising the temperature in the chamber to 55/60°C. A pre-

vacuum is drawn and the chamber pressure reduced to approximately 13 kPa; at the same time water vapour at 55°C is introduced to achieve humidification. This stage takes about 15 minutes depending on the size of chamber.

3. Ethylene oxide 15 per cent and 85 per cent carbon dioxide is fed from the gas cylinder in liquid phase. This is filtered, vaporised, reduced in pressure to about 5.95 kg per cm^2 (586 kPa, 85 p.s.i.), heated to 55°C and fed into the sterilizing chamber until a pressure of 5.74 kg or 1.75 kg per cm^2 (565 or 172 kPa/82 or 25 p.s.i.) is reached. This achieves an EO concentration of 1,200 mg per litre of chamber capacity, and the exposure is maintained typically for 30 minutes at the higher pressure, or 120 minutes at the lower pressure. During this stage the temperature and pressure in the chamber are continuously monitored by the control system.

4. The gas is then released safely to the outside atmosphere and a post-vacuum of approximately 13 kPa is drawn. Then follows a series of sterile air rinses in which heated filtered air is drawn into the chamber held under slight pressure, i.e. 0.4 kg (41 kPa, 7 p.s.i.). During this time air is drawn through a high efficiency filter and through the chamber to 'rinse' out ethylene oxide residues from the load. The total cycle time ranges from 90 minutes for the 100 litre unit to 135 minutes for a 2000 litre unit. (Note: some other non-pressurised processes require extended periods of exposure for sterilization; these may be between 1 and 4 hours. Under these circumstances elimination of toxic residues is proportionally more difficult, and takes a longer time.) Residues extracted from the chamber must be vented to outside the building. The post-vacuum stage and air rinsing for desorption of EO gas residues can be extended for 3 to 6 hours depending on the materials sterilized.

Using the high pressure method of sterilization coupled with a short exposure and adequate post-vacuum, the amount of depth of absorption of ethylene oxide can be reduced (Fischer, 1971). Furthermore, the high diffusion coefficient of the additive carbon dioxide, and the low concentration of a 15 per cent ethylene oxide mixture, helps to reduce the problem still further. By an adequate post-vacuum, powerful filtered air-rinse under vacuum and elevated temperature, the ethylene oxide residues can be reduced to a negligible level. Under these circumstances a 24-hour shelf life before use should ensure desorption of any remaining residues.

Negative pressure machines. An example of this type of EO sterilizer is the Steri-Vac 400C which has a chamber capacity of 115 litres (Fig. 7.19). The gas supply is provided from a 100 per cent ethylene oxide unit-dose cartridge. There are two cycles: a 37°C cold cycle with an EO exposure time of approximately 250 minutes, and a 55°C warm cycle having an exposure time of 100 minutes. The total process times are 330 minutes and 195 minutes respectively.

Once the chamber is loaded and the unit-dose cartridge inserted, the cold/warm cycle selected and the start button pushed, the door locks and the automatically controlled EO process begins. A vacuum is created, a cycle of humidification carried out, and EO is introduced to the chamber which remains at subatmospheric pressure. Exposure to EO 1200 mg per litre is maintained for the appropriate period followed by a continuous filtered air purge. This purging continues until the door is opened.

Practically all materials except metals absorb differing amounts of ethylene oxide. Under normal conditions the desorption of EO is a slow process and for this reason it is recommended that after sterilization goods should be stored on an open shelf for at least 24-hours and sometimes as long as four days before use. This is to allow elimination of the toxic residue by natural diffusion to atmosphere.

A precaution worth taking following any ethylene oxide process is to take care that apparatus is not used with saline or blood products before it has been flushed with oxygen

or sterile water. In these circumstances even a minute amount of EO residue can react with the chlorine radical to form chlorohydrates, the toxicity of which is not entirely understood at present. For similar reasons articles which have been sterilized by gamma irradiation should not subsequently be resterilized by ethylene oxide.

With ethylene oxide there are no means at present of adequately monitoring the actual EO concentration at any given point during sterilization. For this reason it is necessary to rely upon microbiological controls (Doyle, 1971; Oxborrow, 1983). A method in common use is Oxoid prepared *B. stearothermophilus* on filter paper and *B. subtilis* (var *globigii*) 10^6 on aluminium strips prepared to the method of Beeby and Whitehouse (Cunliffe, 1966). Envelopes containing up to ten of these strips are placed at different points in the sterilizer chamber and within all articles where it is considered that penetration could be a problem. The strips are incubated overnight and if no growth is apparent, the sterilizer load is released for use after the aeration period.

Under careful preparation and control the spore test described is a good method of monitoring sterilization. A more simple test utilizing earth spores emanates from Denmark. The Danish State Serum Institute test consists of *B. subtilis*, first immersed in a solution of 0.9 per cent NaCl and then dried on pure quartz sand. The sand is then packed in a paper envelope which is used for test purposes in the normal manner. This is a very severe test due to the presence of salt (in contact with the spore) which tends to inactivate ethylene oxide. In practice it could be regarded as more appropriate to the working situation as some items may not be adequately precleansed.

A chemical indicator can be included with each packet to indicate to the user that it has been through the ethylene oxide process; it is not a direct indication of sterility. A gas indicator green tape with yellow stripes is available. This changes shade after exposure to ethylene oxide. Chemical sachets or impregnated filter papers can be prepared in the laboratory and these change colour after being exposed to the gas (Colquhoun, 1969).

Examples of heat-labile equipment suitable for sterilization by ethylene oxide are: catheters, endoscopes (including cystoscopes), cryoprobes, aortic grafts, ophthalmic instruments, plastic tubing, senoran evacuator, Sengstaken tubes.

Formaldehyde

Although formaldehyde is a very powerful and effective biocide, its use for sterilization has largely fallen into disrepute unless combined with sub-atmospheric steam. Sterilization failures in formalin cabinets have been described for many years and it is doubtful whether the formalin vapour penetrates the lumen of catheters even with control of the humidity in the cabinet. The use of formalin combined with sub-atmospheric steam, has been described on page 192.

Activated glutaraldehyde

This is a 2 per cent aqueous solution buffered to a pH 7.5–8.5 by the addition of 0.3 per cent sodium bicarbonate.

Cidex is a commercial preparation of concentrated glutaraldehyde containing an anti-rust agent. Vegetative bacteria and tubercle bacilli are killed in 20 minutes and some spore-forming species are killed in 10 hours at 20°C (Spalding, 1963; Stonehill *et al.*, 1963; Medical Research Council, 1968). Other brands include Asep and Totacide.

The solution is suitable for sterilizing lensed instruments such as cystoscopes and other

types of endoscopes providing the instrument is clean and partially dismantled. It is also suitable for anaesthesia masks etc.

The in-use dilution is slightly irritant to skin and mucous membranes and severely irritant to the eye. All instruments should be rinsed thoroughly in sterile water before use in surgery.

Once diluted and activated long life Cidex solution is effective for up to four weeks and can be reused a number of times since it is expensive. The length of time which a solution is repeatedly used depends on the amount of contamination with organic matter. Repeatedly used solutions should be changed at least fortnightly.

HEAT DISINFECTION

PASTEURIZATION IN WATER

Pasteurization of endoscopes is carried out by immersion for 10 minutes in a thermostatically controlled water bath at a temperature of 70°C to 75°C (Francis, 1961). This is lethal to all types of micro-organisms except resistant bacterial spores. Clean articles such as cystoscopes can be disinfected in this manner provided precautions are taken to avoid air being trapped in the tubular part of the instruments. Other articles must not be added to interrupt the cycle. The method can be used when treatment with chemicals is contraindicated, but its effect is inferior to sterilization.

COLD DISINFECTION

CHEMICAL SOLUTIONS

We now emphasise the term *disinfection* in preference to *sterilization* because under normal conditions chemicals cannot be relied upon to kill spores. It is a method that is used only when sterilization by heat is impracticable and is ineffective unless the chemicals can reach all parts of the articles, which *must* be free from debris, blood and pus, i.e., as in ethylene oxide sterilization (McCulloch, 1945; Perkins, 1956b; Sykes, 1958; Gardner and Peel, 1986).

It must be realised that although fairly short periods of contact with certain chemicals will ensure the destruction of bacteria these short periods refer only to articles with smooth surfaces, such as scalpels. If an instrument has rather intricate parts or joints, some time will be required for the chemical to penetrate into the indentations or joint surfaces.

If the chemical is used in combination with heat the period for disinfection will be reduced. The importance of using heat for sterilization whenever possible cannot be over-emphasised.

Many new chemicals are now in use in the operating theatre, but the lists on page 204 and the examples mentioned in the text include also some of the older and well-established ones. In all cases the instrument must be thoroughly rinsed before use to remove chemical traces which at high concentrations may prove irritant to body tissues.

Table 7.2 Disinfection by chemicals — bactericides in common use (*The minimum period of immersion for disinfection is 10 minutes unless otherwise stated*)

Agent or proprietary preparation	CLEANSING AND DISINFECTION					DISINFECTION		
	Linen bowls, etc objects (%)	Heavy contamination inanimate (%)	Burns, wounds (%)	Pre-surgical hand disinfection (%)	Pre-Surgical skin disinfection (%)	Anaesthesia equipment e.g (face masks tubes, etc) (%)	Endoscopes, electrodes cables, and instrument lamps (%)	Metal instruments (%)
Phenolics								
CLEAR SOLUBLE								
Printol aqueous	1.25	3	...	...	...	...	3	...
Hycolin aqueous	1	1.5	...	...	...	...	1.5	...
Clearsol	1	2	...	...	...	...	2	...
Stericol	1	2	...	...	...	...	2	...
CHLOROXYLENOL								
Dettol aqueous	...	...	5	...	...	...	...	...
Diguanides								
CHLORHEXIDINE (*glucomate*)								
Hibitane aqueous	0.5	...	0.05 (0.01 irrigation of body cavities)	...	...	...	...	...
alcoholic	...	0.5	...	0.5	0.5	...	...	...
Hibidil	...	...	undiluted	...	...	...	...	...
Cyteal aqueous	...	...	0.05	0.5	0.5	...	...	...
Hibscrub aqueous (0.4%)	...	...	...	undiluted	...	...	...	...
Hibsol alcoholic (0.05%)	...	...	...	undiluted	...	...	...	...
Bacticlens aqueous (0.05%) (*acetate*)	...	...	undiluted	...	...	...	...	...
Chlorasept aqueous (0.05%)	...	...	undiluted	...	...	...	...	...
HEXACHLOROPHANE								
PhisoHex/Ster-Zac DC (3%)	...	...	undiluted	...	...	...	...	...
Quaternary ammonium compounds (QAC)								
CETRIMIDE								
Cetavlon	...	...	0.1	1	...	...	...	...
BENZALKONIUM CHLORIDE								
Roccal/Zephiran	...	...	1 to 0.5	...	...	...	...	...

QAC + Diguanides

Savlon concentrate (cetrimide 15% chlorhexidine 7.5%)	...	1 to 3 3
Savlodil sachets (cetrimide 0.15% chlorhexidine 0.015%)	...	undiluted
Travasept 100 (cetrimide 0.155 chlorhexidine 0.015%)	...	undiluted

Halogens

HYPOCHLORATES

Chloros/Domestos/ Sterite/Kirbychlor	...	1000 ppm 5000 ppm [Hb$_s$ Ag blood spillage]
Presept (sodium dichlorisocyanurate)	...	140 ppm 1,000 ppm (2500–10,000 ppm [Hb$_s$ Ag blood spillage]).

IODINE COMPOUNDS

Iodine 2 percent in alcohol	...	undiluted

IODOPHORS

Betadine antiseptic/ Disadine	...	undiluted
Betadine scrub	...	undiluted

Aldehydes

ACTIVATED GLUTARALDEHYDE

Cidex (solution effective for 14 days after activation	...	Undiluted Undiluted

(20 minute exposure minimum)

Phenolics

Carbolic acid (or phenol in its pure state) and cresol with soap (lysol) are now not used as a disinfectant because there are many derivatives that are more effective and less dangerous to use.

The effect of phenol and its derivatives is not clearly understood but it is thought they act by coagulation and lytic tissue effects on the bacteria. Their action seems to be dependent on selective concentration at all surfaces with desaturation of proteins and increase in cell permeability.

Printol

A clear soluble disinfectant with a phenolic base but rather less corrosive than the lysol type. Its dilution in heavily contaminated situations is 3 per cent but for routine surface disinfection this can be reduced to 1.25 per cent (Kelsey and Maurer, 1967).

Hycolin

This is a balanced combination of synthetic phenols which are less corrosive than lysol. It is used for general purposes at a dilution of 1.5 per cent and this should be increased to 2 per cent for heavy contamination.

Clearsol

Contains 40 per cent of phenols consisting chiefly of the powerful xylenol fraction and a mild detergent system. Suitable for general disinfection at a recommended dilution of 1 per cent.

These three synthetic phenolic disinfectants are effective against all common Gram-positive and Gram-negative organisms including *Pseudomonas aeruginosa* (*pyocyanea*). They are compatible with anionic and non-ionic substances such as soaps, anionic detergents, etc.

Chloroxylenol (Dettol)

This is a relatively non-toxic non-irritant biocide which is active against most organisms, including the streptococcus, but rather less active against certain Gram-negative organisms. The destruction of spores is somewhat doubtful.

Dettol antiseptic contains 5 per cent chloroxylenol, 10 per cent terpineol and about 20 per cent alcohol, and is used at a dilution of 5 per cent for general disinfection purposes, 10 minutes being the minimal period of immersion recommended for disinfection.

It is not advisable to bring chloroxylenol preparations, expecially strong solutions, into contact with plastics as they tend to cause deterioration of the material.

Hexachlorophane (PhisoHex, Ster-ZacDc)

This is a biocide which can be combined with soap in a proportion of usually 2 per cent (Gould et al., 1957; Lowbury, 1961). It can be used for surgical hand disinfection, although the use of iodophors and chlorhexidine have become more common.

Hexachlorophane is more effective against Gram-positive than Gram-negative organisms, but its main value lies in the regular use of a solution or soap containing the chemical. If the surgeons and theatre staff use pHisoHex, or hexachlorophane soap regularly it has been

shown that the bacterial flora of the skin is reduced, (Smylie *et al.*, 1959). However, as the effect is cumulative, it may require repeated applications to be effective. But care must be taken not to use hexachlorophane preparations for regular total body bathing; there is a possible risk of toxicity from absorption of hexachlorophane into the blood stream (Scowen, 1972).

Quaternary ammonium compounds (QACs)

These are cationic (positively charged) surface-acting detergents or amines which are derivatives of ammonium chloride. They have a narrower bactericidal spectrum than the synthetic phenols and chlorhexidine, and their activity is affected by the type of water used for dilution, or contact with anionic-type soaps. Hard, acid or iron-rich water reduces their biocidal effectiveness.

QAC compounds are very active against Gram-positive organisms, but resistant against hydrophilic viruses, acid-fast bacteria, and bacterial spores. They are unreliable against Gram-negative organisms such as *Pseudomonas Aeruginosa*, *Pseudomonas cepacia* and *Achromobacter* or *Serratia*. If these organisms gain access to solutions during preparation, storage or use, they will rapidly multiply and result in contamination of the solution. QACs are popular because of their freedom from toxicity and other undesirable effects.

Cetrimide B.P. (Cetavlon)

This is in effect a biocidal detergent. It is not compatible with soap, but used in a dilution of not less than 0.5 per cent, possesses very useful detergent properties which may be applied for the cleansing of wounds. Although this higher concentration is necessary for detergency, its biocidal properties extend down to 0.2 per cent.

Quaternary ammonium compounds + diguanides

The ineffectiveness of QACs can be overcome to some extent by combining them with diguanides. A combination of cetrimide and chlorhexidine has been found to be more effective against Gram-negative organisms (Maurer, 1985). One proprietary product Savlon is available as a concentrate solution containing 15 per cent cetrimide and 1.5 per cent chlorhexidine.

For general biocidal use, such as cleansing wounds and burns, an aqueous dilution of 0.5 per cent Savlon Hospital Concentrate is used. This can be prepared by using one dose sachets of the concentrate added to an appropriate quantity of sterile water. Alternatively, Savodil sachets containing ready to use chlorhexidine 0.15 per cent cetrimide, and 0.015 per cent chlorhexidine can be used.

Diguanides

Chlorhexidine (Hibitane, Bacticlens, Chlorasept, Cyteal)

This well established biocide has proved to be of great use. Single or infrequent applications to the intact skin of any strength solution will not cause irritation, but repeated applications of a 1 per cent solution may eventually give rise to erythema. The dilutions in common use should not give rise to any irritation of the user's skin (Rose and Swaine, 1956).

Hibitane Hospital Concentrate 5 per cent is a solution of 5 per cent chlorhexidine

gluconate, and an aqueous dilution of 0.5 per cent of the concentrate is used for the surface disinfection of inanimate objects, such as bowls, tables, etc. This dilution of Hibitane concentrate is equivalent to 0.025 per cent effective concentration of the antibacterial agent, chlorhexidine gluconate.

For the prophylactic treatment of wounds a Hibitane concentrate dilution of 1 per cent in water (0.05 per cent effective concentration) is used. Bacticlens and Chlorasept contain a 0.05 per cent solution of chlorhexidine gluconate, and are supplied ready for use in plastic sachets. For pre-surgical skin disinfection, 10 per cent dilution of Hibitane concentrate in isopropyl alcohol (0.5 per cent) with an added dye such as geranine or methylene blue (Lowbury, 1961), Hibitane tincture and Cyteal contain 0.5 per cent chlorhexidine gluconate and are used undiluted for skin disinfection. For the *emergency* pre-surgical disinfection of heat-labile instruments, which are immersed for a minimum of 10 minutes before use, a dilution of 10 per cent of Hibitane concentrate in 70 per cent ethyl alcohol (0.5 per cent); and for the final pre-surgical rinse of hands, 1 per cent dilution of Hibitane concentrate in 70 per cent industrial methylated spirit (0.05 per cent). *Dilutions given in brackets always refer to the effective concentration of the antibacterial agent.*

The Hibitane concentrate is generally supplied coloured a distinctive red, and is effective against a wide range of Gram-positive and Gram-negative organisms. Although as with other antibacterial agents, blood slows down the bacterial activity of Hibitane, it is claimed that in a dilution of 0.4 per cent (0.02 per cent) in 50 per cent blood, considerable bactericidal effect is retained. Hibitane is not effective against tubercle bacilli or bacterial spores and has little activity against viruses, but it appears quite comparable with other similar antibacterial chemicals (Ayliffe *et al.* 1984). Except in the greater dilutions it is not compatible with soaps and should not intentionally be combined with these.

Benzalkonium chloride (Roccal, Zephiran)

This is similar in action to other quaternary ammonium compounds. The B.P. solution contains 50 per cent w/v of benzalkonium chloride; Roccal (Bayer) contains 1 per cent benzalkonium chloride and Roccal concentrate (Roccal 10X) contains 10 per cent. If used at a dilution of not less than 0.5 per cent it has very useful detergent properties which may be utilised for the cleansing of contaminated wounds (Spalton, 1951). Its bactericidal properties extend down to 0.025 per cent for irrigation of the bladder, but for general purposes the greatest dilution is not less than 0.5 per cent.

For pre-surgical skin preparation and the cleansing of contaminated wounds, the aqueous dilutions should be between 1 and 0.5 per cent effective concentration respectively. A 70 per cent isopropyl alcohol may be substituted as the dilutent for pre-surgical skin preparation when a more rapid action is desired. When full detergency is not required, a dilution of 0.5 per cent aqueous (0.05 per cent) is quite adequate for bactericidal purposes, and this dilution should be used for the general disinfection of inanimate objects such as bowls or linen etc.

For the final pre-surgical rinse of hands a dilution of 1 per cent (0.1 per cent) aqueous or in 70 per cent isopropyl alcohol should be used, and at this concentration there should not be any undue irritation to the user's hands.

Roccal or Zephiran can be used for bladder or urethral irrigation in the dilution of 0.05 per cent (0.005 per cent), but for retention lavage this dilution must be increased to 0.025 per cent (0.0025 per cent).

Halogens and halogen compounds

The most widely used of these are the hypochlorites and iodines. Chlorine-based compounds act mainly by oxidation and the liberation of its odours may be objectionable. Iodine acts directly by iodination and oxidation, being able to change into the vapour-state readily.

Hypochlorites and dichloroisocynurates

These have a wide range of bactericidal, fungicidal and virucidal activity. They have rapid action, particularly sporicidal, and at low concentrations are non-toxic. As a solution giving 1 per cent available chlorine it can be used for surface application such as floors, and soaking infected linen. It should not be used for instruments or steel holloware as Chlorine damages the surface. Commercial preparations include Chloros Domestos, Sterite, Milton, Kirbychlor and Presept, which are supplied as a concentrated solution requiring dilution before use. (Bloomfield, 1985).

Iodine and iodophors

Iodine is very insoluble in water and therefore is generally combined with alcohol. As a 2 per cent solution in 70 per cent isopropyl alcohol, combining readily with organic material this is still regarded by many as the ideal pre-surgical skin preparation. It is certainly the most lethal to bacteria of all preparations used for this purpose, but unfortunately it does produce an occasional skin irritation which is disturbing for the patient. If a wound is very heavily contaminated and there has been a lengthy delay of the patient's admission to hospital the use of an iodine pre-surgical skin preparation may be indicated.

Povidone-iodine (Betadine, Disadine)

These are non-stinging, non-staining, film-forming, water-soluble iodine complexes (Marr and Saggers, 1964). Iodophors are not irritating to skin and mucous membranes and unlike iodine tincture can be safely bandaged or applied as a compress. Povidone iodine is a topical disinfectant that retains the unique, non-selective microbiocidal activity of iodine, without the undesirable side effects mentioned above. It kills all organisms including spores and has a more prolonged action than ordinary iodine. Its brown colour can easily be washed off skin as well as cotton, wool and silk and its action is unimpaired by blood, serum, pus or soap.

Betadine is available as an aqueous antiseptic solution which is used undiluted for pre-operative skin preparation and as a surgical scrub. The latter contains a suitable detergent and forms a rich lather which is non-staining and non-irritating. Disadine is available as a topical powder spray for application to wounds and lesions.

Note: Bacterial contamination of dilute solutions such as cetrimide and chlorhexidine and even phenolics can occur under certain circumstances. For this reason cork enclosures or cork liners in screw-cap bottles should not be used as cork appears to nourish and protect organisms. Contamination can occur also with the practice of 'topping up' half-empty bottles or of refilling stock bottles without resterilisation. Another cause may be due to the use of unsterile solutions or glassware or the transfer of bacteria to bottles during use (e.g., from the fingers of nurses contaminated while handling infected articles or patients).

Bottles of disinfectant solutions should be date-stamped and used in rotation. Stocks must be kept at a minimum, and the points made above observed. (Medical Research Council, 1968).

Many hospital authorities have established a policy to limit the number, variety and variations in dilutions of disinfectant in general use. Such a policy ensures that the most effective chemical is chosen and lends itself also to economy.

APPLICATION OF METHODS

It is important to remember that the easiest and most effective method of sterilization is by moist heat, and whenever possible this is the method of choice. If an antibacterial agent is used, a thorough pre-cleansing is as vital as the application of the chemical which should always be given sufficient time to penetrate to all parts of the instrument.

Anaesthesia apparatus and ventilators. Anaesthesia breathing circuits, and mechanical ventilators may be contaminated with *Pseudomonas aeruginosa* or other Gram-negative bacteria. It is recommended that breathing circuits should be changed after use by each patient. Unless fitted with disposable bacteria-impermeable filters which can be replaced, ventilators should be disinfected after use.

Face masks, tubing, reservoir bags, 'Y' pieces and Heidbrink valves, airways and endotracheal or endobronchial tubes should be thoroughly cleansed inside and out. Ideally this should be done with a washing machine using a detergent such as Neodian, Lab-brite, Sumazon XL, Helpex No 1, etc. Alternatively the items are immersed in a solution of the detergent and washed by hand giving particular attention to corrugations. Autoclaving is the most reliable method of decontamination, although the life of these items can be shortened by repeated autoclaving, and disinfection by low temperature steam/formaldehyde or pasteurization in a water bath or washing machine at 70°–80°C is an alternative. Immersion in a chemical disinfectant such as 2 per cent glutaraldehyde (Cidex) is acceptable but less reliable than heat unless incorporated in a suitable machine (Ayliffe *et al.*, 1984).

Before sterilizing or disinfecting a 'cuffed tube', the cuff or obturator bag must be empty. Methods of disinfecting ventilators are described in Chapter 11.

Bougies, catheters, etc. These are dealt with under the appropriate headings, e.g., metal, plastic and rubber.

Electrical apparatus. Quite a large proportion of electrical apparatus used in surgery is now manufactured suitable for sterilization by heat. Care must always be taken to observe the manufacturers' instructions regarding a particular instrument as it is possible for some parts to be heat sterilizable and others not.

A large proportion of electrical leads and illuminated retractors are now made autoclavable, but after use they should be dried very thoroughly to minimise corrosion. Those not sterilizable by high temperatures should be immersed in a 10 per cent aqueous solution of Hibitane (0.5 per cent), for a minimal period of 30 minutes, sterilized by ethylene oxide or alternatively subjected to the sub-atmospheric steam/formaldehyde process.

Diathermy or cautery electrodes may generally be autoclaved. If heat sterilization is contraindicated, *emergency* disinfection may be effected by immersing them in a 10 per cent aqueous solution of chlorhexidine (Hibitane, 0.5 per cent) or 2 per cent glutaraldehyde (Cidex) for a minimal period of 10 minutes.

Several of the more modern electric bone drills and saws may be autoclaved complete; in most cases, however, only the outer motor cover or the flexible drive is sterilizable in this

way. The cable must be covered with a sterilized cotton sleeve before use and care taken to ensure that no moisture has collected on or near electrical contacts.

Generally speaking, electric lamps are damaged by heat and should therefore be sterilized ideally by ethylene oxide, or immersed in a chemical antibacterial agent such as 10 per cent aqueous solution chlorhexidine (Hibitane, 0.5 per cent) or 2 per cent glutaraldehyde (Cidex).

Endoscopes. The same rules apply to endoscopes, including cystoscopes, bronchoscopes, oesophagoscopes, etc., but extra care must be taken with optical attachments such as telescopes, lenses and lighting attachments. (Davies *et al.*, 1984; Leers, 1980; Ridgeway, 1985; Babb *et al.*, 1984).

A rapid increase of pressure of steam may cause cracking of the optical attachments, although in practice with modern apparatus this complication is minimised. Similarly breakage may occur if a hot endoscope is cooled too rapidly in cold water before use. Sometimes only the sheath of an endoscope is heat sterilizable, and if the optical/lighting system is required sterile it must be processed by sub-atmospheric steam/formaldehyde, ethylene oxide, or immersed in a 10 per cent aqueous solution of chlorhexidine (Hibitane, 0.5 per cent) or 2 per cent glutaraldehyde (Cidex) vertically for a minimal period of 10 minutes (or treated in alkaline gluteraldehyde (see above). On no account must instruments containing lenses come into contact with any alcohol-based solutions; it will dissolve the lens-mounting cement.

Pasteurization of endoscopes is carried out simply by immersion for 10 minutes in a boiler thermostatically controlled at 70°–80°C instead of 100°C, and it is enough to destroy vegetative bacteria very rapidly (Francis, 1961). Undoubtedly this is preferable to the use of chemicals when higher temperatures are contraindicated.

Metal ware. This is sterilized by autoclaving at 134°C, 2.25 kg per cm^2 (221 kPa, 32 p.s.i.) for six minutes, little or no drying being necessary. Alternatively the articles are contained within a packet and sterilized with the drapes (p. 150).

Glassware. Generally all glassware may be autoclaved if certain precautions are taken and steam can reach all surfaces of the glass. To avoid breakage it is advisable to pre-heat the articles being sterilized by placing them in the autoclave chamber beforehand.

After sterilization glassware should be allowed to cool slowly, thereby avoiding cracking which may occur if the articles are cooled too rapidly. Glassware should not be sterilized together with metal instruments as the latter can cause unnecessary breakages. Dry-heat sterilization is the method of choice for all glassware.

Linen. Gowns, caps, masks and operation drapes are packed into linen or paper packs. These are sterilized at 126°C, 1.41 kg per cm^2 (138 kPa), 20 p.s.i.) for 30 minutes or 134°C, 2.25 kg per cm^2 (221 kPa, 32 p.s.i.) for three and a half minutes.

Lotions. Normal saline and sterile water for hand lotion use should be prepared as individual glass bottles of $\frac{1}{2}$ or 1 litre capacity, which are autoclaved so that the temperature of each container is maintained at 115°C, 0.7 kg per cm^2 (69 kPa, 10 p.s.i.) for 30 minutes. (British Pharmacopoeia, 1980).

The holding period of sterilization depends upon a number of factors which include type of sterilizer, capacity and load, i.e., $\frac{1}{2}$ or 1 litre bottles. This period should be determined initially by a thermocouple recording the temperature reached inside a bottle of water at the centre of the load. Subsequently the temperature/holding period is checked either by an integrated thermocouple or a black spot Browne's tube suspended in one of the filled bottles. The holding period selected for a load of mixed $\frac{1}{2}$ and 1 litre bottles must be that suitable for the latter.

When sterilizing bottles of liquid in a steam sterilizer certain precautions must be taken. The metal caps must have a well-fitted rubber washer which is renewed regularly; a pre-

vacuum is drawn and steam admitted to the chamber gradually; and after sterilization the steam pressure must be reduced over a period of about 30 minutes, otherwise the liquid may boil violently and the bottles burst. *A post-vacuum must not be drawn.* At this stage some autoclaves incorporate a special fluid cycle with spray cooling after sterilization whilst (Howie and Timbury, 1956) maintaining pressure of air in the sterilizer chamber. This avoids bursting of bottles.

After sterilization the caps of the bottles are sealed with *sterile* cellulose tape or a plastic seal. Once a seal on a sterile bottle has been broken, the stopper removed and the contents exposed to the air, a *sterile* label does not indicate sterility of the contents. Saline or water from a sterile bottle or flask must not be used for injection, infusion or washing of sterile instruments unless the seal of the bottle is unbroken at the time of use.

Once opened and not used, such bottles should be regarded as contaminated and must be discarded. Bottles such as the Matbick type incorporate their own seal.

Metal instruments. These are divided into the heat sterilizable and non-heat sterilizable types.

The heat sterilizable metal instruments are made generally of stainless steel which will not rust if the instruments are dried after use. Such instruments, including scissors, dissecting and artery forceps, metal bougies and catheters, etc., may be sterilized on open trays in an autoclave for six minutes at 130°C, 1.76 kg per cm^2 (172 kPa, 25 p.s.i.).

Non-autoclavable instruments made from carbon steel, such as solid scalpels, twist drills and osteotomes, etc., are better sterilized by dry heat or ethylene oxide.

In the dry-heat process of sterilization the instruments are exposed to a temperature of 160°C for one hour *plus* additional time necessary to allow heat penetration to all parts of the load. This additional period ranges between a half and one and a half hours.

In an emergency a 10 per cent solution of chlorhexidine in ethyl alcohol (Hibitane, 0.5 per cent) will disinfect metal instruments in a *minimum* period of ten minutes, providing that the chemical has access to all parts.

Nail brushes. These should be autoclaved at 130°C, 1.76 kg per cm^2 (172 kPa, 25 p.s.i.) for six minutes, or 134°C, 2.25 kg per cm^2 (221 kPa, 32 p.s.i.) for three and a half minutes. The most satisfactory method is to autoclave the brushes in a metal brush dispenser and keep them in the dry state until needed. A separate clean brush is then used for each person.

The best method for reprocessable suture needles is to prepare the needles as sets in paper bags and sterilize by the dry-heat method or autoclaving. Using the latter method, a small piece of vapour phase inhibitor anti-rust paper should be included with the needles when packing; this applies also to steam sterilization.

It is very important to ensure that debris is not lodged in the eye of a suture needle or at any point along the shaft before sterilization. Suture needles are difficult to clean; and generally pre-sterilized disposable suture needles should be used.

Rubber goods. Some of these, including non-disposable tubing, drainage sheeting, catheters and certain endotracheal and endobronchial tubes can be autoclaved providing the drying cycle is not prolonged.

Macintoshes are treated with an antibacterial agent such as 0.5 per cent aqueous Hibitane, and if heavily contaminated should be autoclaved.

Powders. The only satisfactory method of sterilizing powders to avoid clumping is by dry heat or gamma irradiation. These are available commercially, ready-sterilized.

Plastics. Most non-disposable plastics in common use in the operating theatre may be sterilized by wet heat, but care must be taken as at boiling-point and above they become softened and easily damaged.

Polyvinyl chloride (vinyl Portex, both translucent and ivory Magill variety) and polythene

tubing, etc., should be sterilized in ethylene oxide or pasteurized in sub-atmospheric steam/formaldehyde. Most polyvinyl tubing can now be purchased ready sterilized.

Nylon tubing can be sterilized by this method also, but due to its high melting-point 200°C steam sterilization as recommended for metal instruments can be employed.

Plastic tubing should never be shaken upon removal from a water pasteurizer as it is then very brittle and may break at the point where it is secured with bandage.

It is important to ensure that there are no kinks or air bubbles in the tubing during pasteurization and it is preferable to fill the tubing with water beforehand. Kinks in the tubing will result in flattened sections and air bubbles with inefficient disinfection of the lumen. Plastic tubing which has flattened sections or irregularities following disinfection or sterilization can often be returned to its original shape and section by re-heating and then cooling rapidly whilst maintaining the desired position.

The use of other items of plastic equipment in the theatre is rather questionable due to the danger of static electricity formation (Chapter 4), but all inanimate objects such as arm supports and translucent X-ray cassette holders for fracture tables, etc., are disinfected with a 1 per cent aqueous solution of chlorhexidine (Hibitane) before and after use. Other anti-bacterial agents which may be used for this purpose are Roccal and Zephiran at their recommended dilutions. The usual type of materials used for these articles are perspex and fibre glass.

Suture materials. Most ligatures and sutures available in foil or plastic sachets are presented as sterile peel-open overwrap packets. Unopened inner sachets can be disinfected by immersion in a suitable fluid recommended by the manufacturer for a minimum period of 30 minutes before use.

Plastic envelopes containing sterile catgut are stored in a fluid supplied by the catgut manufacturers which consists basically of isopropyl alcohol.

Monofilament synthetic non-absorbables. These are generally sterilized with the instrument sets but can be autoclaved separately in packets at standard autoclave temperature and times.

Braided, twisted, plated, synthetic or natural non-absorbables, etc. These are wound on to metal, nylon or glass ligature reels and are autoclaved. Sterile peel-open packets are generally used containing various sizes of synthetic non-absorbables or silk.

Metal wire, mesh and suture clips. All are autoclavable before use as described under metal instruments. They may be stored in dry sterilized boxes or packets, but in the case of Cushing's or McKenzie's ligature clips these may be included in the set of instruments.

REFERENCES

ALDER, V. G., BROWN, A. M. AND GILLESPIE, W. A. (1966) *Journal of Clinical Pathology*, **19**, 83.
AYLIFFE, G. A. J., COATES, D. AND HOFFMANN, P. N. (1984) *Chemical Disinfectants in Hospitals*. London: Public Health Laboratory Service.
ASSOCIATION OF OPERATING ROOM NURSES (1984) Proposed recommended practices — Cleaning and processing anaesthesia equipment. *AORN Journal*, **39**, 92–98.
BABB, J. R., PHELPS, M., DOWNES, J. AND AYLIFFE, G. A. J. (1982) Evaluation of an ethylene oxide sterilizer, *Journal of Hospital Infection*, **3**, 385–394.
BABB, J. R., BRADLEY, C. R. AND AYLIFFE, G. A. J. (1984) Comparison of automated systems for the cleaning and disinfection of flexible fibreoptic endoscopes. *Journal of Hospital Infection*, **5**, 213–226.
BLOOMFIELD, S. F. AND USO, E. E. (1985) The antibacterial properties of sodium hypochlorite and sodium dichloroisocyanurate as hospital disinfectants. *Journal of Hospital Infection*, **6**, 20–30.
BOGER, W. (1976) *Hospital Topics*, Sept/Oct. 12.
BOLTON, J. (1966) *British Hospital Journal*, May 13, 867.
BOWIE, J. H. (1961) *Sterilisation of Surgical Materials. Symposium*. London: Pharmaceutical Press.
BOWIE, J. H., KELSEY, J. C. AND THOMPSON, C. R. (1963) *Lancet*, **i**, 586.
BOWIE, J. H., KENNEDY, M. H. AND ROBERTSON, I. (1975) *Lancet*, **i**, 1135.

BRITISH PHARMACOPOEIA (1980) 2.A196. London: HMSO.

BRITISH STANDARDS INSTITUTION (1960) Specification for rectangular metal boxes for use in high vacuum steam sterilizers, *BS381*, BSI.

BRITISH STANDARDS INSTITUTION (1982) Specification for paper bags for steam sterilization for medical use. *BS6254*, BSI.

COLQUHOUN, J. (1969) *British Hospital Journal*, July.

CUNLIFFE, A. C. (1966) *Proceedings Central Sterilising Club*, April 29–30th.

DAVIS, D., BONEKAT, H. W., ANDREWS, D. AND SHIGEOICA, J. W. (1984) Disinfection of the flexible fibreoptic bronchoscope against *Mycobacterium tuberculosis* and *M. gordonae*. *Thorax*, **39**, 785–788.

DEPARTMENT OF HEALTH AND SOCIAL SECURITY (1987) *Health Technical Memorandum No 10 — Sterilizers*. London: HMSO.

DEPARTMENT OF HEALTH AND SOCIAL SECURITY (1987) *Specification for Biological Monitors for the control of Low Temperature Steam and Formaldehyde Sterilization*, TSS/S/330/013.

DEPARTMENT OF HEALTH AND SOCIAL SECURITY (1987) *Specification for Biological Monitors for the control of Ethylene Oxide Sterilizers*, TSS/S/330/012.

DEPARTMENT OF HEALTH AND SOCIAL SECURITY (1987) *Specification for Indicator Test Sheets for use in the Bowie and Dick Test (for porous load steam sterilizers*, TSS/S/330/013).

DEVERILL, C. E. A. AND CRIPS, N. F. (1981) Tests on a low temperature steam and formaldehyde autoclave: the Miniclave 80, *Journal of Hospital Infection*, **2**, 175–180.

DOYLE, J. E. (1971) Sterility indicator with artificial resistance to ethylene oxide. *Bulletin of the Parenteral Drug Association*, **25**, 89–101.

FISCHER, E. (1971) Meeting on ethylene oxide sterilisation, University of Wales, September 6th.

FRANCIS, A. E. (1961) Use of a pasteurising water bath for disinfection of cystoscopes. *Journal of Urology*, **86**, 679–682.

GARDNER, J. F. AND PEEL, M. M. (1986) *Introduction to Sterilization and Disinfection*. Edinburgh: Churchill Livingstone.

GOULD, B. S., FRIGERIO, N. A. AND HOVANESIEN, J. (1957) *Antibiotics*, **7**, 457.

HAMBLETON, R. (1986) A new test pack for the Bowie and Dick test on porous load sterilisers. *Infection Control News*, June, 3M Health Care.

HEALTH AND SAFETY EXECUTIVE, *Guidance Note EH 40 — Occupational Exposure Limits*, HSE.

HOWIE, J. W. (1961) *Journal of Clinical Pathology*, **14**, 49.

HOWIE, J. W. AND TIMBURY, M. C. (1956) *Lancet*, **ii**, 669.

HURRELL, D. J. (1980) Low temperature steam disinfection and low temperature/formaldehyde sterilisation. *Sterile World*, **2**, (4), 13–18, Sutton in Ashfield.

KELSEY, J. C. AND MAURER, I. M. (1967) *Public Health Laboratory Service Bulletin*, **26**, June.

KNOX, R. (1961) *Journal of Clinical Pathology*, **14**, 13.

KNOX, R. AND PICKERILL, J. K. (1964) Efficient air removal from steam sterilisers without the use of high vacuum. *Lancet*, **i**, 1318–1321.

KNOX, R. AND PICKERILL, J. K. (1967) Steam sterilisation: a pre-sterilising stage combining a flush-aided pre-vacuum with bursts of steam above atmospheric pressure. *British Hospital Journal and Social Service Review*, **77**, 2377.

LINE, S. J. AND PICKERILL, J. K. (1973) *Journal of Clinical Pathology*, **26**, 716–720.

LOWBURY, E. J. (1961) *Journal of Clinical Pathology*, **14**, 85, 88, 89.

McCULLOCH, E. C. (1945) *Disinfection and Sterilisation*, 2nd edn. London: Kimpton.

MACKENZIE, S. (1966) *British Hospital Journal*, September 16, 1733.

MARR, M. S. AND SAGGERS, B. (1964) *Nursing Times*, June 12.

MAURER, I. M. (1985) *Hospital Hygiene*, p. 79. London: Edward Arnold.

MEDICAL RESEARCH COUNCIL (1945) *The Sterilisation, Use and Care of Syringes*. War Memo. No. 15. London: HMSO.

MEDICAL RESEARCH COUNCIL (1959) Working Party. *Lancet*, **i** 425.

MEDICAL RESEARCH COUNCIL (1968) Aseptic methods in the operating theatre. *Lancet*, **i**, 763.

MORRIS, C. A. AND EVERALL, P. H. (1975) *Lancet*, **i**, 923.

OXBORROW, G. S., PLACENCIA, A. M. AND DANIELSON, J. W. (1983) Effects of temperature and relative humidity on biological indicators used for ethylene oxide sterilization. *Applied and Environmental Microbiology*, **45**, 546–549.

PERKINS, J. J. (1956a) Bacteriological and surgical sterilisation by heat. In *Antiseptics, Disinfectants, Fungicides, Chemicals and Physical Sterilisation*. Edited by C. F. Reddish. New York: Lea and Febiger.

PERKINS, J. J. (1956b) *Principles and Methods of Sterilisation*, p. 163. Springfield, Ill.: Thomas.

PHILLIPS, C. R. AND KAYE, S. (1949) The sterilising action of gaseous ethylene oxide. *American Journal of Hygiene*, **50**, 270–279.

RENDELL-BAKER, L. (1970) *Hospitals*, October.

RENDELL-BAKER, L. AND ROBERTS, R. B. (1970) *Current Researches in Anesthesia and Analgesia*, November.

RIDGWAY, G. L. (1985) Leading article — Decontamination of fibreoptic endoscopes. *Journal of Hospital Infection*, **6**, 363–368.

ROSE, F. L. AND SWAINE, G. (1956) *Journal of the Chemical Society*, **4**, 4422.

SCOWEN, (1972) *Report of U.K. Committee on the Safety of Medicines*, 'Hexachlorophane', February.

SILLS, G. A. (1986) Sterilization, *Nursing*, **1** (3), 109–110.

SMYLIE, H. G., WEBSTER, C. V. AND BRUCE, M. L. (1959) *British Medical Journal*, **ii**, 606.

SPALTON, L. M. (1951) *Chemist and Druggist*, November 24.

SPALDING, E. H. (1963) *Association of Operating Room Nurses' Journal, U.S.A.*, May/June.

SYKES, G. (1958) In *Disinfection and Sterilisation*, pp. 170–339. Edited by McCulloch. London: Kimpton.

STONEHILL, A., KROP, S. AND BORICK, P. M. (1963) *American Journal of Hospital Pharmacy*, 20, 458.

WALTER, C. W. (1948) *The Aseptic Treatment of Wounds*. New York: Macmillan.

WELLS, C. AND WHITWELL, F. R. (1960) *Lancet*, **ii**, 643.

WESSEX INSTRUMENT CASKET, Feature article. *British Journal*, March.

WEYMES, C. (1966) *British Hospital Journal*, September, 1745.

8

Ligature and suture materials

A suture is a stitch used in surgery to approximate living tissues or structures until the normal process of healing is complete.

A ligature is a suture used to encircle a blood vessel to arrest or control bleeding.

Ligatures and sutures are classified in two main groups: the absorbable and the non-absorbable. These two groups are further subdivided into natural and synthetic materials and can be expressed in terms of a family tree according to source, structure and fate within the body (Fig. 8.1).

Natural absorbable materials such as catgut and collagen are absorbed within living tissue by enzymes and phagocytes. Synthetic absorbables, for example polyglycolic acid and poly-dioxanone, are absorbed by hydrolysis occurring in the body tissues. The strength of all absorbable sutures is lost well before absorption takes place.

Some non-absorbable sutures lose their tensile strength in the tissues relatively quickly, for example silk, linen and even nylon. Others such as polyester, polyethylene, polybutester, polypropylene and stainless steel, retain most of their tensile strength and can be truly described as non-absorbable.

Sutures described as monofilament are made from a single strand or filament which is very smooth and passes easily through the tissues. Multifilament sutures consist of several strands of material twisted or braided together. Although these pass less easily through tissues, this problem can be reduced by coating the surface of the suture material.

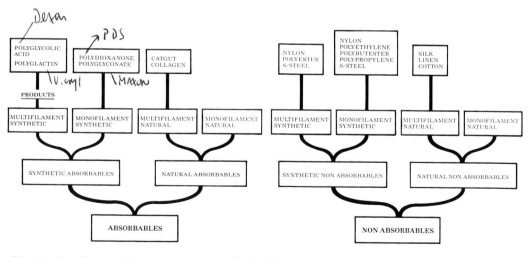

Fig. 8.1 Classification of ligatures and sutures. (Davis & Geck.)

NATURAL ABSORBABLES

Catgut

The most commonly used suture material in this group is still surgical catgut (Stotter *et al.*, 1982). This is substantially pure collagen prepared from the submucosa of animal intestines, normally milk lambs or beef cattle.

The preparation of surgical catgut

The intestines are washed, slit longitudinally into three or four strands, and scraped under a water spray to remove muscle and fat: the process is called sliming. The ribbons of gut may be treated also in alkaline chemical baths to remove the fat by saponification.

According to the diameter of gut required, two or more ribbons may be spun together into a single strand before being dried under tension. The gut is then cut to length and the surface electronically polished to achieve a uniform diameter along the entire length of the strand.

This dried gut is known technically as *plain* catgut. After sterilization, plain catgut is absorbed in muscle tissue in approximately 5 to 10 days, or about a quarter of that time in the peritoneum or serous membrane tissue.

The absorption of catgut in the tissues can be prolonged by immersing the catgut ribbons, following sliming, in a chromic salt solution. As chromic salts are normally colourless, it is usual to add colour to this bath to indicate visually the difference between *plain* and *chromic* (hardened) catgut.

The degree of hardness achieved depends on the composition of the chromic salts and how long the catgut is immersed in the solution. The most generally available is medium *chromic* catgut which, under normal conditions, will persist in the tissues from 15 to 20 days, or a quarter of that time in the peritoneum or serous membrane.

Each of the strands is then graded carefully into six standard metric sizes: from the thinnest to the thickest, 2 (4/0), 3 (3/0), 3.5 (2/0), 4 (0), 5 (1), and 6 (2). (*The ligature or suture sizes quoted refer always to metric gauge, the sizes in brackets are the USP equivalents. The metric size approximates the diameter of the strand in millimetres × 10.*) Although manufacturers generally exceed basic standards, the tensile strength of catgut must reach an average breaking load over either a *surgeon's knot* or *simple knot* as follows:

Size		US Pharmacopeia average minimum tensile strength		European Pharmacopoeia & British Pharmacopoeia average minimum tensile strength	
		Surgeon's knot		*Simple knot*	
2	metric (4/0)	0.77 kgf*	7.55 N**	0.767 kgf	7.51 N
3	metric (3/0)	1.25 kgf	12.3 N	1.27 kfg	12.5 N
3.5	metric (2/0)	2.0 kgf	19.6 N	2.04 kgf	20.0 N
4	metric (0)	2.27 kgf	22.3 N	2.80 kfg	27.5 N
5	metric (1)	3.8 kgf	37.3 N	3.87 kgf	38.0 N
6	metric (2)	4.51 kgf	44.2 N	4.59 kgf	45.0 N

* Kilogram force   ** Newtons

The finished catgut is divided into convenient lengths of about 70 cm (30 in) or 1.52 m (5 ft) to form ligatures or 'needled' sutures. The attachment of non-traumatic suture needles

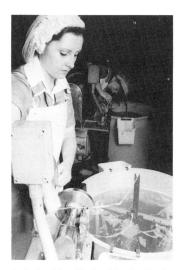

Fig. 8.2 Splitting New Zealand lamb skins into ribbon. (Ethicon.)

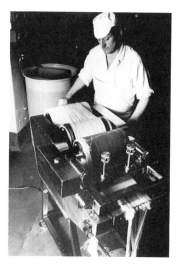

Fig. 8.3 Machine sliming to remove fatty tissue from lamb's intestine. (Ethicon.)

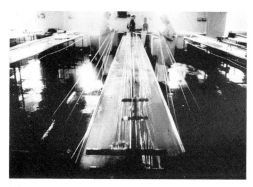

Fig. 8.4 Spinning multiples of ribbon into raw surgical catgut. (Ethicon.)

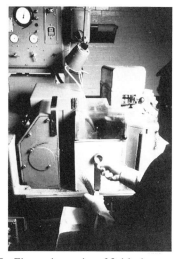

Fig. 8.5 Electronic gauging of finished catgut strands before polishing. (Ethicon.)

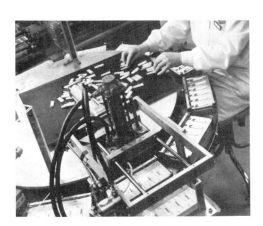

Fig. 8.6 Finished sutures placed in foil inner packets before being sealed in outer packet for sterilization. (Ethicon.)

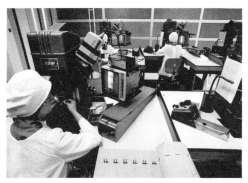

Fig. 8.7 The attachment of non-traumatic needles to strands of suture material with the aid of a TV monitor. (Ethicon.)

is a highly skilled procedure (Fig. 8.7). There are two basic methods of needle attachment. A hole may be drilled longitudinally into the needle shaft, or the needle can be flanged to form a groove (Fig. 8.7). Machines are used to close the needle tightly around the suture material, which is then subjected to a 'pull tester' to ensure that it is firmly attached to the needle (Fig. 8.8).

Under clean, controlled conditions, the finished suture is placed within a support card or on a former in such a manner as to facilitate easy withdrawal without twisting or snagging. A loop or figure of eight winding technique may be used. The suture and support card are then packed in an inner foil envelope containing a solution of isopropyl alcohol, or are first softened to maintain suppleness of the gut and then packed dry. The sealed inner envelope is placed in an outer plastic and paper laminate peel-open envelope (Fig. 8.9), which is then sealed for sterilization, generally by irradiation (Fig. 8.10 and Fig. 7.17).

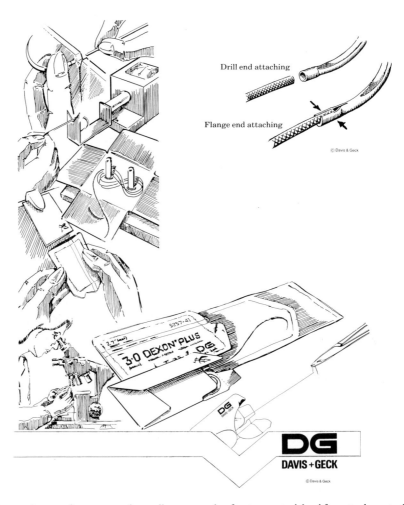

Drill end attaching

Flange end attaching

© Davis & Geck

DG
DAVIS+GECK
© Davis & Geck

Fig. 8.8 The attachment of non-traumatic needles to strands of suture materials. After attachment, the suture is tested on a 'pull tester'. With the finest ophthalmic or micro-needles, the needles are handled under a microscope. The way in which the suture is placed inside the inner support card determines the ease with which it can be dispensed. Larger sizes of suture are machine wound into the support card; fine delicate sutures are hand-wound. Either a loop or figure of eight winding technique may be used. (Davis & Geck.)

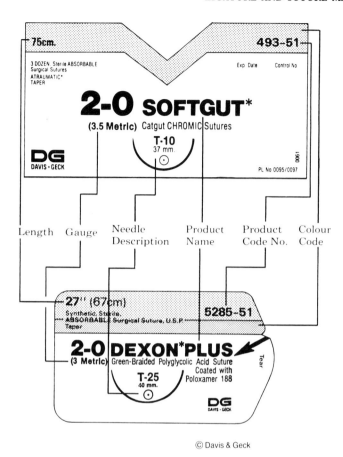

Fig. 8.9 Typical suture packet and suture box labels showing how the essential information is displayed. (Davis & Geck.)

Sterilisation by Ethylene Oxide Gas (ETO)

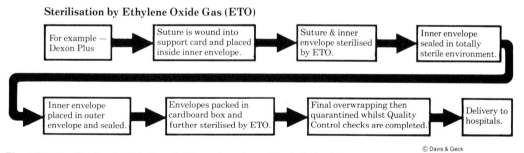

Fig. 8.10 Sterilization by Ethylene Oxide — flow chart. (Davis & Geck.)

Catgut in use

The finest possible size of catgut should be used always; with the continual improvement of tensile strength, the sizes in common use are much finer than those used previously.

For the ligation of small blood vessels 3 or 3.5 (3/0 or 2/0) *plain* catgut is generally sufficient. Large blood vessels and pedicles, such as those requiring ligation in gynaecological surgery, require a stouter *chromic* catgut, size 5 (1) or thicker.

Suture of stomach or bowel in an adult necessitates using size 3.5 or 4 (2/0 or 0) *chromic* catgut, whereas a child will require at least a size smaller, 3 (3/0) for these tissues.

For an adult the peritoneum and muscle can be sutured with *chromic* catgut sizes 5 or 6 (1 or 2); a child will require at least a size smaller, 4 (0).

If subcutaneous tissue is sutured a size 3 or 3.5 (3/0 or 2/0) *plain* catgut is preferred, especially in the case of subcutaneous suture for thyroidectomy.

Some surgeons will use *chromic* catgut throughout an operation, but if *plain* catgut is used it is important that this is not introduced as a suture or ligature into the peritoneum due to rapid absorption, except in very special circumstances, e.g. in the urinary tract.

Homologenous sutures

These are tissue sutures obtained from the patient. The most usual are strips of fascia lata used in Gallie's herniorrhaphy and obtained from the lateral aspect of the thigh. In one method, the strips of fascia, approximately 0.5 cm by 18 cm ($\frac{1}{4}$ in by 7 in), are obtained through a long thigh incision, following which the fascial defect and skin are sutured. It is possible also to remove these strips via two small incisions using a fasciatome, but in this case the fascial defect is not sutured.

The fascial strips are secured on a large-eye Gallie's needle (Chapter 9), either by locking the fascia through itself, or stitching with separate thread sutures before being darned into position over the hernial defect.

Tendons may be used in a similar fashion also, the plantaris tendon of the leg being suitable as its removal results in minimal interference with function.

Collagen tape

Reconstituted chromic collagen tape (Ethicon) can be used as a substitute for homologenous fascia used in various repair operations.

It has advantages over the patient's own fascia in that it avoids an operation on the leg; it ties easily without the need of secondary sutures; it is stronger than fascia of similar mass; and it contains no extraneous tendinous material as that found in beef fascia.

In ophthalmic surgery, collagen tape can be used as a frontal muscle sling for the correction of blepharotosis or ptosis. Ptosis may be congenital or senile, but generally it is acquired by trauma which severs either the levator muscle or the third cranial nerve, or by the invasion of the muscle by a tumour.

In other branches of surgery it can be substituted where fascia would normally have been used. In repair of lacerations of the liver, for example, or in nephropexy, the breadth of the suture is an advantage with these extremely delicate tissues. Collagen tape can be inserted with a suitable needle such as Gallie's or Wright's.

Collagen tape is supplied in cut lengths of 60 cm (24 in) by 3 mm ($\frac{1}{8}$ in) in width.

SYNTHETIC ABSORBABLES

The tensile strength of all synthetic absorbables must conform to the gradings specified in the US Pharmacopeia; at time of writing there was no equivalent European standard. The gradings of average breaking load over a simple knot can be summarised as follows:

Size		US Pharmacopeia average minimum tensile strength	
0.7	metric (6/0)	0.25 kgf	2.5 N
1	metric (5/0)	0.68 kgf	6.7 N
1.5	metric (4/0)	0.95 kgf	9.3 N
2	metric (3/0)	1.77 kgf	17.4 N
3	metric (2/0)	2.68 kgf	26.3 N
3.5	metric (0)	3.9 kgf	38.3 N
4	metric (1)	5.08 kgf	50.0 N

Polyglycolic acid

Dexon (Davis & Geck) is a synthetic polymer of glycolic acid, a naturally-occurring substance. It is absorbed in tissues essentially by hydrolysis and not digested by proteolysis as are gut and collagen. The material is made by extrusion as fine strands which are then braided to form a uniform gauge thread of seven sizes from 0.7 to 4 (6/0 to 1) (Figs. 8.11–8.21). To provide a smooth surface, the strands can be coated with a fine layer of Poloxamer 188, which is an inert absorbable surfactant (Dexon Plus). Tests have shown a minimal absorption in tissue at 15 days, maximum absorption at 300 days, and essentially complete absorption after 60 to 90 days following implantation (Anscombe *et al.*, 1970; Davis & Geck, 1971; Miln *et al.*, 1972; Trimbos, 1985)

Polyglycolic acid sutures are extremely inert and cause minimal tissue reaction (Edlich *et al.*, 1974; Stotter *et al.*, 1982). Size for size compared with catgut they are stronger, are fray resistant and do not become slippery in use. Dexon is supplied in single non-needled lengths of 150 cm, and armed with Atraumatic™ needles in lengths of between 45 and 75 cm. The sutures are sealed in two packets and sterilized by a two-stage ethylene oxide process (Fig. 8.22). With this method, the inner envelope must be sterilized before sealing, which then takes place in a totally sterile laminar airflow environment. Gas can penetrate the outer laminate envelope to complete sterilization, but it is impermeable to micro-organisms.

Because of the increased strength compared with catgut, Dexon and other synthetic absorbables generally enable a size smaller than the examples given for catgut to be used. The main contra-indication is that they should not be used where extended approximation of tissues must be maintained; a non-absorbable material is more suitable for this purpose. As with all sutures, care must be taken with respect to drainage and closure of wounds. Dexon requires special care in placing the first knot; it will not slip and 'snug' down under additional throws. The first throw is always placed exactly where required and knots tied in this way remain secure. As Dexon Plus is surface coated, extra throws are necessary to ensure knot security.

Although Dexon is suitable for deep sutures it can be used as a conventional skin suture or as a subcuticular closure. This technique is particularly suitable for cosmetic surgery where minimal tissue reaction is essential.

Polyglyconate

Maxon (Davis & Geck) is a monofilament synthetic absorbable suture prepared from a copolymer of glycolic acid and trimethylene carbonate. The sutures are available undyed (clear) or coloured green with D & C Green No. 6 to enhance visibility during surgery.

The process of absorption is by non-enzymatic hydrolysis, breaking down into carbon dioxide, B-hydroxybutyric acid and glycolic acid which are excreted in the urine. Approxi-

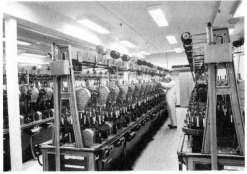

Fig. 8.11 The yarn is twisted together on a braiding machine using a sixteen, twelve, eight filament twist.

Fig. 8.12 The resulting braid is then washed to remove impurities by a process of solvent washing and vacuum sublimation. At this stage, the braid is coated with Poloxamer 188. The braid is then inspected by using a photo electric sensor which shows any imperfections which are then removed.

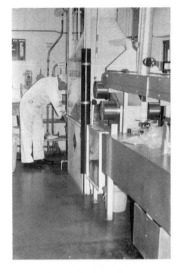

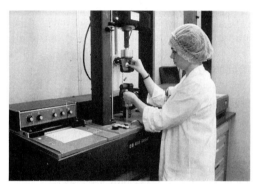

Fig. 8.13 Tensile strength and knot pull tests are carried out to ensure strength exceeds USP standards.

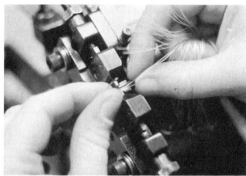

Fig. 8.14 Atraumatic™ needles are attached to the suture material.

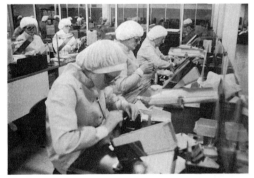

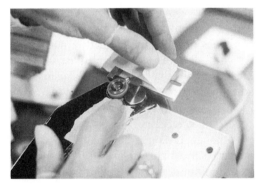

Figs. 8.15–8.16 Sutures are wound and inserted in correct packaging.

Figs. 8.11–8.21 The production of Dexon™ synthetic absorbable suture material. (Davis & Geck.) Production of Dexon begins with chemical processing of glycolic acid; a substance found in fruits, vegetables and the human body. By chemical processing, liquid glycolic acid is polymerised into chains of glycolic acid molecules. These molecules undergo purification including distillation, filtration and crystallisation. The end result is pure polyglycolic acid which is first melted and extruded and then cut into small pellets. These pellets are then melted and extruded through a spinnerette producing filaments of 2 denier. The filaments are gathered into bundles of twelve strands, each bundle is then wrapped on cylinders. The resulting yarn is examined microscopically to ensure uniform filaments with no imperfections. The fibres are then strengthened by controlled heat and stretching.

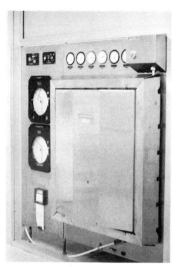

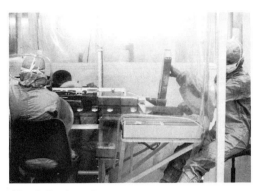

Fig. 8.18 A sterile room where technicians vacuum dry the product to remove moisture and ethylene gas residue. The sterile product is then sealed, and the seal inspected.

Fig. 8.17 Before sealing, packages are sterilized with ethylene oxide. (They are then moved under controlled conditions into a sterile room.)

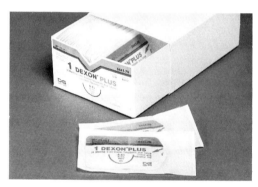

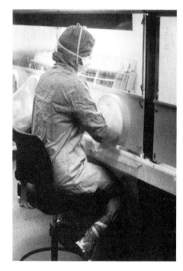

Fig. 8.19 Sterile packaged sutures now receive the outer plastic and paper overwrap and are boxed. Boxed sutures are then sterilized as ethylene oxide gas penetrates and sterilizes both the outside of the inner envelope and the inside of the outer envelope.

Fig. 8.20 Finally, the suture, needle and inner packet are tested to ensure that no microbiological contamination has occurred.

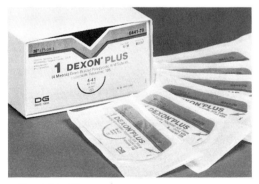

Fig. 8.21 The resultant product — coated Dexon Plus.™

Sterilisation by Irradiation

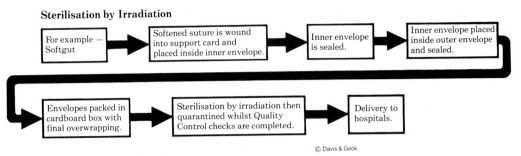

Fig. 8.22   Sterilization by irradiation — flow chart. (Davis & Geck.)

mately 70% of the original suture strength remains 2 weeks after implanation, and approximately 55% of the original suture strength remains 3 weeks after implantation. Absorption is essentially complete 6 months after implantation.

The material is supple and flexible in use, with minimal tissue drag. It is easy to tie, has good knot rundown characteristics, and remains secure once tied. Maxon can be used in most types of soft tissue including skin closure *except* for cardiovascular, ophthalmic, or microsurgery and neural tissue.

Maxon is available in sizes 0.7 (6/0)–3 (2/0) (clear), and sizes 1 (5/0)–4 (1) (green), mounted on atraumatic needles 17 60 mm.

Polydioxanone

PDS (Ethicon) is a monofilament synthetic absorbable suture made from the polyester polydioxanone. During polymerisation, the suture material may be coloured by adding D & C violet No. 2.

PDS sutures are relatively inert. Data obtained from implantation studies show that, at two weeks post implantation, approximately 50 per cent of the suture strength is retained. At eight weeks about 14 per cent of the original strength still remains. Absorption of the suture material generally commences about the 90th post implantation day, and is complete within six months.

The material, available in seven sizes from 0.7 to 4 (6/0 to 1), can be used for procedures in which catgut would be indicated, but it is not suitable when extended approximation of tissues under stress is needed e.g. repair of hernia. Conjunctival, cuticular and vaginal mucosal sutures could cause localised irritation if left in place for longer than 10 days.

Polyglactin 910

Coated Vicryl (Ethicon) is a braided suture prepared from a copolymer of glycolide and lactide, and surface coated with a mixture composed of a copolymer of glycolide and an equal amount of calcium sterate. During polymerisation the suture may be coloured by adding D & C violet No. 2.

Vicryl is a pliable, smooth material, which is made in nine sizes from 0.3 to 5 (8/0 to 2); it allows easy passage through tissue and secure knotting. Data from implantation studies show that more than 55 per cent of the original strength remains at 14 days, and over 20 per cent at 21 days. Absorption of the suture is minimal until about the 40th post-implantation day, and is complete between the 60th and 90th days.

The material can be used for procedures in which catgut would be indicated but it is not

suitable when extended approximation of tissues under stress is needed, e.g. repair of hernia. Conjunctival and skin sutures could cause localised irritation if left in place for longer than 10 days.

Plastafil carbon fibre fixing system

This comprises multiple carbon fibre strands, bollards and toggles. The strands, or tow implant, is made up of approximately 40,000 × 8 micron filaments (Fig. 8.23). The resultant

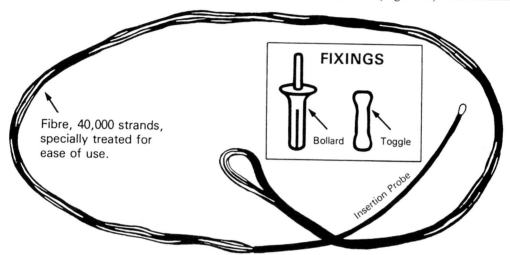

Fibre, 40,000 strands, specially treated for ease of use.

FIXINGS

Bollard   Toggle

Insertion Probe

Fig. 8.23   Carbon fibre implants. (Plastafil, A. W. Showell (Surgicraft) Ltd.)

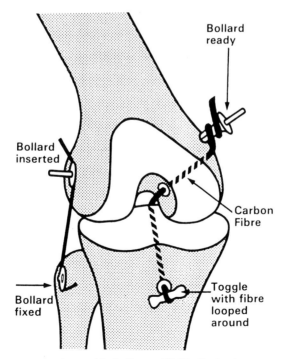

Bollard ready

Bollard inserted

Carbon Fibre

Bollard fixed

Toggle with fibre looped around

Fig. 8.24   Posterior cruciate reconstruction — Mr A. Strover FRCS. (A. W. Showell [Surgicraft] Ltd.)

tow, complete with an insertion probe, is treated with approved surgical gelatine and a bactericide for ease of handling. The bollards and toggles are made from carbon fibre reinforced thermoplastic polymer (iv), biomedically compatible. The implants are supplied sterile, double packed.

The system is used for knee ligament and ruptured tendon repairs. For example, Figure 8.24 illustrates a typical posterior cruciate reconstruction. The tibia has been drilled and threaded with carbon fibre from an anterior approach. The fibre tow is anchored with a toggle, and adjusted with a bollard; the bollard is then locked into a hole drilled in the bone. The carbon fibre acts as a prosthesis and provides a scaffold for the biological reconstruction of the ligament which grows stronger with time.

NON-ABSORBABLE LIGATURES AND SUTURES

Materials in this category may be divided into two classes, those manufactured from natural raw materials, and those which are entirely synthetic. Non-absorbable sutures are not generally used in an infected wound as they may cause sinus formation.

The tensile strength of all synthetic non-absorbables must conform to the gradings specified in the US Pharmacopeia; European Pharmacopoeia and the British Pharmacopoeia. The gradings of average breaking load over a simple knot can be summarised as follows:

Size		US Pharmacopeia average minimum tensile strength		European Pharmacopoeia & British Pharmacopoeia average minimum tensile strength	
0.4	metric (8/0)	0.06 kgf	0.14 N	0.061 kgf	0.6 N
0.7	metric (6/0)	0.2 kgf	1.96 N	0.153 kgf	1.5 N
1	metric (5/0)	0.4 kgf	3.92 N	0.306 kgf	3.0 N
1.5	metric (4/0)	0.6 kgf	5.88 N	0.510 kgf	5.0 N
2	metric (3/0)	0.96 kgf	9.42 N	0.918 kgf	9.0 N
3	metric (2/0)	1.44 kgf	14.11 N	1.53 kgf	15.0 N
3.5	metric (0)	2.16 kgf	21.17 N	2.24 kgf	22.0 N
4	metric (1)	2.72 kgf	26.67 N	2.75 kgf	27.0 N
5	metric (2)	3.52 kgf	34.5 N	3.75 kgf	35.0 N
6	metric (3)	4.88 kgf	47.84 N	5.1 kgf	50.0 N

Silk

This material, generally ivory or black, is braided from numerous gossamer strands of silk. It is supplied on sterilizable spools 20 to 100 m (25 to 125 yds), or in multiple pre-cut lengths ranging from 35 to 45 cm (14 to 18 in), and a single pre-cut length of 1.8 m (72 in).

The sizes available are 0.4 (8/0) (virgin silk), and from 0.7 to 6 (6/0 to 4) or even stronger. The grading in average breaking load over a surgeon's knot can be summarised as follows:

The very fine sizes 0.4 (8/0) blue virgin silk (Surgisilk–Surgicraft), and from 0.7 to 2 (6/0 to 3/0), are useful in vascular and nerve anastomosis, ophthalmic and plastic surgery, and intestinal suturing. sizes from 3 to 4 or 5 (2/0 to 1 or 2) are used for general ligatures and sutures; sizes 5.5 and 6 (3 and 4) are used for large pedicles such as haemorrhoids, etc.

It is important to use serum-proofed silk to reduce capillary attraction which is a peculiarity of plaited or braided materials. Examples of these materials include D & G Silk (Davis

& Geck), Mersilk (Ethicon), and Surgisilk (Surgicraft). The capillary attraction which a non-serum proofed material has is hazardous, as micro-organisms may lodge in the minute spaces of the braiding, becoming a permanent source of irritation and wound infection.

A full range of sterile non-traumatic needled serum proofed sutures are available. Alternatively, if eyed needles are preferred, perhaps for economical reasons, and where many silk sutures are required during operation, it is advantageous to thread several needles before autoclaving as a multipack. In this instance the appropriate needles are threaded with various sizes of silk, and are stitched loosely on to a sponge pad before sterilization. With this method very great care must be taken to check the total number of needles in circulation during operation.

SYNTHETIC NON-ABSORBABLES

Polyamide (Nylon)

Nylon was the first synthetic plastic suture material developed during the 1939–45 war. Since then suture manufacturers have refined the polymerisation process to develop materials which have improved tensile strength and handling properties. These materials have now replaced the use of silkworm gut.

Monofilament

This is a single strand of polyamide supplied in sizes ranging from 0.2 to 2 (10/0 to 2). The grading in average breaking load over a surgeon's knot can be summarised as follows:

The material can be obtained in multiple pre-cut lengths, from 35 cm to 1 m (14 to 40 in); the shorter length is suitable for interrupted skin sutures and the longer length for the 'darn' in herniorrhaphy, or for suturing muscle.

The finest sizes are preferred for face sutures, whereas the strongest are more applicable for 'through-and-through' abdominal tension sutures. A monofilament polyamide suture must be cut at least 10 mm (3/8 in) long, as slight slipping of the knot may occur under certain conditions.

Polyamide as a single strand is relatively inert, can be safely used in the presence of infection (Moloney et al., 1950; Everett, 1970; Edlich, 1974), and may be left in the tissues with very little unfavourable reaction occurring.

Monofilament examples of this material include Ethilon, blue (Ethicon); Surgidek, blue or black (Surgicraft); and Dermalon, white, blue or black (Davis & Geck).

Braided

This is used in a similar manner to braided silk. The sizes available range from 0.7 (6/0) to 2 (5), and the same tensile strengths as braided silk apply. The two colours available, black and blue, do not refer to a particular size but are only preferential colour choices. It is generally supplied in multiple pre-cut lengths of between 35 cm (14 in) and 1 m (40 in), sterile in peel-open packs.

The material is available also armed with non-traumatic needles. Braided polyamide-like monofilament is often used for hernia repair and may be prepared as a mesh which is stitched over the hernial defect.

Sizes 1.5 to 3 (4/0 to 2/0) are used for plastic surgery, skin sutures or fine intestinal sutures; 3 to 4 (2/0 to 1) for ligatures and general muscle sutures; and 5 (2) for herniorrhaphy or large pedicle ligatures.

Examples of this material include Nurolon (Ethicon) and Surgilon (Davis & Geck). A sheathed multistrand polyamide suture is available under the name of Supramid (Surgicraft). The tensile strength of braided sutures is similar to that of monofilament materials.

Polyester

Polyester fibre is supplied as a braided material and is marketed surgically under several trade names including: Dacron (Davies & Geck); Ethibond (Ethicon); Polydek, Sutulene and Tevdek II (Surgicraft); and Ticron (Davis & Geck). Ethibond (green in colour) is coated with polytetramethylene adipate (polybutylate) to ensure smoothness and handling with no risk of flaking or fraying. Polydek (green) is coated with polytetrafluoroethylene (PTFE); Tevdek (green) is impregnated with PTFE; the surface of Ticron (white or blue) is treated with silicones; Sutulene (black) is impregnated with waxes. Dacron (white or black) consists of untreated polyester fibres.

Sizes in common use are 1 to 3 (5/0 to 2/0) for plastic, skin, ophthalmic or intestinal sutures and ligation of small vessels; 3.5 to 5 (0 to 2) for muscle sutures and stout ligatures. The materials available are serum proofed and are handled in a similar manner to braided silk, braided nylon or linen thread. Polyester is also used for the fabrication of cardiovascular prostheses, e.g. bifurcated aortic grafts.

Polybutester

This is a monofilament material supplied under the trade name Novafil (Davis & Geck). It is claimed that polybutester is superior to polypropylene in terms of flexibility, suppleness, and strength. It has an elasticity which permits recovery from elongation and facilitates knot rundown and secure tying.

Novafil is blue in colour and supplied as needled sutures sizes 0.5 (7/0) to 3 (2/0).

Polypropylene

Monofilament polypropylene is available under the trade names Prolene, blue, (Ethicon); Prodek, black (Surgicraft); and Surgilene, clear or cyan blue (Davis & Geck). The material is extremely inert, stronger than monofilament polyamide in most sizes and very malleable; it will crush and deform easily upon knotting. The knot-holding characteristic is said to be superior to other synthetic suture materials.

Polypropylene can be resterilized, but not more than twice by standard autoclaving, otherwise loss of strength will occur.

The material is available in sizes 0.2 to 5 (10/0 to 2), with or without needles. Polypropylene is suitable for where a non-absorbable suture is required.

Metallic wire

Suture wire is prepared mainly from three metals — non-toxic stainless steel BS3531, the alloy tantalum and silver.

All these may be obtained as a single-strand monofilament suture and the first two as several strands, either twisted or braided, known as multifilament wire.

The multifilament wire is more flexible and less likely to kink during handling. The sizes are graded either as metric or SWG (Standard Wire Gauge). The former vary from 1 to 9 (5/0 to 7), and the latter gauge from fine 40 SWG to stout 18 SWG. Tensile strengths of stainless steel wire are graded up to 2 (2/0) in breaking load over a simple knot, and straight pull breaking load for sizes above 3.5 (0). These can be summarised as follows:

Size			US Pharmacopeia average minimum tensile strength		British Pharmacopoeia average minimum tensile strength			
					Monofilament		Plated/twisted	
1	metric (5/0)	40 SWG	0.54 kgf	5.3 N	0.45 kgf	4.41 N	0.36 kgf	0.53 N
1.5	metric (4/0)	38 SWG	0.82 kgf	8.0 N	1.0 kgf	9.8 N	0.80 kgf	7.8 N
2	metric (3/0)	36 SWG	1.36 kgf	13.3 N	1.7 kgf	16.6 N	1.4 kgf	13.7 N
3	metric (2/0)	32 SWG	1.8 kgf	17.6 N	4.3 kgf	42.15 N	3.4 kgf	33.3 N
3.5	metric (0)	27 SWG	3.4 kgf	33.3 N	5.2 kgf	51.0 N	4.4 kgf	43.1 N
4	metric (1)	26 SWG	4.76 kgf	46.7 N	7.1 kgf	70.0 N	5.7 kgf	56.0 N
5	metric (2)	24 SWG	5.9 kgf	57.8 N	11.3 kgf	111.0 N	9.0 kgf	88.2 N
7	metric (5)	22 SWG	11.4 kgf	112.0 N	–	–	–	–
9	metric (7)	20 SWG	15.9 kgf	156.0 N	–	–	–	–
12	metric (10)	18 SWG	22.8 kgf	224.0 N	–	–	–	–

Surgical stainless steel suture wire is used mainly in orthopaedics and thoracic surgery. For tendon sutures, sizes 0.5 to 2 (7/0 to 3/0) or 40 SWG to 30 SWG are suitable, whereas a stouter wire of sizes 3 to 9 (0 to 7) or 29 SWG to 18 SWG would be needed for wiring fragments of bone together.

It may be used also for closing an abdominal incision in the obese or carcinomatous patient, for oesophageal anastomosis, closure of a chest incision or occasionally as a mesh in the repair of hernial defects.

It is very important that wires made from different metals are not used in contact with each other in the tissues, as a reaction may occur resulting in corrosion (Chapter 23).

Fine wire is used for threading tonsil, nasal and aural snares.

Metal clips (ligature)

Ligatures of flattened silver or tantalum wire are used in neurosurgery and chest surgery for arresting haemorrhage from small vessels, or compressing nerve endings by clipping them. One variety is known as Cushing's or McKenzie's clips and is V-shaped, being prepared with a special cutting clamp which bends and cuts the wire in one operation.

The small V-shaped clips, each arm being about 0.45 cm (3/16 in) long, are stored on a stand or galley, and are removed with special forceps, being handed in the forceps to the surgeon. The wire, clamp, gallery and insertion forceps together are sterilized by autoclaving.

The clips are very useful for ligating blood vessels which are too small or inaccessible for hand ligatures.

Commercially prepared and sterilized clips are available in small, medium and large sizes (Ligaclip, Ethicon). The insertion forceps and cartridges are colour coded for easy identification (Fig. 8.25).

LIGACLIP TRADEMARK
LIGATING CLIPS & APPLIERS

The system
Appliers and cartridges are colour-coded; selection therefore is fast and accurate. Each clip is formed and locked in the applier when the applier is inserted in the cartridge. Cross-locking action between serrations in the applier and the clip keep the clip locked in the applier, without slipping, twisting or dropping out, until the occlusion is made. There's no need for the scrub nurse and the surgeon to grasp the appliers by the handle to maintain tension during transfer. Result: no lost clips, no lost time.

Clips
are made of physiologically inert tantalum, packaged in sterile, autoclavable Nylon cartridges. Spring pressure between the clip and the shoulders of the cartridge prevent the clip from falling out. Only six clips to a cartridge means no waste, and it is seldom necessary to sterilise leftovers.

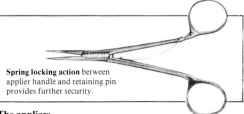

Spring locking action between applier handle and retaining pin provides further security.

The appliers
are made of surgical stainless steel and are colour-coded to match the clips. Sturdily made, they will work reliably even after hours of hard use.

Colour-coding by size
Both cartridges and appliers are colour-coded.
Blue—small; white—medium; yellow—large.

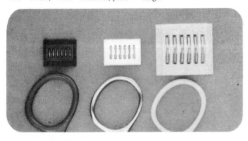

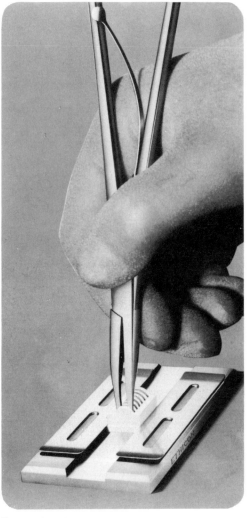

Fast no-ring pick-up
The clip is formed—and locked in place—when the applier is inserted in the cartridge. There's no need to hold the rings during loading.

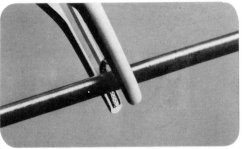

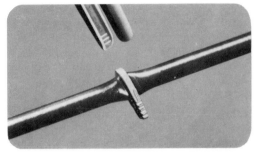

Secure no-ring transfer Nor is there any need for the scrub nurse—or the surgeon—to maintain ring tension during transfer, since the clip is locked in the applier. No lost clips—no lost time. Transfer is fast, positive, sure.

Fig. 8.25 Vascular ligature clips. (Ligaclip, Ethicon.)

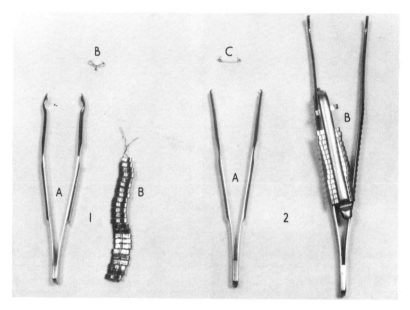

Fig. 8.26   Michel and Kifa skin suture clips. (1A) Insertion and removal forceps (Kifa). (1B) Suture clips (Kifa). (2A) Insertion forceps (Michel). (2B) Clip galley loaded with clips (Michel). (2C) Suture clip (Michel).

Metal clips (suture)

These are metal clips having two sharp points which, when the clip is closed, grip the edges of a skin incision. They are generally used to approximate a wound which heals quickly, e.g. in the region of the neck. They may be used also to close an abdominal incision or thigh incision in conjunction with tension sutures.

The original types in use are Michel and Kifa (Fig. 8.26). Both are loaded on to special insertion forceps, but the Kifa has two projecting lips on its upper surface which allow easy removal after healing has taken place. When these lips are squeezed with forceps the clip opens quite easily.

During the past few years there has been considerable development in the field of suture staples (Jewell *et al.*, 1983; Bucknall and Ellis, 1982). These range from disposable magazines of staples which fit an insertion instrument to completely disposable units. Examples of two of the latter are Proximate II (Ethicon) and Appose (Davis & Geck). A stapler which uses replacement magazines (Precise, 3M) is illustrated in Figure 8.27.

If subcutaneous tissue is sutured, a size 3 or 3.5 (3/0 or 2/0) plain catgut is preferable, especially in the case of a subcutaneous suture for thyroidectomy.

Some surgeons will use chromic catgut throughout an operation but if plain catgut is used it is important that this is not introduced as a suture (or ligature) into the peritoneum due to rapid absorption, except in very special circumstances, e.g. in the urinary tract.

Adhesive skin closures

These are microporous strips of non-woven fabric which are treated on one surface with a chemically inert adhesive. This adheres firmly, is virtually non-irritating, and removes easily and painlessly (Steristrip, Surgical Products/3m Health Care; Suture Strip Plus/Genetic

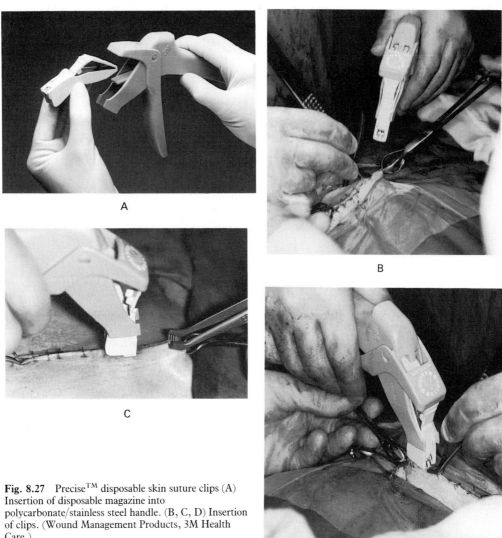

Fig. 8.27   Precise™ disposable skin suture clips (A) Insertion of disposable magazine into polycarbonate/stainless steel handle. (B, C, D) Insertion of clips. (Wound Management Products, 3M Health Care.)

Laboratories Ltd). Steristrip skin closures are sterile strips of Micropore surgical tape, reinforced with polyester filaments, either plain or impregnated with an iodophor, and pre-cut to specific sizes. Suture Strip is an elastic skin closure strip made from non-woven polyester backing coated with an adhesive.

These adhesive tapes are used for a variety of purposes including the primary closure of wounds, as an adjunct to sutures, and to provide support following suture removal. The technique of application is described in Chapter 10, page 289.

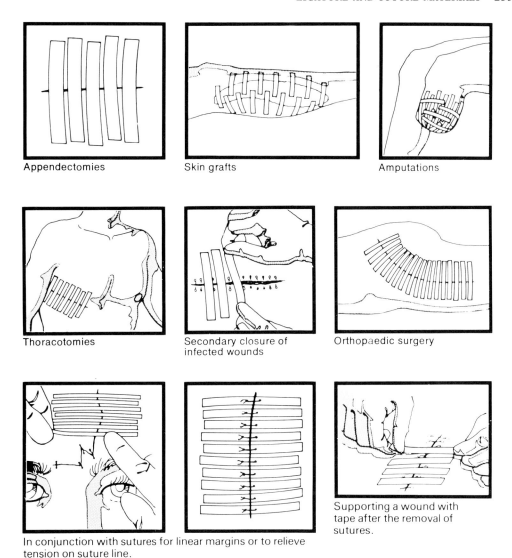

Appendectomies

Skin grafts

Amputations

Thoracotomies

Secondary closure of
infected wounds

Orthopaedic surgery

In conjunction with sutures for linear margins or to relieve
tension on suture line.

Supporting a wound with
tape after the removal of
sutures.

Fig. 8.28 Some uses for 'Steristrip'™ skin closures (Wound Management Products, 3M Health Care.)

REFERENCES

ANSCOMBE, A. R., HIRA, N. AND HUNT, B. (1970) *British Medical Journal*, 57, 108.
BRITISH PHARMACOPOEIA (1980) Vol II. London: HMSO.
BRITISH PHARMACOPOEIA (1986) Addendum. London: HMSO.
BUCKNALL, T. E. AND ELLIS, H. (1982) Skin Closure. Comparison of Nylon, Polyglycolic Acid and Staples.
   Euro. Surg. Res, **14**, 96–97.
DAVIS AND GECK (1971) *Proceedings of a Symposium on Polyglycolic Acid Sutures*.
EDLICH, R. F., PANEK, P. H., RODENHEAVER, G. T., KURTZ, L. D. AND EDGERTON, M. T. (1974) *Journal of
   Biochemical Materials Research Symposium*, **8**, 115.
EUROPEAN PHARMACOPOEIA (1984) 2nd edn, Part II. Council of Europe.
EVERETT, N. G. (1970) *Progress in Surgery (Basel)*, **8**, 14.
FORRESTER, J. C. (1975) *Nursing Mirror*, Jan 16th, p. 48.

Jewell, M. L., Sata, R. and Rahija, R. (1983) A comparison of wound healing in wounds closed with staples versus skin suture. *Contemporary Surgery*, **22**, 29–32.

Miln, D. C. O'Connor, J. and Dalling, R. (1972) *Scottish Medical Journal*, **17**, 108.

Moloney, G. E., Russell, W. T. and Wilson, D. C. (1950) *British Journal of Surgery*, **38**, 52.

Postlethwait, R. W. (1969) In *Repair and Regeneration*. McGraw-Hill: New York.

Stotter, A. T., Kapadia, C. R. and Dudley, H. A. F. (1982) Sutures in surgery. In *Recent Advances in Surgery*. Edited by R. C. G. Russell. Edinburgh: Churchill Livingstone.

Trimbos, J. B. (1985) Knot security of synthetic absorbable suture materials: a comparison of polyglycolic acid and polyglactin 910. *European J. Obstet & Gynae*, **19**, 183–190.

United States Pharmacopeia (1985) *The National Formulary* 16th edn. United States Pharmacopeial. Convention Inc. Rockville, Md

9

Storage and handling of ligature materials and associated instruments

Virtually all sizes and types of ligatures, sutures, scalpel blades and needles etc. can be purchased presterilized. Those items which are more convenient to process at hospital level can easily be presented in sterile pack or boxes (Brigden, 1962). All such sterile supplementary items are stored in dispensers or other suitable containers on trolleys, shelves or in cupboards in the operating suite preparation room.

If ligature materials, e.g. braided materials such as silk and polyester, are sterilized at hospital level, they should be prepared as cut lengths or wound onto cards or metal or nylon spools before sterilization, either with the set of instruments or in packs.

Wire may be stored on metal spools also, but if possible these should be of a larger size to avoid rather small loops of wire which would otherwise tend to kink during the preparation of sutures. Manufacturers also prepare wire lengths and sutures, supplied in sterile packs, and these include 'pull-out' tendon sutures (Pulvertaft).

Scalpel handles, probes, fine dissecting forceps, Michel and Kifa suture clips, suction

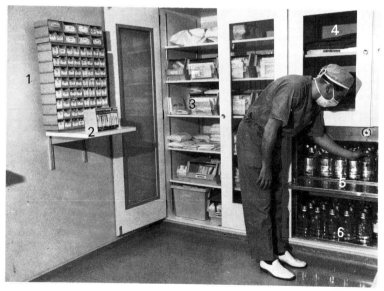

Fig. 9.1 Storage of sterile requisites in operating suite preparation room.
1. Boxes of ligature and suture requirements stored in dispenser.
2. Sterile scalpel blades in dispenser.
3. Supplementary sterile instruments in packs.
4. Preset trays of sterile instruments.
5. Heated cabinet for lotions.
6. Lotions stored at room temperature.

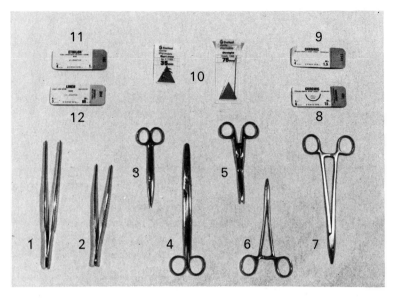

Fig. 9.2 A selection of ligature and suture requirements.

1. & 2. Dissecting forceps, non-toothed.
3. Scissors, stitch.
4. Carless suture scissors.
5. Kilner needle holder.
6. Fine needle holder.
7. Mayo needle holder.
8. Catgut suture — general closure with needle attached.
9. Catgut ligature.
10. Suture needles of appropriate size and shape (see Fig. 9.8).
11. Polyamide — monofilament.
12. Linen thread.

nozzles etc. may be sterilized in packs as supplementary items. These are used in conjunction with ligature requirements and are stored as described previously.

Under clean, dry, storage conditions an intact pack will keep the contents sterile. However, freshly sterilized items should always be positioned behind those already in store and by doing this the use of outdated products should be avoided.

The ligature storage trolley, shelves or cupboards should be given a thorough clean each week. Packets must be inspected for integrity and replaced if there is any doubt in respect of the condition of seals or surface.

General ligature requisites

Suture needles

These are made from plated carbon steel or martensitic stainless steel and occasionally austenitic stainless steel (Chapter 23). The stainless steel needles are to be preferred as they do not rust or snap easily as may the carbon steel variety. The small extra cost is amply compensated by these two advantages.

All needles fall into two principal classes: cutting needles and round-bodied needles.

1. *Cutting needles* have sharp edges, are often triangular in section but include variations such as reverse cutting, hand honed cutting and lancet; these cut a track as they pass through the tissue and are only used on strong tissue which will not be unduly damaged, such as fascia, muscle tendon and skin. Needle shapes such as spatula, lance point and diamond point are used for ophthalmic and microsurgery (Fig. 9.4). The edge of non-disposable

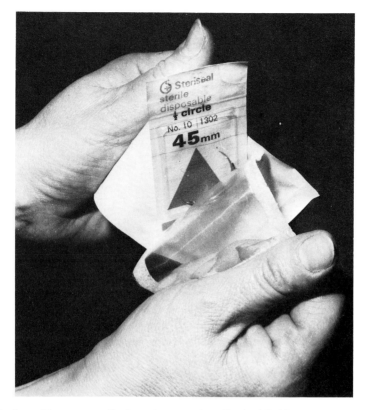

Fig. 9.3 Sterile disposable suture needles in peel-open packet. (Steriseal Ltd.)

'eyed' cutting needles must be sharp, and they must be examined regularly for wear, being discarded when worn as the cost of resharpening would exceed the cost of replacement.

2. *Round-bodied needles* cause less damage and do not actually cut the tissues, but make a puncture which closes very easily afterwards. They are used for suturing delicate tissue such as mucous membrane, fat and intestine.

Almost any style or shape of suture needle may be obtained as a non-traumatic variety; needles into which the catgut or other suture material is fused. This avoids the double thickness of material which is always present when it has been threaded through a needle eye. Round-bodied, non-traumatic needles are used for the closure of intestine, stomach, the ducts of glands, blood-vessels, and for the suture of nerves or any delicate tissue which may become traumatised during suture with conventional needles. Cutting, non-traumatic needles are used in plastic surgery for the suture of the face and other areas of skin, to minimise scar formation. They are used sometimes also for tendon suture, or for conjunctival and corneal suture in ophthalmic surgery.

Suture needles are further subdivided into straight, curved, half-circle, five-eighths circle, and special shapes or types.

Straight cutting needles. Size 65 to 100 mm ($2\frac{1}{2}$ to 4 in) in length, are used for skin sutures. The most common type are called Simm's abdominal needles.

Straight round-bodied needles. These are usually the fine intestinal type. Sizes 40–60 mm are used for intestinal suture or as a fixation needle during nerve and tendon suture. In the latter case, the degree of pull required (upon the proximal and distal segment of the nerve

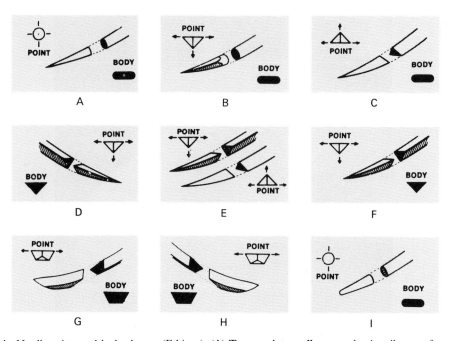

Fig. 9.4 Needle points and body shapes. (Ethicon). (A) **Taper point needle** — used primarily on soft, easily penetrated tissue such as peritoneum, intestine, or the heart. This needle creates the smallest possible hole in the tissue with minimal tissue damage. The body of the needle is flattened and ribbed to improve its stability in the needle holder. (B) **Tapercut**^{TM} needle — designed for use on tough tissue where a narrow bodied cutting pointed needle is required. It has a sharp reverse cutting tip at the point, with the remainder of the needle blending into a taper cross section. All three edges of the tip are sharpened to provide uniform cutting action. (C) **Conventional cutting needle** — has two opposing cutting edges with a third edge on the inside curvature of the needle. The conventional cutting needle changes in cross-section shape from a triangular cutting tip to a flattened body. (D) **Reverse cutting needle** — used to cut through tough, difficult to penetrate tissues such as fascia and skin. It has two opposing cutting edges, with the third cutting edge on the outer curvature of the needle. The reverse cutting needle is made with the triangular shape extending from the point to the swage area, with only the edges near the tip being sharpened. (E) **Precision point needle** — designed for use in plastic or cosmetic surgery, including the emergency repair of facial injuries and for suturing children. The specially honed precision point assures smooth passage through tissue and a minute needle path that heals quickly. (F) **Micro-point**^{TM} spatula needle — is a smooth, sharp reverse cutting edge needle for use in ophthalmic surgery. Each needle is individually honed to extreme sharpness and inspected under high power magnification. (G) **sabreloc**^{TM} needle — a sharp, flat type 'side-cutting' needle designed to split through the layers of scleral or corneal tissue, and travel within the plane between them with virtually no resistance. The needle is flat on top and bottom, thereby eliminating cutting out which would result from a conventional reverse cutting needle. (H) **Micro-point**^{TM} spatula needle — designed for anterior section ophthalmic surgery, the needle specially honed for sharpness, and is thin and flat in profile for ease of penetration. (I) **Blunt point needle** — a taper needle with a rounded, blunt point that will *not* cut through tissue. It is used for suturing of friable tissues, such as liver and kidney. (*Suture Use Manual: Use and Handling of Sutures and Needles* Ethicon Ltd)

or tendon) to allow approximation of the cut ends, is maintained by passing a round-bodied needle through each segment, and this prevents retraction during suture. (An alternative would be to use silk 'stay' sutures for this required pull.)

Curved cutting needles. These are used mainly for the suture of skin, fascia and tendon. Sizes 17 to 50 mm (26 to 9, small) are used on a needle holder, and those 60 mm (5, medium) to 90 mm (0, large) are used by hand (hand needles).

These needles may be obtained in normal or fine gauge, depending upon the wishes of the surgeon, but needles used in the region of the face should always be the very finest possible.

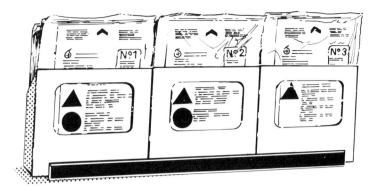

Fig. 9.5 Set of general closure needle packs (Surgicraft.)

Amongst special curved cutting needles the ophthalmic and microvascular types deserve special mention. These are very fine needles ranging from size 3.5 mm to 11 mm and include needles such as the Stallards which is a flattened section corneal needle and others which have reversed cutting edges, etc.

Some surgeons use ordinary cutting needles for the suture of tendons, but most express a preference for the non-traumatic type, such as the Pulvertaft, or multi-filament wire suture. Tendon sutures are generally a single strand, fine stainless steel wire, 1.5 metric (4/O) fused into a curved or straight cutting needle size 26 to 89 mm, supplied pre-sterilized or wound on a card which can be sterilized by autoclaving, or dry heat. The multifilament wire suture is welded in to one end of a similar size needle and packed ready sterilized in a plastic or foil packet. Both of these sutures are available as a single-armed (one needle) or double-armed (two needles) assembly.

Half-circle cutting needles. These are used mainly for the suture of fascia and muscle tendon. Sizes 20 mm (small) to 50 mm (medium) are used on a needle holder and sizes 80 to 110 mm (large) are generally held in the surgeon's hand. Special needles of this type are: the fistula, which are coarse, strong needles; and Lane's which have rather a large eye in comparison to the gauge, which is very useful for threading silk up to size 3.5 (2/0).

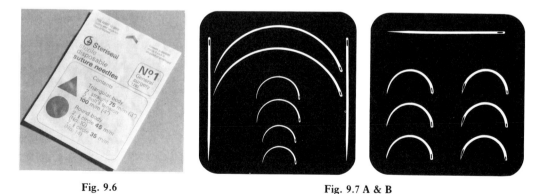

Fig. 9.6   **Fig. 9.7 A & B**

Fig. 9.6 Needle pack. The outer pack is peeled open (Fig. 9.3) and the inner blister illustrated is transferred to the sterile field (Steriseal.)

Fig. 9.7A and B The needles are fixed in a set pattern onto a loose foam pad. Examples of general and gynae closure sets (Steriseal Ltd.)

The fistula needles range from size 19 mm (6, small) to 83 mm (4/0, large), and the Lane's from size 10 mm (⅜ in, small) to 25 mm (1 in, large) to 4 (fine), the larger size being equivalent to size 19 ordinary half-circle needle.

The five-eighths circle or fully curved needle. This is generally of the Moynihan variety. These needles resemble a five-eighths circle as their name implies, and are based upon the idea that nearly every surgical stitch when tied, approximates a circle very closely. In consequence, the more closely the track of the needle follows this, the more evenly will the tension be applied to the tissues.

These Moynihan needles may be round-bodied or cutting edge, which are used for suturing peritoneum or fat, and muscle tendon respectively. The round-bodied type is conventional, but the cutting needle has a flattened lance point, which is rather spear-shaped.

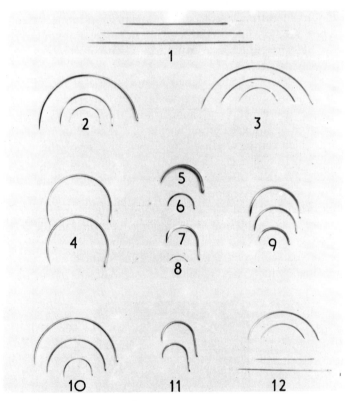

Fig. 9.8 Selection of suture needles in general use.
1. Straight triangular cutting needles (Simm, skin).
2. Half-circle triangular cutting needles (muscle tendon, fascia, etc.).
3. Curved triangular cutting needles (skin).
4. Five-eighth-circle round-bodies and lance-point needles (Moynihan, for peritoneum and muscle respectively).
5. Fascia needle (Gallie).
6. Half-circle triangular cutting needle (fistula).
7. Reversed cutting-edge needle (Hagedorn).
8. Curved triangular cutting needle (non-traumatic, for eye and plastic surgery).
9. Trocar-point needles (Mayo, for muscle and pedicles, etc.).
10. Half-circle round-bodied needles (peritoneum, fat, etc.).
11. Round-bodied fish-hook needles (Symond, for hernia repair, etc.).
12. (*Top*) Curved round-bodied needles (peritoneum, intestine, fat, etc.).
12. (*Bottom*) Straight round-bodied needles (intestine, transfixion ligatures).

There are three sizes, 88 mm ($3\frac{1}{2}$ in, small), 102 mm (4 in, medium) and 114 mm ($4\frac{1}{2}$ in, large), with a smaller round-bodied size about 38 mm ($1\frac{1}{2}$ in), for intestinal suturing.

Special shapes and types. Mayo, Symond's round-bodied fish hook, Hagedorn's reversed, and Gallie's fascia needles are the most popular, all of which are held in a needle holder for use.

The Mayo suture needle. This needle (for catgut), having a large square eye, is a very strong needle used extensively in gynaecology and obstetrics, or where excessive leverage may occur, e.g. during the repair of a hernia.

There are two varieties, the round-bodied and the trocar point (cutting), sizes ranging from 25 mm (6, small) to 51 mm (1, medium).

Symond's fish hook and Hagedorn's reversed. These are both fish-hook in shape and are used for inaccessible suturing. The Symond's needle is round-bodied and the Hagedorn's has a reverse flattened point.

Sizes vary from 19 mm (10, small) to 76 mm (0, large), size 32 mm(6) being useful for hernia repairs.

Gallie's fascia needle is a very broad, flattened needle, with a large eye and a lance point. A strip of fascia lata may be threaded on to this needle and used in hernia repair operations.

Gallie's needles are made only in three sizes, the most commonly used being small 38 mm ($1\frac{1}{2}$ in); the other two sizes are medium 44 mm ($1\frac{3}{4}$ in) and large 60 mm ($2\frac{3}{8}$ in), all of which are half-circle in shape.

It should be pointed out that the sizes of general needles, i.e., curved cutting needles, etc., vary only a little from one size to the other. The nurse will find that many surgeons use alternate size needles in which the difference of size is easily discernible, e.g., 17 mm(26), 19 mm(24), 21 mm(22), 24 mm(20), etc.

Bonney Reverdin needles are special needles which is effect incorporate their own needle holder.

These needles have an eye near to the point which is open on one side. A small, slender shutter may be slid along the handle to close this eye after the suture material has been inserted into it. The closed needle is passed through the tissues first; then the eye is opened; the suture material gripped; the eye closed, and the needle is withdrawn, pulling the suture material through the tissues to complete the stitch.

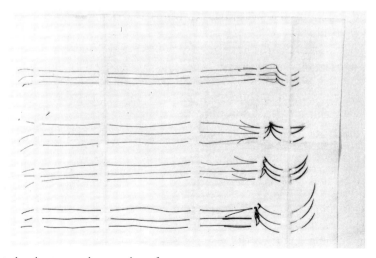

Fig. 9.9 An autoclaved suture pack, opened out for use.

The finer varieties are used by plastic surgeons, e.g., for the repair of a cleft palate, but the most commonly used are the coarser varieties, favoured by gynaecologists, e.g., for uterine suturing.

Disposable scalpel blades and handles

Bard Parker type

The most popular scalpel handle in the United Kingdom is the Bard Parker type which permits the fitting of various sizes and shapes of scalpel blades according to need. There are seven sizes of scalpel handles available; they are sizes 3, 4, 5, 6, 7, 3L and 4L. Of these sizes 3, 4, and 5 or 7 are the most generally used (see Chapter 14, page 405).

Sizes 3 and 4 are the general purpose handles of medium length; sizes 5 and 7 are long slim handles, useful for fine dissection in deep cavities; size 9 is a short slim handle of special use in plastic surgery; and sizes 3L and 4L are long general purpose handles for use in deep cavities.

Of the Swann Morton, Paragon and similar ranges, the most popular sizes of scalpel blades are sizes 10, 11, and 15, which fit handles 3, 3L, 5, 7, and 9; sizes 20, 22, 23 and 24, which fit handles 4, 4L and 6.

Of the Gillette range, sizes D/15, E/11 and 10 fit handles 3, 3L, 5, 7, and 9; sizes A, B/23, C, 20, 21, 22, and 24 fit handles, 4, 4L and 6.

Beaver type

Generally available in the United States and being introduced into the United Kingdom and Europe are the Beaver surgical blades and handles. These provide a wide range of handles including eight general purpose and in excess of twenty three different types of specialised handles. There are well over 125 different shapes and sizes of disposable scalpel blades, ranging from minute blades for ophthalmic and microsurgery, to heavy duty orthopaedic knives. It is not practicable to provide a detailed description of these but a sample range is illustrated in Figure 9.10.

Most manufacturers pack their scalpel blades in grease-free packets, such as the Vapour Phase Inhibitor or metal foil pack. The packet is designed as a sterile peel-open type with the blade ready for use. Individual packets of blades are presented in dispenser boxes which can be stored in a suitable rack.

Skin-graft knives generally incorporate disposable blades available in a sterile peel-open packet. If they are supplied unsterilized these may be coated with a light oil before wrapping in their protective paper cover. This oil should be removed before sterilization, by soaking in a little alcohol, after which the blades should be lifted out and dried carefully. This should not be done in a confined space owing to the vapour liberated.

Skin graft blades can be sterilized by dry heat or alternatively by steam providing they are wrapped in vapour phase inhibitor anti-rust paper.

Solid scalpels

Most of these instruments are made from carbon steel because of the difficulty of obtaining a really good edge with stainless steel.

Under this heading come orthopaedic scalpels, cartilage knives, tenotomy knives, bistouries, etc.

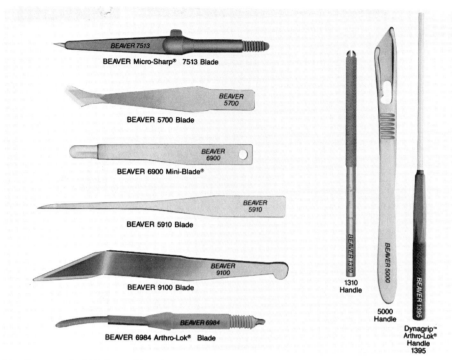

Fig. 9.10   Beaver scalpel blades and handles. (Beaver Surgical Products.)

Orthopaedic scalpels

These vary in size from a small 25 mm (1 in) blade to a 23 cm (9 in) amputation knife and are either straight or bellied in shape. The edges of these should be inspected regularly after use for bluntness, as described in Chapter 6. They are used where there is a risk of breaking a detachable blade, e.g., excising fibrous tissue at a fracture site.

Swann Morton produce a disposable solid type blade and handle, which is similar to the Bard Parker knives but does not snap easily and may be used in all cases where a solid scalpel is required.

Cartilage knives

These are rather a small type of solid knife, the three most popular being the Munro, Smillie and Fairbank.

The Munro has a long handle, with a short blade and a slender stem between the blade and the handle. The Smillie knives have a chisel-type point and are made as a set of three; two with concave edges, one curved for the right and one for the left, and a straight chisel blade for use with a special retractor. The Fairbank knives are made as a set of two; one curved for cutting to the right, and one curved for the left. They have a small blunt probe point with the cutting edge at one side only and are used mainly for meniscotomy as opposed to meniscectomy (Fig. 23.103).

Tenotomy knives

These are long and slender, being used for dividing a tendon through a small puncture

wound. They either have one or two cutting edges, generally with a sharp point. Amongst the most popular are the Parker's double cutting-edge spear-type point, the Jones' single cutting edge and the Adam's set of seven shapes, including blunt and sharp-pointed varieties. There are too many types for individual description, as some surgeons arrange the sharpening of their knives to suit individual tastes.

Bistouries

These are knives which are generally used in conjunction with a special probe or guard for the division of ligaments or fibrous bands of tissue, etc., e.g., during a strangulated hernia operation.

Although there are bistouries with sharp points, the most generally used are those having a probe point which ensures that the cutting is only with the side edge of the knife.

All these knives can be sterilized by dry heat.

Scissors

Although it is better to sterilize those scissors in common use together with the general instruments, it is common practice to store at least the special types of scissors in autoclaved packs.

Scissors may have both points sharp, both blunt, or one sharp and one blunt. They are made from martensitic stainless steel or plated carbon steel, although the latter are not often used in the operating theatre, except perhaps for cutting dressings.

Scissors having both points sharp are generally used for removing sutures, or are of a special type such as fine iridectomy scissors. They may be straight, curved on flat or angled on flat and are mostly of the fulcrum lever principle, although some special iris scissors such as the De Wecker's have a special spring cross action, enabling the surgeon to use them between his forefinger and thumb. It is very useful to reserve ordinary stitch scissors for use during the preparation of ligatures and sutures, so that they do not become mixed with the scissors reserved for the surgeon. Scissors having both points sharp and with serrated edges are available for cutting cartilage, used almost exclusively by the plastic surgeons. Stitch scissors are useful also for cutting fine wire sutures not stouter than 30 S.W.G.

The majority of scissors used for dissection have both points blunt or rounded and are available straight, curved on flat or angled on flat. The most popular are the Mayo scissors or modifications of this pattern, the most usual sizes being from 13 to 20 cm (5 to 8 in) in length. In addition to dissection, these scissors are often used for cutting ligatures and sutures, although it is better to reserve a separate pair for this purpose to give the surgeon the advantage of scissors used exclusively for dissection.

Although Mayo scissors may be obtained in lengths up to 23 cm (9 in), when a long fine pair is required, the surgeon will often prefer a pattern such as the Metzenbaum, McIndoe 18 cm (7 in) or similar. If he requires a heavier pair, his choice may include Nelson's or Mile's which are made in lengths up to 28 cm (11 in), and as straight or curved on flat blades. These longer scissors are of special use in thoracic surgery.

A short fine pair of scissors for use in plastic surgery, peripheral nerve or tendon surgery would be the 13 cm (5 in) Kilner or strabismus scissors, both available as straight or curved on flat blades. The Kilner's scissors have flattened, fine points, which makes them very adaptable for skin dissection.

Scissors having one sharp and one blunt point are useful for cutting dressings although they may be reserved for use by the assistant when he is cutting ligatures and sutures. Some

dressing scissors are made with a blunt platform extending from the tip of the lower blade. This facilitates the introduction of the lower blade under a dressing or bandage, and prevents injury to the patient's skin.

In orthopaedic theatres it may be necessary to store a variety of probes, drills, osteotomes, and gouges, etc., in sterile boxes or packs. The difference between the various types is described in Chapter 23.

Suture clips

These are generally loaded on to a special galley which also forms part of an approximation forceps (Fig. 8.26). The insertion forceps are grooved for the Michel-type skin clips, but are, in addition, bowed for the Kifa type to accommodate the projecting lips.

Drainage tubes, catheters, syringes, and hypodermic needles

A selection of these may be stored in autoclaved packs or purchased ready sterile from the manufacturer.

The handling of ligature and suture materials

It is a totally unacceptable practice to prepare ligatures and sutures for several operations at the beginning of an operation list. Materials so prepared have to be stored on a 'stock' trolley and even with the greatest care it is impossible to maintain sterility.

A separate, small, sterile trolley may be used as an operation ligature trolley for each case, but it is a more convenient procedure to use a corner of the instrument trolley or pre-set tray, placing the prepared materials between two small sterile towels. It is preferable that these towels be of a different colour to the general drapes so that they serve to isolate the ligatures, etc., from the rest of the trolley.

At operation the circulating nurse peels open the outer overwrap cover (Fig. 9.11), and the inner packet is taken by the scrub nurse using long sterile forceps. Alternatively, a 'flip'

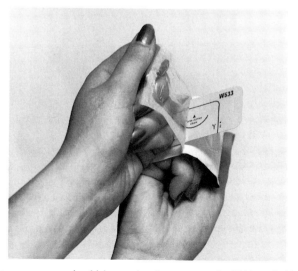

Fig. 9.11 The peel-open overwrap pack which contains the suture pack. (Ethicon Ltd.)

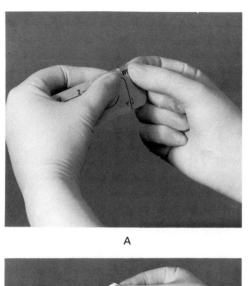

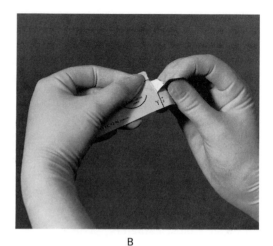

A

B

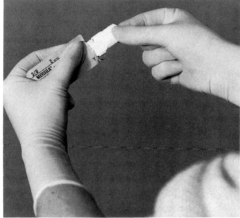

C

Fig. 9.12 Opening an aluminium foil ligature pack. (A) The pack is held with the thumbs together on either side of the notch. (B) Tearing open from the notch along the width of the pack. (C) Removing the ligature. (Ethicon Ltd.)

transfer from the outer wrap to the sterile trolley can be done, but the circulating nurse must take care not to pass her hands over the sterile surface. This method is not ideal.

The inner pack is opened by gently tearing across the V-cut at one side (Figs. 9.12, 9.13). If the suture is packed in alcohol, care must be taken not to squeeze the packet as this done, for fluid may be sprayed out under pressure and may cause damage to the user's eyes.

1. The ligature/suture is removed from the tube or packet with sterile forceps, retaining the size label which is useful for reference, especially when several sizes are in use. It is then withdrawn from the inner pack or 'former', and each end of the strand is grasped with the gloved hands and stretched slightly to remove any kinks (Fig. 9.14 A-C). In orthopaedic surgery this operation may have to be performed using forceps, care being taken to ensure that the suture is not crushed with the forceps except at the end of a strand. A crush mark is the centre of a ligature or suture may cause it to break during handling.

2. The non-needled material may then be threaded on to needles either by hand, or for orthopaedic operations by using a non-touch technique (Fig. 9.14D). The material should be threaded from within the curve of the needle outwards, leaving one end about 5 to 10 cm (2 to 4 in) long; it may be locked in the eye of the needle either by passing through a second time in the same direction or by tying a single knot (Fig. 9.15A). If it is frequently necessary to have a locked suture, it is preferable to use a special needle such as the Paterson or spring-

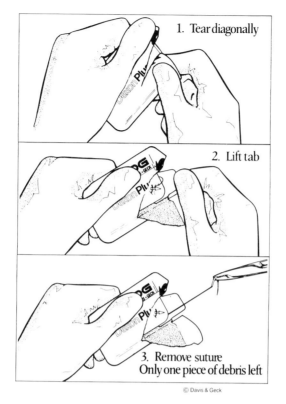

Fig. 9.13 Opening foil suture pack and armed suture. (Davis and Geck.)

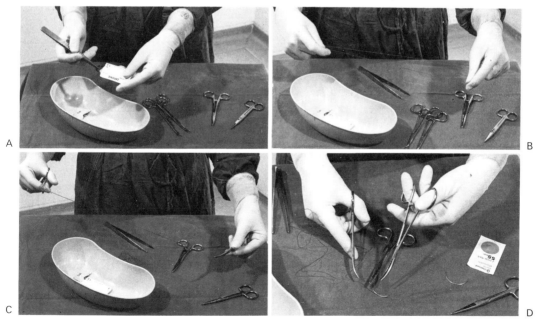

Fig. 9.14 (A) Removing catgut from foil packet. (B) Stretching catgut by hand to remove kinks. (C) Stretching catgut with forceps to remove kinks. (D) Threading a suture needle with forceps.

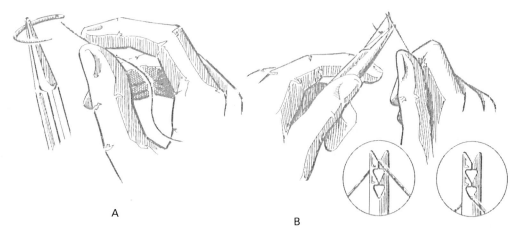

Fig. 9.15 Method of threading a suture needle: (A) Suture material threaded from inside curve. (B) Patterson spring eye needle. (Davis and Geck.)

eye needle, which locks the suture without passing it through the eye a second time or tying a knot (Fig. 9.15B).

Even with Paterson eye or spring-eye needles two strands of suture always pass through the tissues. This creates unnecessary trauma, especially when suturing delicate tissues.

The use of non-traumatic needled sutures is now well established and this obviates the disadvantages of doubling the suture when using a needle having an eye.

Catgut/ synthetic absorbable ligatures and sutures must not be left exposed for any length of time. Ideally the ligature or suture is only removed from the packet just before required, but if prepared previously it must be kept covered with a small sterile towel.

It is very important to ensure that catgut/synthetic absorbables are not soaked before use as this causes the material to swell and increases the speed of digestion in the tissues. Passage once through the tissues will lubricate the suture sufficiently for use. If the surgeon insists on pre-moistening the catgut, it may be drawn *very gently* through a moistened glove or swab.

Care must be exercised when handling ligatures and sutures to avoid fraying, as this will weaken the strand considerably and may cause the breaking of a suture line post-operatively.

The scrub nurse may prepare several ligatures and sutures at the commencement of the operation but should avoid having too many exposed, especially if the operation is lengthy. The length of a ligature should not generally exceed 31 cm (12 in); a continuous suture length ranges between 46 and 61 cm (18 and 24 in), and an interrupted suture length should be between 31 and 46 cm (12 and 18 in).

When tension sutures are being prepared, using thin rubber or plastic tubing to prevent 'cutting in' of the suture after tying, the needle is threaded and a 2.5 cm (1 in) length of tubing passed over the needle point and slid into position overlying the material in the eye. This will prevent the suture material (especially monofilament nylon) from becoming unthreaded, and will simplify positioning the tubing before the suture is tied. The surgeon will require two pairs of artery forceps for each tension suture to secure the ends until he is ready to tie them, after the muscle has been sutured.

Only the end of a needle holder's jaws must be used to grip a needle which is held at a point one-third from the eye and two-thirds from the needle point, the only exception being a fish hook and Gallie's fascia needle. These are gripped at a point about one-quarter from the eye.

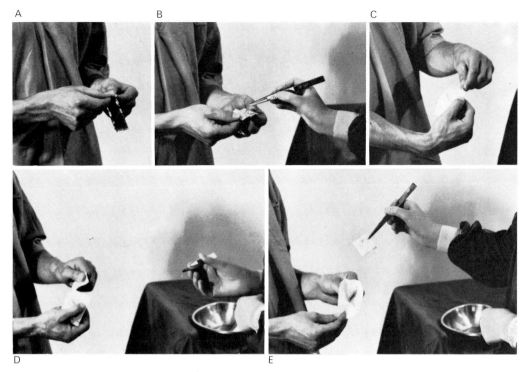

Fig. 9.16 (A) Peeling open a sterile scalpel blade foil packet. (B) Scrub nurse removing sterile scalpel blade from peeled-open packet. (C) Ligature packet in heat-sealed Kraft paper bag. First the bag is nicked, then . . . (D) . . . torn across without touching the torn edge . . . (E) . . . the packet is opened utilising the side gussets and the scrub nurse removes the inner sterile packet with forceps.

Gripping the needle in the one-third/two-thirds position ensures that the surgeon can pass the needle the maximum possible distance through the tissues without further adjustments and with the least possible risk of it snapping at its weakest point, which is near the eye.

When preparing a needle and holder for a right-handed surgeon, the nurse holds the instrument in her right hand and grips the needle with its point facing her left hand. The procedure is reversed for a left-handed surgeon and when the needle is to be used vice versa.

Some needle holders have a cranked handle, and when viewed sideways it will appear that the jaws are at a lower level than the handle. The needle should be gripped so that when it is in the correct position for use the cranked handle is above the level of the jaws and not vice versa when viewed sideways. Suturing of fairly superficial tissues and skin is easier when using this type of needle holder, as the cranked handle remains above the level of the skin even if the jaws are below. This means that the surgeon is able to hold his hand parallel to the skin instead of at an angle, and so avoids obscuring his view of the suture line.

REFERENCE

BRIGDEN, R. J. (1962). Sterile packets for implants and special instruments. *Nursing Mirror*, March 30.

10

Draping operation areas and assisting the surgeon

Although it is the ultimate responsibility of the surgeon to ensure that the operation area is correctly draped following skin preparation, this is frequently left to an experienced member of the operating team.

Furthermore, another doctor usually acts as the surgeon's first assistant, but there are occasions when a theatre nurse may have to act in this capacity. However it must be understood that the duties of theatre staff do not normally include those of first assistant.

Preparing the operation area

1. Elective procedures

Effective pre-operative skin preparation is an important factor in the prevention of post-operative infections; the objectives are:

1. To remove dirt and transient micro-organisms from the skin.

2. To reduce the resident microbial count to as low as possible in the shortest period of time and with the least amount of tissue irritation.

3. To inhibit rapid rebound growth of micro-organisms (AORN, 1983).

The first stages of preparation in the ward may include the removal of hair from the vicinity of the operation site, and a pre-operative bath or shower using an antiseptic combined with a suitable detergent.

Hair removal. Studies have demonstrated that one factor related to the possibility of post-operative infection occurring is the method chosen for the removal of hair pre-operatively. One study reported an infection rate of 0.9 per cent in patients who did not have hair removed before operation; this compared with 2.3 per cent infection rate for patients who were shaved, and 1.7 per cent infection rate for those who had their hair clipped with an electric razor (Cruse and Foord, 1980). Another reference was to the use of a depilatory cream which resulted in a post-operative infection rate of 0.6 per cent, which was the same as in another group of patients who had no shave (Seropian and Reynolds, 1971). Seropian and Reynolds showed, however, that if shaving was carried out immediately before operation the infection rate was only 3.1 per cent compared with 20 per cent if the interval between pre-operative shave and subsequent surgery is prolonged for over 24 hours.

In June 1983, the Lancet Editorial was devoted to the subject of preoperative depilation. The editorial quoted Court-Brown (1981) who had carried out a prospective study on patients undergoing abdominal surgery, comparing the effect of shaving, cream depilation and no preparation on the post-operative wound infection rate. Court-Brown found that the overall infection rates in 406 patients were 12.4 per cent after traditional shaving, 7.9 per cent after cream depilation, and 7.8 per cent with no removal of hair. When only the clean

wounds were considered the infection rate for shaving was 10.4 per cent, against 3.9 per cent and 2.9 per cent for the no preparation group.

Another paper (Wesley *et al.*, 1983) reported the results from a study of 1,013 patients undergoing elective operations. These patients were prospectively randomised to be either shaved or clipped the night before or the morning of operation. The authors found that the infection rate for the clipper method carried out in the morning was 1.8 per cent, less than half that of the other technique for hair removal.

The AORN (1983) recommended that 'the removal of hair from the operation site should be only done as necessary'. The traditional shave appears to increase the risk of post-operative infection, unless it is carried out immediately before surgery. The choice for pre-operative removal of hair would seem to lie between a depilatory cream (example — 3M Surgix) and an electric clipper with a disposable blade assembly (example — 3M Surgical Clipper).

Pre-operative bathing. Patients who undergo vascular, transplant and orthopaedic surgery and prolonged procedures are particularly prone to infection. In these circumstances the pre-operative preparation may include shower/bathing with an antiseptic, such as iodophor, chlorhexidine, or hexachlorophane.

Davies *et al.* (1977) studied the effect of at least three consecutive daily baths with chlor-hexidine (Hibscrub), povidone-iodine, and an unmedicated soap. They found that chlor-hexidine (Hibscrub) achieved the greatest and most rapid reduction of skin micro-organisms; the total count of micro-organisms actually increased after bathing with unmedicated soap. Another study by Brandberg *et al.* (1979) on patients undergoing vascular surgery showed a reduction of post-operative infection rate from 17.5 per cent to 8 per cent after chlorhex-idine (Hibscrub) had been used pre-operatively.

2. Contaminated wounds

Any open wound must have a thorough toilet under anaesthesia before applying the usual skin disinfectant.

Sterilized nylon bristle nail brushes and an antiseptic detergent such as aqueous Savlon 3 per cent are ideal for this purpose. To assist efficient cleansing of a limb, a large, sterile, shallow tray can be placed under the wound area and used as a douche tray.

At least two brushes must be available for this procedure, the first being used for the initial cleansing of skin for a wide area surrounding the wound, and the second in a separate bowl of solution for the wound itself. During initial cleansing, the wound is covered with a sterile swab or towel and it is at this stage that any excess hairs are shaved away.

Although a certain amount of care should be exercised when cleansing a wound, to avoid damage to exposed nerves, etc., it is very important to remove as much debris as possible. The sterilized nylon brushes will be found useful for this, but large fragments of foreign materials or damaged tissue and blood clots which cannot be removed by gentle brushing should be left for removal by the surgeon.

After a thorough toilet, the area is dried with a sterile swab or towel, and skin disinfectant applied before placing the drapes in position.

When a general anaesthesia is not practicable, the surgeon will administer local or regional anaesthesia following minimal cleansing and before wound toilet is commenced.

Draping the operation area

The operation area must be draped to allow free access for the surgeon, but the towels should be so arranged that manipulations do not expose any unprepared skin areas.

Table 10.1 Areas of skin preparation.

Area of Operation	Area of Preparation
Skull	Entire skull, forehead, ears and neck.
Face	Entire face and neck and if necessary including the ears. For eye operations the eyebrows *may* be shaved off, and the lashes are cut with petroleum jelly smeared scissors. This is not necessary if adhesive incise drapes are used.
Chest–Supine	From mid-abdomen to shoulders and neck, extending laterally round loins and thorax, on both sides.
Lateral	From mid-abdomen to shoulders; including the lateral aspects of the thorax and loins on the affected side and extending over the spine.
Abdomen	From the nipples to the upper part of the thighs, extending laterally round abdominal wall and pelvis, on both sides; including the genital region.
Genital region	From the umbilicus to mid-thighs, extending laterally round the pelvis and including the genital and anal regions.
Anal region	The upper part of both thighs, the buttocks, genital region and lower part of the abdomen.
Spine	From the shoulders to the upper part of the thighs, including the anal region and extending laterally round the loins and thorax.
Hand, forearm and upper arm	From the finger tips to the elbow (or shoulder for upper arm).
Foot and ankle	From the toes to knee level for full circumference of the limb.
Lower leg and knee	From the toes to mid-thigh for full circumference of the limb.
Hip and thigh	Whole of the leg, buttocks, and genital region; extending up to the level of the ribs; and over the lateral aspect of the abdomen on the affected side.

If fabric drapes are being used, pieces of sterile water repellent sheet (e.g., Ventile fabric or disposable material) should be placed in position first surrounding the operation area, to prevent contamination should the sterile drapes become damp or soiled.

Methods of towelling or draping are essentially practical procedures, depending upon the wishes of the surgeon, the area, and sizes of towels available. In this chapter we must therefore confine ourselves to general principles, and use these as a basis for practice.

Abdominal and chest operations

One method is first to position four medium size sterile fluid-repellent drapes such as Ventile or other proofed material, so as to form a barrier around the operation site. This is followed by a large fabric laparotomy sheet having a central aperture. More satisfactory is the use of disposable drapes such as Barrier Fabric 450 or Azodrape Azo77 which are inherently fluid-repellent. With this technique, the laparotomy drape is positioned as shown in Figure 10.1 and unfolded to the sides. The drape is then unfolded towards the patient's feet, and finally towards the head. If the patient's arm or arms are abducted on an arm support for transfusion or other purposes, these should be covered with small sterile drapes before commencing the abdominal draping.

Even though preparation is thorough, the skin surface will not remain surgically clean for a prolonged period. If the operation lasts more than half an hour or so, the patient will begin to perspire resulting in surface contamination from micro-organisms from within the sweat pores. Contamination can be minimised by covering the skin with a piece of self-adhesive plastic sheet (Steridrape [polyethylene], Opsite [polyurethrane], Barrier incise sheet, or antimicrobial film such as Loban [iodophor impregnated]). This adhesive plastic incise sheet is stretched over the operation area and with a sterile folded towel or swab, smoothed

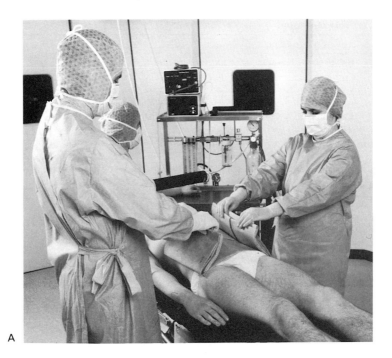

A

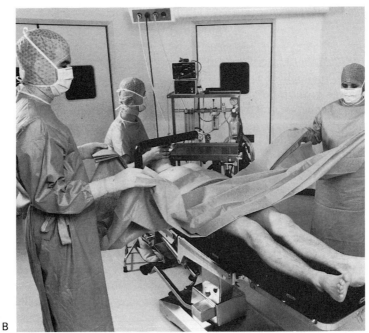

B

Fig. 10.1 Abdominal operation — laparotomy drape. (A) After the skin disinfectant has dried completely, the folded laparotomy drape is placed in position as shown with the aperture over the centre of the abdomen, and then unfolded to the sides. (B) The lower part of the drape is unfolded towards the patient's feet. (C) The drape is unfolded towards the patient's head forming an anaesthesia screen. (D) Draping completed; the drape can be secured with towel clips or adhesive tape strips. (Barrier^{TM} disposable drapes — Surgikos.)

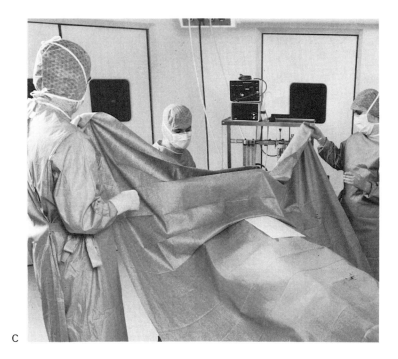

C

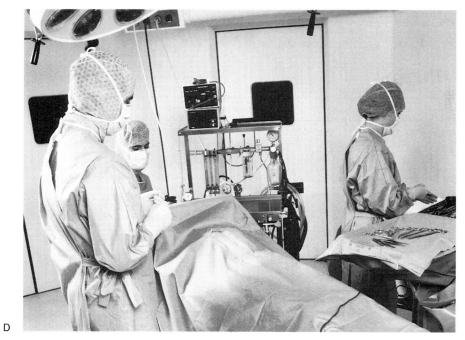

D

Fig. 10.1 (continued)

flat from the centre to the periphery. This ensures positive adhesion and avoids air bubbles being trapped beneath the sheet. The incision is made through the plastic sheet and underlying skin (Figs. 10.2 and 10.3).

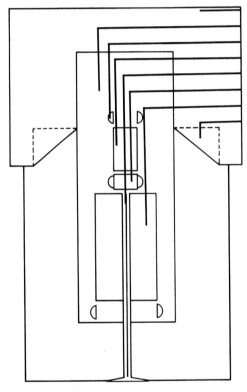

OpSite
S P E C I A L I T Y   D R A P E S

Cardiovascular Drape

PROGUARD Fabric

Reinforcement

Diathermy Clips

OPSITE Window

Leg Gusset

Non-Slip Instrument Pad

Split Leg Window

Arm Gussets

Split Window
The lower incise window is divided into two by a piece of fabric. This split will enable easy manipulation and good conformability to the legs.

Perineal Isolator
An adhesive patch is attached under the drape between the two incise windows. This is designed to isolate the perineum and give extra security. It is waterproof with an absorbent inner layer.

Instrument Pad
A non-slip instrument pad is positioned between the two incise windows.

Diathermy Clips
6 D-shaped diathermy quiver holders are attached to the drape around the incise windows.

Gussets
Gussets are inserted to allow armboards to be used without impeding the fall of the drape.

Anaesthetic Screen
The anaesthetic screen is built into the drape for convenience and security. It is reinforced for additional protection.

Description
A very large T-shaped drape incorporating three incise windows. One of which is for access to the chest cavity and the other is for stripping veins out of the legs. The chest window is the same size as the cardiothoracic drape. The lower window covers the legs from the groin to the ankle.
The drape is designed for cardiovascular procedures where access to the thorax and to the legs is required.

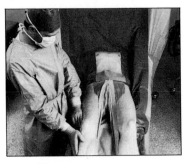

Fig. 10.2 Opsite™ incise surgical drapes — example — cardiovascular drape. (Smith and Nephew Medical Ltd.)

Draping Operation Areas and Assisting the Surgeon

Steri-Drape®2
Surgical Incise Drapes

APPLICATION TECHNIQUE

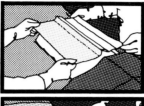

Position drape over patient with liner face down. Grasp liner from underneath and begin peeling liner back.

Peel back liner material, folding liner upon itself. DO NOT REMOVE LINER COMPLETELY. Leave last fold adhered to adhesive area.

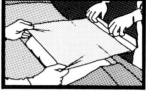

Using folded liner as a "handle bar," stabilize drape over patient. With a folded sterile towel, press and smooth drape to skin, first along planned line of incision. Remove liner completely and incise directly through sterile STERI-DRAPE Surgical Drape.

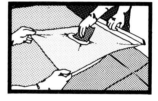

Steri-Drape®
Surgical Towel Drapes

After cutting STERI-DRAPE Surgical Towel Drape in half, unfold the drape. Reach across the surgical site and apply adhesive edge parallel to planned line of incision.

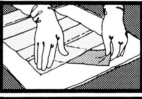

With one hand, slowly peel away protective liner. Use other hand to press adhesive to skin. Repeat procedure for applying other half of drape to opposite side of planned line of incision.

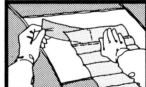

After incision, tuck ends of Towel Drape over wound edge to extend sterile field into peritoneal cavity.

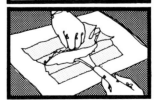

3M and Steri-Drape are trademarks

Fig. 10.3 Application technique for Steridrape™ surgical incise and towel drapes. (Wound Management Products, 3M Health Care.)

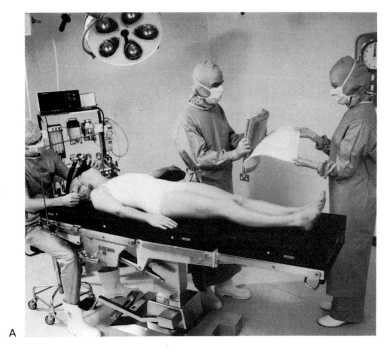

A

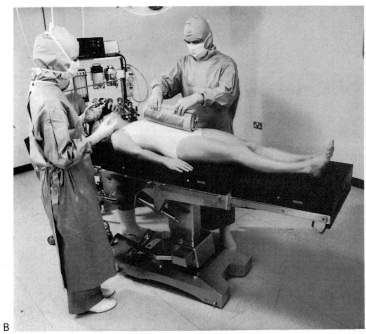

B

Fig. 10.4 (caption on page 262)

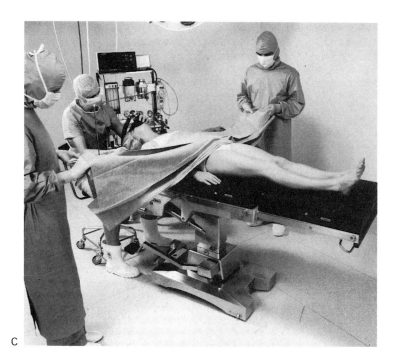

C

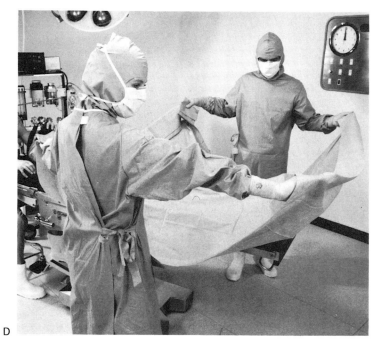

D

Fig. 10.4 (caption on page 262)

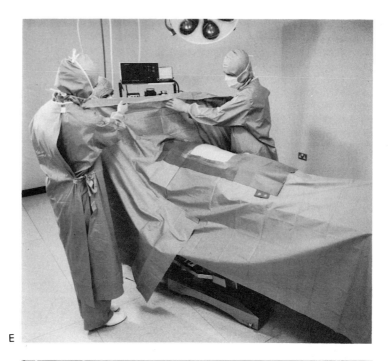

E

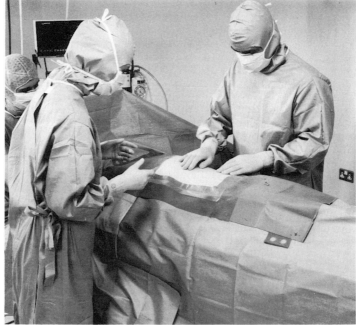

F

Fig. 10.4 Abdominal operation — laparatomy incise drape. (A) After the skin disinfectant has dried completely, the backing paper is removed from the adhesive Barrier incise fenestration at the central aperture. (B) The adhesive fenestration is positioned over the incision site and secured by pressing down firmly on the skin. (C–E) The drape is unfolded first to each side, then towards the patient's feet to cover the end of the operation table, and finally towards the patient's head to form an anaesthetic screen. (F) Built-in arm covers unfold to completely cover arm tables. (Barrier disposable drapes — Surgikos.)

Incise sheets can form a part of a disposable drape. Figure 10.4 illustrates the method of draping for an abdominal operation using a laparotomy/incise sheet (Barrier Fabric 450). This drape also incorporates a biocidal fabric reinforcement around the sheet aperture (Drisite/Microcide) and built-in arm board covers.

A metal wire frame may be fitted to accessory clamps on each side of the operation table near to the head. This can be draped with the upper part of the laparotomy sheet to isolate the anaesthetist from the operation area. It also prevents the drapes from covering the patient's face and obscuring his appearance. The frame is of special use when the patient is conscious and local or spinal anaesthesia has been administered. Care must be taken to avoid the patient's arm from coming in contact with the metal frame, especially if diathermy is being used, as this could result in accidental burns (Fig. 10.5).

If no plastic incise drape has been used, following the incision small skin or surgical towel drapes may be applied to the skin edges. These should be of plastic and not fabric 'tetra towels', which soon become soiled with blood and lose their protective value.

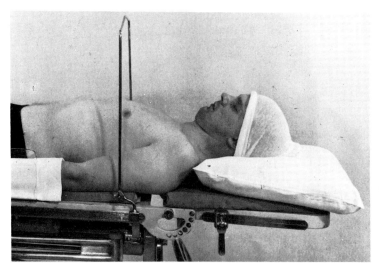

Fig. 10.5 Anaesthesia screen at operation table head. (If the patient is broad, soft pads will be required between the patient's arms and screen uprights.)

Limb operations

It is important that the drapes are secured to withstand any manipulations of a limb during operation.

In addition to small towels, some larger, about 152 cm (5 ft) square, should be available — two for a lower limb, and one for an upper limb.

Only the incision area of the limb should be exposed during operation, unless of course multiple incisions are necessary as for the ligation of varicose veins. Towels may be used to cover the unrequired skin areas, but a sterile stocking made from stockinette is less bulky.

It is very important that all parts of a limb (including the foot) which will be subject to handling by the surgeon must be painted with skin disinfectant.

In orthopaedic surgery, a piece of self-adhesive plastic sheet (Steridrape, OpSite) is generally applied to the skin, thereby providing a drape through which the surgeon makes his incision.

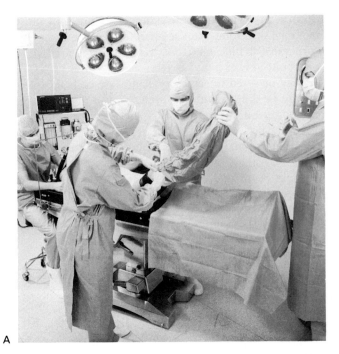

A

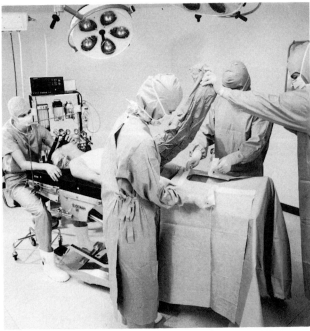

B

Fig. 10.6 Draping lower limb (knee). (A) After the skin disinfectant has dried completely, a large drape is used to cover the non-operative limb. A sterile stocking is then applied to the operative leg and may be secured with a sterile bandage. (B and C) A hinged small split sheet is placed under the operative leg on the sterile field formed by the first drape, and the drape unfolded to the sides and over the end of the operation table. The backing paper is removed from the adhesive edges of the exposed slit as shown. Holding the U part of slit, the tails are secured around the top of the limb and the stockinette. Alternatively, small towels are placed at inner

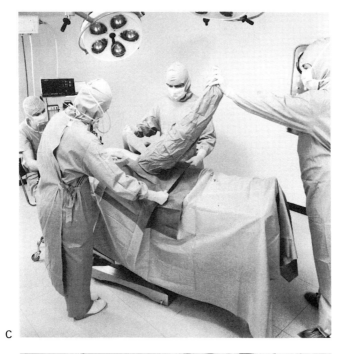

C

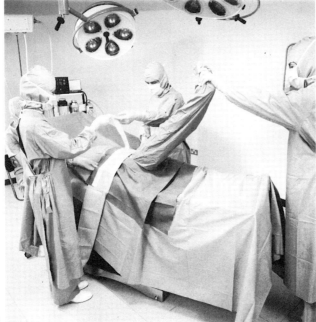

D

Fig. 10.6 (continued)

and outer aspects of the thigh, overlapped above and beneath, and secured with towel clips to form a 'shut off'. (D) A large drape is placed over the upper part of the patient and after removing the backing paper, secured with the adhesive strips by overlapping and folding under the limb. A non-adhesive drape is secured with towel clips. (E and F) The stockinette is fenestrated and if required, an adhesive incise drape is applied to the incision area. (Barrier disposable drapes — Surgikos.)

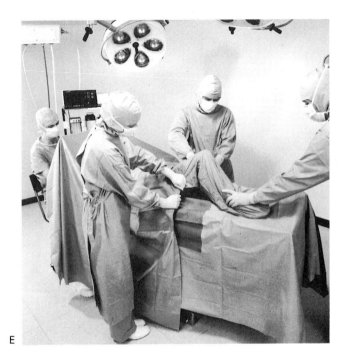

E

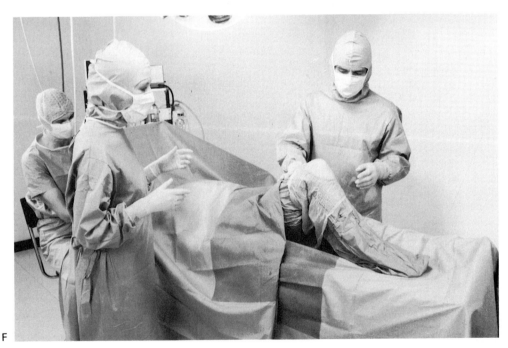

F

Fig. 10.6 (continued)

Using conventional fabric drapes, a sterile water repellent sheet must be placed under the limb before the towels and should extend well about the operation site. For operations on the lower extremities, this means from the foot end of the operation table to mid-thigh, or higher if necessary. When one leg is involved, the water repellant sheet covers the other completely. In the case of upper limb operations, it should cover the arm table and extend well up to the axilla. With the arm across the chest, the water repellent sheet is placed, extending from lower abdomen to axilla.

After covering and overlapping the water repellent sheet with towels, a 'shuff off' towel is used to isolate the prepared from the unprepared areas of the limb. This towel is placed under the limb and crossed over on the opposite side, to be secured with a towel clip or clips.

Alternatively, disposable drapes such as Barrier 450 or Azodrape may be used. The draping procedure includes a split sheet to isolate the perineal area (Fig. 10.6). Draping for hip operations follows a similar pattern (Fig. 10.7).

Cranial operations

These often last a long time and it is important that the drapes remain secure and sterile throughout the whole period. Furthermore, unless great care is taken, soiling of the towels after incision involves the risk of contamination from the underlying skin.

Supine or prone position. This requires a sterile water repellent sheet to be placed under the head first.

Self adhesive plastic sheet (Steridrape, OpSite) may be applied to cover the scalp (Fig. 10.11). The closed eyelids must be covered with sterile eyepads.

The anaesthetist must have access to the patient's airway during operation and further drapes should always be placed with this in mind. A sterile water repellent sheet or disposable drape such as Barrier 450 or Azodrape extending from the scalp and across the chest is draped over a large instrument table or wire screen placed about 31 cm (12 in) above the patient and at shoulder level.

The final towel is placed around the head, first draped over the water repellent sheet (covering the instrument table or wire screen), and then over transfusion stands at each side of the operation table (Fig. 10.12).

This method of draping will ensure complete isolation of the anaesthetist from the operation area, and by forming a tent over the patient provides good access to the patient's airway and lower extremities.

The neurosurgical sitting position. This position with the head flexed and immobilised by a cranial support, requires first a sterile water repellent sheet and towel placed across the shoulders extending from neck level to cover the chair back.

The draping is then completed as previously described, but the towels are draped first over an instrument table positioned just in front of the patient's forehead, and then over transfusion stands at each side of the operation table (Fig. 10.12, p. 275).

Spinal operations (including laminectomy, sympathectomy, decompression, excision of pilonoidal sinus, etc.)

The prone position. A patient placed in the prone position (or the knee/elbow flexed rabbit position), for lumbar, sacral, or mid-thoracic approach, may be draped as for abdominal operations, utilising the 'holed' laparotomy sheet.

High cervical areas. These can be draped similarly, but in addition the head may be isolated with a self-adhesive plastic sheet (Steridrape, OpSite), or covered first by using

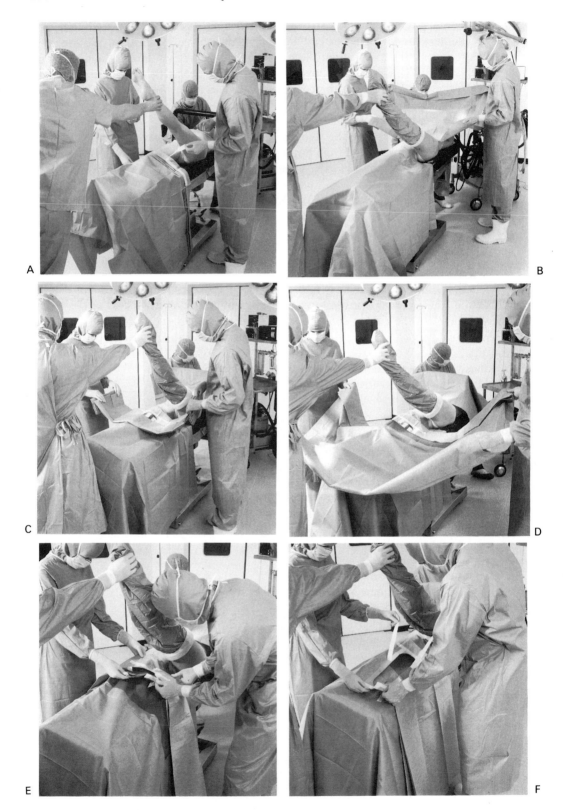

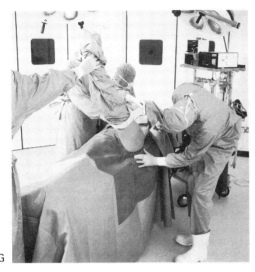
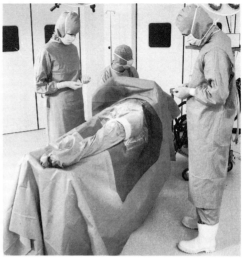

G   H

Fig. 10.7 Draping the hip. (A) After the skin disinfectant has dried completely, the operative leg is held above the operation table, and a large drape unfolded over the non-operative leg exposing the protected adhesive edge. (B) The backing paper is removed from the adhesive edge which is pressed firmly into position across the top of the non-operative leg. (C) Stockinette is applied over the operative leg to mid-thigh, and a large drape placed across the upper part of the patient and unfolded to form an anaesthesia screen. (D and E) A large orthopaedic split sheet is placed on the sterile field formed by the first drape, and unfolded to each side and over the end of the operation table. (F and G) The two folds of the orthopaedic split sheet are grasped and pulled out to expose the U shape of the split. The backing paper is removed to expose the adhesive surface. (H) The U of the split is positioned below the incision line and pressed firmly on to the skin across the top of the operative limb. The draping procedure completed: adhesive incise drape may be applied to the incision area (see Fig. 10.3). (Barrier disposable drapes — Surgikos.)

the two-towel technique described for ENT operations. The cross-over point of the towels should be at the occiput.

Pieces of sterile cotton-wool tucked in at each side of the neck will prevent soiling due to blood trickling down during operation.

Lateral position. These should be draped similarly to abdominal or chest procedures, using four separate water repellent sheets and towels.

Ear, nose and throat operations

In all cases the upper part of the head and hair may be draped in almost the same way.

Two opened towels and a water repellent sheet are placed under the patient's head, the upper towel is crossed over a point above the operation area and secured with a towel clip, i.e., for operations on the eyes, at a point in the centre of the forehead; for operations on the mouth or nose, at a point over the nose bridge after covering the closed eyelids with a sterile (coloured) swab, etc.; and for operations on the ear, superior to the ear on the affected side.

This method of draping will ensure that the hair is always covered and, in addition, the sterile towel underlying will cover the area beneath the head.

The draping is completed by covering the lower part of the patient with a sterile water repellent drape and one or more towels extending from just below the operation area, or a large disposable drape, such as Barrier 450 or Azodrape. For operations on the eyes

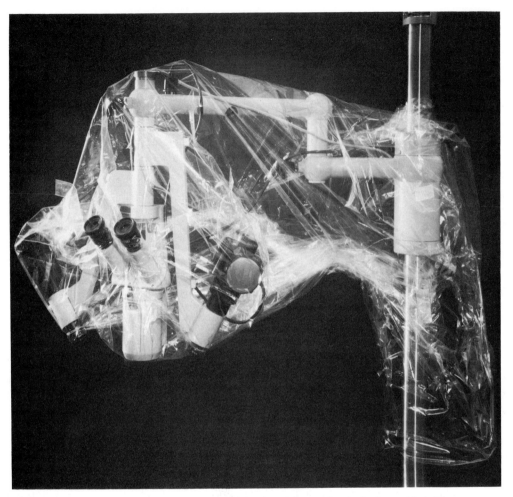

Fig. 10.8 Operating microscope showing method of draping with a sterile plastic sleeve. (Carl Zeiss [OberKochen] Ltd.)

or ears, the lower half of the face, including the nose, should be covered; for those on the mouth or nose, the lower drapes extend from the chin.

Operations on the neck

The head is covered as above, but the towel is crossed over at the centre of the chin.

A pad of sterile wool can be tucked in at each side of the neck to absorb any blood which may trickle down during operation. This is followed by a sterile water repellent sheet across the chest and one or more towels to cover this and the lower extremities. Alternatively a large disposable drape can be used.

The use of towel clips to secure towels in this region is often avoided, due to the difficulty of applying towel clips to the chin for it is very irritating to find that these clips frequently pull away during the course of operation. The alternative is to use three or four monofilament nylon sutures at each point and these cause very little trauma. The sutures are cut out before removing the drapes.

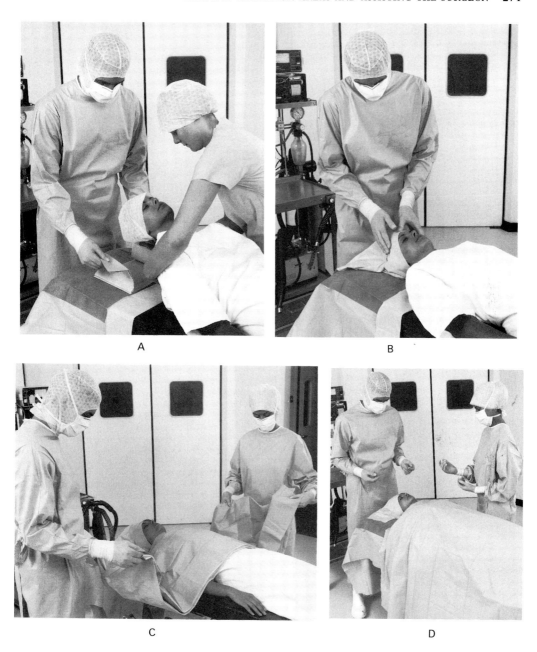

Fig. 10.9 Draping procedure for neck and ear. (A) The circulating assistant lifts the patient's head off the table. The 'scrub' nurse or surgeon either lays two drapes, or a Barrier composite drape on the table under the head, which is lowered to the drapes. (B) The uppermost drape is folded over the patient's head turban fashion and either secured with towel clips or the adhesive strip (Barrier). (C) A large drape is placed on the patient; it is then partially unfolded to the side, and if using a Barrier drape the backing paper removed from the adhesive strip, being at the patient's head end. (D) The upper end of the drape is unfolded and fixed firmly around the neck leaving as much of the face exposed as required. (E) For an operation on the ear a split sheet is used in preference to a large patient drape. This is positioned on the patient's chest and then unfolded to the sides and then over the end of the table. (F) The tails of the split sheet are unfolded to expose the full U-shape of split and the backing paper removed from the adhesive edges. (G) The split sheet is positioned around the operative site and secured to the patient and head drape. (Barrier disposable drapes — Surgikos.)

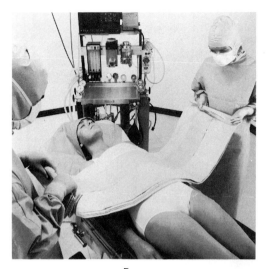

F

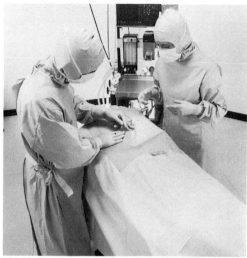

G

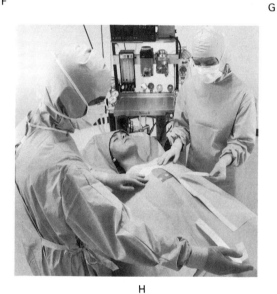

H

Fig. 10.9 (continued)

Operations on the eye

Using a conventional technique the hair is covered as for ENT operations, but the towel is crossed over the forehead just below the hairline. The draping is completed by covering the lower part of the patient with a sterile water repellent drape and large fabric drape, extending from just below the operation area. The simplest method of draping is to use a disposable drape which incorporates a self-adhesive incise drape (Fig. 10.10). This eliminates the need for clipping eye lashes and extends the sterile field up to the eyeball itself.

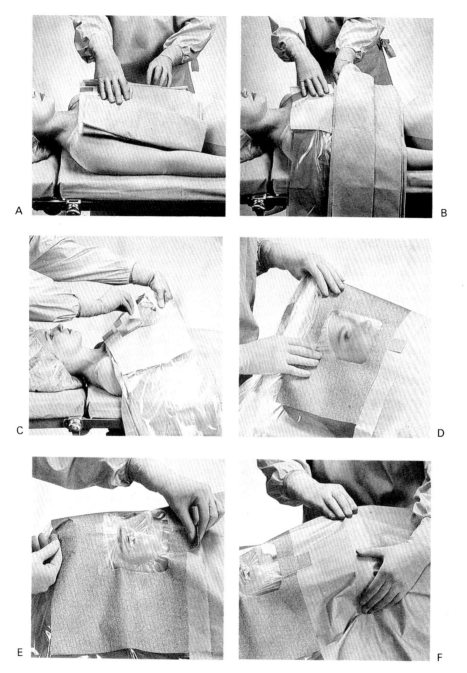

Fig. 10.10   Draping for eye operations — adhesive fenestration. (A) The ophthalmology drape is placed on the patient's upper chest — directional arrows indicate the proper positioning of the sheet for opening. (B) The lower part of the drape is unfolded towards the feet. (C) The white paper strip is removed from the adhesive film. (D) The folds of the clear plastic are gathered in one hand until the adhesive film is under the finger tips for control. The adhesive film is fenestrated as required and gently pressed onto the patient's eye ensuring that it adheres completely to the orbit to maintain a sterile field. (E and F) The remainder of the clear plastic is unfolded to cover the patient's head completely. The underlying aluminium strip is bent to lift the drape from the patient's lower face and used to secure anaesthetic tubing or an air supply. (Barrier disposable drapes — Surgikos)

Steri·Drape®2
Surgical Incise Drapes

APPLICATION TECHNIQUE

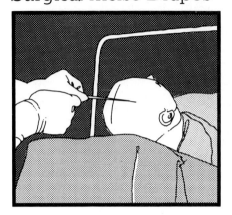

Orientation markings may be applied to the dried, prepped skin.

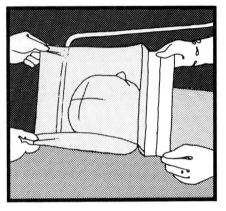

Position drape over scalp with liner face down. Grasp liner tab from underneath and begin peeling back.

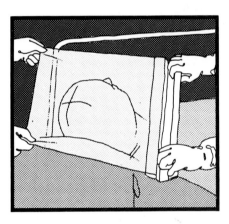

Peel back liner material, folding liner upon itself as you go along. DO NOT REMOVE LINER COMPLETELY. Leave last fold adhered to adhesive area.

3M and Steri-Drape are trademarks

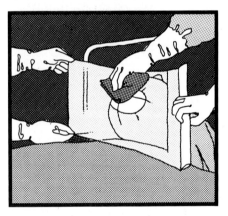

Using folded liner as a "handle bar," stabilize drape over scalp. With a folded sterile towel, press and smooth drape to scalp, first along planned line of incision. Remove liner completely and incise through sterile drape surface.

Fig. 10.11   Application technique for Steridrape used for neurosurgical operations. (Wound Management Products, 3M Health Care.)

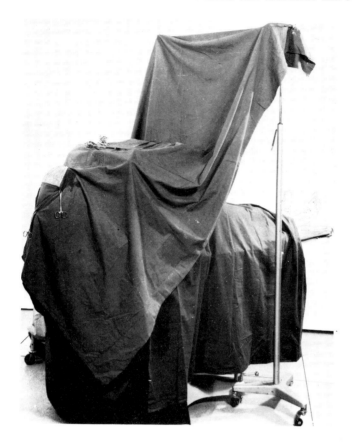

Fig. 10.12 Drapes completed for neurosurgical operation.

Perineal operations (vaginal, rectal, cystoscopy, urethral operations, etc.) in the lithotomy position

Using a conventional technique the first stage is placing a sterile water repellent sheet under the buttocks. This is important, as it prevents contamination from the lower part of the operation table which would otherwise become rather wet during the course of the operation.

A 'holed' water repellent sheet or plastic adhesive drape is used to isolate the operation area from surrounding unprepared skin and this is followed by a special drape having two lateral leg 'bags' stitched to either side of a central slit. The central slit is adjusted around the operation area and the 'bags' cover both legs and operation table stirrups. The upper and lower ends of the 'holed' towel cover the abdomen and lower end of the operation table respectively.

Alternatively, using disposable drapes such as Barrier 450 or Azodrape, the legs are first covered with leggings (Fig. 10.13A), followed by a cystoscopy or similar 'holed' sheet (Fig. 10.13B & C) over the operation area, and sides secured around each leg and stirrup.

A sterile douche tray may be added after the drapes have been positioned correctly.

Synchronous combined excision of the rectum performed simultaneously from the abdominal and perineal route by two surgeons, requires complete draping of the two areas.

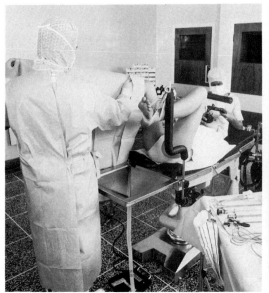

A

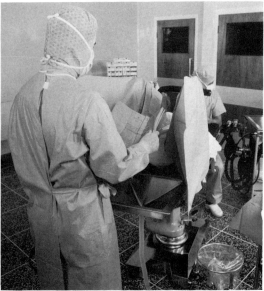

B

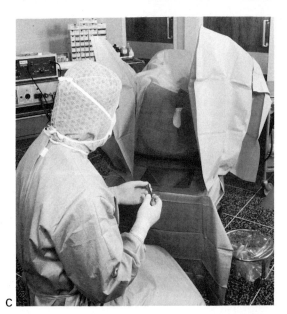

C

Fig. 10.13 Draping for lithotomy position. (A) Using the protective cuff, the legging is slid on to one leg to completely cover both the leg and stirrup. The procedure is repeated for the second leg. (B) The patient is covered with a 'Cysto' fenestrated sheet, the fenestration being adjusted around the operation area, and the mesh screen over fluid collection bucket or operation table extension. (C) The draping procedure completed. (Barrier disposable drapes — Surgikos.)

This is achieved by using a drape as previously described, but having a slit which will extend from the anus to the umbilicus. A small towel is placed to cover and isolate the genitals.

Many surgeons operating in the perineal region appreciate a towel draped as a trough between the patient and themselves. One edge of this towel is secured just below the operation area and to the towel covering the leg and stirrup on each side, the other edge

being clipped to the surgeon's gown. This method will prevent dropped instruments from slipping to the floor and will provide the surgeon with a 'shelf' for his swabs, etc., if he should so desire. Alternatively a narrow table placed transversely may be used and is placed in position before draping.

Assisting the surgeon

It would be very presumptuous to even suggest that the technique, of assisting the surgeon either as first assistant, second assistant or scrub nurse, can be learned from a book. This, like draping the operation area, can be perfected only by careful practical study supervised by an experienced surgeon or senior theatre nurse. There are, however, certain basic points which are fairly universal and common to assisting in general.

The scrub nurse

The development of logical thinking plus a silent technique, whereby metal instruments may be picked up or put down with minimal noise, cannot be over-emphasised (Ginsberg et al., 1967; Willingham, 1971).

The instrument or Mayo trolley is prepared by laying out only those instruments which will be required in the early stages of the operation. These instruments are replaced with others when necessary and as the operation progresses. The instrument trolley should not be crowded as this only leads to confusion, especially at a later stage of the operation.

It is important that the instruments should always be laid out in the same order, not only for tidiness, but because many valuable seconds can be lost searching for a vital instrument. A standard method of preparation of this and other trolleys used in the operation area will reduce delays, especially during critical periods.

The majority of surgeons appear to prefer the order of instruments whereby those required first are placed on the right-hand side of the instrument trolley facing them. This is, of course, a very flexible rule and must be adapted to suit the needs of a particular surgeon, but once established should be strictly adhered to.

The suggested order of instruments would be: at the front of the trolley from right to left, scalpels, dissecting forceps, scissors, artery forceps; at the back of the trolley, retractors, tissue forceps, etc., and any special instruments which may be required at that particular time. If the trolley has a raised edge, the handles of the instruments should project slightly

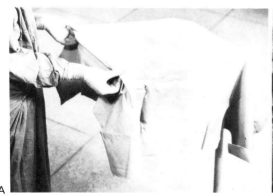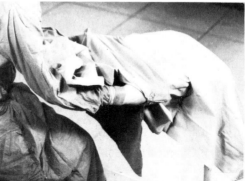

A   B

Fig. 10.14   Preparing the Mayo trolley.

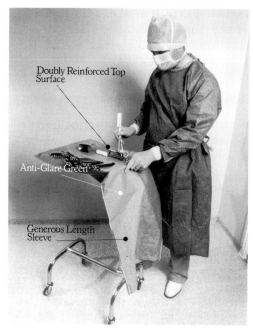

Fig. 10.15   Mayo trolley draped with a disposable reinforced cover which obviates the need for an additional water repellent sheet underneath. (Azodrape^{TM} — Vernon Carus.)

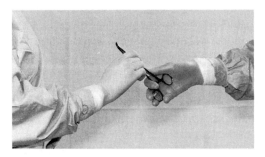

Fig. 10.16   Method of passing an artery or similar forceps.

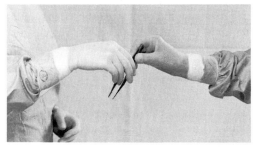

Fig. 10.17   Method of passing a dissecting forceps.

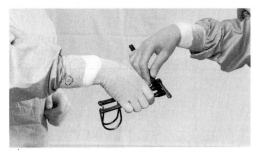

Fig. 10.18   Method of passing a self-retaining retractor.

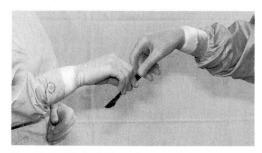

Fig. 10.19   Method of passing a scalpel.

over this edge. Accidental contamination of these projecting instruments is unlikely as the Mayo trolley should be positioned well within the sterile operation area. Some people will disagree with this statement, but it is much easier to pick up an instrument, silently and correctly, when placed in such a manner.

Instruments having sharp points, such as scissors and scalpels, etc., must be placed with their cutting edges or points away from the surgeon.

Soiled instruments should be cleansed before replacing them on the instrument trolley.

Sharp instruments (indeed any instruments) must not be left lying on drapes covering the patient. If the surgeon requires the scalpel conveniently at hand, it should be placed in a small kidney dish and may be held by an assistant.

When passing instruments, they are placed firmly into the surgeon's hand, and it should not be necessary for him to reach for them. Most instruments such as artery forceps, tissue forceps, towel clips, scissors, etc., are always handed in the closed position, on the first ratchet when that is applicable. An instrument should always enter the surgeon's hand so that it may be used without further adjustment. With artery forceps, especially of the curved type, this means the point at the correct angle required by the surgeon, viz., generally upwards.

Self-retaining retractors are also handed for use in the closed position; but self-retaining bone clamps, dissecting forceps, and multiple joint cutting forceps should generally be open when handed to the surgeon.

These are, of course, only a few of the many instruments which the nurse will handle, but it is her duty to determine the correct way to handle a particular instrument *before* operation.

Naturally, the method of passing instruments will depend upon the way in which the surgeon is accustomed to taking them, i.e., if a surgeon extends his hand for a scalpel with the palm uppermost, the scalpel is placed with the blade horizontal, pointing towards the instrument nurse and with its cutting edge facing in the same direction as the extended finger tips. As he closes his fingers on the handle, the cutting edge will be in the correct position for use.

The non-touch technique of passing instruments is now virtually obsolete for it is logical that as the surgeon handles the instruments with his gloved hands there seems no reason why the scrub nurse should not do likewise. However, in orthopaedic surgery care should be taken to avoid touching sterile implants or the points of instruments with the gloved hands.

The preparation and threading of suture needles has been dealt with in the previous chapter, but we must now consider the correct way of handing the prepared suture to the surgeon.

If the needle has been mounted on to a needle holder, this instrument should be handed to the surgeon so that as he takes it, the needle is facing in the correct direction for immediate use (Fig. 10.20). A right-handed person will require the needle facing his left hand, and a left-handed person vice versa. The long end of the suture material is held by the nurse either with her fingers or with forceps, whichever is applicable, until the assistant takes over or the surgeon has completed his first suture.

A large curved or hand needle is held by its mid-shaft, between the index finger and thumb, with the eye facing the nurse and the point towards the surgeon. A straight needle is held between the index finger and thumb but with the eye facing the surgeon and the point towards the nurse. Presenting the needle in this way will allow the surgeon to complete his first suture without further readjustment.

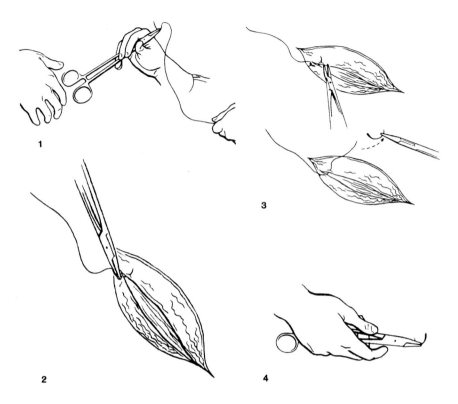

Fig. 10.20 Method of passing a suture. (Ethicon.)
1. Surgeon receives needleholder with needle point toward his thumb to prevent unnecessary wrist motion. Scrub nurse controls free end of suture to prevent dragging across sterile field.
2. Surgeon begins closing with swaged suture.

3. Needle is passed into tissue. Surgeon releases needle from holder and reclamps holder near point end to pull needle and strand through tissue. Eyed or *control release* needle is released from suture.
4. Surgeon leaves *control release* needle or empty eyed needle clamped in same position and returns it to nurse. She passes another prepared suture to him immediately. (Note: Keeping up with needles is easiest if done on a 'one-for-one' basis.)

Ligatures are handed to the surgeon, grasped taut between the fingers of each hand, grasped between forceps, in ligature eggs or on reels. When ligatures are tied by hand, the nurse must ascertain with which hand the surgeon is accustomed to tie. If he uses a left-hand tie, the nurse should face the surgeon, holding the ligature taut, with one end in her right hand and the centre in her left. He will generally take the ligature with his right hand, so that the short end is ready for grasping with his left (Fig. 10.21). This procedure is reversed for a right-hand tie. When the surgeon adopts an 'instrument tie', the length of ligature held between two pairs of forceps should not exceed 31 cm (12 in) (Fig. 10.22).

Ligature eggs or reels are lifted from the nurse's extended palm (Fig. 10.23). Care must be taken to ensure that there is sufficient ligature material protruding from the egg or reel, for if it is too short it may slip back through the ligature egg hole or become locked within strands on the reel. After use, the egg or reel is returned to the scrub nurse by dropping it back in her hand.

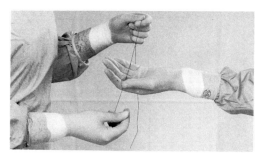

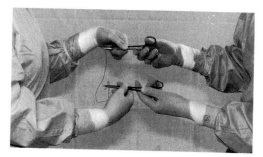

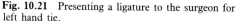

Fig. 10.21 Presenting a ligature to the surgeon for left hand tie.

Fig. 10.22 Presenting a ligature for instrument tie.

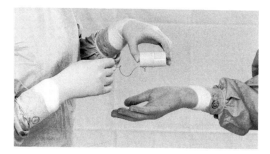

Fig. 10.23 A ligature egg or reel is presented to the surgeon in this manner.

The most important point regarding *all* instruments is that they must be given a rapid final check before handing to the surgeon or his assistant. Special attention is paid to adjustable screws, ratchets, scalpel blades, their edges, and any moving parts on a particular instrument. Although instruments should always be checked by a responsible person before sterilisation, this rapid final check should *never* be overlooked.

The position of the scrub nurse in relation to the surgeon is dependent upon his wishes, and also the area and type of operation. The most logical place is that facing him, for in this position she can follow the surgeon's movements, anticipating his requirements. Some surgeons, however, prefer the scrub nurse a little to the side and behind their operating hand which is extended back as the instruments are required.

It is very difficult to make hard and fast rules regarding this, but readers will find the following to be of general application.

For operations on the face, neck, chest, abdomen or thighs, with the surgeon standing at the right-hand side of the operation table, the nurse should be opposite his right hand and with the instrument trolley at her left. A surgeon standing at the left-hand side of the operation table will require the scrub nurse opposite his left hand and her trolley at the right.

During operations on the lower limbs the nurse may adopt a similar position as above, or stand at the foot of the operation table facing the surgeon, and with the instrument trolley in front of her.

When a surgeon is at the operation table head, i.e., during craniotomy, the best position for the scrub nurse is opposite his right hand with her instrument trolley or neurosurgical table placed over the patient. If the surgeon is left handed the position may be reversed.

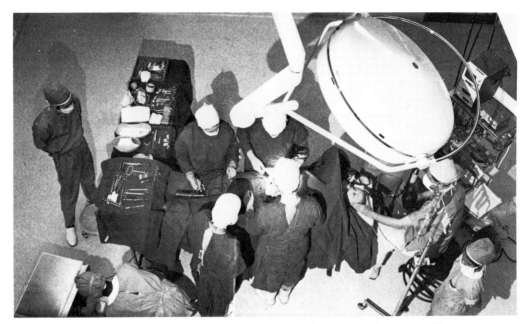

Fig. 10.24   An abdominal operation correctly draped, showing relative positions of surgeons and instrument nurse, etc. (Northwick Park Hospital, London.)

A similar position is adopted at the other end of the table when the knee is flexed over the foot end of the table which is lowered or removed, as during excision of torn meniscus.

An operation performed on the arm table is best served by the nurse standing behind her instrument trolley, facing the patient, and with the surgeon at her right or left, with his assistant opposite.

Occasionally the nurse will be compelled to stand behind and a little to the side of the surgeon owing to the nature of the operation. This is often necessary, for example, during Smith Petersen pinning for fractured neck of femur, where X-ray apparatus occupies considerable space normally required by the scrub nurse.

Whichever position is adopted, the nurse should always be able to observe the surgeon's movements and be capable of handing him his instruments with the minimum of inconvenience (Pearce, 1967).

Finally, it is the duty of the scrub nurse to keep a very careful check on the instruments, needles and swabs or packs, etc., used in the operation, and she should be able to account for *all* at any stage of the operation. She should always inform the surgeon of their correctness before being asked, and must obtain acknowledgment in every case.

The surgeon's first assistant

Occasionally it becomes necessary for a member of the nursing staff to act as first assistant. The purpose of an assistant is to help the surgeon as required, and it is only he who can decide to what extent this assistance is necessary. As the practical knowledge of his assistant increases, so the surgeon will permit him or her to assist more fully. It must be understood that the assistant's duties are to follow the surgeon's wishes exactly, and to perform only those actions which the surgeon expects or requests.

This obvious statement is, of course, only a repetition of that made at the beginning of this chapter, for we must realise that a good assistant is trained in a particular surgeon's ways and methods by practical guidance, and certainly not from a book. The following suggestions are meant as a basis for the embryo assistant, but will be of some help to those who may be called upon suddenly to assist the surgeon.

The assistant either faces the surgeon, standing at the opposite side of the operation table, or is placed at the surgeon's side opposite to the place occupied by the instrument nurse or second assistant.

The main duties of a first assistant are to keep the operation field unobscured and free from blood, either with a suction tube or gauze swabs, using with the latter a 'dabbing' action rather than wiping which may disturb minute blood clots and increase bleeding. Where excessive bleeding is anticipated from the incision, the surgeon may require pressure to be applied at each side of the wound as the incision is made. This applies particularly to operations on the cranium, due to the vascularity of the scalp.

If the assistant is permitted to apply haemostats to severed vessels, care should be taken to grasp only the vessel and a minimum of surrounding tissue with the forceps tip. Excessive tissue clamped with a vessel will require an unnecessarily stout ligature with consequent risk of slipping, and furthermore, resultant necrosis of the tissue may affect healing.

Whenever possible the surgeon will apply forceps to vessels, after dissection from surrounding tissue and before division. He will apply his forceps across the vessel first, followed by the assistant who places his in close proximity. The vessel will be divided by scissors or if the forceps are very close, with a scalpel.

During ligation of a vessel the forceps are held by the assistant in such a manner that they may be re-applied immediately should the ligature slip. After the ligature has been placed around the forceps, the handle is depressed, and the points elevated towards the surgeon, avoiding excessive leverage. It should not be released until he indicates (usually by saying 'off') and care must be taken to do this comparatively slowly in order that the first hitch of the ligature may be tightened on the vessel.

Deep vessels do not generally permit the elevation of forcep points, but they should always be directed towards the surgeon unless he indicates to the contrary.

When cutting a ligature the scissors are held by the thumb and third finger, with the index finger extending along the shanks to the joint, thereby steadying the instrument. As far as possible, the scissor points only are used for cutting, for if the whole length of the blades is used, more than the ligature may be divided, possibly with disastrous results. Ligatures should be cut fairly short, about 6 mm ($\frac{1}{4}$ in), except for the larger vessels which the surgeon will indicate.

In order to avoid the contamination of clean instruments the used instruments should always be returned to the scrub nurse, and not dropped on the drapes covering the patient or on the instrument trolley.

Incise drapes or surgical towel drapes may be applied in various ways but the best method is illustrated in Figures 10.2–10.3. The use of fabric skin or tetra towels is now an outdated practice because they soon become soaked with blood and lose their protective value.

Deep retractors are placed by the surgeon and should *not* be removed by the assistant unless he or she is requested to do so. Superficial retractors, on the other hand, require some alteration of position during the initial dissection and a good assistant will, if the surgeon permits, learn to follow him in this respect without any effort on the surgeon's part. The retractors will be moved to provide the surgeon with the greatest possible access in the particular area which he is working but this is dependent on the degree of retraction permissible.

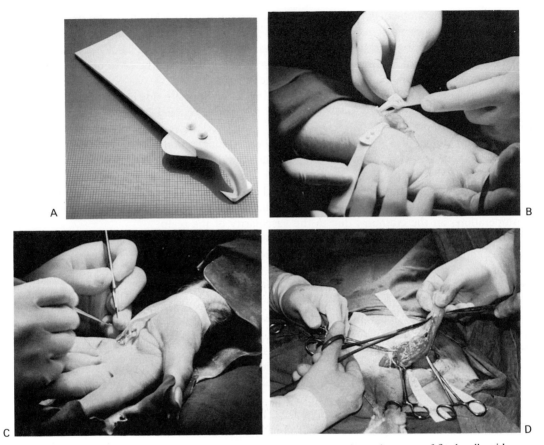

Fig. 10.25 Disposable self-retaining retractor. (A) Retractor, adhesive underneath surface of flat handle with protective peel-off cover. (B) Claws of retractor inserted under skin edge, tension applied and adhesive surface exposed; handle is pressed on to skin and drape surface to maintain traction. (C & D) Exposure of wound. (Steritractor™, Wound Management Products, 3M Health Care.)

The care with which a retractor must be used cannot be over-emphasised and undue force must be avoided owing to the trauma which can result. The surgeon will decide the degree of retraction possible and this must not be exceeded, the tendency being for the retractor to be *held* and not *pulled*. An example of a disposable self-adhesive superficial retractor is shown in Figure 10.25.

Any form of retractor used in the location of a delicate organ such as the liver or lungs, requires some form of pack or swab between it and the organ concerned. A pack should never be obscured by a retractor without the knowledge of the surgeon and instrument nurse, and the assistant should ensure that used packs and swabs are returned to the scrub nurse rather than dropped on to the floor, to assist her in the location of packs and swabs after the operation.

Small swabs or sponges should not be removed from sponge-holding forceps by the assistant, owing to the danger of these swabs being mislaid, especially when large quantities are being used. It is the duty of the scrub nurse to change these swabs when necessary so that a very careful check can be made of the total in circulation.

Any swab or sponge used as a pack must have a tape attached which is always visible and must have a haemostat clipped to it.

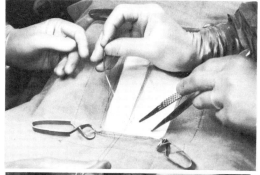
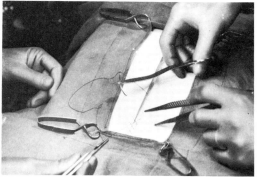
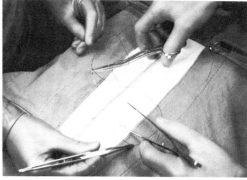

A

B

C

Fig. 10.26 Following the surgeon's suture. (A) Simple continuous suture. (B) Simple continuous suture — 'non-touch' technique. (C) Continuous 'blanket' suture, 'non-touch' technique.

Soiling of the drapes which can occur when opening the bowel, etc., is avoided by using additional towels or packs just before the incision is made. These may be a distinctive colour, often red, and are placed to isolate the bowel from the general drapes. Instruments used for the procedure should remain on these towels or in a separate kidney dish, and are discarded with the towels when the bowel closure is complete.

The surgeon and his assistant change their gloves before concluding the operation and whilst the soiled drapes are being removed.

Hot saline packs prepared by the scrub nurse are replenished when necessary, unless the surgeon indicates that a particular pack should remain in position. This maintenance of moisture and warmth is particularly applicable to exposed bowel which should be kept covered whenever possible.

Sutures are cut in a similar manner to ligatures, but a continuous suture requires the assistant to follow the surgeon, keeping each loop taut as it is made.

After the first knot has been tied, the continuous suture should be held about 8 cm (3 in) from the first loop, pulling the strand a little towards the side of the incision. As the surgeon passes his needle through the tissues and makes each loop, the strand is released. It is then grasped again and the loop held taut, the process being repeated until the surgeon has sutured the entire length of the wound. The degree of tension varies but should be sufficient to prevent each loop slipping, without drawing the tissues together tighter than required by the surgeon.

Where a non-touch technique is operable, this procedure must be performed with forceps, preferably of the non-toothed variety or those specially designed for the purpose. Care must be taken to avoid crushing the material, for if this occurs in the middle of a strand, it may break during suturing or at some stage post-operatively.

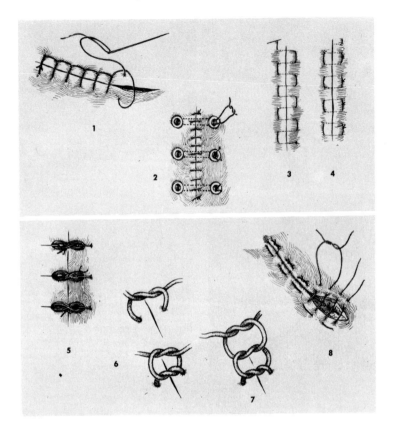

Fig. 10.27   Types of sutures.
1. The blanket or continuous locked suture.
2. Continuous suture and method of using perforated buttons to support tension sutures.
3. Continuous mattress suture.
4. Interrupted mattress suture.
5. Figure-of-eight sutures around pins.
6. Method of placing first and second half-hitches in the square or true knot.
7. The square knot reinforced by third half-hitch.
8. The Halsted interrupted mattress suture.
(From *Manual of Operative Procedure*. Ethicon Ltd.)

Certain continuous sutures, such as the blanket type, require the assistant to hold the material in the correct position for the surgeon to catch each loop with minimum delay. Various methods are illustrated.

Skin sutures are cut at least 13 mm ($\frac{1}{2}$ in) long for subsequent removal. Tension sutures, or those retaining drainage tubes are always left longer than those used for general closure, for easy identification. A different colour of suture material is also very useful for these special sutures which are often removed at different intervals to the skin sutures.

Adhesive skin closures are a method of closing skin incisions which is gaining popularity. Many surgeons use Steri-strip skin closures either alone or as an adjunct to suture. Since 1962, the technique has been used for thousands of major surgical procedures such as appendectomies, thoracotomies and orthopaedic procedures. The non-reactive nature of the tape and adhesive backing makes the material very suitable for plastic procedures such as skin grafts and the secondary closure of infected wounds.

Success of the technique is dependent upon careful adherence to the method of application which is illustrated in Figure 10.31.

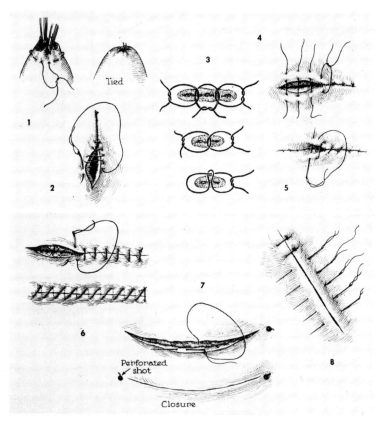

Fig. 10.28 Types of sutures.
1. Purse-string suture around open stump.
2. Closing stump by Cushing stitch.
3. Methods for ligation of pedicles with anchored ligatures.
4. Interrupted Lembert inverting stitch.
5. Continuous Lembert stitch.
6. Two methods of continuous over-and-over closing sutures.
7. Subcuticular suture for closure of skin incision. Perforated buckshot used to anchor suture.
8. Interrupted skin sutures — multiple needle technique.

(From *Manual of Operative Procedure*, Ethicon Ltd.)

The surgeon's second assistant

This duty is frequently delegated either to a nurse or dresser who requires experience before assisting in the capacity of instrument nurse or first assistant. During major operations it may be essential to have a fully experienced person in this position.

Generally the second assistant helps the first by holding extra retractors and performing the duties which the surgeon may indicate.

The correct application of dressings may be supervised by the first assistant, although this task is completed by the scrub nurse, except in special circumstances.

The infected case

Measures must be taken to avoid cross infection and minimise hazards to staff following an infected operation (Medical Research Council, 1968). Of special concern are patients who are carriers of Hepatitis B (Waterson and Batterson, 1977; Hackshaw and Hackshaw, 1975) or who are infected with the human immunodeficiency virus (HIV — AIDS) (Royal College

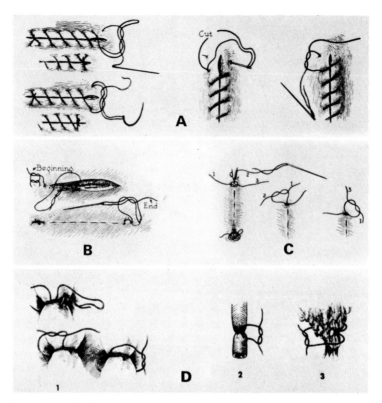

Fig. 10.29 Types of sutures. (A) Variety of methods for securing the ends of completed continuous sutures. Technique for securing ends of both double and single sutures demonstrated. Note method of dividing suture to avoid double thickness of knot. (B) Method of beginning subcuticular suture by placing square knot lateral to incision. Method of ending suture at opposite end of incision. (C) Alternate method for the completion of subcuticular continuous suture by placing a holding knot around end of subcuticular suture. (D) Methods of placing transfixing ligatures to prevent slipping 1. Transfixing ligature of pedicle. 2. Method of placing transfixing ligature in vessel. 3. Tying transfixing ligature of omentum or of hernial sac.
(From *Manual of Operative Procedure*. Ethicon Ltd.)

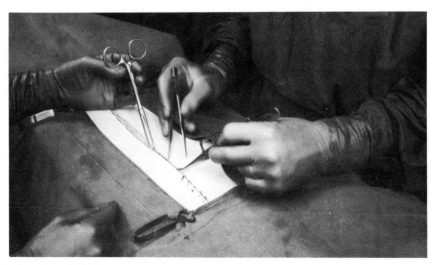

Fig. 10.30 Insertion of Michel suture clips.

Steri-Strip™
SKIN CLOSURES

Basic preparation and application techniques

1. Clean and dry skin for at least 2½ inches around the wound, making sure to remove skin oil or exudate. For best results, use a sponge moistened with either alcohol or saline followed by a firm wipe with a dry sponge. A thin coat of Tr. of Benzoin may be helpful in certain cases. Be sure gloves are dry before handling the tape.

2. Grasp package tabs and peel back.

3. With sterile precautions remove card, break on perforated line and tear off the card tab. Remove strips as needed.

4. At midportion of the incision, apply one-half of the first strip up to one wound margin and press firmly into place.

5. Appose skin edges exactly using fingers or forceps. Press the free half of the tape firmly into place.

6. In large wounds apply additional strips at intervals in the same manner. This eases separation stress and facilitates wound edge approximation.

7. Should the skin surfaces become moist with perspiration, blood or serum, wipe dry with sponge before applying the next strip.

8. Complete the closure with additional strips spaced approximately ⅛ inch to allow for drainage.

9. If, as sometimes happens in large wounds, the skin has gapped under the first strip or two due to initial stress, remove these strips and reapproximate the wound edges with fresh strips.

Note: The correct application of STERI-STRIP Skin Closures requires careful attention to instructions. As in all suturing, ease of application can be attained with STERI-STRIP Closures only after several uses.

3M and Steri-strip are trademarks

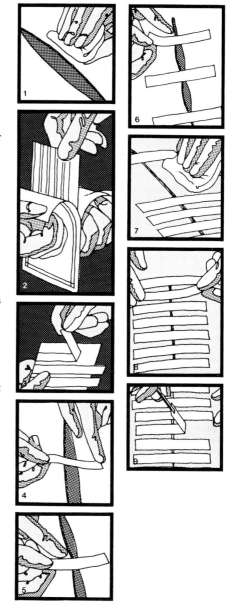

Fig. 10.31 Method of preparing skin and application of Steristrip skin closures. (Wound Management Products, 3M Health Care.)

1. Redistribute stress. Apply additional strips approximately ¼ inch from and paralleling the wound (ladder pattern) to redistribute the tension. This variation gives added protection against unusual disruptive stress.

2. Action areas. For wounds over joints, or in other areas where motion may cause "scissoring" of apposed edges, a criss-cross application gives greater security.

3. Unusual laceration. With V-shaped lacerations, the point of the V is anchored with the forceps and strips applied across both legs of the V.

4. When applying Surgical Dressing, or any other dressing, make sure it completely covers the ends of the tape strips.

Contraindications. When proper steps of application and follow-up are observed, no anatomical regions (except those extremely limited in size) are contraindicated.

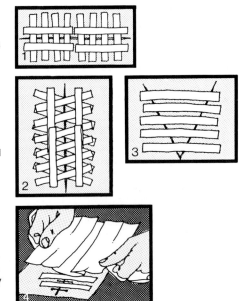

Fig. 10.31 (continued)

of Nursing, 1986). The safety procedures which should be adopted in both situations are virtually identical.

Patients who are suspect carriers of Hepatitis B (serum hepatitis, Australian antigen positive) include those with liver disease, patients in renal units, drug addicts, the tattooed, patients who have received repeated blood transfusions, and those receiving immuno-suppressive drugs. Patients found to be positive for HIV antibodies are considered to have been previously in contact with the virus, presumed to be currently infected and capable of transmitting the infection. It is likely that the hepatitis and HIV viruses can be present in blood, saliva, urine, faeces, bile and vomit. For this reason it is important that staff take measures to avoid contact with body fluids from such patients undergoing operative procedures.

The most important principle is to ensure that all members of the surgical team are aware of the infection hazards and the infection control measures which should be taken. A Royal College of Nursing working party has issued nursing guidelines on the management of patients suffering from AIDS. The following guidelines for operating departments form the basis of good practice (RCN, 1986).

General principles

1. The operation should be scheduled to allow time for adequate cleaning of the theatre and decontamination of equipment.
2. If hair removal is essential, the use of depilatory creams is recommended.
3. The operating team should be limited to essential staff only.
4. Avoid the use of equipment which cannot easily be decontaminated.
5. Disposable theatre gowns and patient drapes are recommended. All theatre personnel should wear a disposable plastic apron under their surgical gown.

6. For wounds which require post-operative drainage, a closed drainage system should be used.
7. At the end of the operation, blood should be removed from the patient's skin, and the wound covered with an impervious dressing that will contain the exudate.
   The following should be available for use:
8. Disposable gowns, drapes and plastic aprons.
9. Face visors or goggles.
10. Adequate supplies of an appropriate chemical disinfectant (Hypochlorite).
11. 'Sharps' disposal container.
12. Plastic bags for disposable items and linen.

Preparation of the theatre and equipment

13. Clear rooms of all non-essential equipment.
14. The anaesthesia machine should be stripped of non-essential items. Autoclavable or disposable breathing circuits should be used.
15. A measured quantity of hypochlorite solution should be put into suction bottles (see Chapter 7, page 204).
16. The operation table and patient trolley should be protected by a water-repellent laminate or equivalent.

Procedures during and after the operation

17. A runner should be available outside the theatre to avoid the necessity of a member of the operating team having to leave the theatre.
18. In keeping with good practice, all blood soaked swabs should be handled with forceps. After counting, they must be put into bags for incineration.
19. At the end of the operation, all staff should remove their disposable protective clothing before leaving the theatre. Used instruments should be handled as little as possible before being sent for processing and sterilization.
20. The contents of suction bottles, urine and other body fluids must be carefully emptied down the sluice hopper, taking care to avoid personal and environmental contamination. (A closed disposable suction system [Receptal] is illustrated in Figure 3.35, page 105).
21. All disposable suction and anaesthesia tubing should be sent for incineration.
22. Non-autoclavable equipment should be dealt with in accordance with agreed local practices.
23. Spillages of blood or any other body fluids should be dealt with using hypochlorite or the recommended chemical disinfectant before routine theatre cleaning (Chapter 7, page 209).
24. After surgery the patient should be allowed to recover in the theatre.

These guidelines (reference in parathesis) can be further amplified as follows:

Patients should be brought to the operating department on their bed, or on a trolley covered with a water repellent sheet (16). The patient should be taken directly into the theatre, *not* through the anaesthetic room.

Preparations before operation include the removal of extraneous equipment and furniture from the theatre (18), but retaining sufficient supplementary items such as suture materials and strapping, etc. to avoid unnecessary 'fetching' during operation (17). Adequate supplies of hypochlorite solution or the recommended chemical disinfectant should be available (Chapter 7, page 209).

A large 'sharps' container should be available for used syringes, needles, scalpel blades etc. (Fig. 10.32). A plastic or enamel tray containing a little hypochlorite solution etc. should be placed on a plastic sheet on the floor; this is for used swabs which can be laid out in order for counting before transfer to plastic bags.

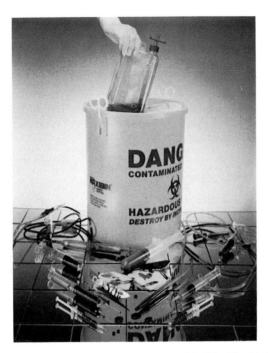

Fig. 10.32   Sharps container for used syringes, scalpel blades etc. (Maxibin, Daniels Healthcare.)

After operation, the scrub nurse, still wearing gown and gloves, carefully bundles up the drapes and other disposable items and places them in their respective plastic bags. She then transfers these to outer disposable bags which are stapled by another person wearing clean gloves. This person then labels the bags with appropriate stickers and removes them for disposal. Similarly, used and unused instruments are securely wrapped within the pre-set tray drapes and returned in sealed bags to the SDU for processing and sterilization. If, exceptionally, any fabric drapes or towels are used and are not blood stained, they are soaked in hypochlorite solution for three hours before sending to the laundry as infected linen. Linen which is blood stained must be incinerated.

Suction traps should be fitted between all suction lines and the machine or vacuum terminal unit. These are discarded for destruction after operation. If blood is spilt at any time it must be wiped up immediately with a paper towel soaked in hypochlorite solution; plastic or rubber gloves must be used (23).

Yellow or other clearly designated labels should be available for identifying specimens. The specimen containers after closing should be wiped over with hypochlorite solution, and then with *clean* gloved hands dropped into a plastic bag which is then sealed.

The scrub nurse and other members of the surgical team remove their gown gloves and plastic apron, taking care not to contaminate hands. Staff, still wearing gown and gloves, clean the equipment and theatre thoroughly using hypochlorite solution. The theatre should be left for an hour before further use (Fig. 10.33).

Afterwards all personnel involved, either in the operation or cleaning the rooms, should leave their potentially contaminated clothing and overshoes in appropriate disposal bags at the door, stepping into a clean gown before going to the changing rooms to shower and obtain clean protective clothing.

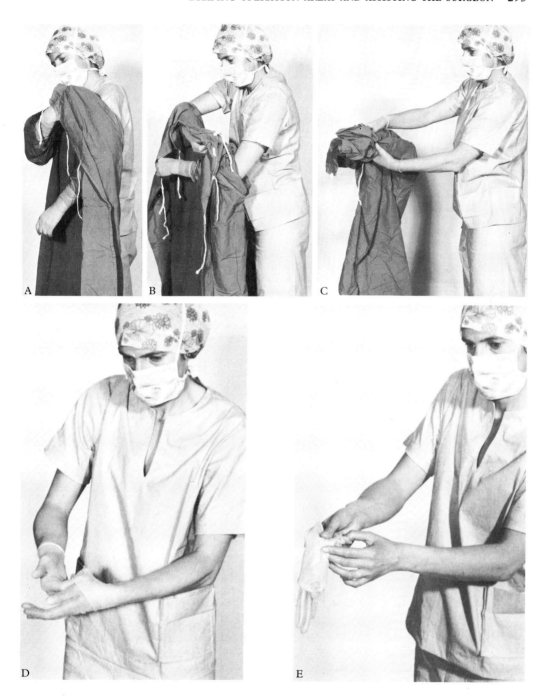

Fig. 10.33   Removing soiled gown and gloves (Royal Berkshire Hospital, Reading). (A) To protect scrub suit and arms from contamination with bacteria which is present on outside of gown; the gown is peeled off one side of body, using the opposite hand, and the inner side of the gown is turned outward. (B) The outer side of the soiled gown is turned away from the body, keeping elbows flexed and arm away from the body, so that the soiled gown does not touch the arms or scrub suit. (C) To prevent outer surface of gloves from contaminating hands, the gloved fingers of one hand grip the outer surface of the cuff and pulls off the glove inside out. (D) and (E) To prevent contamination of the ungloved hand, the person grasps the inner part of the cuff and pulls the remaining glove off the hand.

REFERENCES AND FURTHER READING

ALEXANDER, J. W., FISCHER, J. E., BOYAJIAN, M., PALMQUIST, J. AND MORRIS, J. (1983) The influence of hair-removal methods on wound infections. *Archives of Surgery*, **118**, March, 347–352.

ASSOCIATION OF OPERATING ROOM NURSES INC. (1983) Recommended practices for preoperative skin preparation of patients. *AORN Standards and Recommended Practices for Perioperative Nursing*, AORN, Denver USA.

BAILEY, H. (1967) *Demonstrations of Operative Surgery*, 3rd edn. Edinburgh: Livingstone.

BALLINGER, W. F., TREYBAL, J. C. AND VOSE, A. B. (1972) *Alexander's Care of the Patient in Surgery*. St. Louis: Mosby.

BRANDBERG, A., HOLM, J., HAMMARSTEN, J. AND SCHERSTEN, T. (1970) Paper II in *Problems in the Control of Hospital Infection*, The Royal Society of Medicine International Congress and Symposium Series No. 23, London, Academic Press Inc. Ltd and The Royal Society of Medicine.

COURT-BROWN, C. M. (1981) Preoperative skin depilation and its effect on postoperative wound infections, *Journal of the Royal College of Surgeons*, Edinburgh, **26**, 238–241.

CRUSE, P. J. E. AND FOORD, R. (1973) A 10 year prospective study of 62,939 wounds. *Surgical Clinics of North America*, **60**, February, 27–40.

DAVIES, J., BABB, J. R., AYLIFFE, G. A. AND ELLIS, S. H. (1977) *Journal of Antimicrobial Chemotherapy*, **3**, 473.

GINSBERG, F., BRONNER, L. S. AND CANTLIN, V. L. (1967) *A Manual of Operating Room Technology*. Philadelphia: Lippincott.

HACKSHAW, M. AND HACKSHAW, J. E. (1975) *Nursing Times*, October 16, supp. IX.

LANCET EDITORIAL (1983) Preoperative depilation. *Lancet*, June.

SEROPIAN, R. AND REYNOLD, B. M. (1971) Wound infections after pre-operative depilatory versus razor preparation. *American Journal of Surgery*, **121**, 251–254.

LINTON, J. (1974) Occasional Papers. *Nursing Times*. July 4, 11, 18.

MEDICAL RESEARCH COUNCIL (1968) Aseptic Method in the Operating Suite, *Lancet*, i, 763.

PEARCE, E. (1967) *Instruments, Appliances and Theatre Techniques*, 5th edn. London: Faber.

PUBLIC HEALTH LABORATORY REPORT (1965) *British Medical Journal*, i, 1251.

WATERSON, S. AND BATTERSON, P. (1977) *Natnews*, January, 8.

WESLEY, J. A., FISCHER, J. E., BOYAJIAN, M., PALMQUIST, J. AND MORRIS, M. J. (1983) The influence of hair-removal methods on wound infections. *Archives of Surgery*, **118**, March 347–352.

WILLINGHAM, J. (1971) *Operating Theatre Techniques*. English Edition.

11

Anaesthesia and the anaesthesia room

Anaesthesia is a complex, highly developed science.

So vast is this clinical field that it would be quite impossible to describe in this chapter all the equipment and techniques which are available today. For further information the reader is advised to consult a textbook dealing specifically with anaesthesia.

The anaesthesia nurse or operating department assistant must familiarise herself with the basic principles of apparatus and the use of drugs in the particular theatre in which she works. It would be wrong to suggest that it is necessary to know all the mechanisms of anaesthesia apparatus, or all the effects and complications of certain drugs, but an intelligent and sensible understanding of the basic principles involved is essential in order to give efficient assistance to the anaesthetist.

The maintenance of anaesthesia apparatus is the task of an expert, and the anaesthesia assistant should not tamper with complicated mechanisms about which he or she knows nothing, for it is the anaesthetist's ultimate responsibility to ensure that the apparatus is working correctly before use. However, minor servicing described in this chapter can easily be accomplished by the experienced anaesthesia assistant in co-operation with the anaesthetist. The anaesthesia nurse or operating department assistant who has a natural aptitude for dealing with things mechanical may obtain further information from the technical booklets applicable to a particular anaesthesia machine. The design of the anaesthesia room is described in Chapter 1 (page 46).

Types of anaesthesia

Although methods of anaesthesia can broadly be grouped into several main types, it is important to realise that they are not separate entities, for each may be and often is used in conjunction with the others.

The main types are given below. (Note. The names of drugs when given first time refer to the *British Pharmacopoeia* nomenclature, those following in brackets refer to the brand names.)

1. General anaesthesia, induced by inhalation of gases or the vapour of volatile liquids which vaporise readily at normal room temperatures. These include:

Nitrous oxide. Stored in cylinders in a liquid form, under pressure, often referred to simply as 'gas'. Nitrous oxide is a weak anaesthetic agent of which high concentrations (50–60 per cent) are used in conjunction with other anaesthetics and oxygen.

Cyclopropane. A potent gas stored in cylinders in a liquid form, which is useful as an induction agent particularly for children, but because of its expense and explosive characteristics it is falling into disrepute. The gas must not be used in the presence of cautery or diathermy.

Ether. A volatile liquid which is rarely used now has a wide margin of safety, although prolonged inhalation can cause post-operative vomiting and depression, has an unpleasant, irritant smell, is flammable and explosive when mixed with oxygen.

Halothane (Fluothane). A volatile liquid which is neither flammable nor explosive. Its characteristics include lack of irritation of the respiratory tract; effectiveness in low concentration; rapid recovery after administration; absence of side effects such as vomiting.

Enflurane (Ethrane, Alyrane). A clear colourless, non-flammable liquid with a pleasant ethereal smell. The characteristics of enflurane include pleasant induction, as the vapour is non-irritant, and rapid recovery. The agent is particularly useful for reducing the incidence of awareness during Caesarian section.

Isoflurane (Aerrane, Forane). This is an isomer of enflurane, and although able to produce a more rapid induction than halothane, is more irritant which reduces its usefulness.

Trichloroethylene (Trilene). A blue coloured liquid rarely used in clinical anaesthesia, having a relatively slow rate of vaporisation. Trilene has a predominantly analgesic effect and is used to supplement the gaseous anaesthetics. Used alone as a 0.5 per cent mixture in air it can be administered in small amounts in childbirth to relieve pain without loss of consciousness, must not be used in a closed circuit as it is incompatible with soda lime.

2. General anaesthesia induced by the intravenous administration of drugs such as the short acting barbiturates. The most commonly used in this class are thiopentone sodium (Pentothal, Intraval), methohexitone sodium (Brietal); and non-barbiturates such as etomidate (Hypomidate), ketamine hydrochloride (Ketalar), and midazolam (Hypnovel).

Other drugs, although they may not necessarily be anaesthetics in themselves, are often used intravenously in combination with those listed above. Drugs in this class include analgesics such as pethidine, phenoperidine (Operidine), pentazocine (Fortral), fentanyl (Sublimaze), alfentanil (Rapinfen) and papaveretum; 'competitive blocker' muscle relaxants such as curare (Tubarine), gallamine triethiodide (Flaxedil), pancuronium bromide (Pavulon) alcuronium (Alloferin), atracurium (Tracrium) and vecuronium (Norcuron); depolarising muscle relaxants such as suxamethonium (Scoline); hypotensive agents such as trimetaphan (Arfonad) and pentolinium (Ansolysen). In addition there are antidotes and stimulants which are discussed on pages 345 and 362.

3. Local anaesthesia induced by surface application, local infiltration, regional nerve block and epidural or subarachnoid spinal injection of drugs such as procaine, lignocaine (Xylocaine, Eticaine), prilocaine (Citanest), bupivacaine (Marcain). Cocaine is used for surface application only, e.g., ophthalmic surgery.

4. Induced hypothermia is a state of lowered body temperature produced by physical cooling of patients who are under the effect of a general anaesthetic, and the so-called lytic cocktail of which the most important element is chlorpromazine (Largactil, Megaphen).

5. Neuroleptanalgesia is a state of indifference and insensitivity to pain induced by the intravenous administration of a potent analgesic drug combined with a tranquilliser, e.g. phenoperidine (Operidine) or fentanyl (Sublimaze) combined with a butyrophenone tranquilliser such as droperidol (Droleptan) or haloperidol.

The patient is easily rousable with a normal blood pressure and when awakened remains quiet. He is in a state of apathy and mental detachment in which he is mildly sedated and uncaring about his surroundings.

ANAESTHESIA APPARATUS — BOYLE TYPE

1. The gas cylinders and soda lime canister, etc., on the anaesthesia machine are checked by an experienced anaesthetic nurse or technician (if permitted to do so), and reserves of these, together with bottles of halothane (Fluothane), trilene, enflurane (Ethrane, Alyrane) and isoflurane (Aerrane, Forane) are kept nearby.

2. The anaesthesia nurse also sets out instruments and apparatus required by the anaesthetist. She or he prepares trolleys and trays when necessary for intravenous anaesthesia, endotracheal intubation, and local, regional or spinal analgesia.

The anaesthesia apparatus

Although there are many varieties of anaesthesia apparatus, the principles involve the supply of anaesthetic gases to the patient, either alone or in conjunction with the vapour of volatile anaesthetic agents. Most operating theatres are now supplied with piped gases, but nevertheless each anaesthesia apparatus must be fitted with oxygen and nitrous oxide cylinders for emergency use in case of failure of piped gas supplies.

Anaesthetic Gas Cylinders are coloured in accordance with a British Standards Institute code. Oxygen cylinders are painted black with a white top and O_2 printed in black; nitrous oxide are blue with N_2O printed in black; cyclopropane are orange, with C_3H_6 printed in black; and carbon dioxide are painted grey with CO_2 also in black.

These colour codings, together with some others which are *not* generally used on anaesthesia apparatus, are described on Ohmeda charts.

Regulators are attached to each cylinder to reduce the high-pressure gases, thereby making delivery easily adjustable through individual rotameters which control the amount of gases flowing into the apparatus and to the patient. There is a cylinder contents gauge either for each cylinder, or fitted between two cylinders of the same gas. Nitrous oxide gauges do not accurately give an indication of quantity until virtually empty, i.e., pressure is constant as long as there is liquid nitrous oxide in the cylinder.

Before connecting a new cylinder, after the protective cap has been removed, the valve should be opened momentarily to expel any dust which may have lodged in the valve seating. Failure to observe this may cause grave damage to the delicate gauges on the apparatus. The procedure is known as 'cracking the cylinder'.

Modern anaesthesia apparatus incorporate cylinders which have valves of the 'pin index type', which cannot be connected to the incorrect regulator. The washer between the cylinder and cylinder yoke or regulator yoke must be changed regularly, as it becomes worn.

The cylinder valve must be centred correctly with the cylinder yoke or regulator yoke, and the holding screw turned carefully into its location on the back of the valve, using *hand pressure* only. A leak at this point when the valve is opened usually indicates a worn or absent washer or the gas cylinder being connected to the wrong pin index yoke (Fig. 11.1).

With the male fitting type of valve, used for large oxygen and compressed air cylinders, the bullnose regulator or reducing valve is screwed into the valve seating by hand, and is further tightened with a spanner unless it carries an 'O' ring seal in which case it should be tightened by hand only. If a leak is apparent which cannot be cured by tightening the hexagon nut, the regulator should be replaced at the earliest opportunity, after trying another cylinder. Sometimes a leak may be due to a damaged cylinder valve seating.

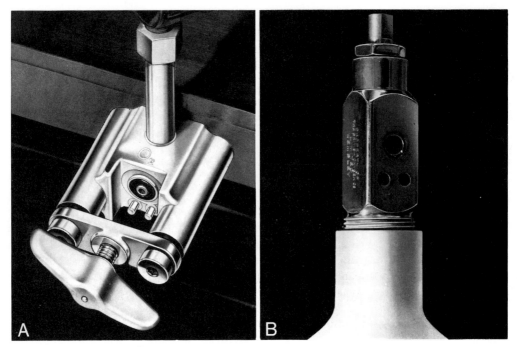

Fig. 11.1   Pin index system. (Ohmeda.)

Important. On no account must *any* grease be used on cylinders, regulators or connections, for the friction produced by the gas may ignite the grease and cause an explosion. Cylinder capacities and pressures are listed in the Appendix.

There are many different types of anaesthesia apparatus. Fundamentally, these machines consist of three main groups: (1) a semi-closed circuit Boyle's type to which can be added a closed circuit; (2) similar to (1) but incorporating a self-contained carbon dioxide absorption circle (closed) circuit; (3) similar to (2) but with electro-mechanical integration. For purposes of clarity the basic characteristics of a Boyle's type anaesthesia apparatus will be described followed by specific reference to particular models.

Basic Boyle's type anaesthesia apparatus

These are designed to use pipeline gas supplies; plus reserve cylinders or just cylinder gas supplies. For pipeline gas supplies the apparatus is connected to the pipeline outlet by colour coded reinforced plastic hoses incorporating self sealing Schrader connectors. The colour coding is white for oxygen, blue for nitrous oxide, black for medical air, and yellow for medical vacuum. In addition the machines are generally fitted with two nitrous oxide cylinders, two oxygen cylinders and one carbon dioxide cylinder. The extra gas and oxygen cylinders are reserves. There may also be provision for cyclopropane (C_3H_6), but the gas cylinder should be removed from the apparatus when not in use to eliminate the fire/explosion hazard due to its explosive properties. (Cyclopropane and ether should never be used or handled in the presence of electromedical equipment including high frequency electrosurgical apparatus — diathermy, and anaesthesia machine related patient monitors.)

The high-pressure gases pass through regulators or reducing valves to the rotameters and thence into a common supply tube either direct to the patient, or are diverted through the

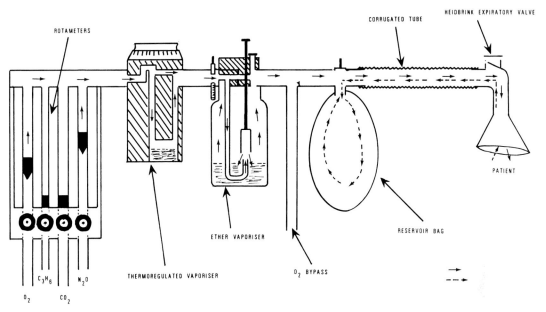

ROTAMETERS

CORRUGATED TUBE

HEIDBRINK EXPIRATORY VALVE

PATIENT

RESERVOIR BAG

ETHER VAPORISER

THERMOREGULATED VAPORISER

O₂ BYPASS

C_3H_6 N_2O

O_2 CO_2

Fig. 11.2   A semi-closed anaesthesia circuit (diagrammatic).

halothane (Fluothane), trilene or other vaporizer, and thence to the reservoir bag. From this bag the gases are carried via the corrugated rubber tube, angle piece and face mask or endotracheal tube to the patient (Fig. 11.2). Adjustment of an expiratory valve situated between the corrugated tube and the face mask enables expiration and excess gases to escape.

Regulators or reducing valves on anaesthesia apparatus are usually spring loaded rubber or metal diaphragm types, and they reduce the high gas pressures to 344 to 689 mB,* 34.47 or 68.95 kPa, 5 or 10 p.s.i.

This enables easy delivery of the gases through individual high-pressure rubber tubes or soldered metal tubes to the control flowmeters (rotameters).

A separate regulator is used for each gas cylinder. An aneroid gauge attached to the regulator indicates the pressure of the cylinder contents.

Rotameters have now superseded other forms of flowmeters for anaesthesia use, due to their greater accuracy.

A rotameter is an accurately made conical glass tube containing a 'float' or 'bobbin' which rises and rotates as the flow of gas increases. The flowmeter must be set perfectly vertical, otherwise the float will not spin round. If not vertical, friction will be caused between the float and the glass wall, and the reading will be inaccurate. A non-spinning float usually requires the flowmeter to be realigned and cleaned by the maintenance engineer.

Rotameters are individually calibrated according to the type and quantity of gas used. These calibrations are shown in the Appendix. The flow of gases is controlled by a fine adjustment needle valve on the rotameter.

The three or four rotameters are grouped together, feeding gases into the apparatus. The oxygen flowmeter is always placed at the extreme left of the 'flowmeter bank', but modern international standards require this gas to be 'preferred', that is, the last gas to enter the mixed gas flow to the patient. This is usually achieved by a tube which loops the oxygen

*millibar

flow over the top of the other gas flows. The position of the oxygen flowmeter is followed by those for cyclopropane, carbon dioxide and nitrous oxide on the extreme right. An oxygen bypass lever supplies emergency oxygen when an increased flow of pure oxygen is required.

Vaporizers are of two types:

(A) The standard Boyle type with an unknown percentage of vapour delivered which changes with time of use and many other factors too numerous to control.

(B) The thermo-compensated type with a known percentage of vapour delivered within various ranges of temperature and gas flows.

The Boyle type. This incorporates a valve or slotted drum which allows the anaesthetist to divert a portion or all of the fresh gases above the surface or through the volatile anaesthetic agent before passing to the patient. The proportion of gases not diverted into the vaporizers passes directly to the patient.

The gases enter the vaporizer via a U-shaped tube over which there is positioned a plunger holding a cylindrical hood. This plunger may be lowered over the open end of the U-tube to increase the vapour concentration. When preparing the machines this plunger must be kept up, except when filling the bottles with anaesthetic agent. It is then lowered to cover the U-tube to prevent liquid entering this tube, which would lead to a dangerously high concentration of vapour.

Both the ether and trilene vaporizers on the Boyle's anaesthesia apparatus are practically identical, the only difference being that the trilene bottle is smaller. The ether vaporizer utilises copper tubing to prevent decomposition of ether by sunlight.

The vaporizers are situated outside the closed circuit — this is known as V.O.C. (vaporizer outside circuit) and in no circumstances do the patient's respirations pass through it.

The vaporizers are filled with anaesthetic agent through the filler cap, a small plastic funnel being found very useful for the purpose. The trilene bottle should not be filled above the 100 ml (4 oz) level and the ether above the 150 ml (6 oz) level. Ether or *any* anaesthetic agent must be put into the bottle either by the anaesthetist *only* or *directly under his supervision*.

Trilene is dyed blue, ether is colourless and with the advent of halothane (Fluothane) which is also colourless very great care must be taken to avoid mistakes.

Before the anaesthesia is commenced, the control levers of the vaporizers are placed in the closed position and the plungers set at their highest level.

Thermo-compensated vaporizers. These have virtually superseded the Boyle's vaporizer and enable known percentages of anaesthetic vapour to be added to the fresh gases of any standard continuous flow anaesthesia apparatus. The patient's respirations are not diverted through the vaporizer as dangerously high concentrations of anaesthetic agent would result.

For example, the Fluotec 4 (Fig. 11.3) provides any concentration of halothane (Fluothane) between 0.5 and 5 per cent, chosen by rotating a calibrated control dial to the appropriate setting. The delivered percentage concentration of anaesthetic vapour is almost independent of factors which have a marked effect on the performance of a Boyle's vaporizer, i.e.:

1. Ambient temperature.
2. Cooling of the liquid by evaporation.
3. Duration of use.
4. Level of the liquid.
5. Variation in the total flow of fresh gases.
6. The effect of jarring or shaking of the vaporizer.
7. Pressure fluctuations due to use of ventilators.

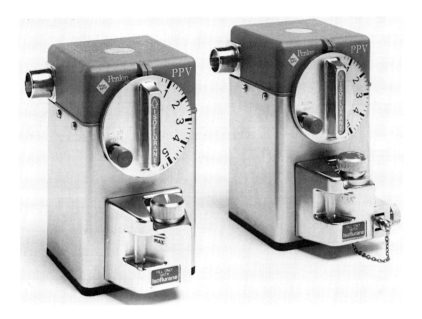

Fig. 11.3 Fluotec 4 vaporizer; Tech 4 vaporizers for other anaesthetic agents have a similar appearance. (Ohmeda.)

Variable temperatures are compensated for by a temperature-sensitive valve fitted in the vaporizer chamber. Vaporizers are calibrated at 21°C and at elevated temperatures. The vaporizer responds very slowly to changes in ambient temperature, and (to prevent the valve closing completely) as a safety feature the temperature sensitive valve does not respond below the range of 12–15°C approximately. At temperatures below 12°C the percentage output is likely to be lower than that indicated on the dial. Depending on the anaesthetic agent, higher temperatures may result in unpredictably high percentage outputs. The flow rate of fresh gases can also effect the percentage output (Fig. 11.4).

Generally, steady and fluctuating back pressures imposed by ventilators do not affect the vaporizers. The greatest effects are observed at combinations of very low flow rates and low dial setting with large and rapid fluctuations. These become progressively less important as the dial setting and flow rate increase and the magnitude and rate of cycling of the pressure fluctuations decrease.

Small effects can occur when the carrier gas composition is changed from oxygen to air or nitrous oxide/oxygen mixture. These are usually of negligible clinical significance.

Figure 11.5 shows a schematic diagram of the Tec 4 vaporizer in the 'ON' position. The vaporizer comprises a vaporizing chamber, sump and sump cover fitted between a cover base and a safety interlock block. The gas duct system lies within the sump cover; above this is the rotary control valve, the lower part of which has ducts and a curved vapour control channel machined into its surfaces. The spindle of the rotary valve passes through the interlock block to the control valve.

When the control dial is turned *on*, the carrier gas splits into two streams — a bypass flow and a flow through the vaporizing chamber which eventually joins the bypass flow to emerge at the vaporizer outlet. In the *off* position, the rotary valve makes a direct link between the 'inlet' and 'outlet' ports within the vaporizer.

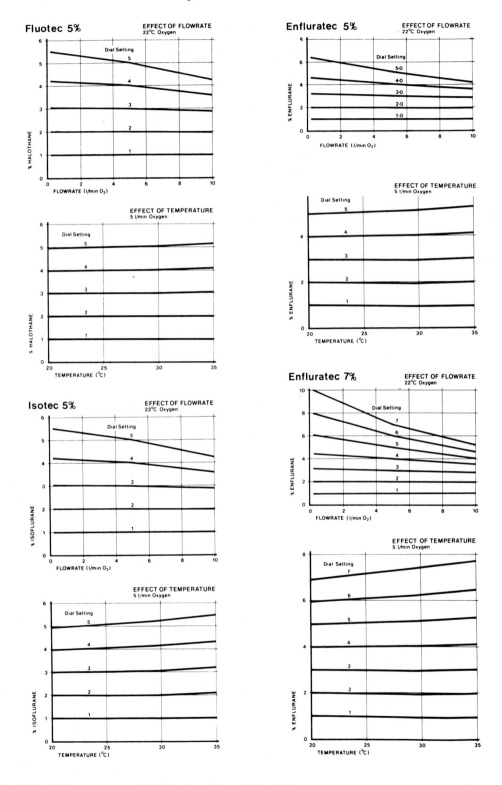

Fig. 11.4   Performance curves for Tech 4 vaporizers. (Ohmeda.)

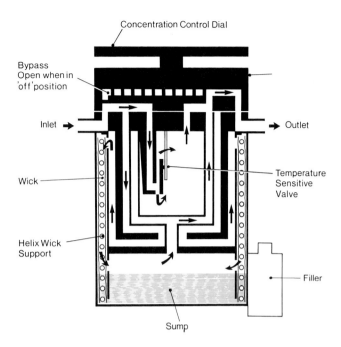

Fig. 11.5 Tech 4 vaporizer schematic diagram. (Ohmeda.)

The vaporizing chamber is lined by two concentric wicks which enclose a nickel-plated copper helix so that the space is converted to a long spiral outlet channel. The wicks, dipping into the liquid, ensure that the vapour is maintained at saturation concentration in the gas leaving the vaporizing chamber. The amount of anaesthetic agent picked up in the vaporizing stream will vary due either to variation in room temperature or to the cooling which takes place when an anaesthetic agent is vaporized. Each causes changes in the effective vapour pressures of the anaesthetic agents. Unless some form of compensating device was used, the output of the vaporizer for a given flow of carrier gas and control dial setting would change with temperature.

The compensating device in the Tec 4 consists of a thermostat which utilises a bi-metallic strip. This metallic strip deflects according to its temperature and controls the proportion of carrier gas entering the vaporizer chamber. If the temperature of the vaporizer falls, the thermostat closes and more carrier gas is allowed into the vaporizing chamber. If the temperature increases, the thermostat opens and less carrier gas is allowed into the vaporizing chamber. In this way the output of the vaporizer remains constant under conditions of changing temperature.

Mention was made previously of the safety interlock block. Firstly, this device ensures that only one vaporizer can be turned on when two or more Tec 4's are used on a compatible Selectatec quick change vaporizer mounting system (Fig. 11.6). The Tec 44 can only be turned *on* when the locking lever is turned to the 'lock' position. This ensures that the vaporizer inlet and outlet ports seal correctly and that no gross leakage occurs. Secondly, with the vaporizer turned *on* it is not possible to unlock and remove it from the Selectatec manifold. Thirdly, the interlock mechanism automatically isolates the vaporizer from all anaesthetic circuits when it is turned *off*. This means that any flow of fresh gas from upstream flowmeters completely by-passes the vaporizer, and there is no possibility of trace

concentrations of anaesthetic agent being picked up. The action of turning *on* the Tec 4 vaporizer automatically reconnects it to the fresh gas supply and to the anaesthesia machine outlet.

The liquid capacity of the Tec 4 is 125 ml; the wick system retains 35 ml. The vaporizer has a single port keyed filler system.

Tech 4 vaporizers are available for use specifically with halothane (Fluothane), enflurane

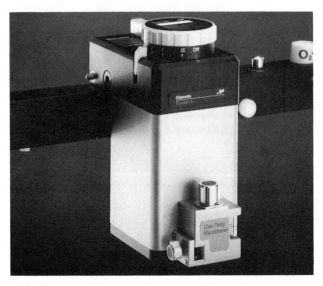

Fig. 11.6   Selectatec quick change vaporizer mounting system. (Ohmeda.)

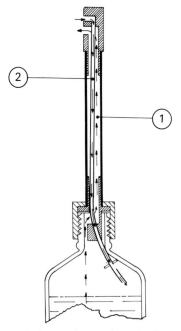

Fig. 11.7   Keyed filler system for anaesthetic vaporizers, schematic diagram of filler tube: (1) outer tube, pin safety unit; (2) inner tube, pin safety unit. (Ohmeda.)

(Ethane), isoflurane (Aerane, Forane) and ether. Another verison of a thermo-compensated vaporizer which also utilises a keyed filler system is the Penlon PPV illustrated in Figure 11.6.

Keyed filler system. As mentioned previously (page 300), great care must be taken to ensure only the correct anaesthetic agent is added to a vaporizer. Ohmeda/Cyprane have developed a safety keyed pin system for use with thermo-compensated vaporizers. This consists essentially of non-interchangeable bottle units which fit the combined filler and drain port of the vaporizer.

The bottle adaptor incorporates a cap which will fit only a specific anaesthetic agent bottle (Fig. 11.7). Attached to this cap is a flexible tube containing two channels. On the delivery end of this tube is attached a plug which fits into the filler/drain port of the appropriate vaporizer. The filler/drain socket is normally sealed with a blank plug (Fig. 11.8B). The procedure for filling illustrated in Figure 11.8 A–F is as follows:

A. Keyed filler adaptor is attached to the bottle of anaesthetic agent.

B. Filler control is closed fully clockwise, the clamp screw is loosened and the plug removed.

C. Keyed end of the bottle adaptor is inserted fully into filler/drain port, and the clamp screw tightened to secure adaptor; the anaesthetic agent bottle is raised above filler/drain port.

D. The filler control is opened by turning fully clockwise, and liquid is allowed to flow into vaporizer until the required level shows on the level indicator glass.

E. The filler control is turned fully clockwise to close, and the bottle lowered to a level below the filler/drain port. Liquid remaining in the bottle adaptor tubing is allowed to flow back into bottle before loosening clamp screw, removing bottle adaptor from receiver and reinserting blanking plug.

F. To drain, steps 1–3 are followed, but keeping the bottle below filler/drain port; the filler control is then opened fully and fluid allowed to run into bottle until flow ceases.

The reservoir bag made of thin anti-static rubber is generally of a 4.5 litre (1 gal) capacity. The anaesthetic gases enter this bag via a drum valve, which is generally a permanently-open 'T' junction.

This bag should be tested regularly for leaks by inflating and submerging in water. There is a tendency for cracks to appear in the folds. The bag should be cleaned and sterilized frequently.

The corrugated tube, made of anti-static rubber and having a wide bore, is joined to the machine at one end and the angle piece at the other by slightly conical metal or hard rubber unions. The union at the angle piece incorporates an expiratory valve.

The tube must be checked regularly for punctures as there is a tendency for deterioration to occur in the corrugations. After use it should be stretched and suspended straight for a period, to release condensed moisture which is often lodged in the corrugations and then sterilized after each operation.

British Standard 3849 (1965) specifies certain sizes of joint fittings on anaesthesia apparatus. Basically it requires that the delivery end of the anaesthesia apparatus shall have a male conical fitting, and the face mask a female conical fitting. The conical fittings on all components of adult size from the male delivery end of the anaesthesia apparatus shall be in the sequence male-female in the direction of gas flow (Fig. 11.9).

The nominal size of adult cone and socket joints is 22 mm diameter. For paediatric use the size is reduced to a nominal 15 mm diameter except that the female connector to the machine outlet, the male conical fitting leading to the mask and the female conical fitting of the face mask should be of adult size (22 mm).

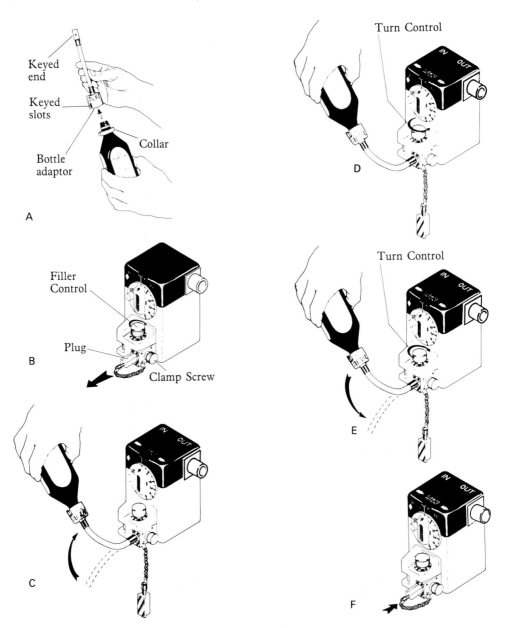

Fig. 11.8 (A–F)   Keyed filler system in use with PPV vaporizer. (Manufactured by Penlon Ltd under licence from Ohmeda.)

The expiratory valve on modern apparatus is usually of the Heidbrink type. This is a spring-loaded valve upon which tension may be adjusted to create a slight resistance against the patient's expirations. When closed circuit is used the valve is completely closed and it is necessary to cut the gas flow down to basic oxygen requirements. Modern valves now have an exhaust port to allow the connection to an anaesthetic gas scavenging system (Fig. 11.10).

Other expiratory valves such as the Coxeter or Magill type may be in use, but basically they are also spring-loaded valves which act in a similar manner.

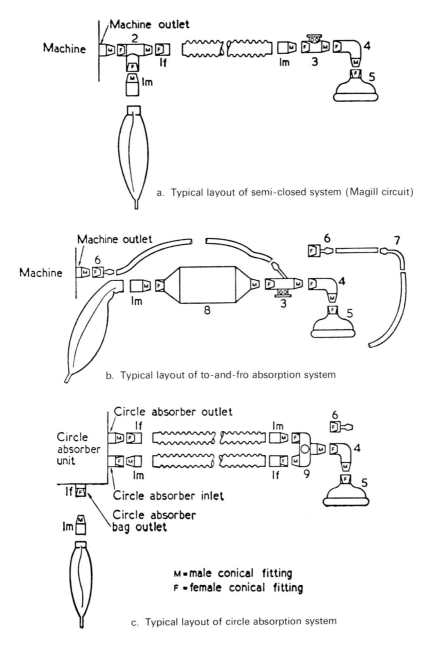

a. Typical layout of semi-closed system (Magill circuit)

b. Typical layout of to-and-fro absorption system

M = male conical fitting
F = female conical fitting

c. Typical layout of circle absorption system

Fig. 11.9 Typical layouts for breathing attachments of anaesthesia apparatus — BS3849.

During operations on the head and neck it may be inconvenient to have the expiratory valve inaccessible under the patient drapes. In these circumstances a breathing circuit such as Bain's may be utilised (Figs. 11.11 and 11.12). This is a tube which has two channels for separate flow of patient's inspirations and expirations; it enables the reservoir bag to be positioned conveniently.

The metal angle piece connects to the face mask, made from anti-static rubber manufac-

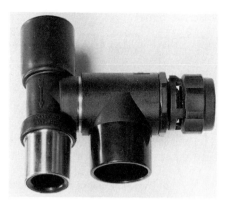

Fig. 11.10 Anti-pollution valve which replaces the standard Heidbrink valve in the Magill anaesthesia breathing circuit. A similar anti-pollution valve is available for Boyle-type circle absorbers. (Ohmeda.)

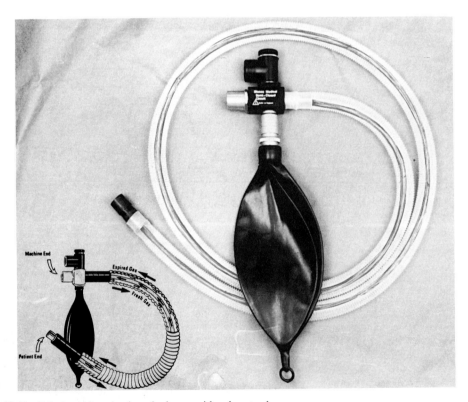

Fig. 11.11 Bain breathing circuit and adaptor with exhaust valve.

tured in a modified funnel shape which, when applied to the patient's face, moulds with the facial contours forming an airtight fit.

The two basic types are (a) those having a solid or moulded lip of suitable design and (b) those having an inflatable cushion.

Although the cushion type (b) must not be over-inflated, even when not in use it should

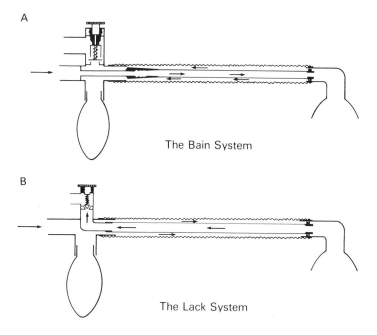

Fig. 11.12 Coaxil anaesthesia breathing systems (A) the Bain System, (B) the Lack System. (Reproduced with permission from *A Textbook of Anaesthesia*: Smith and Aitkenhead.)

contain a proportion of air to avoid deterioration of the inner surface of the rubber. A small plug blocks the air inlet after inflation, and the mask should be stored on the connecting flange with the cushion upwards or on horizontal pegs as in the Gerrard-Reading dispenser (Fig. 1.39).

An anti-static rubber harness may be used by the anaesthetist to maintain the face mask in position.

The Clausen and Connell head harness are the two in common use. Both are attached by two or three hooks, either fixed to the face mask or on a ring which fits over it. The Clausen

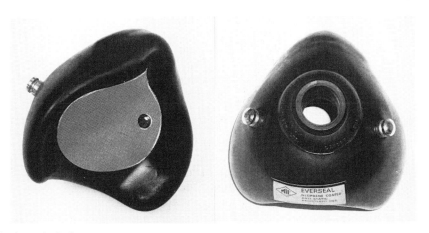

Fig. 11.13 Anaesthesia facemask, padless. (Everseal.)

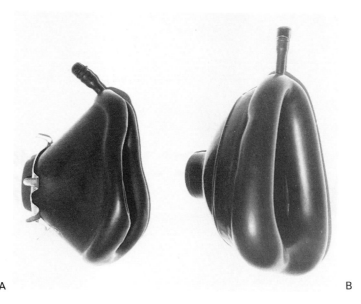

A   B

Fig. 11.14   Anaesthesia facemask, inflatable pad, (A) McKesson, (B) Essex.

harness has three limbs with several perforations, which may be suitable attached to the three hooks. The Connell has only two specially designed loops which are adjustable and maintain a friction hold on the two limbs.

All rubber items used on anaesthetic apparatus with the exception of endotracheal tubes and some airways have anti-static properties (see Chapter 4).

An endotracheal tube and connection may be attached directly to an expiratory valve and the corrugated tube by substituting a Magill catheter connection for the angle piece and the face mask. In this case the corrugated tube and expiratory valve are supported carefully, to avoid pulling on the endotracheal tube after insertion. This is achieved by using adhesive strapping, Sellotape, or a specially designed head harness such as the Connell, after placing a pad of gauze or sponge rubber between the expiratory valve mount and the patient's face. Under BSI standard the Magill or similar connection must have an internal diameter of not less than 11 mm. This also applies to the machine end of the endotracheal tube connections.

An airway may be used in the patient's mouth to prevent the tongue from falling back (impeding or obstructing respirations), and also prevent teeth clenching an endotracheal tube. There are many varieties, but all are a curved moulded shape which fits comfortably in the pharynx, holding the base of the tongue forward. A metal insert prevents compression of the airway by the teeth if it has been manufactured from a soft material. They may be made from rubber, thermoplastics (vinyl) or less commonly from metal. The most generally used are the Phillips rubber type in six sizes, and the Guedel rubber or plastic in four sizes plus two extra small sizes for infants.

The Heirsch airway is similar to the Phillips, but has an oxygen feed tube fitted to the metal insert, which is of special use in children.

Where the Phillips metal insert has side perforations, it is intended that these perforations remain above the level of the rubber or plastic moulding. This is a safety arrangement whereby the patient's airway would not become obstructed should the main aperture become accidentally blocked, e.g., with the edge of the sheet or blanket.

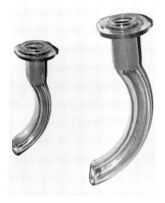

Fig. 11.15 Guedal airways, pvc, 7 and 11 mm.

The carbon dioxide absorption circle closed circuit added to the basic Boyle's apparatus

In the circle apparatus two corrugated tubes are used, one for the delivery of gases to the patient through a one-way inspiration valve, and another through which the expiratory gases are directed into the rebreathing bag via another one-way expiration valve. The patient's expirations, from the reservoir bag, pass through the soda lime canister and a selected proportion of carbon dioxide is removed. The expirations then mix with fresh gases from the rotameters which may have been passed through the vaporiser. It is possible also to pass the patient's expirations through a special vaporizer although this is not common practice. (This is then termed vaporiser in circuit.) This gas mixture is directed through the inspiration valve and along the corrugated tube back to the patient, thereby completing the circuit (Fig. 11.16).

The soda lime will only absorb a certain amount of carbon dioxide before it becomes exhausted, but modern methods of manufacture have produced a substance which will allow several hours of use before exhaustion is apparent.

The Ohmeda Series 5 carbon dioxide absorber 4. This is designed to use a 2 kg capacity soda lime canister connected to a control head by means of an external corrugated tube which is screwed into the head with a large plastic hand nut. The canister is made of transparent acrylic material to enable the colour change of indicating soda lime to be seen easily. Unidirectional inspiratory and expiratory valves in the control head incorporate transparent Visidisks, each featuring a coloured 'pip'. These are readily visible, giving immediate confirmation that both discs are in position. The control head of the Series 5 absorber is of simple one-piece construction. The control lever that allows gases to flow through, or by-pass the canister, has a positive spring-loaded action. A manometer can be fitted which plugs into the control head.

The transparent canister is divided centrally by a perforated metal baffle which effectively reduces 'channelling' of gases (bypassing the soda lime). In use, the gases are routed down through the central tube and up through the soda lime, so that the soda lime in the lower chamber becomes exhausted first. When the colour change in the lower chamber is complete, the soda lime in the chamber may be replaced and the canister refitted with the freshly filled chamber uppermost. When used in conjunction with the Boyle's anaesthesia apparatus, the absorber can be mounted in four different positions on either side of the table

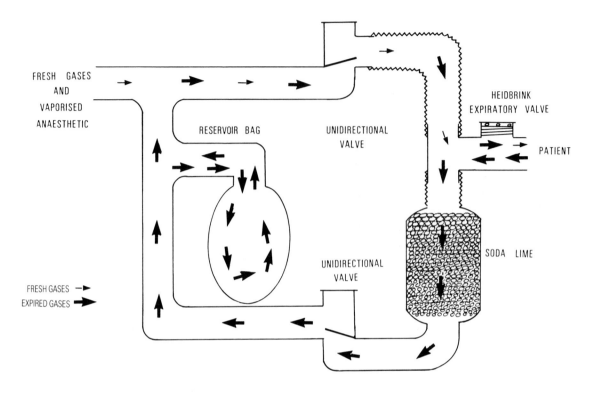

FRESH GASES
AND
VAPORISED
ANAESTHETIC

RESERVOIR BAG

UNIDIRECTIONAL
VALVE

HEIDBRINK
EXPIRATORY VALVE

PATIENT

UNIDIRECTIONAL
VALVE

SODA LIME

FRESH GASES →
EXPIRED GASES →

Fig. 11.16 A closed or circle circuit (diagrammatic.)

frame, above or below the instrument table. The fresh gas supply tube is plugged into the anaesthetic gas outlet on the manifold panel.

Fresh gases are supplied from the main part of the Boyle's anaesthesia apparatus and enter the absorber through an inlet at the back.

After filling or changing of the soda lime canister, special care should be taken to ensure that the replaced canister is properly fitted to its seal and is leak-proof. From time to time a 'flush through' of the head and empty canister to remove collected moisture is advisable.

Soda lime of 4/8 mesh having little or no dust should be used. After refilling the canister, it should be blown through if possible with oxygen, to remove any dust which may have accumulated in the packing.

Modern soda lime preparations such as Medisorb (Ohmeda) contain a coloured indicator, which retains its colour so long as the soda lime remains active. After four to six hours' use, Medisorb changes from a pink to a cream colour and should be replaced. Calona indicates exhaustion by a change from green to brown. Many machines are now fitted with transparent absorber canisters which permit the colour of the soda lime to be easily observed.

The canister should always be filled to the top with soda lime to utilise the full effect of carbon dioxide absorption.

Trilene should not be used in a circle circuit because it reacts with heated-up soda lime to form a highly toxic agent di-chloracetylene, which in susceptible patients may cause palsy of various cranial nerves or fatal encephalitis and necrosis of the liver.

The Waters' canister 'to and fro' method of carbon dioxide absorption consists of a cylindrical metal or plastic canister containing soda lime, a reservoir bag, conical

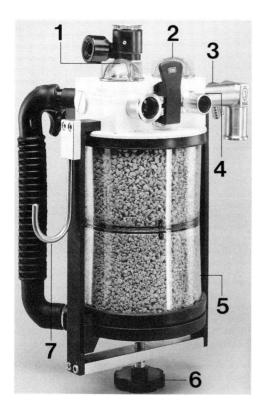

Fig. 11.17 Carbon dioxide absorber for closed circuit anaesthesia. (Series 5, Ohmeda.)

1. Visidisk coloured pip system provides at a glance confirmation that the transparent uni-directional valves are fully operational.
2. Valve cover domes facilitate cleaning and servicing.
3. Fresh gas entry port located at a point just above the reservoir bag attachment port. This ensures that as much fresh gas as possible enters the bag (or alternatively the extension tubing/ventilator connecting tube).
4. An additional entry port for fresh gas provides flexibility in the positioning of the fresh gas feed.
5. The canister design ensures effective gas channelling, which reduces resistance to breathing, extends soda lime life, and results in lower operating costs.
6. A simple hand-operated clamp screw locking device enables rapid removal of the canister or cleaning and re-charging with fresh soda lime.
7. Hook for storing patient circuit detachables not in use.

mount/expiratory valve with side tube for fresh gases and angled mount for face mask, or Magill mount for endotracheal tube.

The canister is placed as close to the patient as possible. The patient's respirations pass through the canister twice and it is an efficient method of carbon dioxide absorption, although the heavy canister is rather difficult to secure in position.

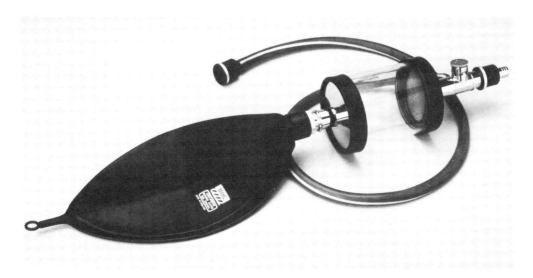

Fig. 11.18 Waters' 'to and fro' carbon dioxide absorption canister.

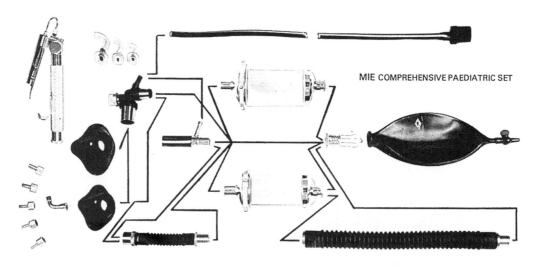

MIE COMPREHENSIVE PAEDIATRIC SET

Fig. 11.19   Paediatric anaesthesia set with 85 g (3 oz) soda lime canister. (M & I.E. Ltd.)

A circle or closed circuit has many advantages, including the conservance of expensive anaesthetic vapours or gases such as cyclopropane and halothane (Fluothane); the very accurate control of anaesthetic agents and degree of anaesthesia using minimal anaesthetic (especially useful with the poor risk patient and long operations); the conservance of body moisture and heat.

The Boyle 2000 international anaesthesia apparatus

This enables the anaesthetist to structure an anaesthesia apparatus to his own requirements. The basic trolley is constructed on a bolt together principle for simple, compact transportation and permits the full range of anaesthetic accessories to be accommodated. Forty different cylinder/pipeline gas supply configurations are available, including cylinder or pipeline models with pin index or overseas yokes. Figure 11.6 (page 304) shows a Selectatec back bar which is designed so that one or two vaporisers can be fitted without the removal of any other components.

Another version of the Boyle-type anaesthesia apparatus is the Cavendish 500 illustrated in Figure 11.21.

ANAESTHESIA SYSTEMS WITH ELECTRO-MECHANICAL INTEGRATION

As a process of evolution rather than revolution, a new generation of anaesthesia apparatus is emerging. These anaesthesia systems feature improved patient and operator safety; improved ergonomics, i.e. system layout and accessibilty to the anaesthetist; improved engineering and reliability; and increased use of electro-mechanical control. Two examples are described.

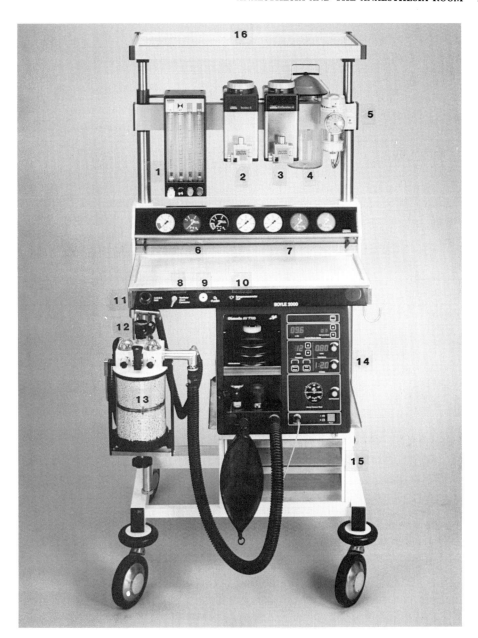

Fig. 11.20 Anaesthesia apparatus. (Boyle 2000, Ohmeda.)

1. Bank of 4 rotameters, O_2 (preferred gas), Air, CO_2 and N_2O.
2. Isoflurane (Forane, Aerane) Tech 4 vaporizer.
3. Interlocked Enflurane (Ethrane) Tech 4 vaporizer.
4. Suction receiving jar.
5. Pipeline suction unit.
6. Pipeline supply status gauges.
7. Cylinder supply status gauges.
8. Connection for pressure-based ventilator alarm unit.
9. Oxygen flush button.
10. Connection for sphygmomanometer.
11. Connection for anaesthetic gas scavenging system.
12. Swivel common gas outlet.
13. Series 5 carbon dioxide absorber unit.
14. OAV electronic anaesthesia ventilator.
15. Double drawer storage unit.
16. Top monitoring equipment shelf.

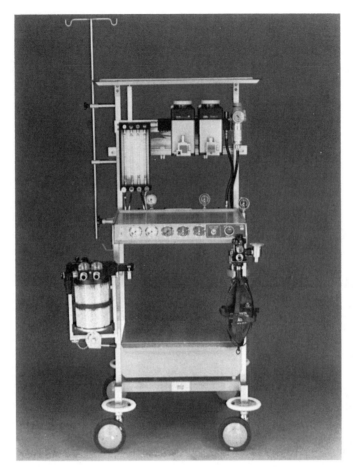

Fig. 11.21   Anaesthesia apparatus. (Cavendish, M & I E Ltd.)

The Ohmeda Excell range of anaesthesia apparatus incorporates the following features:

Patient safety

Safety link 25. This is a physical connection between the O_2 and N_2O gas flow control valves that prevents the delivery of less than a nominal 25 per cent O_2 (tolerance 21–29 per cent) in O_2/N_2O mixtures.

CO_2 *maximum gas flow rate limitation.* Conventional Boyle's type anaesthesia systems allow the delivery of up to 35 litres per minute of CO_2 when the gas flow control valves are fully opened, and therefore negates the efficacy of any safety link between O_2 and N_2O. The Excel anaesthesia apparatus features a physical stop on the gas flow control valve to prevent the delivery of CO_2 gas flows of greater than 2 litres per minute.

Pin-indexing of flow tube modules. This is provided to prevent transposition and reversal of the gas flow tubes during service and maintenance.

Preferential oxygen. Although the oxygen flow module is on the extreme left of the flow-meter bank, the design ensures that oxygen is always the last gas to enter the mixed gas flow to the patient. This minimises the risk of inadvertent delivery of hypoxic mixtures caused through oxygen leaking from cracked or displaced flow tubes.

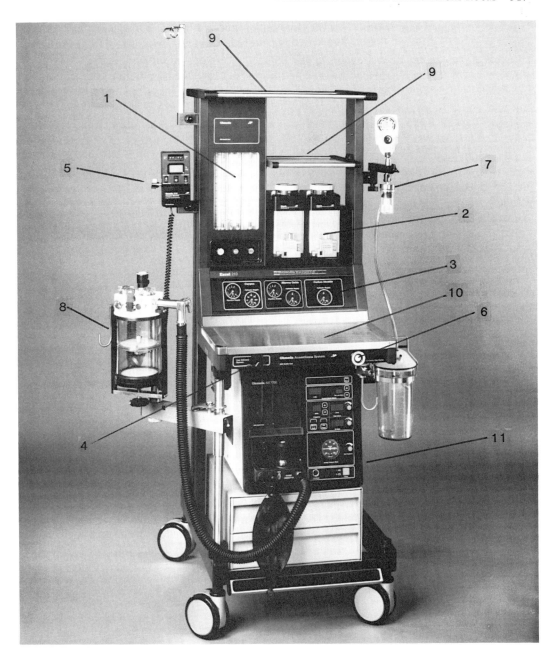

Fig. 11.22 Anaesthesia apparatus. (Excel, Ohmeda.)

1. Three gas flowmeter block including safety link between O_2 and N_2O. Flow control valves ensure a nominal 250 ml O_2 in O_2/N_2O mixtures, and CO_2 flow limited to a maximum of 2 litres per minute.
2. Tec 4 vaporizers with safety interlock mechanism.
3. Cylinder and pipeline supply pressure gauges.
4. System ON/OFF master switch.
5. Oxygen monitor.
6. O_2 flush button.
7. Pipeline medical vacuum controller
8. Series 5 CO_2 absorber fitted on adjustable mounting bracket.
9. Monitoring equipment shelving.
10. Work surface.
11. OAV anaesthesia ventilator.

Oxygen failure warning system. This provides an audible indication of oxygen supply failure when the supply pressure falls to below half of normal operating pressure. The device also shuts off all remaining gases flowing to the patient and opens an air entrainment valve.

System on-off switch. The apparatus must be physically 'switched on' before use. Switching on activates a base flow of oxygen of nominally 200 ml/minute. This is the basis of the safety link and ensures that the 25 per cent nominal minimum O_2 can be guaranteed across all selected O_2/N_2O flow rates; and even with exceptionally low flows below 1 litre minute volume, some oxygen is always flowing.

The *on-off* switch also activates an audible pneumatic self-test, which will not sound if there is a gross leak in the pneumatic system. Finally, the *on-off* switch will activate any integrated equipment if fitted, including monitors such as inspired oxygen, minute tidal volumes, breaths per minute, and circuit pressure; and an integrated ventilator monitor such as the OAV 7750.

Selectatec vaporizer back bar mounting system. This is the same safety feature described previously for the Boyle 2000.

System ergonomics

Integrated, separated, anaesthesia ventilator. As an option the apparatus can be fitted with an integrated ventilator in which the bellows or gas delivery module is physically separated from the control/monitoring module. The control module is fitted at eye level, to allow easy recognition of key ventilatory parameters (volume, frequency, pressure and inspired O_2 concentration), whereas the bellows module can be positioned to suit individual needs and techniques.

Full length, side rail, vertical accessory mounting system. This is to permit a large range of accessory items exactly where the user requires. Such items would include anaesthetic gas scavenging, suction systems, humidifiers etc.

Improved engineering

The Excel apparatus utilises a unique machined brass block in which all the high pressure in the pneumatic system is contained. Both the anaesthetic gas inputs(cylinder and pipeline) and outputs from the block are non-interchangeable. The gas regulators used are all metal diaphragm types, containing no perishable parts. This should provide improved regulator reliability and longevity.

The Penlon AM 1000 anaesthesia apparatus incorporates a number of improved design and safety features.

Patient safety

Vaporizer interlock system which allows fitting of up to three vaporizers to the apparatus, but allows the use of only one vaporizer for delivery of anaesthetic agent. Although designed for use with Penlon PPV vaporizers, other makes can be fitted.

Control of gas output in conjunction with a gas cut-off system is achieved with a para-magnetic oxygen analyser. This prevents mixtures containing less than 25 per cent oxygen being delivered to the patient. The accuracy and response time of this type of analyser is excellent and the system will run without maintenance, under normal operating conditions, for the life of the whole anaesthesia apparatus. There are no battery or fuel replacement

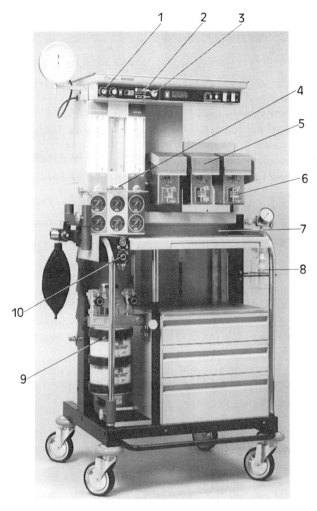

Fig. 11.23 Anaesthesia apparatus. (AM 1000, Penlon Ltd.)
1. O_2 alarm.
2. O_2 display.
3. Paramagnetic O_2 analyzer.
4. Interlocked N_2O and air rotameter selection.
5. Interlock system which allows use of only one vaporizer at a time.
6. PPV anaesthetic vaporizer.
7. Work surface.
8. Anaesthetic gas scavenging system.
9. CO_2 absorber.
10. Common gas outlet.

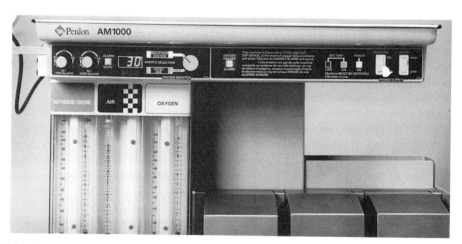

Fig. 11.24 In-sight in-use display. (AM 1000, Penlon Ltd.)

requirements; the battery back-up system provides emergency power for the oxygen analyser and alarm systems.

System ergonomics

In-sight in-use principle displays the combination of gas/anaesthetic agent subduing other options, thereby effectively minimising irrelevant visual detail from the work area.

Height adjustable work surface for procedures which require standing or sitting. The work surface includes a pull-out writing tablet, on which is inscribed a pre-operative check list.

The reader is reminded again that little detail has been given regarding the maintenance of these anaesthesia apparatus. It is the responsibility of the anaesthetist to ensure that the machines are in good working order, and the degree of simple maintenance by the anaesthetic nurse or technician depends upon his or her experience, mechanical ability and, above all, the anaesthetist's orders in this matter. There should be a routine planned maintenance either by the manufacturer or a specially trained service engineer.

Scavenging systems

Mention was made in Chapter 1 of the need to reduce the level of pollution due to waste anaesthetic gases in the operating theatre atmosphere (page 32). Typical sources of pollution are:
  a. Excess gas from expiratory valves.
  b. Polluted discharge from ventilators, which may or may not include the driving gas.
  c. Expired air from the patient.
  d. Leaks from equipment, poorly fitting face masks, etc.
  e. Spillage e.g. due to filling vaporizers.
  f. Diffusion through tubing(this is thought to be negligible).

An anaesthetic gas disposal system (scavenging system) can remove the pollution from sources a and b, and specifically from c, but has no effect from sources d, e and f. Pollution from these latter sources can only be removed by adequate room ventilation. It has been found that pollution can be significantly reduced to a small fraction of the uncontrolled level by a combination of:
  1. A properly designed and commissioned scavenging system.
  2. Adequate room ventilation.
  3. Prevention of leaks from equipment, face masks, etc.

There are two basic forms of scavenging system, passive and active. Passive systems use the patient as the air mover; active systems use a mechanical air mover. Passive systems are only suitable for a spontaneously breathing patient, and cannot remove the polluted discharge from some ventilators.

The performance of passive systems depends on factors such as outside wind conditions, length of vertical pipe run, etc. and is therefore unpredictable. Moreover, because they are unlikely to meet the exacting requirements for patient safety, passive systems are not generally recommended. Scavenging systems which rely on the extract ventilation system for the method of waste gas disposal are unlikely to be reliable over a long period of time. One reason for this is that lint and fluff liberated in the operating theatre rapidly accumulates in the system, leading to a reduction in performance; the inclusion of a filter is not possible with these systems. The central piped vacuum system, which operates at a high vacuum is generally considered to be unsafe for anaesthetic gas scavenging (DHSS, 1976; Spence, 1978, and Light, 1979).

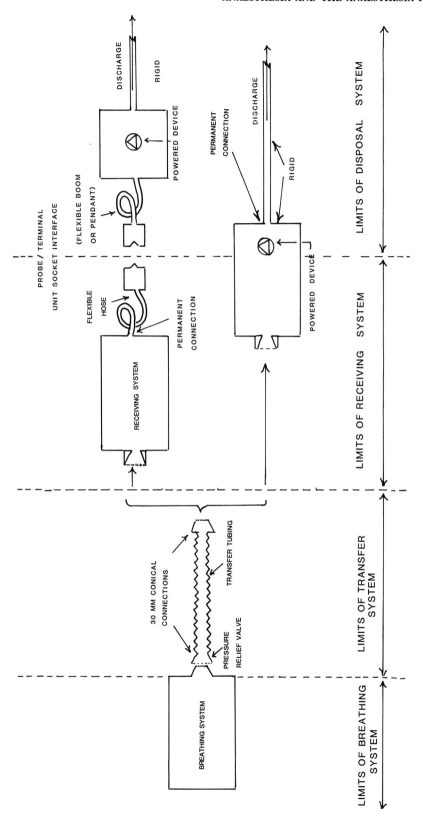

Fig. 11.25 Schematic diagram of an anaesthetic gas scavenging system.

A scavenging system should be capable of removing the polluted discharge from ventilators and an active system is considered most suitable. It should be capable of removing a continuous flow of 80 litres/minute, and a superimposed flow of 40 litres/minute for a period of one second in each successive 4 second period. The requirements for patient safety are that, in the event of failure or obstruction of any tubing of the system, the maximum pressure in excess of that imposed by the anaesthetic breathing system should not exceed 1 kPa at 30 litres/minute and 2 kPa at 90 litres/minute. In addition, the system must not induce a flow from the breathing system of more than 0.5 litres/minute.

A draft British Standard is currently being prepared which covers the design and safety requirements of anaesthetic gas scavenging systems. The principles are shown schematically in Figure 11.25.

In order to connect an anaesthetic gas scavenging system (AG system) to a breathing system, the exhaust port of the breathing system has to be provided with a 30 mm male conical connection (Fig. 11.10). This male connector is attached to the inlet of the AGS transfer system. The transfer system includes a pressure relief valve (1 kPa at 30 litres/minute) at its inlet, and transfers waste and/or excess anaesthetic gases to the receiving system (Fig. 11.25), which is usually attached to the anaesthesia breathing machine. The receiving system incorporates an air break which provides the means of limiting induced flow in the event of a failure in the disposal system, and allows excess or waste gases to escape into the operating theatre. It also includes a simple flow indicator and filter, and acts as a reservoir to match the intermittent flow from the breathing system to the continuous flow in the disposal system. The receiving system is connected, either via a flexible tube or directly to the fixed point of the disposal system, by means of a standard probe and socket connector; this permits local choice in the selection of components. The disposal system provides the means of discharging the gases to a safe place and includes a powered device, flow controls, and a warning system to provide an alarm in the event of failure.

VENTILATORS

It is now commonplace to use controlled respiration during anaesthesia or following traumatic conditions such as head injuries. This may be accomplished simply by rhythmically squeezing the anaesthetic reservoir bag or by mechanical ventilators.

Many types of ventilator have been developed; some are specifically for use during anaesthesia, whereas others are suitable for mechanically assisted artificial ventilation, particularly in the intensive care unit situation. There are others which can be used for both purposes, utilising air or a mixture of air and oxygen.

Basically ventilators could be divided into three main groups:

1. *Flow generators.* A *fixed volume* of gases (taken from a constant flow) is delivered into the lungs. A wide *variation in the pressures* reached at the end of inspiration (or inflation) may be observed on the manometer gauge, e.g., when a patient tries to breathe against the machine, irregular patterns result with high and low values at random.

Fibrosed and stiff or congested lungs, airway obstruction including excessive secretion, foreign body, broncho-spasm, etc. (low compliance), all will require high-pressure values.

Should this pressure reach a certain level, usually 39.226 mB to 68.645 mB (40 to 70 cm) of water, a safety valve blows off a proportion of the given volume.

Any leak will deprive the patient of the comparable proportion of the original delivered volume and therefore the pressure (manometer) gauge will register a suspiciously low value.

2. *Pressure generators.* With these the ventilator produces a selected pressure within the limits of time imposed by the respiratory rate. The amount of gases required for this pressure depends upon the compliance of the lungs and chest; and will need a variable volume of gases to achieve this. The ventilator will compensate for all but the gross leaks by delivering a larger volume of gases.

3. *Ventilators providing a choice of volume or pressure.* Some ventilators are electrically driven (with a manual control for emergency), others convert a continuous flow of oxygen or compressed air from a cylinder or pipeline, into an intermittent flow to the patient. It would be impossible to mention all the ventilators available and we will therefore confine ourselves to a few observations on three: the Manley Pulmovent, Nuffield series 400 and the OAV 7700.

It is possible to utilise almost any type of ventilator with the basic Boyle's apparatus. Figure 11.27 illustrates a Manley Pulmovent anaesthetic ventilator of the flow generator, volume pre-set type .

In conventional ventilator systems, the drive gas exerts pressure directly on the outside of a bellows or bag enclosed within a pressure chamber, to produce the inspiratory phase. This direct approach gives rise to two main problems; it requires a large volume of drive gas — in excess of the minute volume ventilation of the patient, and the servo system is integrated with the ventilation system which presents difficulties in sterilizing the components.

The Manley Pulmovent MPT 2000 (Ohmeda)

This operates on a different principle: the ventilator drive unit is controlled by a fluid logic circuit with the driving gas supply completely separate from the respirable gas to the patient. Any suitable driving gas can be used — the consumption being only a fraction of the patient's minute volume. The inspiratory phase is not determined by the driving gas pressure but by spring-loaded bellows (set at 68.645 mB★, 70 cmH$_2$O) which eliminate the possibility of excess pressure being transmitted to the patient. A relief valve opens automatically if the patient circuit is subjected to a negative pressure of 10 cm H$_2$O. Ambient air is then entrained to prevent gas deficiences to the patient. Non-interchangeable connections ensure that the ventilator components cannot be incorrectly assembled.

The patient's *minute volume* is determined by the actual flow of gases to the ventilator, which remain uninterrupted during the patient's breathing cycle. Gas supplied to the patient, however, is interrupted to define the inspiratory and expiratory breathing phases. There are internal bellows which expand during the expiratory phase to accomodate the continuous inflow of fresh gases until the pre-set *tidal volume* is achieved. At this point the inspiratory phase commences. When the inspiratory phase is completed, the cycle continues into the expiratory phase. The cycle is repeated continuously while ventilation is taking place. Ventilatory frequency is automatically set as the result of the *minute volume* divided by the *tidal volume.*

★ millibar

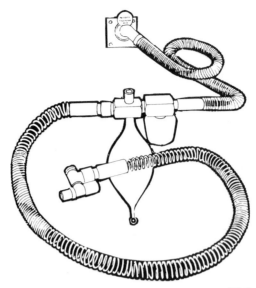

Fig. 11.26 Anaesthetic gas scavenging system with in-line condensate trap. (M & I.E. Ltd.)

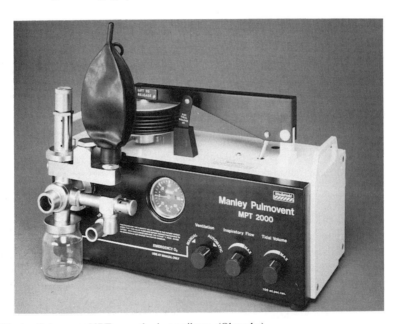

Fig. 11.27 Manley Pulmovent MPT anaesthesia ventilator. (Ohmeda.)

In the inactive condition both ventilator bellows are collapsed, inspiratory valves VI and V2 are closed, expiratory valve 3 is open, and expiratory valves V4 and V5 are closed (Fig. 11.28* and 11.29).

When the gas supply is turned on, if both *automatic/manual* selectors are set to *automatic* ventilation, gas enters the ventilator at the gas inlet and flows directly into bellows B1 which

---

* *Note: all the information and circuit diagrams in this section on ventilators is the copyright of the particular manufacturer and is reproduced by their kind permission. The material should not be further copied, re-reproduced or used without their permission.*

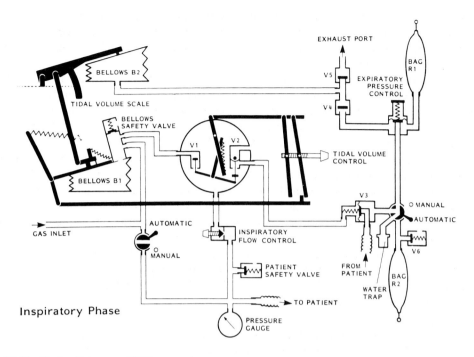

Fig. 11.28 Manley Pulmovent MPT automatic mode schematic diagram inspiratory phase. (Ohmeda.)

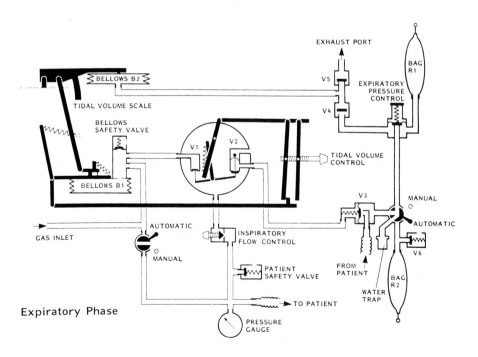

Fig. 11.29 Manley Pulmovent MPT automatic mode schematic diagram expiratory phase. (Ohmeda.)

incorporate a safety valve to relieve any excess pressure. With the *inspiratory flow* control adjusted to give the required *minute volume*, the bellows B1 expand against the action of their return spring, and operate an adjustable mechanical linkage which is connected to the inspiratory valve assembly.

The bellows B2 also expand as they are mechanically linked to bellows B1; this creates a sub-atmospheric pressure which opens valve V4 and ensures valve V5 is fully closed. The mechanical linkage between bellows B1 and the inspiratory valve assembly is adjusted by setting the *tidal volume* control. When the bellows expand to the selected *tidal volume* limit, the linkage then *opens* inspiratory valves V1 and V2.

During the inspiratory phase when valves V1 and V2 are *open*, the contents of the bellows and the incoming gas discharge via valve V1 into the patient breathing circuit. The rate at which this takes place is determined by the setting of the *inspiratory flow* control. Simultaneously the pressure in the bellows flows via valve V2 to *close* valve V3 against the action of its return spring which closes the expiratory circuit. Meanwhile, the contents of bellows B2 discharge to atmosphere via valve V5, and *close* valve V4.

As both the bellows discharge their contents they gradually return to the collapsed condition due to the action of the bellows B1 return springs. As bellows B1 collapse, the mechanical linkage is operated once again to *close* valves V1 and V2.

During the expiratory phase valve V1 *closes* the inspiratory circuit; valve V2 shuts *off* the gas supply to valve V3 and vents all pressure to atmosphere. Valve V3 then opens due to the action of its return spring, and allows expired gases to pass into bag R1 via the *expiratory pressure* control valve. This forms the passive duration of the expiratory phase and it can be positive or atmospheric depending upon the setting of the expiratory control valve. The expiratory phase involves bellows B1 filling with gas, and as they expand the bellows B2 also expand, being mechanically linked to bellows B1; this creates a sub-atmospheric pressure which in turn *opens* valve V4 and *closes* valve V5. Bag R1 now discharges into bellows B2.

For the manual mode, both *automatic/manual* selectors are set to *manual*. When the gas supply is turned on, gas enters at the gas inlet and flows via the *ventilations* selector and the patient outlet directly to the patient. As the gas supply takes the path of least resistance, bellows B1, the inspiratory valve and the *inspiratory flow* control are all by-passed. The *expiratory pressure* control valve, bag R1, valves V4 and V5, and bellows B2 are all shut off by the expiratory circuit *ventilations* selector. Consequently bellows B1 and B2 remain in the collapsed condition, valves V1 and V2 remain closed, and valve V3 remains open.

The patient expires via valve V3 and the expiratory circuit *ventilations* selector into bag R2. Ventilation of the patient is manually controlled by bag R2 and valve V6.

The plug-in patient circuit can be removed quickly and easily for cleansing and sterilization by autoclaving (Fig. 11.30).

The Nuffield Series 400 anaesthesia ventilator (Penlon)

This is intended primarily for use with a CO_2 absorber circle system or co-axial (Bain) breathing system (Fig. 11.31). The ventilator comprises a fluid logic module which automatically controls a 'bellow-in-bottle' unit. Compressed gas, normally air or oxygen at a pressure of approximately 340 kPa (50 lb force per in^2), is used to operate a logic module and to provide the power needed to compress the bellows during controlled ventilation. The design of the unit keeps the driving gas completely separate from the respirable gas supplied to the patient.

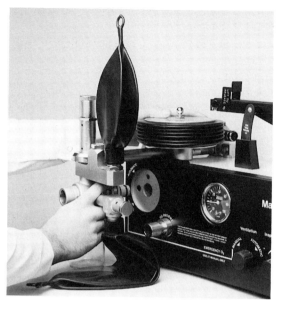

Fig. 11.30 Manley Pulmovent MPT plug in patient circuit. (Ohmeda.)

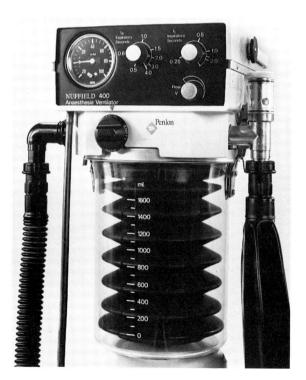

Fig. 11.31 Nuffield series 400 anaesthesia ventilator. (Penlon.)

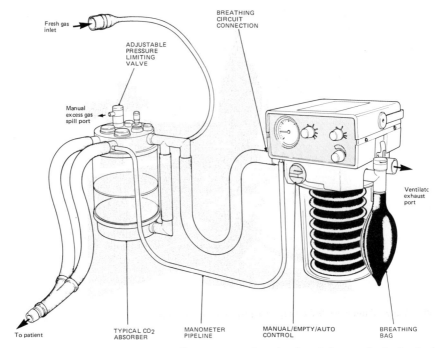

Fresh gas
inlet

BREATHING
CIRCUIT
CONNECTION

ADJUSTABLE
PRESSURE
LIMITING
VALVE

Manual
excess gas
spill port

Ventilatc
exhaust
port

To patient

TYPICAL CO$_2$
ABSORBER

MANOMETER
PIPELINE

MANUAL/EMPTY/AUTO
CONTROL

BREATHING
BAG

Fig. 11.32   Nuffield series 400 anaesthesia ventilator, connected to absorber circle anaesthesia circuit. (Penlon Ltd.)

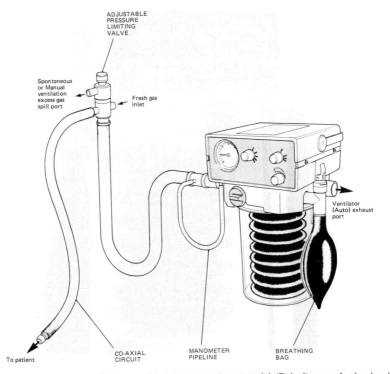

ADJUSTABLE
PRESSURE
LIMITING
VALVE

Spontaneous
or Manual
ventilation
excess gas
spill port

Fresh gas
inlet

Ventilator
(Auto) exhaust
port

To patient

CO-AXIAL
CIRCUIT

MANOMETER
PIPELINE

BREATHING
BAG

Fig. 11.33   Nuffield series 400 anaesthesia ventilator, connected to co-axial (Bains') anaesthesia circuit. (Penlon Ltd.)

The ventilator is a pressure transformer, controlling respiratory rate by means of time cycled, constant flow generation as follows:

1. *Inspiratory phase* — Pressure flow transformer, constant flow generator; time and flow directly pre-set and tidal volume indirectly pre-set.

2. *End of inspiratory phase* — Time cycled.

3. *Expiratory phase* — Atmospheric pressure generator.

4. *End of expiratory phase* — Time cycled.

The ventilator operates as a controller with an atmospheric base pressure wave form; it does not act as an assistor or a *minute volume* divider. Figures 11.32 and 11.33 illustrate the Nuffield 400 used with an absorber circle anaesthesia circuit and co-axial (Bane) circuit respectively.

The patient circuit module of the ventilator comprises an easily autoclavable valve unit with a lid and disc assembly (Fig. 11.34). The bellows (12) (Figs. 11.35, and 11.36) are attached to the disc, the last convolution being stretched over the disc rim to retain the bellows in position. The flanged lid fits on to the rim of the canister which has a silicone seal; cutaways in the lid flange ensure positive location of the lid on each side of the canister fastening hooks.

The valve unit incorporates the anaesthesia (breathing) circuit port (I.S.O 22 mm male connection) (8), *manual/empty/auto* valve (17) and cam (18), spill valve (15), exhaust port (16), and a connection mount for a breathing (reservoir) bag (19). A pressure relief valve (7), pre-set to operate at 60 cm H_2O, is fitted to the unit to give patient protection.

The control module circuit is actuated when the *manual/empty/auto* valve (17) is set to the *auto* position. This action moves the cam (18) to operate valve (1) and supply driving gas to the logic driving circuit via pressure reducing valve (2). The adjustable pressure reducing valve is pre-set during manufacture to protect the circuit from variations in driving gas pressure.

From the reducing valve (2) gas is supplied to the spool valve (3). Depending on the spool position, gas is supplied to either the inspiratory flow control valve (6) and inspiratory timer (4) or to the expiratory timer (5). The adjustable timers provide alternate pulse signals to change the position of the spool valve (3), and so control the inspiratory and expiratory phase times.

The control module is linked to the patient circuit through inflating valve (10) which is actuated during the inspiratory phase, the driving gas moving a spring biased spool, in the valve, to close the exhaust port (20). With the exhaust port closed, driving gas enters canister (13) and compresses bellows (12), displacing the anaesthetic gases through spill valve (15) and into the anaesthesia circuit to the patient's lungs.

During the inspiratory phase, spill valve (15) remains closed to the exhaust port (16) by the driving gas pressure acting on the valve diaphragm through signal line (14).

The fixed setting relief valve (11), connected to inflating valve (10), protects canister (13) against excessive driving gas pressure. Driving gas will continue to flow into the canister at a constant flow rate as determined by the setting of the inspiratory flow control valve (6). The volume displaced from bellows (12) to the circuit is the product of inspiratory time and flow rate, and is indicated on the volume scale engraved on the canister.

On completion of the inspiratory phase, as set by the timer control valve (4), spool valve (3) is switched and the driving gas in the inspiratory circuit is exhausted to atmosphere through exhaust port (20). The expiration phase now starts, and bellows (12) expand under the influence of gravity assisted by a small weight attached to the base of the bellows. During this phase a small negative pressure, approximately 2 cmH_2O, is generated by the bellows and is normally absorbed within the breathing circuit and will not be transmitted to the

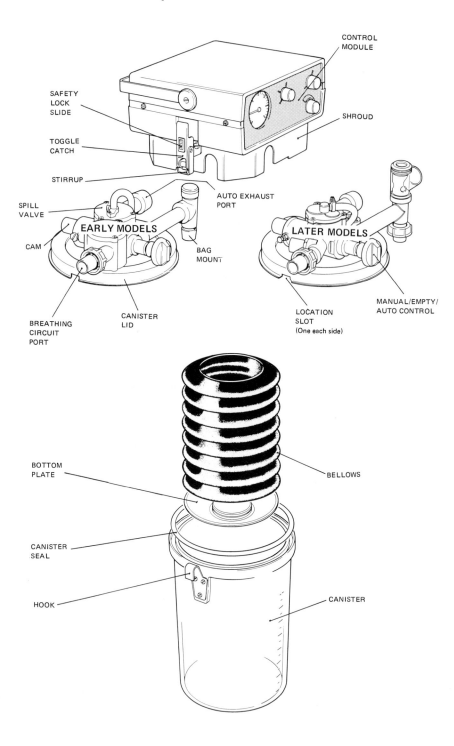

Fig. 11.34 Nuffield series 400 anaesthesia ventilator, disassembly for sterilization. (Penlon Ltd.)

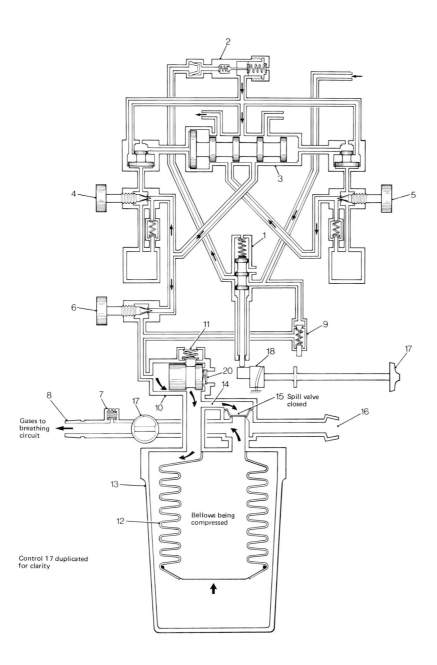

Fig. 11.35 Nuffield series 400 anaesthesia ventiltor schematic diagram of inspiratory phase — auto mode. (Penlon Ltd.)

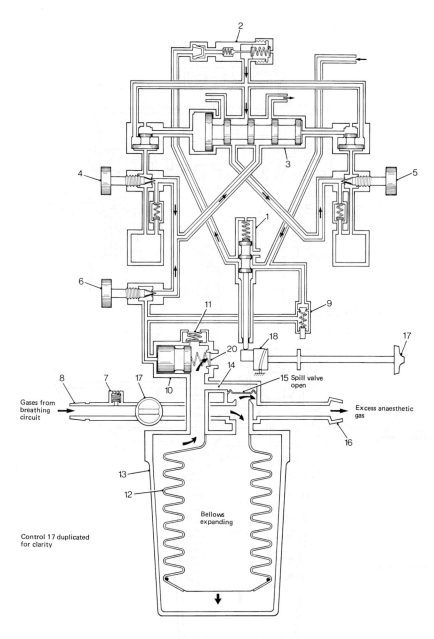

Fig. 11.36 Nuffield series 400 anaesthesia ventilator schematic diagram of expiratory phase — auto mode. (Penlon Ltd.)

Key to Figs 11.35/36

1. Driving gas valve.
2. Pressure reducing valve.
3. Spool valve.
4. Inspiratory timer.
5. Expiratory timer.
6. Inspiratory flow control valve.
7. Pressure relief valve.
8. I.S.O 22 mm male connection.
9. Driving gas bypass valve.
10. Inflating valve.
11. Relief valve.
12. Bellows.
13. Gas canister.
14. Signal line.
15. Spill valve.
16. Exhaust port.
17. *Manual/empty/auto* valve.
18. Cam.
19. Breathing reservoir bag attached to connector 8. (Not shown.)
20. Exhaust port.

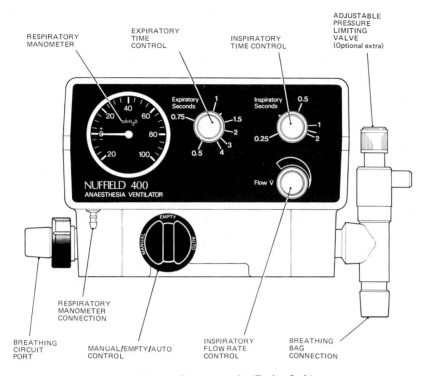

Fig. 11.37   Nuffield series 400 anaesthesia ventilator, controls. (Penlon Ltd.)

patient's lungs. Any excess anaesthetic gas in the circuit during expiration flows out of exhaust port (16) via spill valve (15) now that the valve is no longer pressurised.

The ventilator controls are as follows:

Manual/empty/auto. This combines the function of switching the pneumatic control *on* or *off*, and modifying the ventilator patient circuit to suit a particular mode of operation. The function of the *manual* and *auto* controls are self-evident (Fig. 11.37). The intermediate position marked *empty* is used to compress the bellows and empty them of air before attaching the anaesthesia circuit. Once the bellows have been emptied, the control is left in the *manual* position until the ventilator is required to operate.

Inspiratory flow rate control. This is an uncalibrated control; the knob is turned to the *left* to *increase* flow, and to the *right* to *decrease* flow.

Inspiratory phase time control. Calibrated in seconds, this enables the duration of the inspiratory phase to be set within a range of 0.25 to 2 seconds. It is adjusted until the displacement of the ventilator bellows generates the required *tidal volume* as indicated on the scale marked on the side of the canister.

Expiratory time control. Also calibrated in seconds, this rotary control allows the duration of the expiratory phase to be set within a range of 0.5 to 4.0 seconds. It enables adjustment of the required inspiration to expiration (I:E) ratio and ventilating frequency. The I:E ratio is determined by comparing the settings of the two time controls. The ventilating frequency, in breaths per minute, is determined by dividing the sum of the I and E settings into 60. For example:

I time = 1 sec; E = 2 sec; Total = 3 sec
Frequency = 60/3 = 20 breaths per minute

Displaced volume scale. The scale marked on the bellows canister shows the volume in ml displaced from the ventilator to the breathing circuit. It gives an approximate indication (in ml) of the *tidal volume*. The precise *tidal volume* can only be monitored by a spirometer interposed at the patient connection port of the breathing system. Depending upon the type of breathing circuit used, the *tidal volume* delivered to the patient will be diminished by the internal compliance of the circuit, but augmented by the fresh gas flow.

Respiratory manometer. This gauge is calibrated for -20 to $+100$ cm H_2O. A 'zero' adjustment screw is provided on the gauge dial. Connection to the breathing circuit is made via the external connection nipple provided immediately below the gauge. A 22 mm tee piece is provided for inclusion in the patient circuit.

Anaesthetic gas scavenging system. Automatic Pressure Limiting (APL) valve fitted to breathing system. During automatic ventilation the patient's expired gas is discharged from the ventilator exhaust port (16) which can be easily connected to an anaesthetic gas scavenging system. When operating on manual or spontaneous ventilation, the patient's expired gas is discharged from the APL valve on the breathing system. These two outlets may be joined by hoses to a common receiving system leading to the AGS system (page 321).

APL valve fitted to ventilator. Surplus gas will be discharged from the APL valve during manual ventilation, and from the ventilator exhaust port during automatic ventilation. These outlets may be joined by hoses to a common receiving system.

Safety checks

The following checks should be carried out when the ventilator is dismantled for cleaning and sterilization:

Patient circuit — visual checks:

1. Canister 'O' seal is in good condition and fitted correctly.
2. Bellows are not damaged or deteriorated.
3. Pressure signal hose (canister to spill valve) is not damaged or blocked.

Patient circuit — functional checks. With the patient circuit separated from the ventilator, *auto* mode is selected and the breathing circuit port occluded. The bellows are compressed and allowed to hang freely. The bellows should remain stationary if all joints are leak free. If the bellows fall slowly, the following are checked:

1. Correct fit of bellows to patient circuit.
2. Integrity of spill valve diaphragm.
3. *Manual/empty/auto* valve.
4. Bung used to occlude the breathing circuit port.

The following checks are carried out with the ventilator assembled and cycling with a breathing circuit and test lung connected:

1. A manometer is connected into the circuit and the connection to the test lung occluded. The ventilator relief valve should open and the relief pressure should be indicated on the pressure gauge (60 cm H_2O).

2. The *auto* is switched to *manual* and a check made that the test lung can be ventilated manually.

Patient circuit — Adjustable Pressure Limiting (APL) Valve checks. On ventilators fitted with an APL valve, the following additional checks should be made after cleaning and sterilization:

1. The ventilator is connected to the appropriate anaesthesia circuit and *manual* is selected.

2. The APL valve is closed completely, and the patient connection port of the circuit

blocked. The breathing bag is inflated fully using the fresh gas supply to the circuit. The gas supply is turned off and the manometer or bag watched to see if leakage is apparent.

3. When satisfied that leakage rates are acceptable, the APL valve is opened to ensure that gas leaves the circuit without obstructon. The valve is normally left fully open when passing the ventilator as ready for service.

Pneumatic circuit checks. The control module should not be adjusted in any way. Provided the ventilator is operating smoothly, and the cycling function is as described in the principles of function described previously, the major components do not require any routine maintenance.

The Ohmeda anaesthesia ventilator 7700

This is an electronically controlled, pneumatically operated lung ventilator which can be used in either an open or closed system configuration (Fig. 11.38). Patient ventilation is controlled by the operation of a bellows assembly which is mechanically linked to a pneumatically operated drive unit. The gas supply to the drive unit is controlled by electronically operated valves, therefore the movement of the bellows is determined by the operation of the electronic controls. The bellows gas circuit and the drive unit gas circuit, like the two other ventilators described above, are pneumatically independent from the respirable patient circuit.

The ventilator can be operated either in one of two automatic modes or in a manual mode. The airway pressure display is provided in all three modes, but other displays and facilities vary as follows:

In the primary automatic mode with a flow transducer connected in the patient circuit, the ventilator provides automatic ventilation with breath synchronisation. *Minute volume, tidal volume,* I:E ratio and breath frequency displays are also provided.

In the secondary automatic mode, without a flow transducer connected, the ventilator provides automatic ventilation but *without* breath synchronisation and *without minute volume*

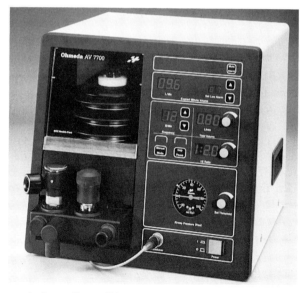

Fig. 11.38 OAV 7700 anaesthesia ventilator. (Ohmeda.)

and *tidal volume* displays. The I:E ratio and breath frequency displays, however, are provided in this mode.

With manual mode selected the patient can be ventilated manually by using the patient circuit rebreathing bag, and, provided that the flow transducer is fitted, the *minute volume* and *tidal volume* displays are provided. If the transducer develops a fault, it can be disconnected and ventilation continued, but without *minute* and *tidal volume* displays.

The Ohmeda AV 7700 incorporates a sophisticated range of safety features shown on the control panel in Figure 11.39 which include:

Ventilator based alarms

Power failure. Battery operated continuous audible tone and illuminated Power Fail red legend. Activated if the electrical supply to any of the ventilator's systems fails.

Gas failure. Continuous audible tone and illuminated gas fail red legend. Activated if the driving gas supply pressure decreases to less than 250 kPa for a one cylinder drive model or to less than 200 kPa for a two cylinder drive model.

Ventilator failure. Continuous audible tone and illuminated Vent Fail red legend. Activated if ventilator develops an internal fault, but if the fault is transitory the ventilator automatically restarts. If the fault clears spontaneously, the settings have to be checked for any variation from those previously set.

Ventilator based warnings

Frequency not as set. Frequency display intermittently illuminated. Activated if the ventilator's delivered frequency is less than the setting of the frequency control. This may be due to the I:E ratio and *tidal volume* controls being set to a condition which is incompatible with the selected frequency, or because the patient's breath is inhibiting the inspiratory phases.

Adverse I:E ratio. The I:E ratio display is intermittently illuminated. Activated if the I:E ratio is less than 1:1.0 at any time.

Patient based alarms

Patient disconnect (Lo Press). Intermittent audible tone accompanied by intermittent illumination of the Patient Disconnect (*Lo Press*) legend. Activated if the airway pressure gauge pointer does NOT cross the set threshold level. Threshold can be set within the range of 5 to 50 cm H_2O; setting indicated by a 'white flag'.

Excess P_{aw} (Hi Press). Audible tone of short duration accompanied by illumination of Excess P_{aw} (*Hi Press*) red legend which remains illuminated until the start of the next delivered breath. The ventilator automatically reverts to an expiratory phase to reduce airway pressure immediately the alarm is activated; it also cancels any Inspiratory Pause selection. Alarm activated if the airway pressure gauge pointer crosses the maximum level which can be set within the range of 25 to 70 cm H_2O; setting indicated by a 'red flag'.

Low minute volume. An intermittent audible tone accompanied by intermittent illumination of the Set Low Alarm display. Activated if the displayed *minute volume* falls below the level indicated on the Set Low Alarm display; can be set within the range of 1 to 30 litres/minute.

To set up the ventilator for closed system configuration, first the fresh gas supply hose is connected to the absorber, and the inspiratory hoses between the absorber and the transducer. The patient supply hose is connected between the absorber and the ventilator Patient

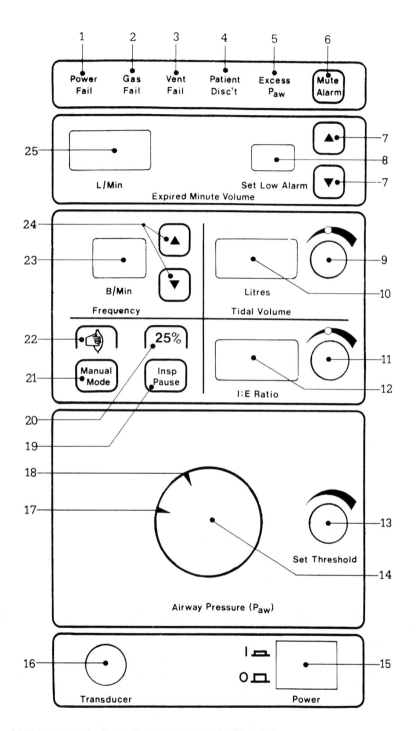

Fig. 11.39 OAV 7000 anaesthesia ventilator, control panel. (Ohmeda.)

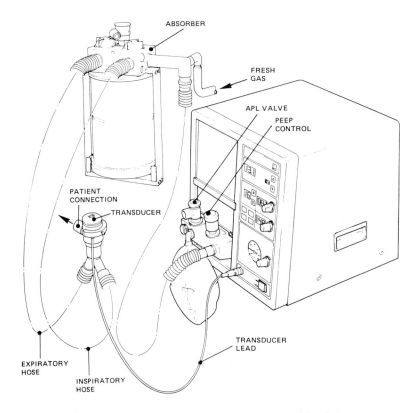

Fig. 11.40 OAV 7000 anaesthesia ventilator, closed system configuration. (Ohmeda.)

Connection port, and the transducer lead to the ventilator front panel connection. The ventilator APL valve is fully opened, the PEEP control turned fully counter-clockwise, and the fresh gas supply set as required (Fig. 11.40).

For an open system configuration, the blanking device from the ventilator fresh gas inlet is unscrewed, the inlet connection fitted, and the fresh gas hose connected. The patient hose and transducer are coupled to the non-rebreathing valve. The non-rebreathing valve outlet is coupled to an AGS system and the transducer lead connected to the ventilator front panel connection. The ventilator APL valve is fully opened and the fresh gas flow set as required (Fig. 11.41).

The electronic start up procedure provides a nominal 16 breaths/minute with a *tidal volume* of approximately 0.8 litres at an I:E ratio of approximately 1:2. The *tidal volume* and I:E ratio values are dependent upon the patient system configuration, airway pressure and fresh gas flow into the system. The procedure is as follows:

1. *Tidal volume* control and the I:E ratio control are set to the 'blue dot' position.

2. Set Threshold control is rotated fully counter-clockwise to set the Airway Pressure 'white flag' to 5 cm H_2O, and the 'red flag' to 25 cm H_2O.

3. Power switch is turned ON, and a check made that the Alarm Tone emits a bleep and that numerical displays illuminate for three seconds as illustrated in Figure 11.47A and detailed as follows:

— that all numerical displays are illuminated and that each individual display, with the exception of the I:E ratio, displays a figure 8 for three seconds; the I:E ratio displays

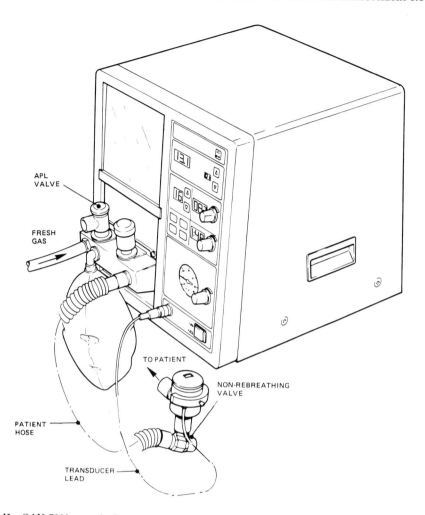

APL
VALVE

FRESH
GAS

TO PATIENT

NON-REBREATHING
VALVE

PATIENT
HOSE

TRANSDUCER
LEAD

Fig. 11.41 OAV 7000 anaesthesia ventilator, open system configuration. (Ohmeda.)

1:8, also for three seconds.

— that the Patient disconnect (*Lo Press*) and Excess P_{aw} (*Hi press*) alarm legends are illuminated for 3 seconds.

— that the Manual Mode and 25% Inspiration Pause legends are illuminated for three seconds.

4. There are six safe start up confirmation checks (Fig. 11.47B):

— that after a three seconds delay the Expired *minute volume* Set Low Alarm displays 01 and all other displays revert to zero.

— that after the bellows is driven for 2 cycles the Frequency display indicates 16, and after the next cycle the I:E ratio is approximately 1:2.0, the *Tidal volume* is approximately 0.80 litres, and the Expired *minute volume* commences to increment. (The *tidal volume* and the Expired *minute volume* do *not* illuminate if the flow transducer is not connected to the front panel socket.)

The patient respiratory circuit can easily be removed for cleansing and sterilization at 134°C for 3 minutes. This is illustrated in Figure 11.48.

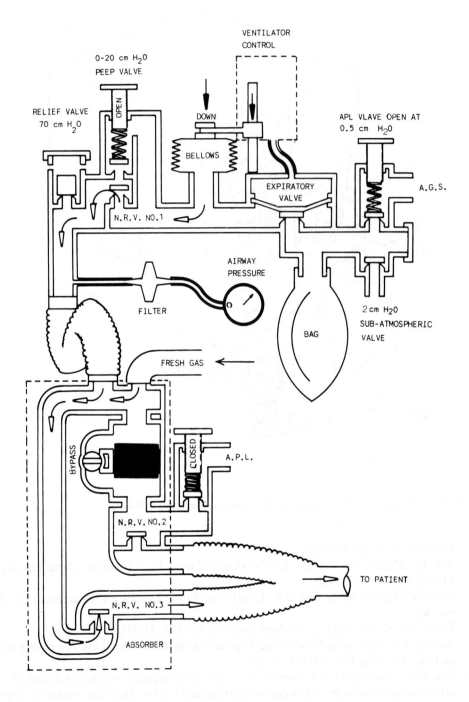

Fig. 11.42 OAV 7000 anaesthesia ventilator, schematic diagram of circle rebreathing system, inspiratory phase. (Ohmeda.)

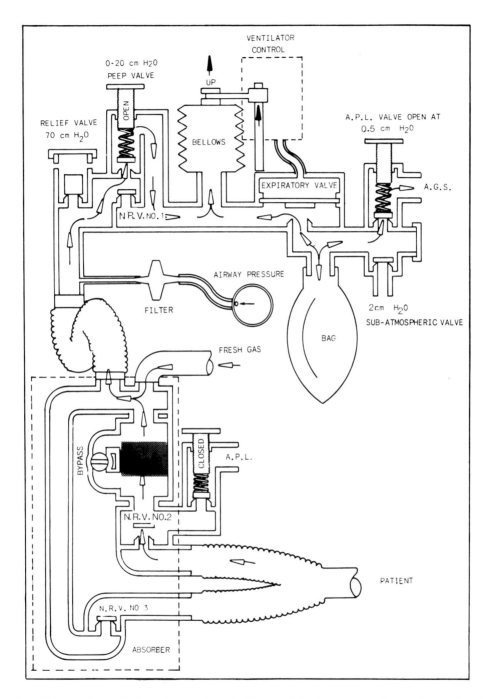

Fig. 11.43 OAV 7000 anaesthesia ventilator, schematic diagram of circuit, start of expiratory phase. (Ohmeda.)

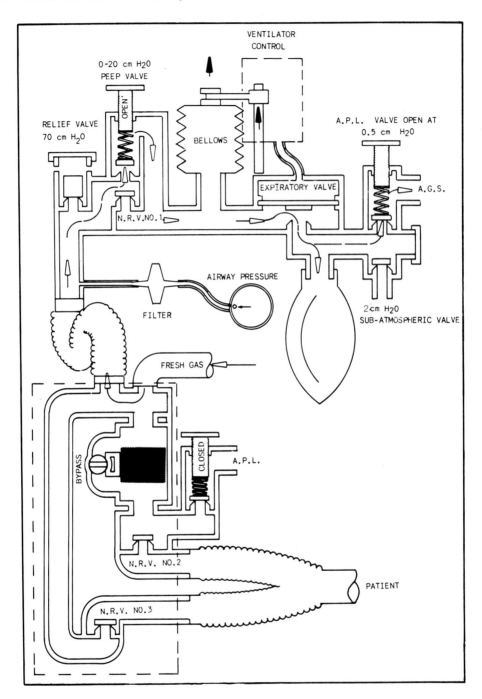

Fig. 11.44 OAV 7000 anaesthesia ventilator, schematic diagram of circuit, mid end of expiratory phase. (Ohmeda.)

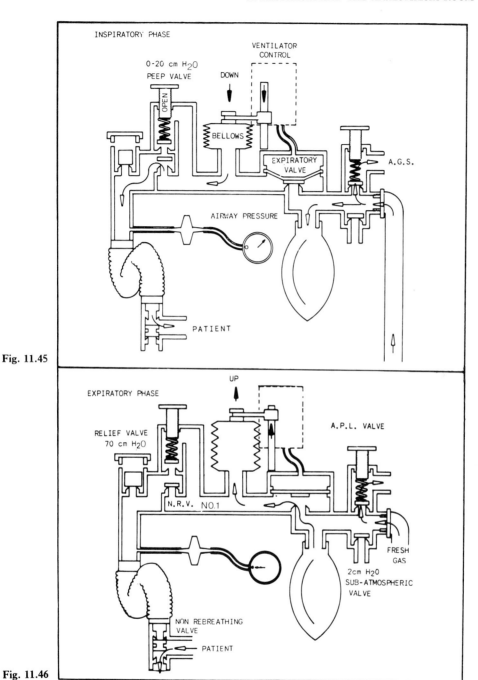

Fig. 11.45

Fig. 11.46

Fig. 11.45 OAV 7000 anaesthesia ventilator, schematic diagram of non-rebreathing system, inspiratory phase. (Ohmeda.)

Fig. 11.46 OAV 7000 anaesthesia ventilator, schematic diagram of non-rebreathing system, expiratory phase. (Ohmeda.)

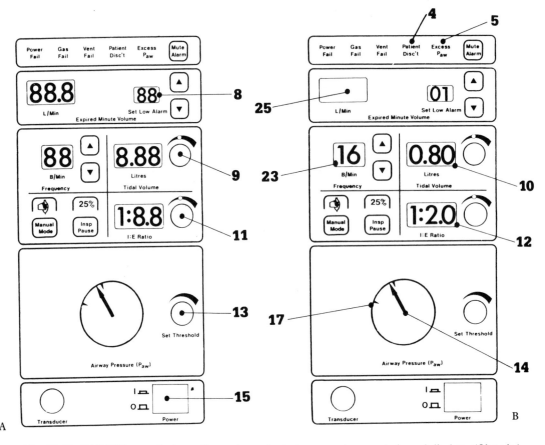

Fig. 11.47 OAV 7000 anaesthesia ventilator, electronic start-up procedure, control panel displays. (Ohmeda.)

4. Patient disconnect warning.
5. Excess P_{aw} warning.
8. Set low alarm indicator.
9. Tidal volume control.
10. Tidal volume indicator.
11. I:E ratio control.
12. I:E ratio indicator.
13. Set threshold control.
14. Airway pressure indicator.
15. Power ON/OFF control.
17. White flag indicator.
23. Frequency indicator.
25. Expiratory minute volume indicator.

Intravenous anaesthesia

A selection of intravenous anaesthetic agents, relaxants, stimulants and antidotes should be clearly labelled and available for the anaesthetist.

The intravenous barbiturates in common use are thiopentone sodium (Pentothal, Intraval sodium) 2.5 per cent, methohexitone sodium (Brietal) 1 or 2 per cent, etomidate (Hypomidate) 2 per cent and Ketamine hydrochloride (Ketalar). A thiopentone 2.5 per cent solution is prepared by dissolving 0.5 g in 20 ml of sterile pyrogen-free distilled water respectively.

Fentanyl (Sublimaze), alfentanil (Rapifen), morphine, and pethidine, are used extensively. Pethidine is often diluted to a 1 per cent solution containing 10 mg per ml.

Relaxants in common use include the 'competitive blocker' muscle relaxants such as tubocurarine chloride (Tubarine), gallamine triethiodide (Flaxedil), pancuronium bromide (Pavulon) and alcuronium chloride (Alloferin); and depolarising muscle relaxants such as suxamethonium chloride (Scoline).

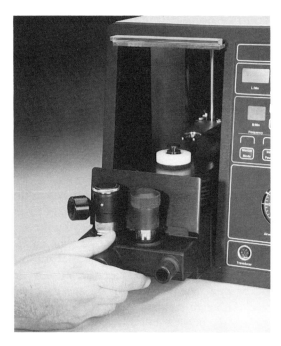

Fig. 11.48   OAV 7700 anaesthesia ventilator, removal of patient circuit for sterilization. (Ohmeda)

Stimulants available should include, aminophylline, methoxamine (Vasoxyl, Vasoxine), metaraminol (Aramine), isoprenaline (Insuprel), noradrenaline (Levophed) and adrenaline. Antidotes commonly needed include atropine, neostigmine (Prostigmine), naloxine hydrochloride (Narcan), doxapram hydrochloride (Dopram), glycopyrronium bromide (Robinol), edrophonium chloride (Tensilon).

It is the anaesthetist's responsibility to prepare these solutions, but if the anaesthesia nurse is permitted to do so, she should check the preparation with a second person, label each syringe and show the anaesthetist the ampoules or bottle from which the injection has been prepared.

A 10 ml or 20 ml disposable sterile syringe is used for barbiturates, and a 2 ml or 5 ml disposable sterile syringe for other drugs, including pethidine, relaxants, antidotes, etc. The integrity of the sterile pack containing the syringe should be checked by trying to squeeze the air gently from the inside.

The sizes of needles used vary with individual choice but for general purposes a size 18 to 21 needle is usual, with perhaps a size 23 for small or delicate veins. The anaesthetist will require a number of 'filling' needles (plastic quills) to aspirate drugs from the ampoules, and larger bore needles for rubber-cap bottles.

For continuous or intermittent intravenous injections, either the syringe and needle are left in position so that small quantities may be injected as required, or a special needle such as the butterfly is left in the vein and the syringe attached to the needle each time injection is necessary.

Continuous intravenous anaesthesia can be maintained by using a very weak intravenous solution, which is administered via a saline infusion, or small quantities of the drug can be injected into the infusion tube, as required.

Where it is the habit of the anaesthetist to prepare several solutions at the same time, he should label syringes to aid identification.

Medico-legally it is the anaesthetist who is responsible for the right drug being injected. Accidents do occur, and so a nurse should never be offended if the anaesthetist does not appear to trust her spoken word. He must be absolutely certain; where life is concerned, personal considerations are of no account. It is not sufficient to check the name on the outside of the ampoule box. The inscription on the ampoule itself is the *only* proof that the correct drug is being given.

Endotracheal and endobronchial intubation

Apparatus for passing an endotracheal tube must be ready before the commencement of any anaesthesia induction, even if the anaesthetist has not requested its preparation. In resuscitation this procedure will be one of the first performed by the anaesthetist, unless a tube is already in position. Laryngoscopes used when introducing an endotracheal tube include the Magill straight-blade, the anatomical shaped blade Macintosh type and the intubating laryngofibrescope which acts as a guide for the insertion of an endotracheal tube.

There are three basic types of endotracheal tubes, the oral type, both cuffed and non-cuffed and the nasal type. Although each is indentical in diameter, the nasal tube is *slightly* softer when pressed between the fingers, and this allows it to comply with the configuration of the nasal space. Some endotracheal tubes are armoured by incorporating a metal or nylon spiral within the tube wall. These tubes have less tendency to become kinked or compressed and are of special use during operations on the skull and chest.

The endotracheal tube is used:

1. When in the opinion of the anaesthetist the airway is liable to be obstructed, e.g., face down, the young and elderly patient.

2. For operations in which it is necessary because of surgical technique, e.g., throat or chest operations.

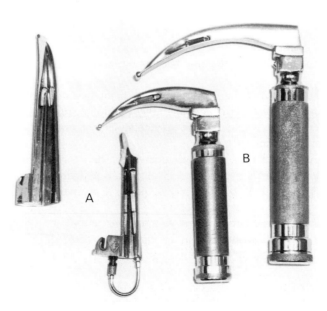

Fig. 11.49 Laryngoscopes, (A) Anderson. (B) Macintosh curved.

3. For upper abdominal operations and artificial ventilation.

4. When the towelling and position of the patient prevents the anaesthetist gaining easy access to the patient's head, and thus guaranteeing a free airway, e.g., craniotomies.

5. To prevent the inhalation of blood or vomit, e.g., emergencies.

6. In the treatment of cardiac arrest.

The anaesthetist generally is likely to use an endotracheal tube which has a terminal cuff which, when inflated with air, impinges upon the tracheal mucosa, thereby sealing the lungs from the upper respiratory passages to prevent the inhalation of blood or vomit. It is important to realise that there is not a fixed volume of air necessary to secure air-tight fitting of the tube within the trachea. The amount may vary between 2 ml and 10 ml of air and this can be tested by the anaesthetist when inflating the lungs (Mackensie *et al.*, 1976).

Nasal tube sizes range from 3 mm to 5 mm internal diameter for a child; 5 mm to 6.5 mm for an adolescent; and 6.5 mm to 9 mm for an adult. Oral tubes range from 3.5 mm to 6.5 mm for a child; 7 mm to 8 mm for an adolescent; and 9 mm to 12 mm for an adult.

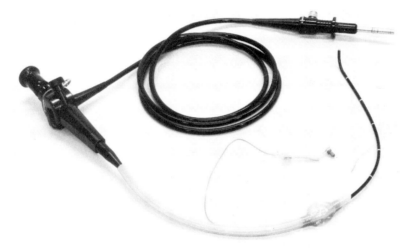

Fig. 11.50   Intubating laryngofibrescope. (Olympus LFI, Keymed.)

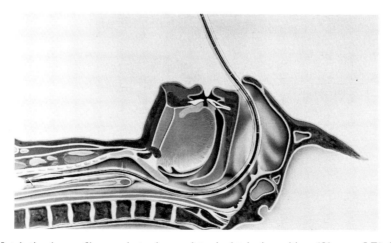

Fig. 11.51   Intubating laryngofibrescpe in trachea, endotracheal tube in position. (Olympus LF1, Key Med.)

The experienced anaesthetic nurse or technician will learn to select the sizes and type of endotracheal tubes required; cuffed tubes must always be tested by inflating the cuff before use by the anaesthetist. All the apparatus should be laid out in the order required, giving special attention to the provision of correct size tube connections, and laryngoscopes in good working order. The electric lamp on the latter must illuminate brightly and if necessary the battery should be changed before use. A second laryngoscope must always be available in case of lamp failure during use. The care of electrical endoscopes has been dealt with in Chapter 3. A tube of lubricant is usually required and this may be combined with a local anaesthetic such as 2 per cent lignocaine (Xylocaine). An example of a non-anaesthetic lubricant is K-Y jelly. A suction machine with long suction catheters is prepared, together with a small bowl of clean water for rinsing the catheters. A surface anaesthetic e.g., 4 per cent lignocaine (Xylocaine) and laryngeal spray may be required.

The endobronchial tube is in effect an extended cuffed endotracheal tube of smaller dimensions, which is passed into the left or right bronchus. Formerly during chest operations, the anaesthetist utilised two tubes, one in the unaffected lung for the purpose of anaesthesia, and one in the other for the purpose of aspiration during operation. Endo-

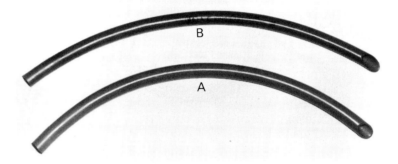

Fig. 11.52   Endotracheal tubes, (A) Magill plain oral 7 mm, (B) plain nasal 7 mm.

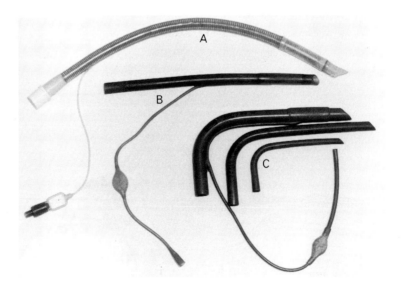

Fig. 11.53   Reinforced endotracheal tubes: (A) nylon/latex, cuffed 7.5 mm; (B) silicone wire, cuffed 8 mm; (C) Oxford cuffed and plain.

bronchial tubes have an inflatable cuff to isolate the intubated lung. It is now common practice to use a divided airway or doubled lumen cuffed tube such as the Carlens: this achieves the same purpose. The anaesthetist will require a bronchoscope of suitable type, in addition to the standard laryngoscope, etc., and may also need a long bronchial spray with a surface anaesthetic, e.g., lignocaine (Xylocaine).

All endotracheal and endobronchial tubes must be cleaned thoroughly with a brush and warm antibacterial detergent solution after use. Those having inflatable cuffs are checked before being stored away, care being taken to avoid water entering the cuff or pilot tube. The tubes are always sterilized after use although absolute sterility cannot be guaranteed during intubation.

After use, laryngoscope handles should be cleaned, and the blade dismantled from the handle, cleaned and sterilized. Most modern instruments have nylon insulation and gold-plated electrical contacts which will withstand autoclaving. If they are the older type either subatmospheric steam/formaldehyde or ethylene oxide should be used.

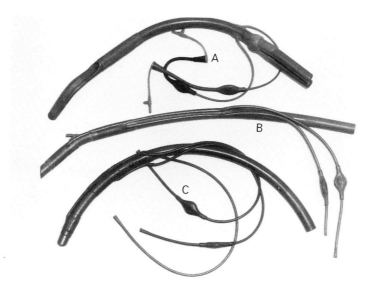

Fig. 11.54 Endobronchial tubes: (A) Robertshaw double lumen, medium left; (B) Gordon Green double cuff 9 mm; (C) Brompton Pallister double cuff 9 mm.

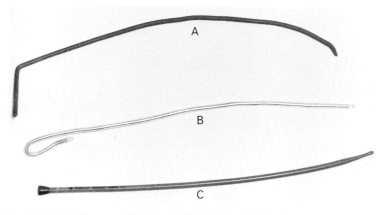

Fig. 11.55 Endotracheal tube directors. (A) Oxford, (B) Satinslin, (C) Neoplex.

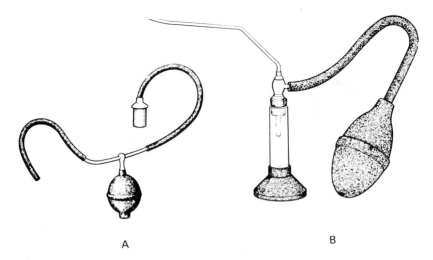

Fig. 11.56   (A) Macintosh spray. (B) Rowbotham spray. (Downs Surgical Ltd.)

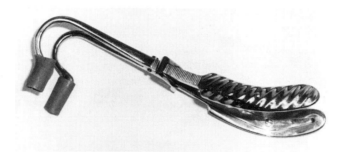

Fig. 11.57   Mouth gag, Fergusson-Acland.

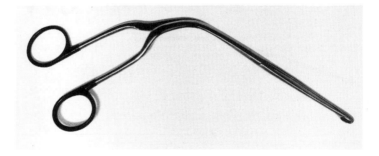

Fig. 11.58   Magill introducing forceps.

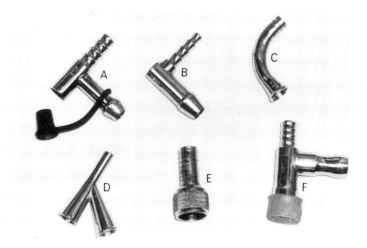

Fig. 11.59   Connectors for endotracheal tubes (corrugated end fits tube). (A) Cobbs, (B) Rowbotham, (C) curved Magill, (D) Magill side inlet, (E) Nosworthy, (F) Magill suction.

Local or regional anaesthesia

This may range from a simple injection for infiltrating a small area, to an extensive nerve block.

Whereas a 10 ml or 20 ml syringe is adequate for a minor procedure, involving the injection of a few millilitres of anaesthetic agent, it is preferable to use a self-filling syringe for larger quantities. The alternative is to leave the needle in position and prepare several syringes filled with anaesthetic agent, using these consecutively.

A fine hypodermic needle of size 23 will be required for the initial 'weal', followed by a longer one of wider bore. A selection of needles should be available, ranging from 5 cm to 10 cm (2 to 4 in) in length, and 20 to 26 B.W.G. in gauge.

Anaesthetists require exploring needles having long bevels and others having short bevels. A short bevel needle is essential for nerve blocks, especially the brachial plexus block, where a long bevel needle may increase the risk of pleural puncture or perforation of a blood-vessel.

Amongst the anaesthetic agents most commonly used are procaine, eticaine, lignocaine (Xylocaine), prilocaine (Citanest), and bupivacaine (Marcain).

A 1.5 or 2 per cent lignocaine is used for the initial infiltration or when only a small quantity is required. Where a larger quantity is necessary, the strength of solution is reduced to 1 per cent or 0.5 per cent and the amount injected limited to the maximum dose of the agent (e.g., the maximum dose of plain lignocaine (Xylocaine) in a normal healthy adult is 13 to 15 ml of a 1.5 per cent solution, 23 ml of a 1 per cent solution or 46 ml of a 0.5 per cent solution). Dosage must be reduced in the ill and elderly.

In order to produce vasoconstriction, and thereby lessen capillary haemorrhage, adrenaline may be contained in the solution of lignocaine. For general infiltration to demarcate tissue layers as in mastectomy, adrenaline solution may be prepared as a 1 in 400,000 to 1 in 100,000 saline solution according to the total amount being injected. This is normally prepared in the pharmacy sterile products unit but a 1 in 400,000 solution may be prepared by adding 1 ml of 1 in 1000 adrenaline to 399 ml of local anaesthetic agent. A 1 in 100,000 solution may be prepared by adding 1 ml of 1 in 1000 adrenaline to 99 ml of anaesthetic agent. A 1 in 100,000 addition of adrenaline also prolongs the action of the local anaesthetic by delaying absorption up to six hours and thereby increases the safety margin for larger doses. In the case of lignocaine the maximum dosage becomes approximately twice that of the plain solution.

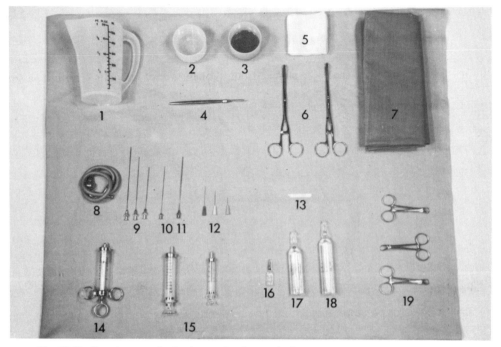

Fig. 11.60 Requirements for local or regional anaesthesia.

1. 0.5 litre measuring jug.
2. Skin antiseptic.
3. Bonney's blue for marking infiltrated area.
4. Skin pen and nib.
5. Green swabs.
6. Sponge holding forceps, Rampley (2).
7. Sterile towels.
8. Self-filling attachment (Pidkin), for Labet syringe.
9. Locking needles (Labet).
10. Brachial plexus needle (Short point).
11. Filling needle.
12. Hypodermic needles (18, 12 and 1).
13. File.
14. Syringes (Labet).
15. Syringes, 10 ml and 2 ml.
16. Adrenaline 1 in 1000.
17. Lignocaine (Xylocaine) 1.5 per cent.
18. Sterile distilled water.
19. Towel clips.

An easy way of preparing a small quantity of 1 in 400,000 adrenaline is to add the contents of a 1 ml ampoule of 1 in 1000 adrenaline to a 20 ml ampoule of saline solution from which 1 ml has been withdrawn, leaving 19 ml; 1 ml of this mixture is added to a second 19 ml ampoule containing anaesthetic solution. Should this be done by the anaesthetist, the nurse's or assistant's watchful eye would make sure that the first ampoule containing the saline is safely discarded after removing 1 ml, so as to avoid accidents.

The computation of local anaesthetic solutions, with or without adrenaline, is entirely the anaesthetist's responsibility, although selected strengths may be prepared by the pharmacist before they are required. If the anaesthesia nurse or assistant is permitted to prepare injections, she should *always* check the preparation with the anaesthetist, retaining all containers for his inspection.

Following operation, when a local anaesthetic has been administered, great care must be taken to avoid injury to areas which may remain analgesic for several hours. This applies especially to the use of hot-water bottles and electric blankets as a post-operative measure.

The topical application of anaesthetic agents such as cocaine to the eyes and lignocaine, etc., to the mucosa of the mouth, pharynx or respiratory tract, requires special after-care. The eyes must always be covered for several hours, as foreign bodies may impinge upon the cornea without the patient feeling their presence. Even with a minor operation, a patient

who has had an application of local anaesthetic to the mucosa of the respiratory tract is not permitted to eat or drink for at least two hours following operation and until he can cough effectively, as the resultant paralysis of the soft palate and epiglottis would allow foreign matter to enter the trachea. Watch also for possible reactions to the local anaesthetic including convulsions. If there is the slightest doubt or history of previous sensitivity a small test dose should be given first.

Spinal and epidural analgesia

Requirements for spinal analgesia should always be autoclaved before use in a special spinal packet.

Spinal analgesia is produced by making a spinal intrathecal injection of a heavy or light solution (in relation to the specific gravity of CSF) of anaesthetic agent such as lignocaine (Xylocaine) and bupivacaine (Marcain). In spinal analgesia the drug mixes with the cer-

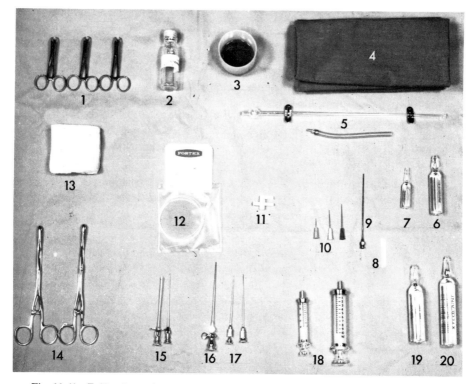

Fig. 11.61 Epidural or spinal anaesthesia requirements prepared as one pack.

1. Towel clips.
2. Sterile CSF specimen bottle.
3. Aqueous skin antiseptic.
4. Sterile towels.
5. Spinal manometer and connecting tube.
6. Bupivacaine (Marcain) with 1 in 200,000 adrenaline (available as separate sterile pack).
7. Prilocaine (citanest).
8. File.
9. Filling needle.
10. Hypodermic needles, size 20, 12 and 1.
11. Three-way tap.
12. Epidural plastic cannula.
13. Green swabs.
14. Sponge holding forceps, Rampley (2).
15. Epidural needles.
16. Spinal needle.
17. Spinal needles.
18. Syringes, 2 ml and 10 ml.
19. Sterile distilled water.
20. Lignocaine (Xylocaine) 1.5 per cent.

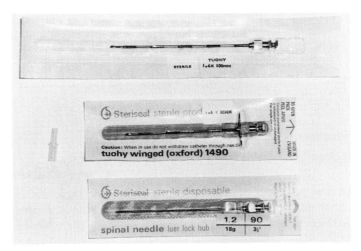

Fig. 11.62 Single use epidural and spinal needles. (A) Howard Jones type 1.2 mm × 90 mm. (B) Tuohy needle 1.6 mm × 1000 mm. (C) Tuohy winged (Oxford) 1.6 mm × 80 mm.

ebrospinal fluid and bathes a portion of the spinal cord and nerve roots, thereby rendering part of the body analgesic as well as paralysing the muscles. The extent of its desired action is determined by the anaesthetist and depends upon the volume of solution, the specific gravity of the solution and the position of the patient during and immediately after injection.

Epidural analgesia is produced by the slow injection of a larger volume of local anaesthetic agent into the epidural space between the ligamentum flavum and the dura. A special needle or cannula is used to facilitate the introduction of an indwelling nylon catheter through which the anaesthetic agent is injected.

For injection, the patient may either be sitting up with his legs over the side of the operation table, and head and shoulders bent forwards; or lying on the side with his legs drawn up, the head and shoulders being bent towards his knees.

Storage of equipment

Rubber equipment, e.g., endotracheal tubes deteriorate and soften with time, therefore over-stocking should be avoided. Rubber should be stored at temperatures below 21°C. No lubricant based on liquid paraffin should be used; it ruins rubber.

Drugs should also be stored at relatively low temperatures. The reserve stock and those particularly sensitive to heat such as suxamethonium chloride (scoline) and heparin should be kept in a refrigerator.

The patient

So far we have dealt with the apparatus and drugs necessary for the induction of anaesthesia and we must now consider the patient himself.

A patient comes to the theatre with a certain amount of apprehension, even although he may be the last person to admit this. The manner in which he is treated may seriously affect the induction of anaesthesia and his subsequent recovery. He should be made to think that he is the centre of attention, and that all possible skill is being used for his welfare.

The patient should always be accompanied to the theatre by a ward nurse, and if possible this nurse should remain with him until the induction of anaesthesia is complete. The psychological effect of this is very good, for the patient feels reassured by the presence of a ward nurse who is often the person responsible for his nursing care after the operation.

The nursing process

Unfortunately, often due to staffing difficulties, it is not possible for a ward nurse routinely to accompany her patient into the anaesthesia room. In an effort to obviate the disadvantages created by this situation, some operating departments have instituted a form of the nursing process or peri-operative care.

Over the past two decades, with the ever increasing complexities of theatre nursing, the theatre nurse has almost disappeared behind the barriers of the operating theatre. Furthermore, theatre nurses are gradually being engulfed with an ever increasing load of machinery and equipment, losing some track of the patient (Shaw, 1977).

The nursing process is an attempt to return more to patient-orientated nursing instead of job-orientated nursing. It is an attempt to ensure that each patient is observed and treated as an individual, rather than a 'case to be carried out second on the list'.

The nursing process is not of course confined to the operating theatre; it is a flexible systematic problem-solving approach to planning all forms of nursing care. Published literature includes reference to its application for the surgical patient and it is a concept which is well established in North America (Coates, 1974; Gruendemann, 1973; Rogers, 1975; Saylor, 1975).

In the operating theatre the nursing process or peri-operative care consists of three main parts; a pre-operative visit related to a nursing assessment of the patient; care of the patient during surgery; post-operative nursing evaluation of the patient.

Any pre-operative visit must be planned carefully, for if it is carried out either in the wrong way, or by wrong person irreparable psychological stress may result. Some anaesthetists question the concept of the pre-operative visit by operating department staff, and argue that it may cause confusion for the patient who also is visited by the anaesthetist. There are others who consider that anxieties can be allayed provided the procedures are well defined (Cox, 1987; Donworth, 1987).

The person visiting should be a qualified nurse and one who is to be directly involved in the care of the patient during surgery. A suitable person might be the anaesthesia nurse or theatre sister participating in the theatre operation list the following day. The nurse must be familiar with the techniques of approaching a pre-operative patient, particularly the psychological responses to be expected. The nurse must have a comprehensive knowledge of surgical procedures, although of course it is assumed that the surgeon has already explained the operation planned. The most important aspect of the visit is to be able to answer questions about pre- and post-operative nursing care. But it does give the opportunity for the theatre staff to introduce themselves, and make the patient aware of those who are to be responsible for his nursing care during surgery.

These objectives are summed up in the paper by Hazel Shaw (Shaw, 1977) as:
1. To collect data
2. to lessen the anxieties that the patient may have towards his operation
3. to improve patient care by knowing the patient and his problems before operation and to enable the theatre staff to anticipate equipment that may be needed for his care
4. to help the patient to understand the procedures and equipment that will be used in his care
5. to improve communication between ward staff, theatre staff and surgeons
6. to involve the theatre nurse more with total patient care and to encourage her to keep up-to-date with new procedures and ideas
7. to re-inforce information that the patient has already been given by ward staff and surgeons (the utmost co-operation is needed here to avoid possible confliction of information)

The second part, relating to care of the patient during surgery, does not alter established procedures. However, the first part of the nursing process should enable theatre staff to give a more efficient service, having a sense of security in knowing that patients are receiving the best possible care.

The final post-operative nursing evaluation should be carried out in a similar manner to the pre-operative visit. The main purpose is to enable the theatre nurse to be aware of continuing total patient care. The opportunity should be taken, if appropriate, to ascertain whether the patient may have any comments which could improve care before the anaesthesia induction period. It enables an evaluation of the pre-operative assessment to be made, and widens the nurse's knowledge of the ward situation.

The introduction of the nursing process requires considerable planning and care to become successful. The aspects described refer only to one approach and the reader is directed to other published literature on the subject.

Assisting the anaesthetist

Some or all of the duties described to assist the anaesthetist may well be performed by the anaesthesia nurse or operating department assistant whichever is most suitable and convenient.

The patient must be accompanied by X-rays, case notes, signed consent for anaesthesia and operation, pathological reports and drug sheet and any other relevant information which will be of use to the surgeon or the anaesthetist. The ward nurse should know the preparation which the patient has had, the time at which food or drink was last taken, the type and amount of pre-operative drugs administered, and the time at which they were given. She is responsible for seeing that any dentures, artificial eyes etc. have been removed, and must know whether the patient has passed urine or has been catheterised, and the time and amount passed, together with any abnormalities detected in routine ward tests.

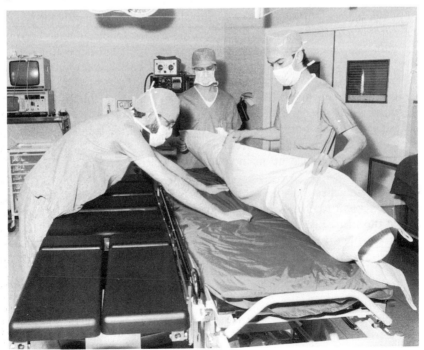

A

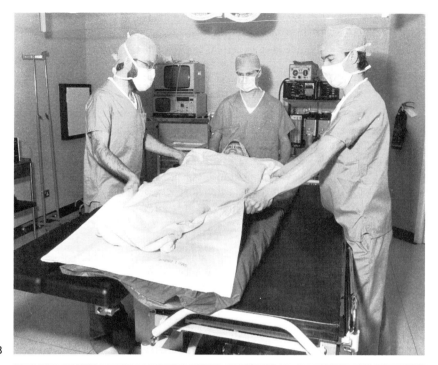

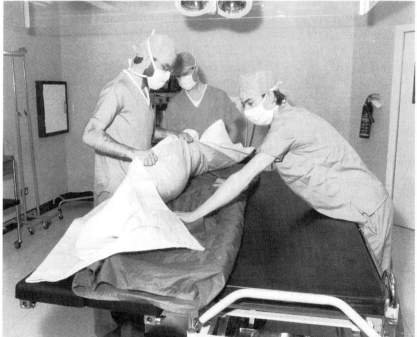

Fig. 11.63 Easyslide™ patient handling system is designed as a simple, quick and easy method of transferring a patient from one surface to another with minimal risk of back strain to staff. It consists of a fibre-filled, nylon-covered tube which is slipped under one side of the patients' body; the gentle frictionless rollering action is used to slide the patient, without lifting, from bed to trolley or operation table. (A) The patient is rolled onto side and the Easyslide tucked under. (B) The patient is then rolled on the Easyslide to new surface. (C) Finally, the patient is rolled onto other side and the Easyslide tube removed. (Nesbit Evans.)

It is now common practice to transport the patient to the operating department on his bed. The patient is then transferred either to a theatre trolley or remains on his bed for transfer to the anaesthesia room (see Chapter 1, page 11). The patient is anaesthetised on the trolley, bed or may be transferred on the underlying canvas stretcher to the operation table in the anaesthesia room. An alternative method is to use a 'fabric' transfer sleeve such as the Easyslide (Nesbit, Evans) (Fig. 11.63).

A patient must *never* be left alone in the anaesthesia room or theatre for he may be confused following the administration of the pre-operative drugs or sedative, and this may lead to accidental personal injury such as a fall from the trolley or operation table. Identification of the patient, his correct operation and correct site is of paramount importance. This procedure starts in the ward where some identification of the patient's name and case number must be attached to him before he is transferred to theatre. The house surgeon must mark the operation site with an indelible marker indicating the correct side or digit. This is especially important with the unconscious patient, aged or child. The identification can either be in the form of a bracelet (only removable by cutting if off) or details written on the patient by means of a skin pen.

On arrival at the theatre the patient's identification is checked against the case notes and operation list. If conscious, he is further asked his name. The anaesthesia and operation consent form must also be checked (Murray Wilson, 1971).

The surgeon should see the patient before anaesthesia is induced and confirm it is the correct patient, operation and site. This is of vital importance if a limb or digit is to be amputated.

The patient should always be made as comfortable as possible in transit and whilst waiting. Unless the patient is unconscious with the attendant dangers of an obstructed airway, it is a simple matter to remove excess pillows just before induction is commenced. The nurse should see that the patient is kept as quiet as possible, and should not encourage conversation unless it is obvious that the patient feels more relaxed doing so.

During induction the nurse stands by in case the patient becomes restless, but if he does she must not attempt to wrestle with him but must apply gentle restraint, with one arm across the legs just above the knees, using the other arm to prevent any wild flinging about of the patient's arms. She should not hesitate to ask for further assistance in dealing with the obstreperous patient and wild alcoholics.

For intravenous injection, the selected arm is extended towards the anaesthetist and either a quick-release tourniquet applied to the upper arm, or the nurse constricts the venous

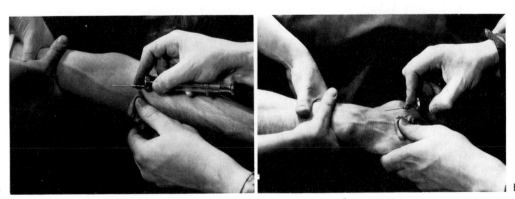

Fig. 11.64   (A) Method of holding upper arm for an intravenous injection, as an alternative to a tourniquet. (B) Method of holding wrist for an intravenous injection, as an alternative to a tourniquet.

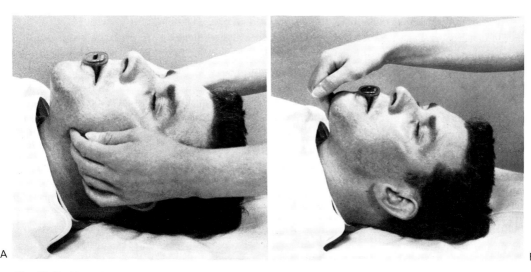

Fig. 11.65 Extension of the neck of an unconscious patient, (A) method one, (B) method two.

return by encircling the upper arm with her hands. The patient clenches his fist to make the veins prominent, and after the anaesthetist has aspirated blood into the syringe which probably indicates that the needle is in a vein, the compression of the upper arm veins is released at the anaesthetist's request. The nurse stands at the head of the trolley or operation table to support the patient's jaw when relaxation is complete. The anaesthetist will then apply pressure over the area of injection, which is continued by the nurse when the inhalation anaesthesia is commenced.

Too many nurses regard the maintenance of a good airway in the unconscious patient as just 'holding' up the jaw. Although this *may* suffice in some cases, the nurses must realise the principles behind any method chosen.

When unconscious, the muscles supporting the lower jaw relax, allowing it to sag. The tongue is also paralysed, allowing it to fall backwards, thereby obstructing the patient's airway.

The basis of keeping an airway clear is extending the neck.

The nurse should place her fingers behind the angle of the jaw on each side, lifting it slightly forwards (Fig. 11.65a). This will pull upon the muscle attachments of the tongue, preventing it from falling backwards and thereby maintaining an unobstructed channel between the mouth and larynx. Alternatively the chin can be lifted forwards in a similar manner (Fig. 11.65b), but this latter method is not so efficient, especially if the patient has a receding chin.

An unobstructed airway is indicated by quiet respirations, noisy breathing is usually a sign of obstructed breathing. The position of the head or lower jaw may require adjustment to achieve this object — so the nurse should use her hands, sense of hearing and observe the patient's colour and respiration.

As the patient loses consciousness, following the i.v. injection of a barbiturate and relaxant, especially in emergency situations it is possible for regurgitation of stomach contents to occur before the anaesthetist has inserted the endotracheal tube. The nurse or anaesthetic assistant may be required to perform the Sellick manoeuvre as soon as unconsciousness intervenes.

The Sellick manoeuvre (cricoid pressure) (Sellick, 1961; Smith and Aitkenhead, 1985)

consists of temporary occlusion of the upper end of the oesophagus by backward pressure of the cricoid cartilage against the bodies of cervical vertebrae. This prevents regurgitation of oesophageal or stomach contents during induction of anaesthesia, and also prevents gastric distension from positive pressure ventilation administered by face mask (or mouth to mouth resuscitation).

Some anaesthetists prefer to inform the patient and apply cricoid pressure just before administration of the intravenous induction agent; others apply it as soon as consciousness is lost. The cricoid is palpated and lightly held between the thumb and forefinger of the right hand. The cricoid cartilage is pressed firmly in a posterior direction, thus pressing the oesophagus between the cricoid cartilage and the vertebral column. As soon as unconsciousness intervenes, firm pressure can be applied without obstructing the airway and this is maintained until the endotracheal tube has been inserted and the cuff inflated. The assistant may be asked to clip off the pilot tube when the anaesthetist has inflated the endotracheal tube cuff so that it just fits the lumen of the trachea. If a pair of haemostats is applied, only the tips are used, and as near the inflating syringe as possible; this reduces wear and tear of the pilot tube. Some endotracheal tubes incorporate a self-sealing valve, thereby obviating the need for forceps.

Hearing may become very acute as unconsciousness develops and it is the last sense to be depressed. It is therefore unwise for anyone to speak during the initial stages of anaesthesia. Bandages should not be touched, or covers removed until the patient is completely unconscious.

The anaesthesia nurse or assistant will hand instruments, etc., to the anaesthetist as required and like the scrub nurse in theatre, will try to anticipate his requirements.

The anaesthetist has many things to watch during the course of anaesthesia, including the colour of the patient, the pulse, respiration, blood pressure, cardiac activity (sometimes by means of an electro-cardiogram), in addition to keeping the general condition of the patient under observation. He *may* assign certain duties to the anaesthesia nurse or technician in this respect, and may require him or her to keep a record of the patient's pulse, and if sufficiently experienced, blood pressure also. He or she will adjust the rate of flow of transfusions, indicated by the anaesthetist, and replace transfusion solutions under his directions.

Guedal describes four stages of anaesthesia which are demonstrable with ether and cyclopropane. However, with the short-acting barbiturates, the patient falls rapidly asleep and excitement is rarely seen.

The first stage is one of analgesia when peripheral sensation is lost, but the nervous system is under control. In the first stage of induction there are frequently swallowing movements, followed by regular respiration and analgesia.

The second stage is one of excitement, with movement of the limbs followed by tonic spasms of the muscles, dilated pupils and roving eyeballs. Quite often this stage is very short and almost absent, especially when anaesthetising the deeply sedated patient.

The third stage is the stage of surgical anaesthesia which may range from moderate to deep according to the type of operation. During this stage, the anaesthetist is on his guard against:

The fourth stage which is respiratory and cardiac arrest.

If the patient collapses on the operation table with acute cardio-circulatory arrest his recovery may well depend upon prompt action by all the theatre staff. Without treatment, irreversible damage may occur in three minutes and a lasting recovery of the brain, and thus the whole body, is impossible after eight minutes.

As the anaesthetist and anaesthetic nurse have a vital part to play, the catastrophe is being dealt with in this chapter.

The following is an outline of the type of scheme most prevalent today.

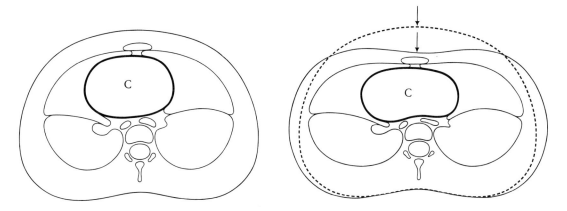

Fig. 11.66 External cardiac massage.

Cardiocirculatory arrest

If this has occurred immediate steps are taken to restore adequate ventilation and circulation. The anaesthesia nurse or assistant will be required to keep a record of the time from the first warning, calling out this time, initially, at 15 second intervals with particular emphasis at each minute.

The anaesthetist, having given warning and noted the time, tilts the operation table head downwards, stops the anaesthetic, ensures that the airway is clear, and administers oxygen under pressure. He may later pass an endotracheal tube if one is not already inserted; time is precious.

At the same time the surgeon commences external cardiac massage. (It is now accepted that circulation can generally be maintained in cardiac arrest without thoracotomy and by rhythmic external manual compression of the sternum which in turn compresses the heart between it and the spine, forcing out blood into the aorta. Relaxation of the thoracic cage releases the pressure on the heart and allows it to fill with blood. This must be done on a rigid surface similar to the operation table, boards under a mattress or on the floor.) The compression on the lower half of the sternum must be by the heels of the hands (not the fingers), one on top of the other, aided by the weight of the body. This pressure should not be exerted on the ribs or epigastrium otherwise fracture of the ribs or rupture of the liver or spleen may occur.

Depression of the sternum should be at least 3 to 4 cm with each stroke, with a frequency of 60 strokes per minute. This should produce a palpable radial pulse with a blood pressure of 8 to 13 kPa (60 to 100 mmHg). Rhythmic compression of the sternum, whilst giving good temporary artificial circulation, does not produce effective ventilation. This must be accomplished either by manual compression of the anaesthesia machine bag, or attachment of the endotracheal tube to a ventilator.

If the patient responds, the surgeon may instruct his assistant and the scrub nurse to complete any vital stage in the operation. Alternatively he will hand over cardiac massage to the assistant and complete the operation himself.

Immediately cardiac massage has been started, the circulating nurse or anaesthesia nurse fetches the cardiac resuscitation set which comprises various drugs, transfusion fluids and equipment, syringes and needles, electrical defibrillator (external or internal) and if possible an electrocardiograph monitor, which should be connected to the patient (Chapter 3).

When ventricular asystole is responsible for the arrest of circulation, external massage may re-establish normal rhythm. If there is no response, intracardiac injections may be tried. The most generally used is adrenaline 1 in 10,000 dosage 3 to 5 ml intracardiac or if a very slow ventricular rate has been established, adrenaline 1 in 10,000, 1 ml per minute intravenously. This is for myocardial stimulation.

Calcium chloride, 10 per cent may be given intracardiac or intravenously in a dosage up to 10 ml, this increases tone in a flabby heart.

These measures may provoke ventricular fibrillation which can then be treated with a D.C. counter shock administered by the defibrillator. A D.C. counter shock may also be tried to provoke ventricular fibrillation (if massage is unsuccessful) which can be treated with a second shock. The shock should be given starting (manual control) at 200 J/2 to 4 millisecond.

If a defibrillator is unavailable, ventricular fibrillation can sometimes be treated by intravenous lignocaine (xylocaine) 200 mg or propranolol (Inderal) 5 mg given slowly.

With cardiac arrest of more than the briefest duration, acidosis, both metabolic and respiratory, is likely. If the period of arrest exceeds 2 minutes or if cardiac massage has been carried out for longer than 15 minutes, the patient should have 200/500 ml of 4.2 per cent sodium bicarbonate intravenously.

The blood pressure should be maintained if necessary by the addition of isoprenaline (Aleudrin) or metaraminol (Aramine) to the intravenous fluid.

If pulmonary oedema is suspected or if the volume of intravenous fluid given has exceeded 1500 ml, a diuretic may be given (e.g., frusemide (Lasix) 20 mg or more intravenously).

If normal consciousness does not return fairly quickly, there may be cerebral oedema (which invariably follows a period of anoxia) which may be treated by intravenous 50 per cent sucrose or Urevert.

Two indications for open thoracotomy and direct cardiac massage are (a) inability to restore a radial pulse and satisfactory blood pressure (e.g., in a stout patient when compression of the sternum is difficult or in chest injuries involving the rib cage) and (b) the absence of a D.C. defibrillator when only an A.C. defibrillator is available for direct application to a fibrillating heart.

General outline of procedure for cardiocirculatory arrest:
1. Arrested heart
2. External massage, controlled pulmonary ventilation
3. No beat; adrenaline given or attempt with D.C. shocks, this causes beat or
4. Fibrillation of the heart
5. D.C. defibrillator applied using large moistened, firmly attached electrodes with a surface area of at least 10 cm and supplying in adults 200 to 400 J D.C. over 2 to 4 milliseconds. All staff take hands off patient to avoid a personal electric shock.
6. Beat recommences
7. Intravenous transfusion of 200/500 ml of 4.2 per cent sodium bicarbonate, plus possibly noradrenaline to maintain blood pressure
8. Endotracheal tube passed at earliest opportunity, artificial ventilation continued until normal respirations recommence
9. If external massage unsuccessful, direct massage via a thoracotomy may be considered. If the chest is opened, antibiotics should be given.

Cardiac-respiratory arrest trolley. It is prudent to assemble together the apparatus and drugs required for the treatment of cardiac-respiratory arrest. This may consist of a simple trolley for use within the operating suite or a more complex unit designed to transport the equip-

Table 11.1 Essential contents of a cardiac resuscitation trolley.

Airways: Sizes 4–00.	Connections (3)	
Laryngoscopes: Adult Blade.	Ambu Bag to Endotracheal.	
Child Blade.	Strapping: 12 mm (0.5 in).	
Pen Torch.	Scissors: Small straight Mayo's.	
Mouth Gag.	Sterile Intracardiac Needle.	
Magill's Forceps.	Butterfly needles and infusion sets	
20 ml Syringe.		
Defibrillator.	*DRUGS ON TROLLEY*	
Electrode Jelly.	Calcium Chloride 10%	10 ml.
Suction Unit with Yankauers Sucker.	Atropine Sulphate	600 micrograms/ml
Oxygen Cylinder.		
Ambu Resuscitator.		
Cardiac Arrest Board.	Dextran 40, 70 and 110 (Rheomacrodex, Macrodex, Dextraven) plasma substitute	500 ml
Endotracheal Tubes. Sizes from 9.5 to 5.5 with connections.		
Spencer Wells Artery Forceps.	Gelatin (Haemacel) plasma substitute	500 ml
Sphygmomanometer.		
Needles: 4 No. 15.	Adrenaline	1/10.000.
4 No. 1.	Ketamine (Ketalur)	10 mg
Syringes: 2×1 cm^3.	Pentazocine (Fortral)	30 mg/ml
2×5 cm^3.	Naloxone (Narcan)	400 microground/mlmicrogram
2×2 cm^3.		
Elastoplast 75 cm (3 in).		
i.v. Cut down set.	Diazapam (Diazemuls)	5 mg/ml
Disposable Giving Set.	Hydrocortisone	100 mg/ml
Intracath.	Lignocaine 1%	10 ml.
i.v. Needles.	Propranolol	1 mg/ml in 2 ml.
Stethoscope.		
Receiver with suction catheters.	Sodium Bicarbonate B.P.	8.4% or 4.2%

ment to other parts of the hospital. In the latter case, in addition to laryngoscopes and endotracheal tubes with their connections, Ambu resuscitator, the trolley should contain, a portable suction device, bronchoscope, defibrillator, ECG monitor and equipment for setting up a transfusion.

The drugs most likely to be needed in the treatment of cardiac arrest are:

Cardiac arrest. Adrenaline (epinephrine) 1 in 10,000 10 ml

Calcium chloride 10 per cent 10 ml

Lignocaine (Xylocaine) 1 per cent 10 ml

Sodium bicarbonate 8.4 per cent i.v. (equivalent to 1 mEq/ml) dosage 100 ml initially after 30 seconds arrest or 4.2 per cent dosage 200 ml initially.

Supportive cardiac therapy. Isoprenaline 200 micrograms/ml diluted to 500 ml with a 5 per cent dextrose solution i.v.

Potassium chloride (1.5 g in 10 ml) diluted to 500 ml with a 5 per cent dextrose solution i.v. (20 mEq potassium)

Myocardial failure. Digoxin (Lanoxin) 250 micrograms/ml i.v.

Oubain (Ouabaine Arnaud) 250 micrograms/ml.

Frusemide (Lasix) 10 mg/ml i.v.

Cerebral dehydration and diuresis. Mannitol solution 20 per cent (dose 1 to 200 ml)

Respiratory complications

Adrenaline 1:10,000

Aminophylline 250 mg per 10 ml i.v.

Naloxone (Narcan) 100

Hydrocortisone 100 mg/ml i.v.

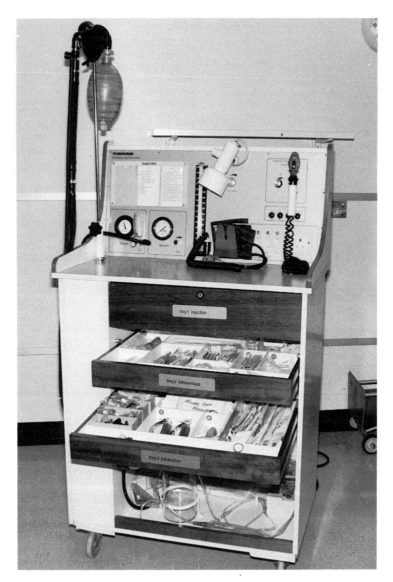

Fig. 11.67   Cardiac arrest trolley.

When the operation is completed the anaesthetist will give instructions to the nurse accompanying the patient back to the ward. Under no circumstances must the patient leave the theatre suite until the anaesthetist is satisfied that he is fit to do so.

A good airway must be maintained in the manner described earlier but if there is any doubt regarding this or the possibility that the patient may vomit, he should be placed on his side with the underlying limb flexed, and the shoulders supported.

The patient is transferred carefully to the trolley or bed with minimal movement, and covered with blankets before leaving the theatre suite. After returning him to his bed, if it is necessary to roll him to recover, this must be done very gently, not only to avoid injury to the operation area, but also because a sudden rapid movement of the unconscious patient can cause cardiac arrest.

A tray containing mouth gag, tongue forceps, boxwood wedge, small towel, and vomit bowl or kidney dish should be carried with the patient during transit between the theatre and recovery ward. These instruments must remain by the bed until the patient has recovered consciousness.

An airway or endotracheal tube left in position by the anaesthetist post-operatively should not be removed until the patient attempts to reject it. Attempts at rejection by the patient reveal that his swallowing reflex has returned and that unless there is any clinical contra-indication, the tube may be removed.

Oxygen administered post-operatively to an unconscious patient should be given by means of a suitable catheter, mask or oxygen tent. On rare occasions, if an endotracheal tube is *in situ*, oxygen may be given via a catheter passed into the lumen of the tube for a few inches. The oxygen flow in this latter case should not be above 3 litres per minute. The recovery of a patient in the recovery ward may be prolonged depending on the anaesthetic used. The awakening from natural sleep is generally quite different to the patient's experience in recovering from anaesthesia (Asbury, 1974). For further information on recovery nursing the reader is referred to textbooks devoted to this subject (Norris and Campbell, 1985; Campbell and Spence, 1983; Buxton Hopkin, 1970).

REFERENCES

ASBURY, A. J. (1974) *Nursing Times*, January 24, 106.
BUXTON HOPKIN, D. A. (1970) *Anaesthesia, Recovery and Intensive Care*. London: English University Press.
CAMPBELL, D. AND SPENCE, A. A. (1983) *Norris and Campbell's Nurse's Guide to Anaesthetics, Resuscitation and Intensive Care*, Edinburgh: Churchill Livingstone.
COX, H. (1987) The peri-operative role (a personal view), *NATNews*, **24**, No. 1, 15–16
COATES, L. (1974) *AORN Journal*, **19**, 1091–1104.
DEPARTMENT OF HEALTH AND SOCIAL SECURITY (1976) Pollution of operating departments by anaesthetic gases, HC 76/38.
DONWORTH, G. (1987) On the road to recovery, *NATNews*, **24**, No. 1, 12–14
GRUENDEMANN, B. J. (1973) *The Surgical Patient: Behavioural Concepts for the O.R. Nurse*. St. Louis: Mosby.
HAID, B. AND HOSSLI, G. (1956) *Cardiac and Respiratory Arrest*. Roche Products Ltd.
JUDD, P. A., TOMLIN, P. J., WHITBY, J. L., INGLIS, T. C. M. AND ROBINSON, J. S. (1968) *Lancet*, ii, 1019.
LIGHT, S. (1979) *Nursing Mirror*, January 11, 20.
LUMLEY, J. (1976) *British Journal of Anaesthesia*, **48**, 3.
MACKENSIE, C. F., KLOSE, S. AND BROWNE, D. R. G. (1976) *British Journal of Anaesthesia*, **48**, 105.
MILLINGTON, C. (1976) *NATNews*, **13**, 18–22.
MURRAY WILSON, A (1971) *Nursing Times*, November 11, 1406.
NORRIS, W. AND CAMPBELL, D. 1985 *Anaesthetics, Resuscitation and Intensive Care*, Ethedn. Edinburgh: Churchill Livingstone.
NORTH-WEST THAMES REGIONAL HEALTH AUTHORITY (1980) Personal communication.
ROSE, M. (1978) Vacuum pipelines for anaesthetic pollution control. *British Medical Journal*, 21st January, p. 176
ROGERS, P. M. (1975) *AORN Journal*, **21**, 1278–1288.
SAYLOR, D. R. (1975) *AORN Journal*, **22**, 624–636.
SELLICK, B. A. (1961) *Lancet*, ii, 494–496.
SHAW, H. (1977) The Nursing Process, the Operating Theatre and Patient. Unpublished paper; Theatre Nursing Education and Research Fellowship Fund.
SMITH, G. AND AITKEN HEAD, A. R. (1985) *Textbook of Anaesthesia*. Edinburgh: Churchill Livingstone.
SPENCE, A. A. AND KNILL-JONES, R. P. (1978) *British Journal of Anaesthesia*, **50**, 713.
STEVENS, H. R. (1969) *Lancet*, i, 732.
SYKES, M. K. (1946) *British Medical Journal*, i, 561.
VESSEY, M. P. AND NUNN, J. F. (1980) Occupational Hazards of Anaesthesia, *British Medical Journal*, **281**, 696–698

12

Operating microscopes

(The illustrations in this chapter, unless indicated otherwise, have been provided by Carl Zeiss (Ober Kochen) Ltd.)

Binocular operating microscopes have become indispensable equipment for an increasing range of surgical procedures. A great number of new surgical interventions that were previously impossible have evolved from the continued application of microsurgical techniques.

Microsurgery in its present form is thought to have started with Dr Karl Nylen, Assistant Medical Director of the University of Stockholm Ear Clinic in 1921, when he used for the first time a low power monocular microscope for ear surgery. He then took a Zeiss Slit Lamp in 1922, added a light source and suitable support, and thereby created the first true binocular operating microscope.

In spite of this success, binocular loupes and loupes mounted to spectacle frames predominated over the use of compound microscopes for three decades until, in 1953, the first complete operating microscope, designed primarily for ear surgery, was introduced by Carl Zeiss in West Germany to the design of one of its scientists, Dr H Littmann.

Some thousand operating microscopes of this type were in use in otology before it was adopted in other surgical disciplines. In 1966, the introduction of large computers made possible the solving of complex optical problems in the design of 'zoom' type microscopes and the first motorised zoom instrument appeared. These were more suited to ophthalmology, and the use of the microscope rapidly spread through peripheral nerve surgery, vascular surgery and reconstructive surgery. The advent of double microscopes enabled the use of an assistant in hand surgery. There is now hardly a surgical discipline which does not make use of the microscope.

BASIC PRINCIPLES

The operating microscope achieves two purposes. The first is to provide a magnified image of small objects, and the second is to provide a magnified view of larger areas upon which more precise surgery can be performed.

The operating microscope consists of a stereo microscope, which in principle is two monocular microscopes placed side by side. Each of the monocular systems provides a slightly different angular view of the object, thereby providing a three dimensional image. This three dimensional image is essential for providing depth perception, so that the surgeon may place his instruments and sutures accurately on the required spot.

Most operating microscopes consist of four basic components (Fig. 12.1):
1. the binocular tube, which contains the eyepieces, attached to
2. the main body of the instrument, which incorporates

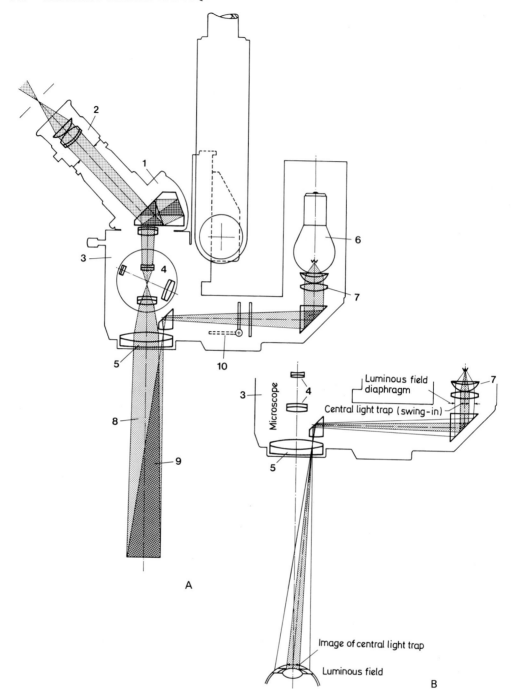

Fig. 12.1 A. The component parts and optical paths of an operating microscope.

1. Binocular tube
2. Eyepieces
3. Body
4. Magnification changer
5. Objective
6. Illumination
7. Collector lens system for illumination
8. Observation beam path
9. Illumination beam path
10. Swing-in filters.

B. The principle of the swing-in pupil eclipsing device for ophthalmology, which protects the patient's macula from excessive radiation during long surgical operations.

3. optics for varying the magnification, and screwed into this on the lowest part
4. is an objective or lens, which can be interchanged.

In addition to this viewing unit, an illumination system is attached. This allows light from a suitable source to be fed onto the operating area, either via the microscope body and through the lens, or additionally/alternatively at an angle onto the operating site.

The whole of the viewing and illuminating system is attached to a fine focussing slide which is carried on some form of support or stand by means of couplings that will vary according to the type of surgery being performed. The most common system is the mobile floor stand which can be wheeled up to the operation table. However, this can impinge on the space around the operation table required for surgeon/s, assistants, scrubbed nurse, trolleys for instruments, peripheral equipment and the anaesthesia team. A solution to this problem is to have the microscope mounted on a ceiling suspension unit, thus clearing the theatre floor. These units can be mounted onto a track system, so that when not in use, the microscope can be parked out of the way against the theatre wall.

THE OPERATING MICROSCOPE

Bodies

There are two basic types of operating microscope, with several variations upon each, depending upon the surgical specialty involved (Fig. 12.2). The first is the manual type, featuring fixed magnification steps and manual focus. It is normally favoured in ENT surgery, where routine microsurgical techniques at a standard magnification are regularly used. The usual instrument features five magnification steps of $\times$ 0.4, 0.6, 1.0, 1.6, 2.5.

The second type is the zoom system; this has the advantage of offering stepless magnification through the whole of its range, which can be in the ranges of 1:4, 1:5, or 1:6 depending upon the model. This is applicable to the more sophisticated types of microsurgery for the following reasons:

1. The precise magnification required for any task can be selected.
2. By zooming, the user can continuously monitor the whole operating area at low magnification and complete the detailed work at high magnification.
3. The zoom action can be motorised and controlled by a foot switch, freeing the hands completely for the microsurgery.
4. For documentation recording, it enables the detail on film or television to be precisely determined.

Objectives

An objective for an operating microscope is described by its focal length, i.e. a 200 mm objective focusses at this distance from the operation site. Because an objective is a 'thick' lens made up of several lens elements cemented together to achieve the necessary high image quality, this focal length is always slightly greater than the working distance. The focal length of the objective is one factor in determining the overall magnification obtained, and this is one reason for selecting a given objective, the other is the required working distance. It would be no good selecting a focal length too great (the user would be too stretched to be comfortable) nor too small (no room for access of instruments). A range of objectives for the operating microscope are available from 50 mm to 2000 mm, the extremes of this range being for specialised purposes; for normal microsurgery the range extends from 150 mm to 400 mm in 25 mm steps.

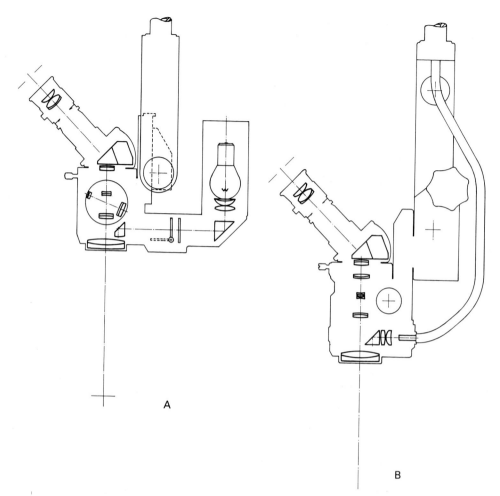

Fig. 12.2 Design principles of operating microscopes. (A) With 5-stage magnification changer, manual operation. (B) With zoom system and integral fibre-optics illumination, motorised zoom operation.

Binoculars

These too have a focal length (f = 80 mm, 125 mm, 160 mm, 170 mm) and also affect the overall magnification. Their design varies with the surgical requirements (Figs. 12.3 and 12.4). They are made 'straight' where the predominant use of the microscope is horizontal or angled at up to 45°, 'inclined' where the predominant use is vertical, or in an 'inclinable' variation where it is essential that the microscope can be used at any angle. The inclinable version also has the advantage that surgeons with different back lengths can adopt a comfortable operating position. All binoculars have the ability to adjust to the user's inter-pupillary distance.

Eyepieces

These come in varying magnifications, classifically: 8 x, 10 x, 12.5 x, 16 x and 20 x. Modern versions screw into the binocular tubes rather than push-in as in earlier versions. This ensures that incorrect positioning of the eyepieces in the binocular is avoided.

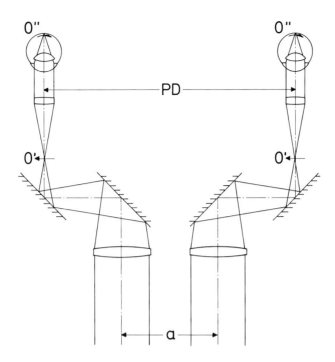

Fig. 12.3 The inter-relationship of binocular tube and eyepiece (schematic) O' = intermediate image plane; O'' = image on the retina; PD = interpupillary distance; a = stereo base of binocular and microscope body.

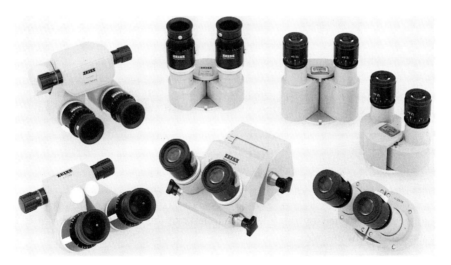

Fig. 12.4 Range of binocular tubes.

For many years eyepieces have accommodated spectacle wearers, but in the past few years prescription spectacles have become fashionably larger, resulting in an increased back vertex focal distance; the image of the latest wide field eyepieces is formed further away from the eyepiece lens. One of the commonest mistakes in using the microscope is incorrect positioning of the eye in relation to the image formed by the eyepiece: it is essential that

the head is in the correct place to avoid the 'keyhole' effect that can occur. Eyepieces also include a dioptre setting with lock, in the range of + or − 8 dioptre. Ametropes within this statistically most frequent range can work without their spectacles if they wish, provided the ametropia requires only spherical and not cylindrical correction of astigmatism. In the latter case, it is imperative that the prescription spectacles are worn and that the dioptre setting of the eyepieces is put at 0.

Magnification/field of view

It will be seen from the above that the final magnification (and corresponding field of view) will vary depending upon the combinations chosen. Whilst this information is always given in the operating instructions supplied by the manufacturer, it is worthwhile to be aware of the formula used in the calculation.

VM = total magnification of an operating microscope

$$VM = \frac{fT}{fO} \times y \times VE$$

Where
  fT = focal length of binocular
  fO = focal length of objective
  y   = engraved factor on knob of manual microscope mag. changer or magnification factor displayed in the window of a zoom microscope.
  VE = magnification of eyepiece.
  e.g. Manual microscope, bino f = 125
      objective f = 200
      magnification changer 1.6
      eyepiece 12.5 x

$$\text{Final magnification} = \frac{125}{200} \times 1.6 \times 12.5 \, x = 12.5 \, x$$

The *Field of View* (FV) is the diameter of the area seen magnified expressed in millimeters. In the case of Zeiss microscopes, this is arrived at from the formulae:

A. Older type binoculars

$$FV = \frac{200}{VM}$$

Where:
  200 is a constant formed by the internal diameter of the binocular, and VM is the total magnification of the microscope.

  e.g. $\frac{200}{12.5} = 16$ mm.

B. New wide angle binoculars

Where:
  220 is a constant and VM the total magnification.

  e.g. $\frac{220}{12.5} = 17.6$ mm.

Stands

Several factors have combined over recent years to necessitate redesign of the old type of microscope floor stands. The microscope has in many cases become more sophisticated, sometimes with several different motorised controls (focussing, zoom, x-y movement, motorised slit illuminators) and more accessories (Fig. 12.5). These include surgical lasers that can be directly attached to the microscope, and closed circuit colour television for those members of the team who can't actually see the operation being performed through the microscope.

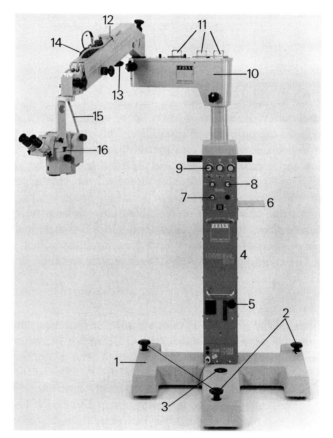

Fig. 12.5 The Carl Zeiss operating microscope stand S3B

1. Stable base on 5 double castors
2. Levelling feet for locking movement
3. Spirit level (*by adjustment of feet* [2], *allowance can be made for unevenness of theatre floor*)
4. Column, containing electrical assemblies for functions of microscope
5. Sockets, for insertion of foot or hand control switches
6. ON-OFF switch
7. Control knob for built-in bi-polar coagulator (*output socket adjacent*)
8. Variable speed controls for zoom and focus
9. Rheostat controls for up to three lighting systems, with selectors for illumination type
10. Horizontal arm rotatable 285°, with knobs for setting the ease of motion and locking the joints
11. Integrated fibre-optic illumination system for 1 or 2 lamps, with spare slide-in module
12. Articulated suspension arm for counterbalancing microscope weights from 3 kg to 18 kg
13. Safety slider for patient protection
14. Outlets for all functions of microscope and accessories
15. Fibre-optic cable for 'cool light' co-axial illumination
16. Operating microscope.

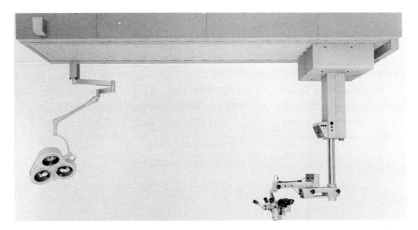

Fig. 12.6 Ceiling-mounted operating microscope on electro-mechanical track. When not in use, the microscope can be parked out of the way against the wall of the theatre.

Modern floor stands offer the ability to carry more weight, have a longer reach on the carrying arm and remove the problems of instability. The more complex versions have such facilities as built-in bi-polar coagulators and multi-illumination outlets.

Ceiling suspension units have the same sort of facilities and the added advantage of clearing floor space. The tracked versions have motorised movement across the theatre for parking (Fig. 12.6).

The particularly intricate positioning of the microscope in neurosurgery has led to the production of specialised floor and ceiling stands, where the complete instrument is balanced to move easily in any conceivable direction and then instantly locked in that position by magnetic switches. These can be activated by finger trigger controls, or a mouth switch.

Controls

In the case of the manual microscope, all controls such as focussing, magnification change and tilt of the microscope are done by hand knobs. These can be covered with sterilizable rubber caps, or the complete instrument can be draped with a sterile plastic drape (Fig. 10.8, Chapter10).

With motorised microscopes, the functions are normally controlled by a foot switch, or the controls built into a specially designed operating chair (Fig. 12.7). They can alternatively be controlled through a hand switch, which can be inserted into a sterile plastic bag before use.

The complexity of the modern microscope means that an ophthalmic instrument can provide 14 functions, and to find all these switches on one panel needs lots of practice. This has led to the development of the Voice Activated Microscope. Through a microphone attached to the binocular, the operator gives instructions to the control unit (fitted to the stand), which responds audibly to confirm that the function is understood; all the functions are then controlled from one foot switch.

The unit is available in several different languages and can be programmed to respond to the surgeon's voice pattern after a short training session. It is possible to store in memory the voice patterns of up to 15 different users, each of whom must enter his code number before starting the operation. The voice control will then ignore words spoken by other members of the team and respond only to the user.

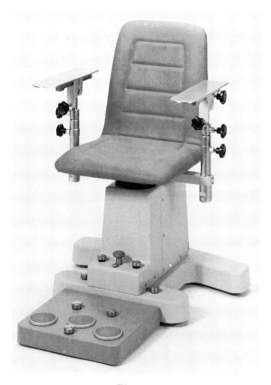

Fig. 12.7

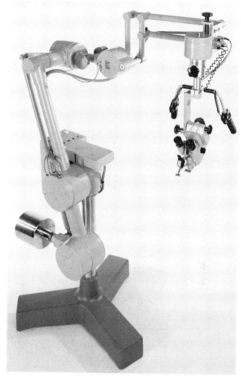

Fig. 12.8

Fig. 12.7 Motorised operating chair, with adjustable arm supports and foot switches controlling all microscope functions.

Fig. 12.8 The Contraves stand for micro-neurosurgery. The complete microscope is balanced for weightless manoeuvrability in any conceivable direction and locked by magnetic switches activated by trigger controls or mouth switch.

Illumination

Whilst co-axial illumination still remains the most commonly used (essential for deep surgery, as in ENT), a wide choice now exists. It can be of moderate intensity — 6 v 30 w tungsten, high intensity — 12 v 100 w halogen quartz: both in integral lamp housings at the rear of the body. Alternatively, illumination can be provided by a remote source 12 v 100 w halogen quartz fibre-optic light generator mounted in the arm of the stand. The latter has the advantage of lowering the temperature of both the microscope and the operation site, and of enabling a fused lamp to be replaced quickly, away from the immediate areas of the operation. For neurosurgery the fibre-optic light source can be 250 w metal halide. Additionally, inclined illumination and a motorised slit lamp is available for ophthalmology.

Hazards of light

It has been demonstrated in recent investigations that direct high intensity illumination on to a patient's macula in eye surgery can result in permanent damage to the retina. For this reason occlusion discs can be fitted to older microscopes; these swing into the light path and protect the patient (Fig. 12.1a). Modern fibre-optic systems for ophthalmology usually provide a switchable change from co-axial to oblique illumination, so that direct light is only

offered to the patient's retina for the brief period necessary to check the cleanliness of the posterior capsule.

Additionally, swing-in filters are provided in newer instruments to protect both the patient and the eyes of the surgeon from the so-called 'blue light hazard', by removing the violet/lower blues end of the spectrum from the illuminated field.

Co-observation and assistants' microscopes

Many different, and at first sight confusing, systems are in use to enable someone other than the surgeon to view what is happening during microsurgery.

It is important to understand the difference between co-observation and assistants' microscopes. The previous paragraph, entitled 'Basic principles', describes how a three-dimensional image is formed by the two telescopes that form an operating microscope. The 'stereo base' upon which this principle is constructed, is the separation of the two separate beams of the microscope (Fig. 12.3). This distance is normally 22 mm (Carl Zeiss, West Germany). By the introduction of a beam splitter (Fig. 12.9), the image can be split 50/50 between the main microscope and two side ports (for co-observation and/or image recording). In one of these ports ca be fitted either a monocular or binocular co-observation system. Thus, by viewing through one of these systems, another member of the team, e.g. scrub nurse, can follow the operation closely. In the case of the binocular system, the view obtained will be a true three-dimensional image. However, in this case, the stereo base is not formed from two beams, but by splitting only one of them; the stereo base is 7 mm. This reduces the stereoscopic impression considerably, and together with the increased overall distance from the operation site, makes this system unsuitable for direct co-operation in the operation.

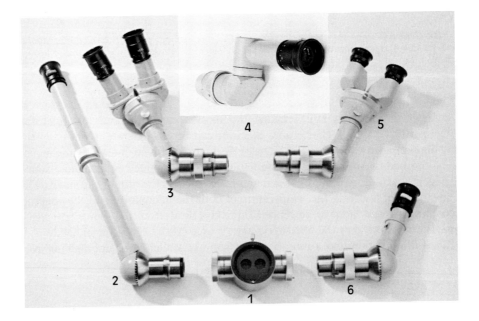

Fig. 12.9 Co-observation tubes
1. Beam splitter into which are fitted: camera, television or the following:
2. Long monocular
3. Bino (*inclined*) observation
4. Multi-angle short monocular
5. Bino (*straight*) observation
6. Short monocular.

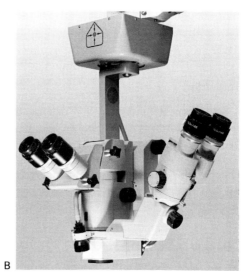

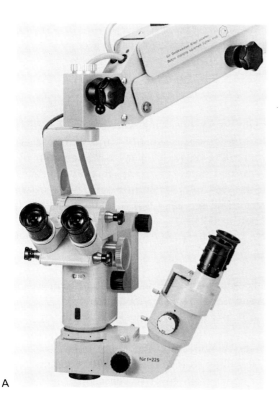

A

Fig. 12.10 Assistants' microscopes: (A) 8°, (B) 0°.

An assistants' microscope, on the other hand, has the same stereo base as the main microscope (Fig. 12.10). It can be equipped with its own independent three step magnification changer, so that the assistant can select a different magnification from the surgeon.

Constant development over the years has reduced the angle at which an assistants' microscope looks at the operation site in relation to the main instrument. The early ones had an angle of 27°, followed by 19° and more recently 8°. In 1986, Carl Zeiss introduced their latest assistants' microscope, the 0° version. This shares exactly the same view as the main microscope, around which it can be rotated, and, for example, makes possible for the first time the involvement of an assistant in vitreous body surgery.

Documentation

Early camera systems for the operating microscope were very much of the hit and miss variety, and the excellent photographs produced by some users really demonstrated their skill as photographers. The introduction of high speed artificial light colour films, and 35 mm cameras with automatic exposure control, has simplified documentation recording enormously. It is also possible now to equip the microscope with co-axial flash equipment, controlled by a sensor in the modern 35 mm camera, for the more difficult situations sometimes experienced.

Cine cameras adapted for the microscope have been around for a number of years, but the relatively high cost of cine film and the introduction of low priced, high quality colour television cameras, together with video recorders, has led to a decrease in the use of cine film and an increase in colour video recording.

In documentation recording, it is imperative that one eyepiece (preferably the one on the same side as the camera) is equipped with a focussing aid graticule to obviate accommodation errors.

Television

It is possible to mount a TV camera on virtually every operating microscope. A ceiling mounted microscope will accept even extremely large broadcast quality cameras, but in the last few years many excellent, light weight, single tube colour cameras have come on the market. These, together with the even more recent solid state, very compact and inexpensive cameras, are revolutionising microsurgery from the viewpoint of theatre staff. Whereas no-one but the surgeon and possibly the scrub nurse could see what was happening, now it is feasible for the whole team to follow the operation in detail.

Care and maintenance

Despite the complexity of the modern operating microscope, its care and maintenance as far as theatre staff are concerned is a relatively simple matter, provided that:

a. At least two members of staff are given total responsibility for checking, setting up and storing the instrument.

b. Those members have received adequate instruction from the manufacturer of the microscope (whose representatives will always be willing to give the necessary training).

c. They have read the appropriate instruction books from cover to cover.

d. The staff know precisely what adjustment and maintenance may be carried out by themselves, and when it is necessary to call in a specialist service engineer.

e. Ample supplies of spare parts, such as lamps, fuses and sterilizable caps or disposable drapes are always kept in stock.

f. It is realised by all that an operating microscope is a precision instrument that is expensive and must be treated with care. The cost of a manual operating microscope is about as much as a new car in the medium price bracket, and a sophisticated motorised instrument can cost as much as a new house.

Preparation of the microscope ready for the operation

To set up the microscope for an operation, the following tasks must be carried out:

1. Position the microscope for the specific operation and the comfort of the surgeon, bearing in mind the space requirements of the assistant, scrub nurse, anaesthesia team and the necessary equipment and sterile trolleys.

2. Check the path of the mains lead from the wall socket, ensuring that it does not constitute a hazard and that it will not be run over by heavy equipment.

3. Check the security and tighten, if necessary, the safety locks between microscope and couplings and couplings and stand.

4. Ensure that where different objectives and binocular tubes are available, the correct ones are fitted for the particular operation.

5. Check the cleanliness of objectives and eyepieces and clean if necessary, not forgetting any assistants' microscope or observer tube.

6. Switch on the microscope, first at the wall socket, second at the stand and lastly, switch on the lights (after the operation this procedure must be reversed — first switch off lights,

next stand, lastly wall). This prevents a sudden surge of current through the lamps, shortening their life.

7. Check that all the lights on the microscope are working and replace faulty lamps.

8. Check that all the functions of the microscope are working. These can include focus, zoom, x-y movement, motorised slit lamp movement, and bi-polar coagulator in respect of motorised microscopes, focussing, magnification change and geared couplings in manual instruments.

9. Check the balance of the microscope with the accessories to be used and adjust as necessary.

10. Adjust the tension on the various movements of the microscope arms etc. to match the requirements of the individual surgeon.

11. Bring the microscope to the working position and set the angle of the body (vertical, horizontal or inclined) perpendicular to the pathology of the particular operation site.

12. Set the inclination of the binocular (if variable), the dioptre setting of the eyepieces, and the inter-pupillary distance of the binocular to the user's requirements. A card record kept for each surgeon will simplify this procedure. Alternatively this may be done by the surgeon himself prior to scrubbing.

13. Ensure that the focussing, and if fitted, the x-y coupling are at the centre point of their travel (nothing is more frustrating for a user than needing to move the microscope and finding it is at the extremity of its range).

14. If sterilizable caps are being used (these are available for all controls that need to be handled by scrubbed personnel), check that enough sets are to hand to last until they can be re-autoclaved. In addition, make sure that you have one or two individual spares; they may be accidentially pulled off and dropped to the floor.

Problems with the microscope

It is important that the user is fully aware of how to set up the microscope to suit his or her own eyes. Most problems that occur are associated with incorrect setting up procedures. An incorrectly set up microscope will result in its use being both tedious and unsatisfactory. The check list that follows should be used:

Interpupillary distance (PD). The distance between the two pupils of the eye varies between 48 mm and 76 mm. The binocular tube can be narrowed or widened to match. When correctly set up, the PD can be read from a scale on most modern binoculars (Fig. 12.11).

To determine individual PD, the binocular should be set to maximum PD and an attempt made to look through the microscope; only one eye will see an image. The PD should be closed whilst continuing to look; two images will appear as the correct PD is approached, the distance between these two images must be reduced until they coincide. This value, which is the individual's PD, is read off and noted.

Eyepieces

(*a*) *Dioptre setting.* As already mentioned (see Basic principles, eyepieces) spectacle wearers can keep their glasses on and dial 'O' at the dioptre setting. But the image seen down a microscope is an 'infinity' image, which means that only distance spectacles should be worn, not reading, bi- or multi-focal lenses.

If spectacles are not worn it must not be assumed that the dioptre setting is automatically

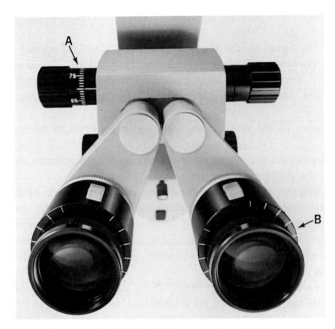

Fig. 12.11 Adjusting the microscope for individual vision correction. (A) Interpupillary adjustment scale. (B) Dioptre setting adjustment scale.

'O', it may be + or − a little, and each eye may be different. To determine an individual's dioptre setting (Fig. 12.11), proceed as follows:

(i) Set eyepieces to 'O'.

(ii) Set coarse focus of microscope, at lowest magnification, by means of arm of stand onto a piece of graph paper, or onto a cross drawn on a piece of paper.

(iii) Set zoom or manual magnification changer to highest magnification. Carefully focus the microscope with foot or hand control.

(iv) Without changing the focus, change the magnification down to its lowest position.

(v) Adjust each eyepiece to bring the cross/graph paper into sharp focus. Do this by starting at the maximum + dioptre setting and turning the eyepiece clockwise; if the sharpest focus position is passed, it should be returned to fully anti-clockwise setting and clockwise movement started again. The focussing of the microscope should not be adjusted at all during this operation.

(vi) Steps (iii), (iv) and (v) are repeated.

(vii) A note is made of the dioptre setting for each eye and kept for future reference.

If the dioptre setting is correct, then after focussing the microscope at high magnification, it will still be in focus when changing down through the magnification range.

(b) Pushed in? With push-in eyepieces, check that they are pushed fully home into the binocular.

Relationship of eye to eyepiece. As well as an observation beam path, the microscope has an illumination beam path; the latter comes into focus as an 'exit pupil'. Only if the exit pupil of the microscope is brought into the pupil plane of the eye will the microscope be properly usable. Failure to achieve this will result in two faults:

1. The full field of view offered by the microscope is not seen. As if looking through a keyhole, the head must be turned to change the viewing direction. Under these conditions a stereoscopic impression may never be gained.

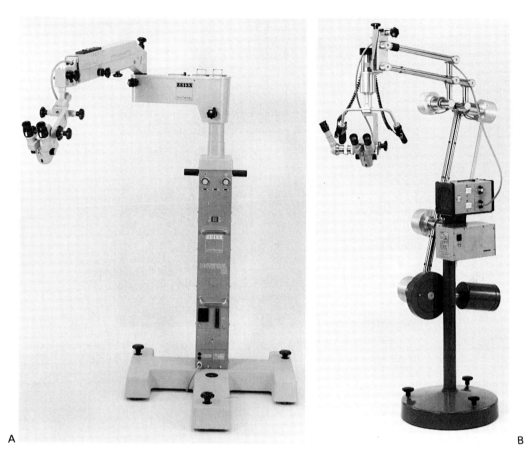

A   B

Fig. 12.12 ENT operating microscope, which has the following characteristics:
(i) Manual focus and five step magnification changer
(ii) Cool light fibre-optic illuminaton
(iii) Straight biocular tube and objectives 200 mm for middle ear surgery, and 400 mm for laryngeal procedures. (A) Microscope mounted on a standard counterbalanced floor stand. (B) Microscope mounted on weightless balance Contraves stand.

2. A decrease in image brightness will be found, as only a fraction of the light rays will reach the user's retina. This is often the cause of complaints that the microscope hasn't enough light, and requests to the staff to increase the intensity.

In practice, the user's eyes are likely to be not close enough to the eyepieces: only very rarely are users too close. People with deep set eyes should fold back the rubber eyecups, or slide in the adjusting tubes of the eyepieces.

The plane of the eyepieces' exit pupil can easily be found by holding a sheet of white paper behind the eyepieces in a dimmed room; site and lateral extension of the microscopes' exit pupil are given by the narrowest point of the light bundle emitting from the microscope.

Comfort and relaxation

a. The user should be seated as comfortably as possible, sitting with a straight back and not a curved spine. As much support as possible should be provided for the forearms, wrists and hands, and the microsurgery performed with the fingers unstressed. This can be

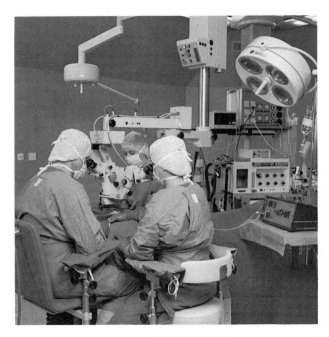

Fig. 12.13 Ophthalmic operating microscope. The OpMi 6CFCXY instrument, controlled from an operating chair, is mounted on an electro-mechanical ceiling suspension unit, and has the following features:
  (i) Fully motorised focus, zoom (1:6 ratio) and X-Y movement.
 (ii) Inclinable binocular.
(iii) Cool light fibre-optic illumination, both co-axial and oblique.
 (iv) Swing-in pupillary stop for patient protection.
  (v) Swing-in blue light.
 (vi) 200 mm objective and additional 8° microscope for assistant.

achieved at some expense by a proper operating chair with adjustable arm rests. If this is impossible, then use can be made of sandbags, folded towels or even by resting the hands and forearms with care on the patient.

b. Instruments should be handed to the surgeon, or placed so that he can find them without taking his eyes from the microscope. Remember again that the microscope image is at infinity; if the user looks sideways he will need to focus his eyes and not leave them relaxed.

c. Beware of accommodation. It is easy, particularly in the younger surgeon (senile presbyopes for once have an advantage), to subconciously focus his eyes through the microscope on to where he perceives the operation site to be. During a long procedure, the user should occasionally zoom up and down, or change the magnification manually between high and low; this will help to relax the eyes. Allowing this involuntary accommodation to occur will result in unnecessary strain and subsequent tiredness.

d. Microsurgery is tiring, due mainly to the unnatural immobility of the eyeballs. In a long operation, this can be exacerbated by holding the head in a fixed position and putting strain on the neck muscles. This can be alleviated by altering the angle of the inclinable binocular (if fitted) during the procedure, thus putting the head into a different position. If this accessory is not fitted, it may be possible to alter slightly the inclination of the microscope.

e. Only as much magnification as necessary should be used. At higher magnifications the decrease in depth of focus can make constant re-focussing a chore.

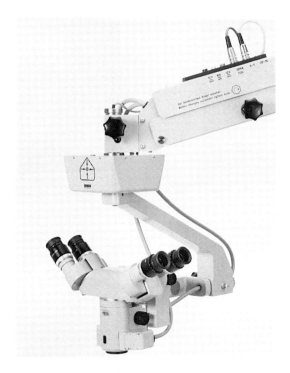

Fig. 12.14 Operating microscope for plastic/hand/reconstructive surgery. This double-headed microscope, the OpMi 6SDFC, is designed for two surgeons to operate together and has motorised focus, zoom and X-Y movement. The Cardian X-Y coupling allows tilting of the microscope in both East-West and North-South directions. Cool light fibre-optic illumination is provided through twin co-axial prisms. The instrument can be mounted either on a rollable floor stand or ceiling support, and is controlled through foot, hand or operating chair-mounted switches. As shown here, it is fitted with two straight binocular tubes, one or both of these being exchangeable for inclinable tubes to compensate for surgeons of differing heights.

f. The lowest comfortable level of illumination should be selected. More is not seen if the light is too bright; the pupils merely close to compensate. A low level of light is better for the user, the life of the lamps and (in ophthalmology) the patient.

MAINTENANCE

The operating microscope should preferably be the subject of a maintenance contract with the manufacturer, when once a year a trained specialist engineer will carry out a complete service on the optical, mechanical and electrical functions.

Routine maintenance by the theatre staff consists of the following easily accomplished tasks:

a. Immediately after surgery, bone fragments, blood spots and saline splashes should be removed with a soft cloth soaked in a surface-active, luke warm detergent. If splashes of saline are not removed from the surface of the objective immediately after surgery, they form a film which destroys any anti-reflection coating.

b. Painted surfaces of the microscope and stand should be cleaned regularly with a soft cloth or brush. Contaminated areas should be cleaned with ethyl alcohol or de-mineralised methylated spirit, never acetone or ether.

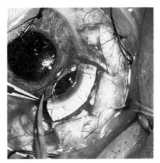

Fig. 12.15   Tumour of cilliary body. (Freiburg University Eye Clinic.)

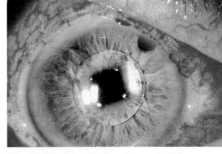

Fig. 12.16   Iris clip lens inserted. (Ulm University Eye Clinic.)

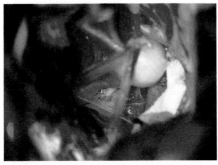

Fig. 12.17   Large aneurysm on basilar artery. (Professor Gruss, Wurzburg Neurosurgical Clinic.)

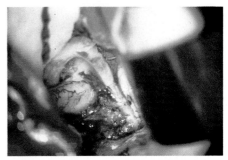

Fig. 12.18   Anterior aneurysm. (Professor Gruss, Wurzburg Neurosurgical Clinic.)

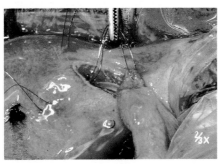

Fig. 12.19   Tubo-uterine implantation. (Dr Cognat, Lyon.)

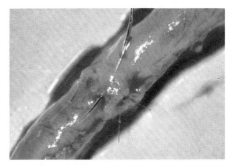

Fig. 12.20   Anastomosis of vas. (Dr W. Werber, Munich.)

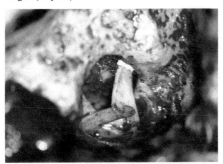

Fig. 12.21   Tympanoplasty after previous radical operation; replacement of stirrup bone. (Dr H. Schobel, St Polton.)

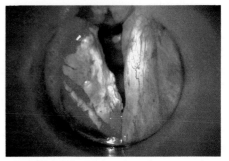

Fig. 12.22   Removal of the right vocal cord with neoplasm in situ. (Dr C. Naumann, Wurzburg University ENT Clinic.)

c. Only the outside optical surfaces of eyepieces and objectives should be cleaned. This can be done with a soft, grease-free brush (rinsed in ether before use and allowed to dry), or an air blower. Finger prints and similar contamination can be removed with a cotton wool bud, soaked in ethyl alcohol, or in very stubborn cases, acetone.

d. Dust is a great enemy. The microscope should be kept covered when not in use and never left without objective, binocular tube or eyepieces fitted. If cameras are kept locked up for security reasons, the dust cap should be replaced in the beam splitter outlet port.

e. All accessories, especially spare objectives and eyepieces, should be kept in dust proof containers.

13

Fibre-optic endoscopy

Fibre-optics

Fibre-optics have replaced, to a great extent, the conventional optic and light systems in endoscopes. Fibre-optic instruments are available for many applications; the use of specific instruments such as cystoscopes and arthroscopes is included in the appropriate chapters. However, it is opportune here to describe the basic principles of fibre-optic endoscopy, relevant to the field of gastroenterology, where the most significant advances have been made in endoscope design. In addition, the basic principles of handling, care and maintenance of fibrescopes remains the same for all applications. This includes their use for bronchoscopy and the newly emerging fields of flexible sigmoidoscopy, cystoscopy and intubating laryngoscopy (Chapter 11, page 347).

Fibre-optics is a term applied to a system for transmitting light and images through thin fibres of optical glass by the phenomenon of total internal reflection (Hollanders, 1979). Remarkable efficiency has been achieved in optics with present instruments, but there have been limitations to the degree of perfection obtainable, and these include:

1. Limitation of light transmission of fibres, amounting to 70 per cent of the individual fibre diameter.

2. Up to 10 per cent loss of light intensity for each 30 cm length of fibre bundle from the light source.

3. Good transmission of red and green light through the fibres, but poor transmission of blue light, an important consideration when selection materials for colour photograhy.

4. Resolution depends on diameter of fibre and packing density.

5. Some fibres will inevitably break during use, and users have to adapt to the effect of a few 'black' spots in the image formed.

The latest generation of fibrescopes use more advanced fibre-optics which reduce these limitations somewhat. Also the development of video endoscopes, which use miniature electronic 'imaging chips' to transmit the image electronically to a television monitor, has eliminated the image guide fibre bundle altogether (Fig. 13.1). At time of writing, it remains to be seen how widely this technology will be applied to the wide range of endoscopic procedures.

The fibre-optic endoscope system consists of three basic parts: the light source or generator unit, the insertion tube and optical image guide bundle, and the instrument or endoscope control section.

The light source. The light is supplied by a high-intensity lamp which has an in-built parabolic reflector. This reflector, which although focussing the visible light rays into the optical bundle, allows the long (or hot) infra red rays to pass through. This ensures relatively cold light is passed to the instrument or endoscope. Special lamps such as quartz iodine,

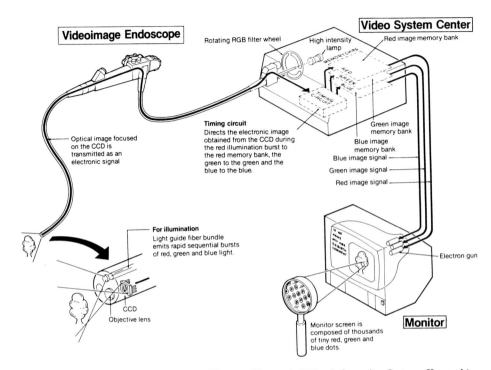

Fig. 13.1 Videoimage endoscope principles. (Olympus Electronic Video Information System, Keymed.)
Rather than through a fibre bundle, videoimage endoscopes obtain their image via an electronic microchip called a CCD. The image captured by the objective lens is relayed to the CCD face at the endoscope tip. The CCD transmits the image (black and white) along the endoscope body to the video system control in the form of electronic signals proportional in strength to the intensity of the various portions of the image.

A rotating red, green and blue filter wheel inside the video system control causes light emitted from the tip of the videoimage endoscope to be short, rapid sequential bursts of red, green and blue light. During each burst of colour, the CCD records a black and white image of the area being viewed as it appears under the particular colour of illumination, and images are sequentially stored in memory for each 'colour' image. The output of the memory banks are sent simultaneously to a colour monitor, where each signal activates an electron gun which illuminates only its own colour of phosphor dot on the monitor screen. The colour additive effect of the thousands of tightly packed red, green and blue dots produces a colour television picture.

metal halide and xenon have been developed to give a high intensity of light up to 500 watts, which overcomes some of the optical limitations described previously.

The light guide or fibre light bundle. This is connected at one end to the light source and at the other to the endoscope; it contains up to 20,000 flexible optical fibres which are incoherent (not capable of carrying an image). The bundles transmit a pre-focused light of high intensity and even density to the endoscope; they are sheathed in metal and PVC, and are extremely flexible (Carr-Locke, 1, 1977; Hollanders, 1979).

The intensity of light output at the patient end of the optical bundle varies with the working distance from the object. This may be as high as 5,000 ft candles at 25 mm (1 in) distance, but generally averages 1,600 to 2,800 ft candles intensity. The degree of intensity can be adjusted.

The instrument or endoscope. This is optically continuous with the fibre cable for the purpose of illumination. In addition, a separate set of up to 36,000 coherent optical fibres terminating proximally at an eyepiece, and distally at an appropriate lens, carry an image through the scope (Fig. 13.2). Both these sets of optical glass fibres are contained in a

Optical System

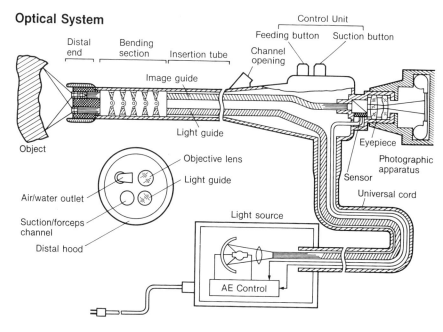

Fig. 13.2 The principles of a fibre-optic endoscope. (Olympus, Keymed.)

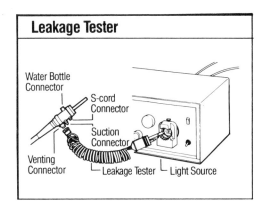

Fig. 13.3 Leakage test for OES fibrescopes.

The totally sealed construction of the OES fibrescopes makes it possible to check very simply the integrity of the whole fibrescope, including checking for pin holes in the bending section rubber. This should be done to reduce the incidence of major repairs by revealing leaks before they have an opportunity to damage the internal components of the fibrescope.

The test is carried out as follows:

1. Plug leakage tester into the output socket of an Olympus light source or OES maintenance unit.
2. Turn on pump and make sure there is no air coming out from the connector.
3. Connect the end of the flexible tube to the venting connector on the fibrescope.
4. The bending section rubber will expand due to the increase in internal pressure.
5. Totally immerse the fibrescope. The presence of a stream of small bubbles indicates a fluid leak. (A few initial bubbles due to air trapped in the control knobs, etc, is of no concern.) If a leak is detected, the instrument should be sent for repair before further use.
6. Remove the instrument from the water.
7. Disconnect the leakage tester from the light source. Wait for 30 seconds for pressure to equalise, and for bending section rubber to return to normal.
8. Disconnect leakage tester from fibrescope

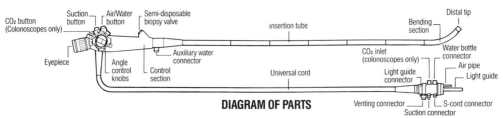

CO₂ button (Colonoscopes only) · Suction button · Air/Water button · Semi-disposable biopsy valve · insertion tube · Bending section · Distal tip · Eyepiece · Angle control knobs · Control section · Auxiliary water connector · Universal cord · CO₂ inlet (colonoscopes only) · Light guide connector · Water bottle connector · Air pipe · Light guide · Venting connector · Suction connector · S-cord connector

DIAGRAM OF PARTS

ONLY TOTALLY IMMERSE OES FIBERSCOPES DISTINGUISHED BY BLUE BAND AROUND THE EYEPIECE

A

USE THIS PROCEDURE IMMEDIATELY AFTER EACH EXAMINATION.
FAILURE TO DO SO MAY RESULT IN A MALFUNCTION OF THE INSTRUMENT.

YOU WILL NEED:—
*Cleaning solution *Compatible disinfectant solution *Clean or distilled water
*Suitably sized containers for disinfectant and water *Gauze swabs
*Scrub brush (soft) *Cotton-tipped applicators
*Special OES cleaning brush *Olympus OES adaptor for channel cleaning (MB-19)
*Olympus OES A/W channel cleaning adaptor (MB-107)
*Olympus OES all-channel irrigator (CW-1 or CW-2) with 30cc syringe
*ETO cap *Rubber gloves *Silicone oil *30% alcohol *Leakage tester (MB-155)

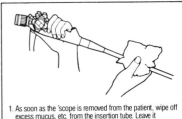

1. As soon as the 'scope is removed from the patient, wipe off excess mucus, etc. from the insertion tube. Leave it connected to the light source and suction pump.

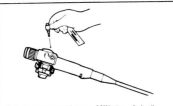

2. Turn off air pump and remove A/W button, placing it separately in cleaning solution. Insert A/W channel cleaning adaptor.

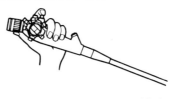

3. Turn air pump back on and operate A/W channel cleaning adaptor to feed air and water alternately for approximately 10 seconds each. Turn off light source.

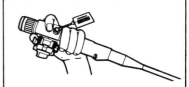

4. Place distal tip in water and aspirate through suction channel for approximately 10 seconds. Alternate aspiration of water and air several times. Turn off suction pump and disconnect suction line from light guide connector.

5. Remove A/W channel cleaning adaptor, suction button, biopsy valve(s), distal hood and CO₂ button (colonoscopes only) and place with air/water button in cleaning solution for separate cleaning.

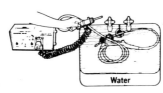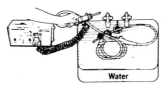

Water

6. Disconnect water bottle, remove 'scope from light source and perform leak test procedure.

Cleaning Solution

7. Ensure 'scope is detached from light source and immerse entire instrument in cleaning solution.
CAUTION NOTES:
1) The light guide plug may be extremely hot after removal from the light source — DO NOT TOUCH.
2) Before immersion, ENSURE ADAPTOR AC10-S HAS EITHER BEEN LEFT ATTACHED TO THE LIGHT SOURCE, OR REMOVED FROM THE 'SCOPE.

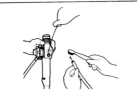

8. Insert special OES cleaning brush through channel opening to brush the 'dead space,' then through suction button hole into instrument channel to tip of 'scope and clean carefully with a soft brush on emerging.

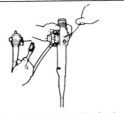

9. Repeat down universal cord suction channel, again cleaning brush with soft brush before withdrawal.

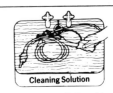

Cleaning Solution

10. Clean insertion tube and control body carefully using gauze swabs and soft brush with the cleaning solution, to remove all debris. Clean distal end with soft brush. On duodenoscopes clean forceps raiser mechanism with soft brush.

B

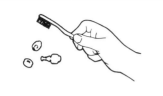

11. Thoroughly wash and rinse in clean water all accessories including suction and air/water buttons (and biopsy valve(s) if to be re-used).

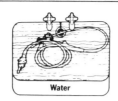

12. Discard cleaning solution, place 'scope in clean water, and rinse.

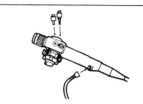

13. Replace air/water and suction buttons (and CO₂ button on colonoscopes). Attach adaptor for channel cleaning to channel opening.

14. Reconnect suction line to 'scope and turn on suction pump. Holding the control section out of the water and ensuring the free end of the adaptor for channel cleaning remains in the water, aspirate water for approximately 10 seconds.

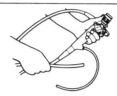

15. Remove entire instrument from water and continue to aspirate air for approximately 30 seconds.
Turn off suction pump and detach suction line from scope. Remove adaptor for channel cleaning.

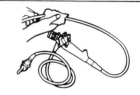

16. Dry 'scope carefully using disposable paper towels. Replace biopsy valve. CAUTION: ENSURE LIGHT GUIDE CONNECTOR IS COMPLETELY DRY BEFORE RECONNECTING TO AC10-S OR LIGHT SOURCE.

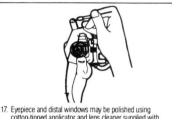

17. Eyepiece and distal windows may be polished using cotton-tipped applicator and lens cleaner supplied with the instrument.

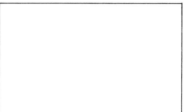

18. Check air and water flow on reconnection to the light source, prior to re-use.

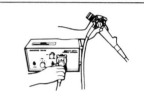

19. Prior to storage, disconnect water bottle from light guide connector, cover water bottle connector with finger and depress air/water button to expel all residual water.

Some instruments contain extra channels, for instance:

Some OES 'scopes incorporate an auxiliary water channel.
OES duodenoscopes incorporate the forceps raiser mechanism through a raiser control wire channel.
OES colonoscopes incorporate a CO₂ insufflation line.
These channels may be cleaned, disinfected and rinsed with the aid of a syringe during the routine procedures. Where necessary, supplementary cleaning tubes are included with the standard OES set.

LUBRICATION

(a) Before storage, the rubber seals of the suction and air/water buttons should be lubricated sparingly, using the silicone oil provided in the standard OES set.

(b) On OES duodenoscopes, also lubricate the forceps raiser mechanism before storage.

C

Fig. 13.4 Method of cleaning Olympus OES Fibrescopes. (Keymed.)

protective sheath, which generally incorporates additional channels for suction, gas infla-
tion/irrigation, and the passage of flexible biopsy or operative forceps and electrodes.

Care of fibre-optic endoscopes. The principles for the care of rigid endoscopes have already
been described in Chapter 5, but it is important to emphasise the special care required for
fibre-optic instruments after use. It can be said that 'the useful life of endoscopic instruments
is inversely proportional to the number of people using them'.

Fibrescopes are exceptionally expensive but comparable with their complexity; in 1988
a gastroscope cost in the region of £8,500. It is therefore essential to adhere to the manufacturer's instructions regarding cleaning and maintenance (NATN, 1979).

IMPORTANT: DO NOT ATTEMPT DISINFECTION UNTIL THE CLEANING PROCEDURE DESCRIBED ABOVE HAS BEEN CARRIED OUT.

The OES design allows total access to all internal and external surfaces for disinfection solution. The effectiveness of the disinfection procedure depends upon:

a) Rigorous mechanical cleaning to remove all organic debris prior to disinfection.
b) Removal of internal air bubbles which may prevent access of the solution to the internal surfaces.

CAUTION
Although the OES range has been designed for total immersion in both detergent and disinfectant solutions, routine, regular, long term immersions are not recommended, otherwise disinfectant odour may linger. Disinfectants are available which are effective against vegetative organisms within 30 minutes.
Follow the manufacturer's instructions and if required, ask your bacteriologist to check your disinfecting procedure. Use only disinfectants that have been tested for compatibility with fiberscopes.
If the fiberscope has been seriously contaminated, you may wish to immerse in disinfectant for longer periods, but do not exceed 10 hours.
DO NOT AUTOCLAVE YOUR OES FIBERSCOPE OR CLEAN WITH CHEMICAL SOLVENTS OR ULTRASONICS.

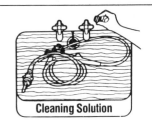

Cleaning Solution

1. Clean 'scope thoroughly as shown above. Ensure light source adaptor AC10-S has been removed from the 'scope.

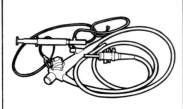

2. Remove air/water and suction buttons, and biopsy valve(s). On colonoscopes, also remove CO_2 button. Connect all-channel irrigator.

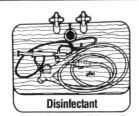

Disinfectant

3. Immerse the entire instrument and irrigator until covered by disinfectant. The suction, air/water and CO_2 buttons and biopsy valve(s) should also be immersed in the disinfectant.

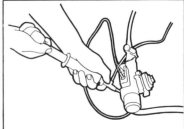

4. Flush air/water and suction/biopsy channels to remove air.

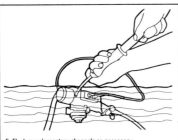

5. Flush supplementary channels as necessary.

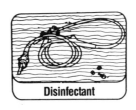

Disinfectant

6. Disconnect all-channel irrigator and leave instrument immersed for the recommended time in accordance with disinfectant manufacturer's instructions.

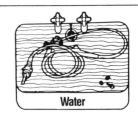

Water

7. On completion of disinfection period, remove the 'scope, buttons, and valves from the disinfectant. Rinse by immersing in clean water.

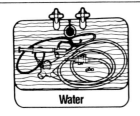

Water

8. Reconnect all-channel irrigator to 'scope.

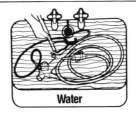

Water

9. Flush all channels, including supplementary channels, thoroughly with water to remove disinfectant.

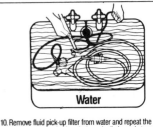

Water

10. Remove fluid pick-up filter from water and repeat the flushing process forcing air through all channels to expel the water.

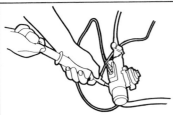

11. Remove the instrument, complete with irrigator, from the water and place on a clean, dry surface. Again, pump the syringe to remove internal water from all channels.

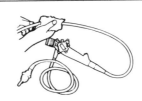

12. Remove all channel irrigator from 'scope and dry 'scope carefully, paying special attention to eyepiece and distal lenses, light guide connector, electrical terminals in eyepiece. Dry all valves and replace them, ready for use.

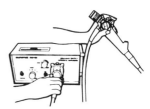

13. Prior to storage, disconnect water bottle from light guide connector, cover water bottle connector with finger and depress air/water button to expel all residual water.

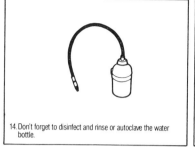

14. Don't forget to disinfect and rinse or autoclave the water bottle.

CLEANING AND DISINFECTION OF ACCESSORIES

NOTE: Only those accessories identified by green colour coding or marked "autoclave," may be autoclaved.
1. Meticulous mechanical cleaning, followed by 5 minutes of ultrasound (at 40 kHz or higher), is mandatory prior to sterilisation by autoclaving (refer to autoclavable accessory instructions for details).
2. Standard autoclave cycles, including "flash," may be used provided the temperature does not exceed 132°C (270°F).
3. Accessories may also be boiled for up to 30 minutes.
4. Accessories may be disinfected by immersion in cold fluid disinfectant for a period of time as recommended by the solution manufacturer. Ensure accessories are rinsed thoroughly in clean water after disinfection.
5. Always lubricate operating wires and mechanisms with silicone oil before storage or re-use.

Fig. 13.5 Method of disinfecting Olympus OES fibrescopes. (Keymed.)

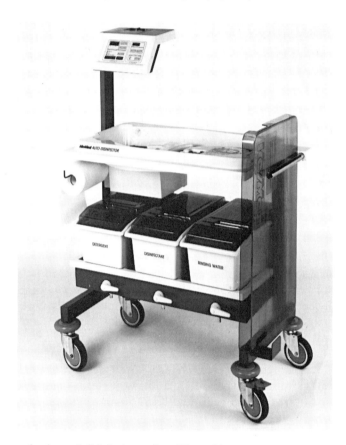

Fig. 13.6 Endoscope cleaning and disinfecting trolley. (Keymed.)

Debris and mucus must be removed from the instrument and channels immediately after use using a mild detergent such as Savlon 1 per cent, followed by copious rinsing in warm water. After thorough cleaning, in early models the insertion tube only of the endoscope can be terminally disinfected by immersion in a chemical fluid such as glutaraldehyde (Cidex). The new generation of OES fibrescopes and electronic endoscopes is fully immersible for more efficient cleaning and disinfection. Moreover these instruments allow regular 'leakage testing' to avoid fluid penetration (Fig. 13.3). If the instrument has been used on

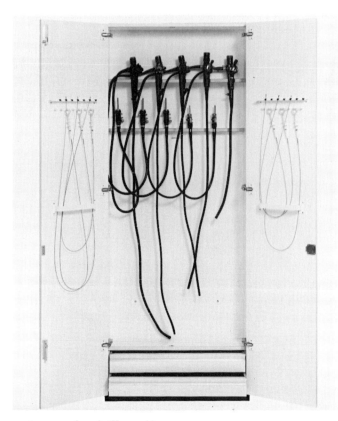

Fig. 13.7 Endoscope storage cupboard. (Keymed.)

a patient known or suspected to have a viral disease such as hepatitis or Acquired Immune Deficiency (AIDS), it will have to be subjected to total immersion (if of the immersable type) or exposure to ethylene oxide (Chapter 7). After cleaning and disinfection, flexible fibrescopes should be stored as shown in Figure 13.7. Care must be taken not to drop or damage the fibrescope as this will cause individual fibres to shatter, and lenses to crack.

Endoscopes used for operative procedures or penetrating tissues, i.e., laparoscopes, arthroscopes, thorascopes, choledocoscopes etc., must be used in a sterile condition. Although some rigid instruments may be compatible with steam sterilization, the others will have to be processed by soaking in cold fluid disinfecting agents or by the ethylene oxide method described in Chapter 7, page 198.

Gastrointestinal fibrescopes (including gastroscopes, duodenoscopes and colonoscopes)

Before the advent of fibre-optics, the rigid instruments available had many limitations. Fibre-optics enabled the development of endoscopes which not only have a flexible shaft, but give an operator the ability to manoeuvre the tip of the instrument by changing its configuration.

There are three basic types of instruments:
1. Forward or oblique (foreoblique) viewing for examination/biopsy.
2. Side or lateral viewing for examination/biopsy/operative procedures in the duodenum.

3. Forward viewing with two channels for complex operative procedures.

The first type of instrument is suitable for examining the oesophagus, most of the stomach and the upper part of the duodenum, and serves 90 per cent of situations.

The second type, side or lateral viewing instrument, is needed in 10 per cent of cases, when full examination of oesophagus, stomach, duodenum and biliary system is required. This includes the fundus of the stomach and fornices of the duodenal bulb.

The third type of instrument is generally larger in diameter than the previous two (although there are exceptions), which enables suitable dimension of channels to be incorporated for operating instruments. A wide range of procedures can be undertaken. All three types of instruments can be obtained from several manufacturers, although for simplicity only one will be mentioned: The Olympus Optical Co. Ltd (marketed by KeyMed in the United Kingdom).

Examples of type 1 are the Olympus GIF-Q10 (diameter 11 mm, forward viewing, suitable for examination/biopsy), and the GIF-K10 (diameter 11.4 mm, foreoblique viewing, for therapeutic procedures such as injecting oesophageal varices); type 2 includes Olympus TJF-10 (therapeutic duodenoscope, 4.2 mm channel, suitable for carrying out retrograde cholangio-pancreatography by cannulation of the papilla of Vater and advanced biliary therapy); an example of type 3 would be the Olympus GIF-2T10 (diameter 12.6 mm, forward viewing, suitable for advanced therapy such as haemostasis or the removal of polyps from the stomach).

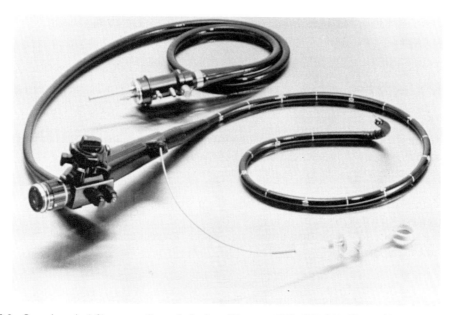

Fig. 13.8 Gastrointestinal fibrescope, forward viewing. (Olympus OES, GIF-Q10, Keymed.)

Upper gastrointestinal endoscopy

Definition

The examination of the interior of the oesophagus, stomach or duodenum, using a fibrescope.

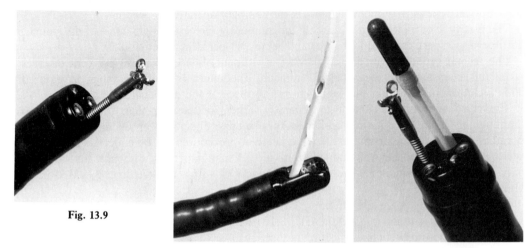

Fig. 13.9

Fig. 13.10   Fig. 13.11

Fig. 13.9 Distal tip of gastrointestinal fibrescope, biopsy forceps emerging. (Olympus OES, GIF-Q10, Keymed.)

Fig. 13.10 Distal tip of therapeutic duodenal fibrescope, 4.2 mm instrument channel and 12 Char biliary stent. (Olympus OES, TJF-10, KeyMed.)

Fig. 13.11 Distal tip of therapeutic forward viewing gastrointestinal fibrescope, with twin 4.2 mm instrument channels, with heater probe and biopsy forceps emerging. (Olympus OES, GIF-2T10, Keymed.)

Position

Left lateral or sitting.

Instruments

    Suitable fibrescope (e.g., forward, or side viewing depending on whether
        oesophagus/stomach/duodenum are to be examined)
    Fibreoptic light source/diathermy power supply
    Plastic mouth guard
    Biopsy forceps (these include those suitable for cutting, grasping, taking cytology
        specimens etc., Fig. 13.13)
    Accessories for endoscopic diathermy (e.g. snares, knives, electrodes, Fig. 13.14)
    Angled tongue depressor
    Pharyngeal spray
    Topical anaesthetic, e.g., 1 per cent lignocaine (Xylocaine)
    Lubricant e.g., Lignocaine (Xylocaine) gel
    Oesophageal bougies and tubes sizes 16 and 18 Charriere gauge may be required
    Water container/irrigator
    Medical vacuum
    Camera
    Endoscopy trolley.

Outline of procedure

The patient is usually sedated with intravenous diazepam or diazemuls; a calm atmosphere and gentle technique can do much to reduce anxiety, complications and the need for heavy

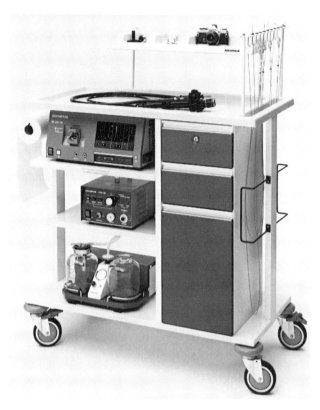

Fig. 13.12   Endoscopy trolley. (Keymed.)

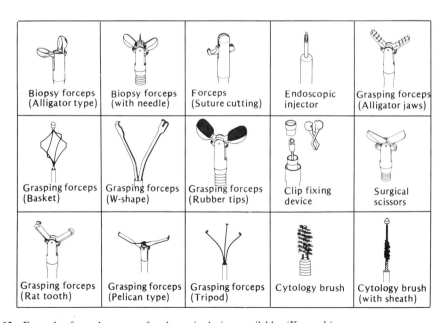

Fig. 13.13   Examples from the range of endoscopic devices available. (Keymed.)

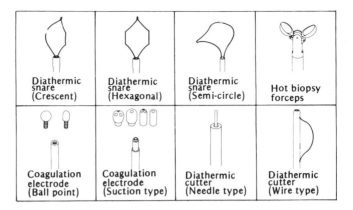

Diathermic snare (Crescent)	Diathermic snare (Hexagonal)	Diathermic snare (Semi-circle)	Hot biopsy forceps
Coagulation electrode (Ball point)	Coagulation electrode (Suction type)	Diathermic cutter (Needle type)	Diathermic cutter (Wire type)

Fig. 13.14   Accessories for fibrescope diathermy procedures. (Keymed.)

sedation. In addition, a topical anaesthetic is applied to the pharynx (1 per cent lignocaine spray). An assistant stands behind the patient (who is sitting or lying on his left side), supporting his head, and encouraging him to bend his neck forward to relax his neck muscles and to avoid moving his head from side to side (Hollanders, 1979).

A plastic mouth-guard is then placed between the gums and teeth, the lubricated fibre-scope is passed through the guard and over the tongue, and the patient is asked to swallow. This usually opens the upper oesophageal sphincter (cricopharyngeus) so that the instrument can be advanced into the oesophagus. If, because of severe retching, the instrument cannot be passed, an attempt may be made to pass it under direct vision. If this fails a small oesophageal dilator may be passed in order to relax the cricopharyngeus sufficiently to permit passage of the instrument. No force should ever be employed in this procedure as perforation of the oesophagus can occur. If the patient is in a sitting position, when the instrument is well past the cricopharyngeus, the patient is placed on his left side for completion of the examination.

Examination of the oesophagus. The patient's head is elevated 10–50° and a partial exam-ination is carried out as the instrument is advanced towards the stomach. Complete exam-ination is usually left until the end of the endoscopy procedure, unless obvious pathology is found in the oesophagus.

The examination is started by inflating the oesophagus with air until a view of the lumen is obtained. Successful examination requires nearly continuous use of air, water and suction to keep the lens clean and the oesophagus distended. The operator keeps the fibrescope in the centre of the lumen by co-ordinated use of the angle control knobs and flexible tube rotation.

Special care is exercised to avoid mucosal trauma when passing the instrument through the hiatus and into the stomach. In case of strictures, when the hiatal opening is visualised, a biopsy forceps is passed through the suction channel into the stomach and the scope is gently passed over the forceps safely into the stomach. The forceps are then withdrawn.

At the end of the procedure, a more complete inspection of the oesophagus is carried out as the instrument is withdrawn. This would include relation of the gastro-oesophageal mucosal junction to the diaphragmatic hiatus (possible hiatus hernia); state of oesophageal mucosa (possible sophagitis, varices and tumours). If necessary, biopsy forceps are intro-duced into the suction channel and specimens taken for histology; brush cytology specimens may also be taken.

Examination of the stomach. The patient's head may be tilted downwards 10–15°, and the instrument is then passed through the hiatus 2–3 cm into the stomach. Sufficient air is inflated to open up the body of the stomach, the objective lens is rinsed and the scope is positioned in the centre of the gastricumen. Combined with intermittent suction to remove secretions and the air inflation the instrument is manoeuvred along the greater curvature of the stomach to the pylorus. It may be necessary to place the patient on his back in order to pass the instrument through the pylorus into the duodenum and if difficulty is experienced a similar procedure to that described for entry to the stomach may be carried out, utilising a biopsy forceps as a guide.

Examination of the duodenum. As with the oesophagus and stomach the duodenum is best examined as the fibrescope is withdrawn. The organ is inflated with air and the scope manoeuvred into the second part of the duodenum. During a slow withdrawal of the instrument, a careful examination is carried out, and if necessary biopsy or brush cytology specimens are taken. Duodenal ulcers are generally shallow and small, and tend to be found in the folds of the duodenal cap. Retrograde cholangiopancreatography and other operative procedures can be undertaken by cannulation of the papilla of Vater (Figs. 13.17 and 13.19) (Schiller and Peachey, 1978).

When examination of the duodenum is completed, a detailed examination of the stomach is carried out as the instrument is withdrawn. The objective is to achieve complete examination of the stomach, paying special attention to areas which can easily become 'blind' spots in the examination, e.g. the lesser curvature, severe cascade deformities of the stomach wall, the cardia and fundus. Operative procedures may include biopsy with forceps and brush cytology; removal of foreign bodies; diathermy excision of polyps. The biopsy forceps is a delicate precision instrument which must be used with great care. Biopsies are torn off as opposed to cutting with the forceps to avoid using force to close the jaws when the biopsy is taken, which may separate the attachment of the pull wire from the forceps tip. The endoscopist will manoeuvre the forceps in and out, operating the controls of the fibrescope, whilst an assistant opens or closes the forceps jaw as required.

Withdrawal of instrument. When examination of the oesophagus has been completed the angle free control is released and the instrument gently withdrawn. The operator may inspect the larynx, possibly the trachea, and the pharynx before the instrument is completely removed.

Lower gastrointestinal endoscopy

Definition

The examination of the interior of the colon using a fibrescope.

Position

Usually left lateral

Instruments

Colonofibrescope
Fibreoptic light source/diathermy power supply
Biopsy forceps (these include those suitable for cutting, grasping, taking cytology
  specimens etc. (Fig. 13.13)

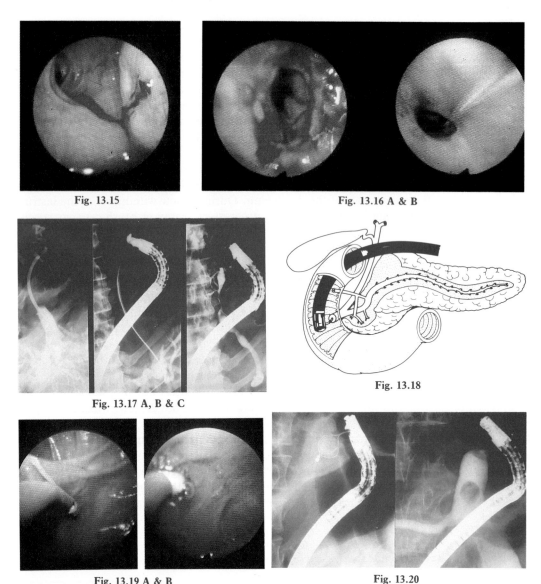

Fig. 13.15

Fig. 13.16 A & B

Fig. 13.17 A, B & C

Fig. 13.18

Fig. 13.19 A & B

Fig. 13.20

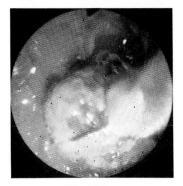

Fig. 13.21

Fig. 13.15   Stigmata of recent haemorrhage; active oozing from ulcer base.

Fig. 13.16   Oesophageal stricture. (A) Passage of guide wire through benign oesophageal stricture. (B) Stricture after balloon dilatation.

Fig. 13.17   (A) Cholangiogram showing malignant stricture in distal common bile duct. (B) Passage of guidewire and guiding catheter through the obstruction with the prosthesis advancing through the stricture. (C) Final position of prosthesis draining the obstructed biliary system.

Fig. 13.18   Diagrammatic view of ampullary cannulation. (Courtesy, Dr D. L. Carr-Lock and *Nursing Times*.)

Fig. 13.19   (A and B) Endoscopic view of guiding catheter inserted through papilla of Vater, and prosthesis advancing over catheter.

Fig. 13.20   Cholangiogram showing biliary stone engaged in dormia basket.

Fig. 13.21   Biliary stone extracted by dormia basket.

(Figs. 13.15–17 and 13.19–21; Courtesy Dr J. Leung, Combined Endoscopy Unit, Prince of Wales Hospital, Hong Kong.)

Accessories for endoscopic diathermy (e.g., snares, cutter, electrodes (Fig. 13.14)
Colon stiffening tube
Lubricant e.g., lignocaine (Xylocaine) gel
Water container/irrigator
Carbon dioxide gas source
Medical vacuum
Camera.

Outline of procedure

Good colonoscopy is a procedure which requires good pre-operative radiology with adequate double contrast barium enema pictures of the whole colon. The most common indication for colonoscopy examination is to clarify an abnormality revealed radiologically by barium enema; colonoscopy may also be carried out for persistent symptoms such as rectal bleeding, passage of mucus or colonic pain despite negative investigations such as sigmoidoscopy and barium enema.

Thorough preparation of the bowel is essential if the operator is to achieve a complete examination. Although such preparation is not a part of this operative description it is useful to note that this preparation may consist of a low residue diet for two days before examination and the administration of purgative enemas. (Carr-Locke, 2, 1977.) Therapeutic

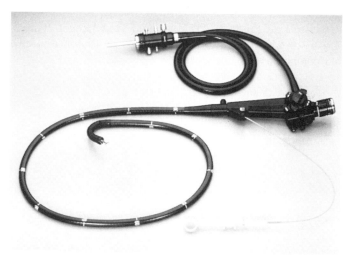

Fig. 13.22 Colonoscope. (Olympus OES, CF-IT10, Keymed.)

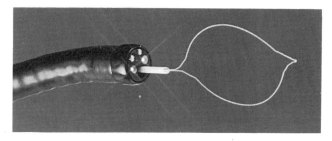

Fig. 13.23 Polypectomy snare emerging from distal end of colonoscope. (Olympus OES, CF-IT10, Keymed.)

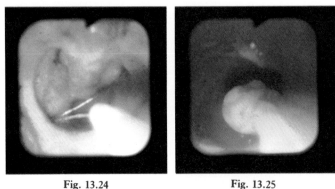

Fig. 13.24   Fig. 13.25

Fig. 13.24   Snare approaching colonic polyp. (Courtesy Dr D. L. Carr-Locke.)

Fig. 13.25   Just after colonic polyp has been excised by diathermy. (Courtesy Dr D. L. Carr-Locke.)

colonoscopy often includes the removal of polyps (polypectomy). The colonoscope has the facility for blowing in carbon dioxide so that explosive gas mixtures do not form in the bowel whilst polyps are being removed by diathermy. Complete colonoscopy requires X-ray screening facilities, although left-sided examinations can be done without.

The patient may be sedated with diazepam or diazemuls; if discomfort or pain is left during the procedure this may be supplemented by intravenous pethidine or inhaled nitrous oxide 50 per cent with oxygen 50 per cent (Entonox). The patient at first lies on his left side but may find it more comfortable to turn prone as the examination proceeds.

A well-lubricated colonoscope is introduced into the rectum and gently advanced along the centre of the bowel under direct vision. Great skill is required to manoeuvre the scope along the sigmoid colon and through the various bends into the ascending colon. However, it is safe to progress if the bowel mucosa is seen to slip past the instrument tip. Examination of the whole colon can take up to two hours.

As with upper gastrointestinal endoscopy, the best views of the interior of the colon are usually obtained on withdrawal of the instrument. It is at this stage that biopsies or cytology specimens are taken and polypectomy performed. For polypectomy the bowel gas is replaced with carbon dioxide and a diathermy snare loop passed through the suction/biopsy channel. With a special diathermy power source and appropriate precautions (Chapter 3, page 92), a diathermy current is applied to the snare which has been tightened around the base of the polyp which is cut away without bleeding. The cut polyp can be removed with biopsy holding forceps and sent for histology. The angle controls are returned to normal and the instrument gently withdrawn.

Proctoscopy and sigmoidoscopy

Definition

An examination of the rectum or sigmoid flexure of the colon, using an illuminated endoscope passed per anum. (The fibre optic aspect would consist only of the illumination device.)

Position

Left lateral, lithotomy or kneeling.

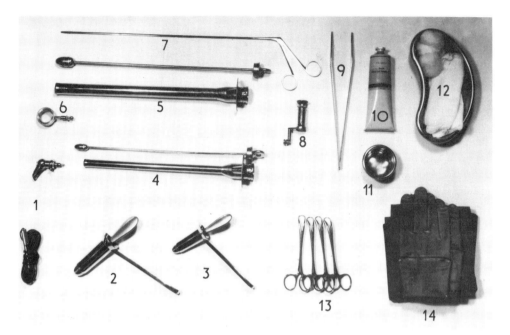

Fig. 13.26   Proctoscopy and sigmoidoscopy.
1. Sigmoidoscope light lead and light attachment.
2 and 3. Large and small proctoscope (Kelly).
4 and 5. Large and small sigmoidoscopes (Norton Morgan.)
6. Eyepiece for sigmoidoscope.
7. Biopsy forceps, cutting jaws (e.g., Brunings cup, Yeoman, etc.).
8. Telescope attachment.

9. Dissecting forceps, non-toothed.
10. Soft paraffin lubricant.
11. Gallipot containing Savlon 1 per cent.
12. Wool and gauze swabs.
13. Towel clips.
14. Gloves and dressing towels.

Not illustrated:
Double inflation bellows, and battery or transformer.

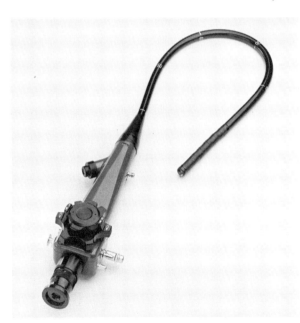

Fig. 13.27   Sigmoidofibrescope, used as an alternative to the instruments illustrated in Figure 13.22. (Olympus OSF 2, Keymed.)

Instruments.

As Figure 13.26.

Outline of procedure

The lubricated endoscope is passed via the anus. When the surgeon uses a sigmoidoscope, the walls of the colon are kept separate by inflating with air. Small pledglets of cotton-wool are held with the long forceps to swab the area in view, and the biopsy forceps may be used to obtain a specimen of tissue for histology. Sometimes a rectal or colonic polyp may be diathermised and in this case the indifferent electrode is applied to the patient's leg, observing the precautions listed in Chapter 2. The active electrode is inserted through a special attachment at the proximal end of the endoscope.

REFERENCES AND FURTHER READING

CARR-LOCKE, D. L. (1977) Gastrointestinal endoscopy — 1. *Nursing Times*, **73**, 1348.
CARR-LOCKE, D. L. (1977) Gastrointestinal endoscopy — 2. *Nursing Times*, **73**, 1403.
NATIONAL ASSOCIATION OF THEATRE NURSES (1979) *A Report on the Care and Sterilisation of Fibre Optic Endoscopes. Staffing and Training Sub-Committee*, September.
SCHILLER, K. F. R. AND PEACHEY, J. (1978) Gastrointestinal fibre-endoscopy. *Nursing Mirror*, November, 30.
HOLLANDERS, D. (1979) *Gastrointestinal Endoscopy*. London: Baillière-Tindall.

14

General instruments

There are two methods of instrument selection: (*a*) enough instruments are prepared for a particular operation; (*b*) basic instrument sets are used and specialised instruments are added to these as required.

In this book method (*a*) is used only for highly specialised or very minor procedures. Method (*b*) is used extensively, for it ensures that the instruments to which the surgeon is accustomed are always at hand and is a method which is suited to the pre-set tray system of sterilization. Also, by arranging the instruments in groups, teaching is simplified.

Except in minor procedures or when only a few instruments are needed, the more common instruments are not illustrated. This is to allow greater prominence to the special instruments described.

The general set (Figs. 14.1 to 14.28)

The general set of instruments is selected according to the kind of operation, and preference of the surgeon; but this set should include sufficient basic instruments for the majority of general procedures. However, the instruments listed, indeed any of the operation sets described in the following chapters, are intended to act only as a guide and must, of course, be adjusted in type, size or number to suit a surgeon's individual requirement.

A basic general set of instruments could consist of the following:
Scalpel handles Nos. 3 and 4, with Nos. 10 and 20 blades (Bard Parker), 2.
Dissecting forceps, toothed, small (Lane), 2.
Dissecting forceps, toothed, large (Bonney), 2.
Dissecting forceps, non-toothed, small and large, 2.
Scissors, curved on flat, small and large (Mayo), 2.
Scissors, straight (Mayo).
Scissors, straight, stitch.
Artery forceps, curved on flat (Kelly Fraser/Dunhill/Halstead), 10.
Artery forceps, straight (Moynihan), 10.
Artery forceps, straight 20 cm (8 in) (Spencer Wells), 5.
Dissector (MacDonald/Durham/Watson-Cheyne).
Aneurysm needle.
Photoclips for anchoring soiled dressing bag, diathermy leads or suction tubing etc., 3.
Curetting spoons, medium and large (Volkmann), 2.
Probe, malleable silver.
Sinus forceps.
Sponge-holding forceps (Rampley), 5.
Needle holder, large (Mayo), 2.

Needle holder, small (Kilner), 2.
Towel clips (Backaus), 5.
Tissue forceps (Lane), 5.
Tissue forceps (Allis), 5.

Retractors, single hook, sharp and blunt, 2.
Retractors, double hook, blunt, 2.
Retractors, medium (Langenbeck), 2.
Retractors, large (Morris), 2.

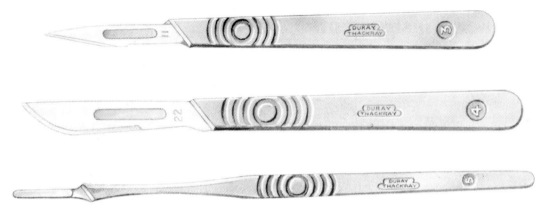

Fig. 14.1   Duray scalpel handles sizes 3, 4 and 5.

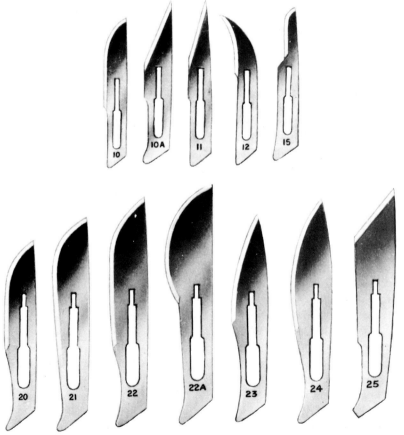

Fig. 14.2   Disposable scalpel blades sizes 10–25. (See also Fig. 9.10 page 245.)
(Chas. F. Thackray Ltd)

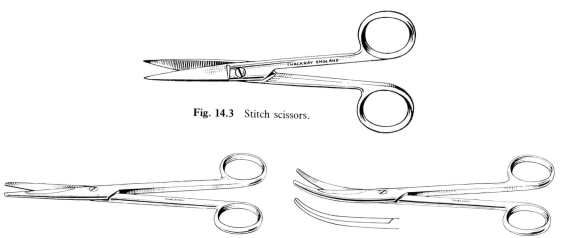

Fig. 14.3   Stitch scissors.

Fig. 14.4   Mayo scissors (straight).

Fig. 14.5   Mayo scissors (curved).

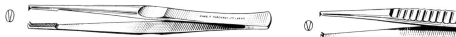

Fig. 14.6   Lane toothed dissecting forceps.

Fig. 14.7   Treves toothed dissecting forceps.

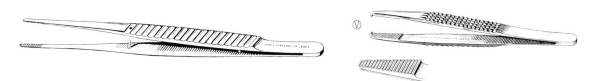

Fig. 14.8   Non-toothed dissecting forceps.

Fig. 14.9   Bonney toothed dissecting forceps.

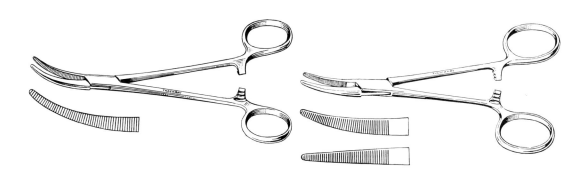

Fig. 14.10   Crile artery forceps.

Fig. 14.11   Dunhill artery forceps.

(Chas. F. Thackray Ltd)

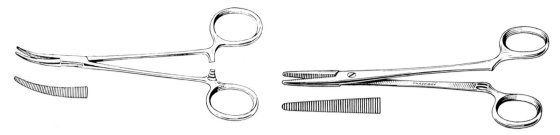

Fig. 14.12   Halstead Mosquito artery forceps.

Fig. 14.13   Spencer Wells artery forceps.

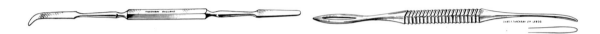

Fig. 14.14   MacDonald dissector.

Fig. 14.15   Durham dissector-raspatory.

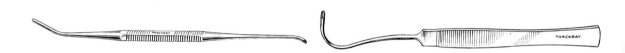

Fig. 14.16   Watson-Cheyne dissector.

Fig. 14.17   Syme aneurysm needle.

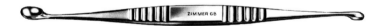

Fig. 14.18   Volkmann curetting spoon. (Double end. Four sizes A, B, C and D. Biomet Ltd.)

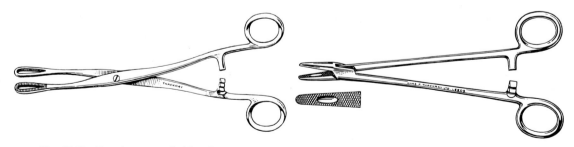

Fig. 14.19   Rampley sponge-holding forceps.

Fig. 14.20   Mayo needle holder.

(Chas. F. Thackray Ltd)

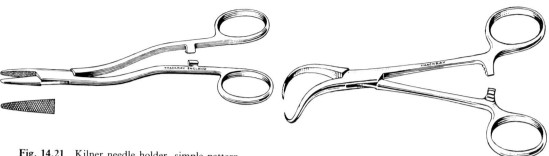

Fig. 14.21 Kilner needle holder, simple pattern.

Fig. 14.22 Mayo Backhaus towel forceps.

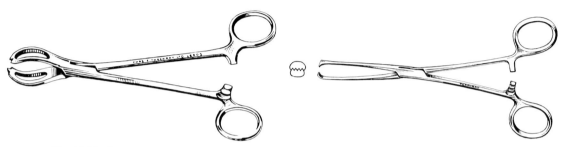

Fig. 14.23 Lane tissue forceps.

Fig. 14.24 Allis tissue forceps.

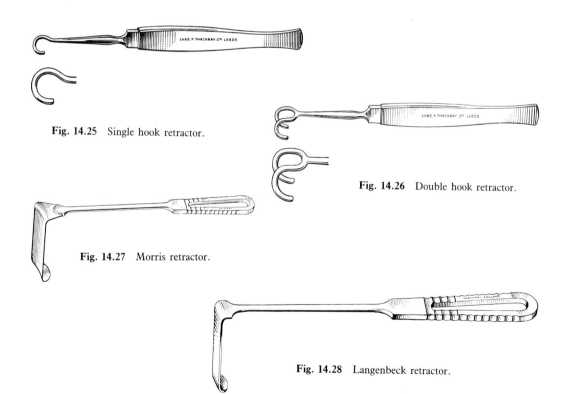

Fig. 14.25 Single hook retractor.

Fig. 14.26 Double hook retractor.

Fig. 14.27 Morris retractor.

Fig. 14.28 Langenbeck retractor.

(Chas. F. Thackray Ltd)

15

General operations — the abdomen

The laparotomy set (Figs. 15.1–15.7)

Combined with the general set, this is the basis for all major operations on the abdomen and is suitable for a midline, paramedian, transverse or elliptical incision. Bowel clamps and special instruments are added as required.

Gall-bladder forceps, curved on flat (Moynihan), 6.
Long tissue forceps (Lane), 6.
Artery forceps, curved on flat (Kelly Fraser), 25.
Long scissors, curved on flat (McIndoe).
Hernia director (Key).
Hernia bistoury, curved.
Aneurysm needle, large (Moynihan).
Artery forceps, straight 20 cm (8 in) (Spencer Wells), 25.
Deep retractors, curved narrow blade (Deaver), set of 4.
Retractor, self-retaining abdominal (Gosset/Denis Browne).
Deep retractor, right-angled narrow blade (Kelly).

Not illustrated:
2.5 and 3 (2/0 and 0) Chromic catgut or synthetic absorbable for ligatures.*
2.5, 3, 4, and 5 (2/0, 0, 1 and 2) Synthetic absorbable for ligatures.
4 or 5 (1 or 2) Chromic catgut, synthetic non-absorbable or silk on large half-circle, round-bodied needles for peritoneum, and large half-circle cutting needles for rectus or linea alba. (Proportionally smaller for children.)
5 (2) Monofilament synthetic non-absorbable (strong) on curved cutting needles for tension sutures (optional).
2.5 (2/0) Synthetic non-absorbable or silk on curved or straight cutting needles for skin.
Fine rubber tubing or buttons for tension sutures.
Michel or Kifa skin clips or disposable skin staples (optional).

Types of central abdominal incisions

High midline incisions

These are used for operations on the stomach, liver, gall-bladder, spleen, etc. A vertical

---

* In all the following chapters, suture sizes are described in metric sizes followed by the original BPC sizes in parentheses. The term synthetic absorbable ligatures and sutures embraces materials such as polyglycolic acid (Dexon), Polydioxanone (PDS), and Polyglactin 910 (Vicryl). Synthetic non-absorbables include polyamide (Nylon), polyester (Dacron, Ethibond, Polydek, Sutulene, Tevdek II, and Ticron), Polybutester (Novatil), polypropylene (Prolene, Prodek and Surgilene), and stainless steel wire.

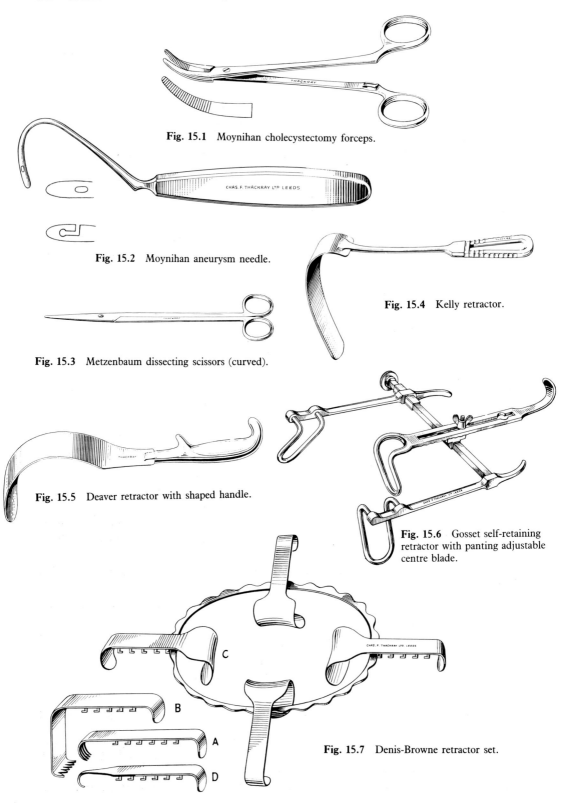

Fig. 15.1   Moynihan cholecystectomy forceps.

Fig. 15.2   Moynihan aneurysm needle.

Fig. 15.3   Metzenbaum dissecting scissors (curved).

Fig. 15.4   Kelly retractor.

Fig. 15.5   Deaver retractor with shaped handle.

Fig. 15.6   Gosset self-retaining retractor with panting adjustable centre blade.

Fig. 15.7   Denis-Browne retractor set.

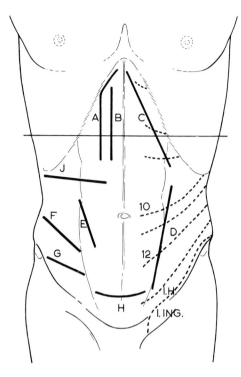

Fig. 15.8 An outline drawing of the anterior abdominal wall in which the course of the nerves are shown by interrupted lines and the position of some of the commoner incisions are indicated by continuous lines. (A) Mayo-Robson's (hockey stick) modified paramedian incision for biliary tract operations. (B) Right supra-umbilical paramedian incision (for stomach and duodenum). (C) Kocher's sub-costal incision for stomach and spleen, and on the right side for biliary tract. (D) Left pararectal incision for colon. (E) Battle's incision for appendectomy. (F) Right iliac gridiron incision for appendectomy. (G) Lanz incision for appendectomy. (H) Transverse incision for subrapubic cystotomy. (J) Upper quadrant transverse. (I.H.) Iliohypogastric nerve. (I.ING.) Ilio-inguinal nerve. (Bruce. Walmsley and Ross.)

midline incision is made through the skin, extending from just below the xyphisternum to the umbilicus where it curves outwards to avoid this landmark. The incision is continued through the linea alba to expose the peritoneum, which is picked up with forceps and incised.

Low midline incisions

These are used for operations on the lower bowel, bladder, uterus and rectum, etc. A vertical midline incision is made through the skin, extending from the pubis to the umbilicus where it curves outwards. The anterior rectus sheath is split following the line of the linea alba, and the peritoneum is picked up with forceps and incised.

Paramedian incisions

These are used primarily to gain access to one side of the abdomen and are placed accordingly. A vertical skin incision is made 2 cm from the midline. The extent of the incision depends upon the operative procedure; e.g., for caecal or lower colon operations the incision would extend from just above the level of the umbilicus to the pubis, for gastric or gall-

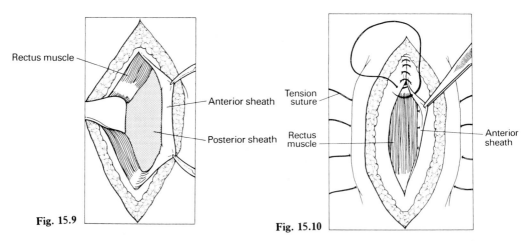

Rectus muscle

Anterior sheath

Posterior sheath

Tension suture

Rectus muscle

Anterior sheath

Fig. 15.9

Fig. 15.10

Fig. 15.9 (above left) Paramedian incision. The rectus mucle has been retracted laterally to expose the posterior sheath, which is then incised together with the peritoneum.

Fig. 15.10 (above right) Closure of paramedian incision. The rectus muscle covers the suture line in the posterior sheath. Tension sutures have been inserted. The anterior sheath is being repaired by a continuous suture. (Rintoul: *Farquharson's Textbook of Operative Surgery.*)

bladder operations the incision would extend from just below the costal margin to the umbilicus. For extensive procedures the incision would be a combination of both types just given.

The anterior rectus sheath is incised 2 cm from the midline and the rectus muscle retracted laterally or split between its fibres. The posterior rectus sheath and peritoneum together are picked up with forceps and incised.

Transverse (Kocher's type) incisions are not often used as there is danger of damage to the nerves supplying the rectus muscle. An oblique skin incision is made below the costal margin. The rectus muscle, external oblique and underlying internal oblique and transversus muscles are divided across in line with the skin incision, and the peritoneum is opened in the usual manner.

Pfannenstiel transverse elliptical incision

This is favoured by the gynaecologists. The skin is incised elliptically just above the pubis. The anterior rectus sheath is incised transversely in line with the skin incision, and is retracted to expose the rectus muscles which are freed from the sheath. The rectus muscles are separated from the midline and the peritoneum is picked up with forceps and incised vertically.

Closure of central abdominal incisions

The peritoneum and posterior rectus sheath are sutured with a continuous chromic catgut or synthetic absorbable on a round-bodied needle. Non-absorbable tension sutures on curved cutting needles may be inserted in midline and paramedian incisions. These tension sutures pass from one side of the incision through the skin, figure-of-eight manner through the muscle, and out through the skin again on the opposite side of the incision. The sutures are tied over a button or thin rubber tubing after the muscles have been approximated.

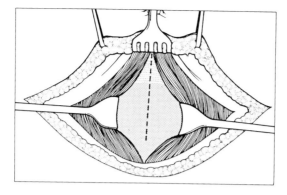

Fig. 15.11 Lower abdominal transverse incision with vertical separation of the recti. The incision is curved so as to lie in the skin creases. After the anterior sheaths have been incised, and the superior flap elevated upwards, the recti are separated and held apart by retractors. Transversalis fascia and peritoneum are then incised in a vertical direction. (Rintoul: *Farquharson's Textbook of Operative Surgery.*)

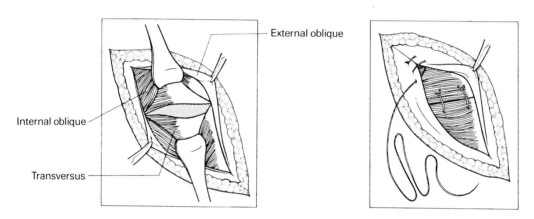

External oblique

Internal oblique

Transversus

Figs. 15.12 (left) and **15.13** (right)   Gridiron incision, in which the muscles are not divided, but are split in the line of their fibres — external oblique in the line of the skin incision, internal oblique and transversus in a more or less transverse direction. The muscles are held apart by retractors, to expose transversalis fascia and peritoneum, which are then incised as one layer. The method of closing the incision is shown. (Rintoul: *Farquharson's Textbook of Operative Surgery.*)

Alternatively, several interrupted sutures of non-absorbable synthetic material may be inserted to approximate the muscles before using chromic catgut.

For midline and paramedian incisions, the anterior rectus sheath or linea alba is sutured with interrupted or continuous chromic catgut, a synthetic absorbable or synthetic non-absorbable material, on a cutting or lance point needle.

Kocher's incision is closed by approximating the muscles with interrupted mattress sutures of chromic catgut or a synthetic absorbable, which are left long and tied when all have been placed.

The skin is closed with interrupted or continuous synthetic non-absorbable or silk on a curved or straight cutting needle, sometimes used in conjunction with Michel, Kifa skin clips or disposable staples (lower midline incisions especially).

Appendectomy

Definition

Removal of the appendix.

Position

Supine.

Instruments

> General set (Figs. 14.1–14.28)
> Bowel-holding forceps (Hamilton Bailey)
> Long artery forceps, curved on flat (Moynihan gall-bladder or Gordon Craig artery forceps), 5
> Suction tubing, nozzles and tube anchoring forceps
> 2.5 and 3 (2/0 and 0) Chromic catgut, synthetic absorbable or non-absorbable, or silk for ligatures
> 2.5 (2/0) Chromic catgut or synthetic absorbable on a non-traumatic curved or straight intestinal needle for purse-string suture
> 3 or 4 (0 or 1) Chromic catgut or synthetic absorbable on a small half-circle round-bodied needle for peritoneum and first muscle layer
> 3 or 4 (0 or 1) Chromic catgut or synthetic absorbable on a small half-circle cutting needle for muscle aponeurosis
> 2.5 (2/0) Synthetic non-absorbable or silk on a medium-curved or straight-cutting needle for skin sutures (Michel or Kifa skin clips or disposable skin staples may be required)
> (Medium-sized tube drain or corrugated drain may be required).

Outline of procedure

Incisions used for this operation include the McBurney 'grid iron', the Battle type and the right lower paramedian. (If a paramedian approach is used, the instruments for laparotomy are selected.)

The centre of a McBurney incision lies in the right iliac region, situated over a point which is at the junction of the outer with the inner two-thirds of an imaginary line joining the umbilicus with the anterior superior iliac spine. It is about five or seven cm in length, and is approximately parallel with the inguinal ligament. The aponeurosis of the external oblique is incised in line with the skin incision. The underlying fibres of the internal oblique and transversus muscles are separated at right angles to the external oblique to expose the peritoneum. The peritoneum is picked up with forceps and incised.

A Battle incision is made more towards the midline, and the rectus muscle is retracted medially to expose the peritoneum which is picked up with forceps and incised.

The caecum is identified and the appendix grasped with a pair of tissue forceps. The meso-appendix is ligated with chromic catgut, a synthetic absorbable or silk, and the base of the appendix is crushed and ligated with chromic catgut or a synthetic absorbable. A purse-string suture is placed around the appendix base, the appendix is removed and the stump invaginated before tying the purse-string suture. All instruments which have come in contact with the transected stump are discarded before the operation proceeds.

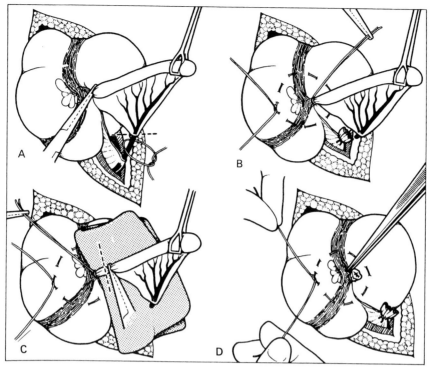

Fig. 15.14 Technique of appendectomy (A) Meso-appendix clamped and divided; base of appendix crushed with forceps. (B) Meso-appendix tied off; appendix ligatured at base; purse-string suture inserted. (C) Appendix clamped distal to ligature and about to be divided against swab. (D) Appendix stump about to be invaginated before tightening of purse-string suture. (Rintoul: *Farquharson's Textbook of Operative Surgery.*)

When the appendix is adherent in a retrocaecal position, the surgeon may divide it and invaginate the stump before ligating the meso-appendix.

The wound is closed by suturing the peritoneum with continuous chromic catgut or a synthetic absorbable on a round-bodied needle, the internal oblique and transversus muscles with similar (but interrupted) sutures and the external oblique with a continuous chromic catgut or a synthetic absorbable suture on a cutting needle. Finally the skin is closed with interrupted synthetic non-absorbable, or silk sutures on a cutting needle or by inserting skin clips or disposable skin staples.

If the appendix has perforated, the surgeon may insert a drainage tube through a separate stab incision before closing the wound.

Drainage of an intrapelvic abscess

Definition

The establishment of a temporary drainage tract for an intraperitoneal pelvic abscess.

Position

Supine.

Instruments

> General set (Figs. 14.1–14.28)
> Artery forceps, straight, 20 cm (8 in) (Spencer Wells), 5
> Deep retractors, narrow blade (Deaver), 2
> Suction tubing, nozzles and tube anchoring forceps
> Long plastic drainage tubing and wound suction apparatus (Redivac, Portovac)
> Ligatures and sutures as for appendectomy (or laparotomy).

Outline of procedure

A long plastic sump drainage tube (a narrower suction tube placed within a wider tube with perforations) is inserted into the pelvis through a McBurney or lower paramedian incision and connected to a wound suction apparatus. The wound is closed in the usual manner for that particular incision.

OPERATIONS ON THE GALL-BLADDER AND COMMON BILE DUCT

Cholecystostomy

Definition

An opening made into the gall bladder to establish drainage of bile.

Position

Supine, with liver bridge elevated (optional); operation table tilted sideways 15° towards the patient's right.

Instruments

> General set (Figs. 14.1–14.28)
> Laparotomy set (Figs. 15.1–15.7)
> Liver retractor (Nuttall)
> Gall-stone forceps (Desjardin)
> Common bile duct probes (Bake)
> Intestinal occlusion clamp, curved (Doyen)
> Gall-stone probe (Desjardin), 3 sizes.
> Malleable scoop and probe (Moynihan)
> Catheters, self-retaining (De Pezzer and Malecot, sizes 16 and 18 Charrière gauge), page 783.
> Catheter introducer, page 783
> Gall-bladder trocar and cannula
> Long plastic drainage tube
> 'T' drainage tubes (Kehr), assorted sizes
> Haemostatic agent (gelatine sponge)

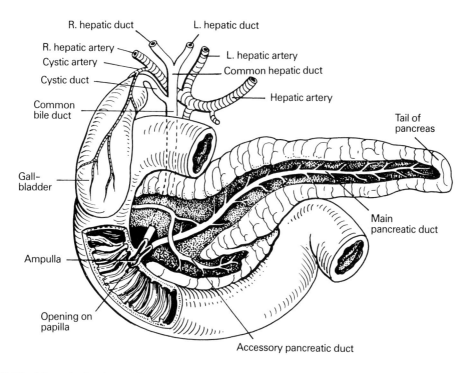

R. hepatic duct
L. hepatic duct
R. hepatic artery
Cystic artery
Cystic duct
Common bile duct
Gall-bladder
Ampulla
Opening on papilla
L. hepatic artery
Common hepatic duct
Hepatic artery
Tail of pancreas
Main pancreatic duct
Accessory pancreatic duct

Fig. 15.15 Schematic drawing to show the relations of the gall bladder and bile ducts to the duodenum and head of pancreas. (Rintoul: *Farquharson's Textbook of Operative Surgery.*)

10 ml syringe and exploration needle
Suction tubing, nozzles and tube anchoring forceps
Laparotomy ligatures and sutures
2.5 (2/0) Chromic catgut or a synthetic absorbable on a small curved non-traumatic
    intestinal needle for purse-string suture.

Outline of procedure

Through a right paramedian, right upper quadrant, transverse Kocher's subcostal or upper
midline incision, a purse-string suture is placed in the tip of the gall-bladder. A trocar and
cannula is inserted at a point in the centre of this purse-string suture and the bile evacuated.
Desjardin's forceps may be used through the stab opening to extract any gall-stones. A long
drainage tube is inserted and secured by tying the purse-string suture.

The wound is closed in the usual manner and the drainage tube connected to a sealed
bottle or disposable plastic bag.

Cholecystectomy

Definition

Removal of the gall-bladder.

Fig. 15.16   Desjardin gall-stone probe.

Fig. 15.17   Moynihan gall-stone probe and scoop.

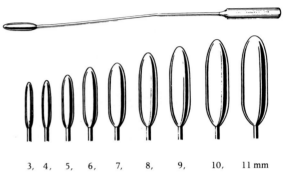

Fig. 15.18   Bakes common bile duct dilators.

3,   4,   5,   6,   7,   8,   9,   10,   11 mm

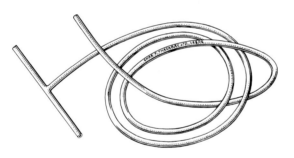

Fig. 15.19   Kehr 'T' tube. Sizes available: 12, 15, 18, 21, 24 and 27 Charrière gauge. Rubber or plastic.

Fig. 15.20   Ochsner gall-bladder trocar.

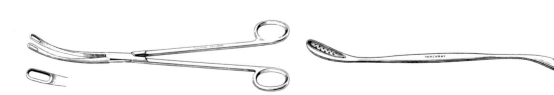

Fig. 15.21   Desjardin gall-stone forceps.

Fig. 15.22   Moynihan gall-stone scoop.

Position

Supine, with the liver bridge elevated (optional); operation table tilted sideways 15° towards the patient's right.

Instruments

(As above).

Outline of procedure

The incision is as above; the cystic duct and artery are identified, clamped, ligated with chromic catgut, a synthetic absorbable or non-absorbable, or silk, clamped distally, and divided. The gall-bladder is freed from the liver and removed. The raw surface of the liver may either be sutured over with 2.5 (2/0) chromic catgut or a synthetic absorbable on a small curved non-traumatic intestinal needle, or a haemostatic agent (e.g., gelatine sponge or Surgicel) applied.

A long drainage tube is inserted and the wound closed in the usual manner.

Choledochotomy

Definition

An incision into the common bile duct, usually for the extraction of gall-stones.

Position

Supine, as for cholecystectomy.

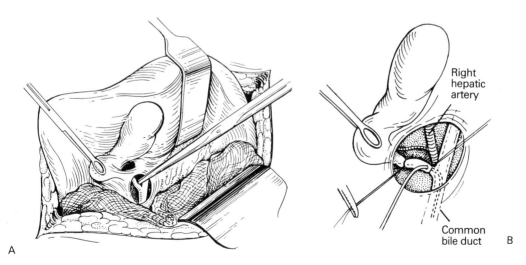

Fig. 15.23 (A) Cholecystectomy by the retrograde method — exposure of the cystic duct at its junction with the common hepatic duct, in the right free border of the lesser omentum. (B) Cystic duct divided between ligature and clamp, and cystic artery displayed. (Rintoul: *Farquharson's Textbook of Operative Surgery*.)

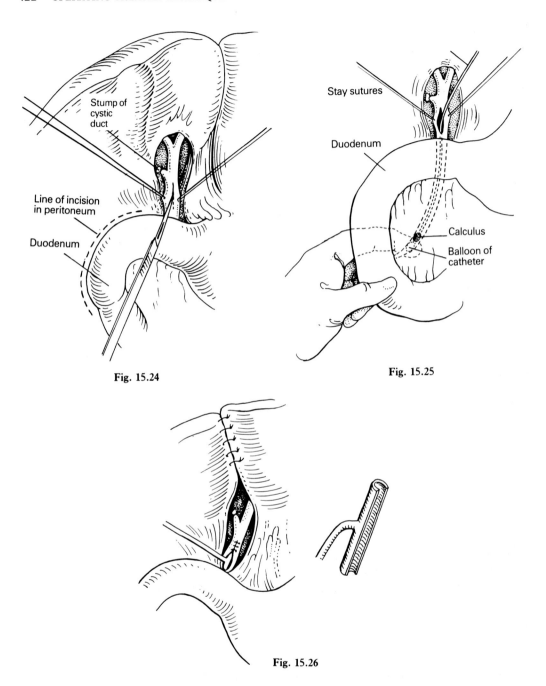

Stump of
cystic
duct

Line of incision
in peritoneum

Duodenum

Fig. 15.24

Stay sutures

Duodenum

Calculus

Balloon of
catheter

Fig. 15.25

Fig. 15.26

Fig. 15.24 (above left) Method of opening the supra-duodenal part of the common bile duct by an incision between stay sutures.

Fig. 15.25 (above right) Removal of a calculus in the lower part of the common bile duct using a Fogarty biliary catheter.

Fig. 15.26 (left) T-tube drainage of the common bile duct. The incision in the duct is sutured *above* the emerging limb of the tube in order to avoid any drag on the suture line when the tube is withdrawn. (Rintoul: *Farquharson's Textbook of Operative Surgery*.)

Instruments

As above, plus malleable probes, bougies, irrigation syringe, catheter and warm saline.

Outline of procedure

The incision is as above; the common bile duct is identified and two long 'stay' sutures of 2.5 (2/0) chromic catgut or a synthetic absorbable on a small (20 mm) non-traumatic intestinal needle are inserted. The duct is opened between these sutures, suctioned and explored with probes and Desjardin's forceps. The duct may be irrigated with saline before inserting a Kehr's T-tube; and the incision in the duct is sutured with further 2.5 (2/0) chromic catgut or a synthetic absorbable sutures, *above* the emerging limb of the tube in order to avoid any drag on the suture line when the tube is withdrawn.

An additional long drainage tube is placed in the vicinity of the duct and the wound is closed in the usual manner.

Cholecystogastrostomy

Definition

Anastomosis between the gall-bladder and the stomach.

Position

Supine.

Instruments

(As above)

Outline of procedure

The incision is as above; the gall-bladder is drained with a trocar and cannula and then approximated to the stomach. Curved occlusion clamps are applied and an anastomosis made with two layers of 2.5 (2/0) chromic catgut or a synthetic absorbable sutures on a small or medium cuved non-traumatic intestinal needle. A long drainage tube is inserted in the vicinity of the anastomosis and the wound closed in the usual manner.

Cholecystoenterostomy

Definition

The procedure is as above but the anastomosis is made between the gall-bladder and the jejunum, often with jejuno-jejunostomy.

Pancreatic duodenectomy (Whipple's procedure)

Definition

The head of pancreas, duodeum, part of the jejunum and stomach are resected, together with the lower half of the common bile duct and part of the pancreatic duct.

Position

Supine.

Instruments

>   General set (Figs. 14.1–14.28)
>   Laparotomy set (Figs. 15.1–15.7)
>   Gall-bladder set (Figs. 15.16–15.22)
>   Gastrectomy set (Fig. 15.32)
>   Suction tubing, nozzles and tube anchoring forceps
>   Diathermy leads, electrodes and lead anchoring forceps
>   Laparotomy ligatures and sutures
>   2, 2.5 and 3 (3/0, 2/0 and 0) Chromic catgut or a synthetic absorbable on small and medium half-circle and curved non-traumatic intestinal needles for anastomoses
>   2.5 (2/0) Synthetic non-absorbable or silk on small curved non-traumatic intestinal needles.

Outline of procedure

Through a midline incision a partial gastrectomy, duodenectomy, partial jejunectomy, pancreatectomy and choledochectomy is performed. The stump of the pancreas is joined to the remaining portion of the jejunum (pancreaticojejunostomy) as an end to end anastomosis. The end of the common bile duct is anastomosed to the jejunum (choledochojejunostomy), using interrupted synthetic non-absorbable or silk sutures in both cases. The stomach is anastomosed to the jejunum (gastro-jejunostomy) in the usual manner and the wound is closed.

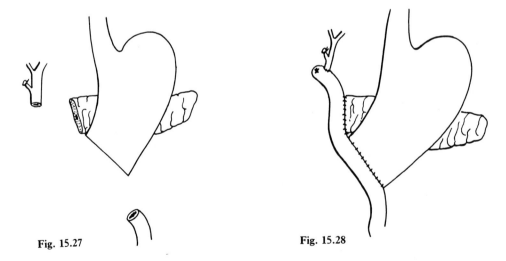

Fig. 15.27   Fig. 15.28

Fig. 15.27   Structures remaining after pancreaticoduodenectomy.

Fig. 15.28   Reconstruction following pancreaticodudenectomy (Rintoul: *Farquharson's Textbook of Operative Surgery.*)

Ramstedt's operation

Definition

An operation performed for the relief of congenital pyloric stenosis and which consists of division of the circular muscle fibres of the pylorus.

Position

The patient is placed in the supine position or immobilised on a padded crucifix if local anaesthesia is being used.

Instruments

Sponge-holding forceps (Rampley), 5
Towel clips, 5

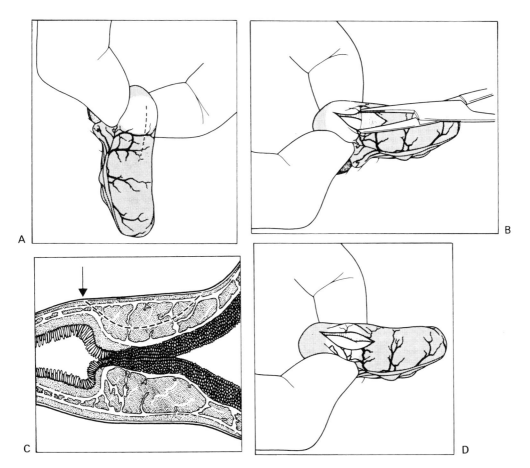

Fig. 15.29 Ramstedt's operation; pyloromyotomy for congenital pyloric stenosis. A. The posterior part of the tumour is pinched with the finger and thumb to stretch the anti-mesenteric border. Dotted line indicates incision. B. Mosquito artery forceps are introduced into the incision and spread so as to split the hypertrophied muscle. C. Cross-section of hypertrophied pyloric muscle and line of incision. Arrow indicates the point where special care must be taken to avoid penetration of the mucosa. D. Pylorotomy completed. Intact mucosa bulges into base of incision. (Rintoul: *Farquharson's Textbook of Operative Surgery.*)

Scalpel handles No. 3, with Nos. 10 and 15 blades (Bard Parker), 2
Fine dissecting forceps, toothed (Gillies), 2
Fine dissecting forceps, non-toothed (McIndoe), 2
Scissors, straight, 13 cm (5 in) (Mayo)
Scissors, curved on flat, 18 cm (7 in) (Mayo)
Long scissors, curved on flat (McIndoe)
Sinus forceps
Blunt dissector (Watson Cheyne)
Blunt dissector (MacDonald)
Fine artery forceps, curved on flat (mosquito), 5
Fine artery forceps, straight (mosquito), 5
Small retractors, double hook, 2
Medium retractors (Czerny), 2
Fine tissue forceps (McIndoe), 5
Skin or tetra towel forceps (Moynihan), 4 for the sides of the wound and 2 for the ends
   of the wound (Optional)
2 and 2.5 (3/0 and 2/0) Chromic catgut or a synthetic absorbable for ligatures
2.5 and 3 (2/0 and 0) Chromic catgut or a synthetic absorbable on small half-circle round-
   bodied needles for peritoneum and muscles
2 (3/0) Synthetic non-absorbable or silk on a small curved or straight cutting needle for
   skin sutures.

Outline of procedure

Through a small midline or paramedian incision, the pylorus is delivered into the wound
and an incision made through the tumour wall into the circular muscle fibres, care being
taken to avoid incising the mucosa. These fibres are stretched with artery or sinus forceps
until the mucosa herniates into the muscle incision. The wound is closed in the usual
manner.

Gastro-jejunostomy

Definition

The establishment of an opening between the stomach and the jejunum.

Position

Supine.

Instruments

General set (Figs. 14.1–14.28)
Laparotomy set (Figs. 15.1–15.7)
Intestinal occlusion clamps, straight (Doyen), 2
Intestinal occlusion clamps, curved (Doyen), 2
Twin occlusion clamps (Lane), optional
Fine tissue forceps (McIndoe), 5
Fine artery forceps, straight (mosquito), 5

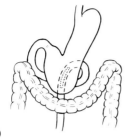

Fig. 15.30 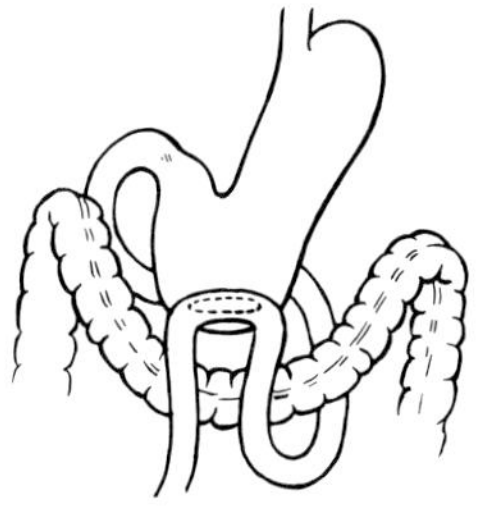   Fig. 15.31

Fig. 15.30 Posterior gastro-jejunostomy. The jejunum is brought through an opening in the transverse mesocolon, and is anastomosed to the posterior wall of the stomach. (Farquharson and Rintoul: *Textbook of Operative Surgery, 6th Edn.*)

Fig. 15.31 Anterior gastro-jejunostomy. The jejunum is brought round as a long loop below the transverse colon, and is anastomosed to the anterior wall of the stomach. (Farquharson and Rintoul.)

Suction tubing, nozzles and tube anchoring forceps

Laparotomy ligatures and sutures

2.5 and 3 (2/0 and 0) Chromic catgut or a synthetic absorbable on medium or small curved non-traumatic intestinal needles for anastomosis

2.5 (2/0) Synthetic non-absorbable or silk on small curved non-traumatic intestinal needles for anastomosis.

Outline of procedure

Through a left paramedian or midline incision an opening is made in the avascular space of the transverse mesocolon. The posterior wall of the stomach is grasped with tissue forceps on the lesser and greater curvatures at each end of the proposed line of anastomosis. The jejunum is grasped with tissue forceps also, and occlusion clamps applied to the stomach and jejunum. A continuous 2.5 (2/0) chromic catgut or a synthetic absorbable suture or interrupted silk sutures are used for the posterior seromuscular layer joining the stomach and bowel. The stomach and jejunum are then opened and gastric contents evacuated with the suction tube. The second posterior row of sutures consists of a continuous 2.5 or 3 (2/0 or 0) chromic catgut or a synthetic absorbable through and through all layers of the stomach and bowel, and this is continued around the stoma to form the first anterior layer. If a continuous absorbable has been used for the first posterior layer, this suture is continued to form the second seromuscular layer of the anastomosis; alternatively, interrupted silk sutures are used. The opening in the mesocolon is sutured to the stomach before wound closure. This operation is often combined with vagotomy.

Partial gastrectomy

Definition

Resection of a portion of the stomach with anastomosis between the remaining portion of the stomach and the duodenum or jejunum.

Position

Supine.

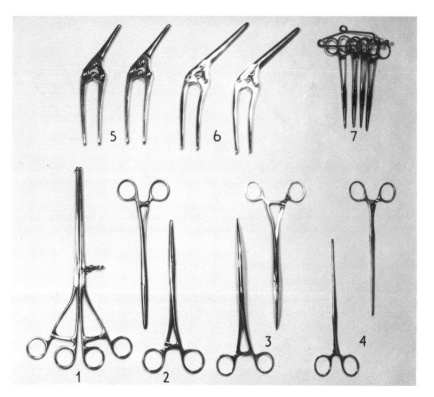

Fig. 15.32 Gastrectomy and resection of bowel.
1. Twin occlusion clamp for stomach or intestine (Lane).
2. Intestinal crushing clamps (Joll), 2.
3. Intestinal occlusion clamps, curved (Doyen), 2.
4. Intestinal occlusion clamps, straight (Doyen), 2.
5 and 6. Intestinal crushing clamps, double action, small and large (Payr), 2 of each size.
7. Fine tissue forceps (McIndoe), 4.

Instruments

General set (Figs. 14.1–14.28)
Laparotomy set (Figs. 15.1–15.7)
Gastrectomy set (Fig. 15.32)
Automatic bowel stapler
Fine artery forceps, straight (McIndoe), 5
Suction tubing, nozzles and tube anchoring forceps
Laparotomy ligatures and sutures
2.5 and 3 (2/0 and 0) Chromic catgut or a synthetic absorbable on small and medium curved and half-circle non-traumatic intestinal needles for anastomosis
2.5 (2/0) Synthetic non-absorbable or silk on a small curved or half-circle non-traumatic needle for anastomosis.

Outline of procedure

There are several variations in the technique of gastric resection but basically the initial dissection is the same. The incision may be right paramedian or midline and possibly transverse.

The Billroth I or Schoemaker Operation. The omentum on the greater curvature of the stomach is dissected free down to the duodenum, clamping, dividing and ligating the blood vessels in the process. The right gastric vessels on the lesser curvature of the stomach are identified and divided between stout ligatures of chromic catgut, synthetic absorbable or silk. A crushing clamp is placed across the duodenum at its junction with the stomach, and then alongside this but just distally an occlusion clamp is also applied. The duodenum is divided with a scalpel, which is then discarded. The left gastric or coronary vessels and the vessels in the omentum on the upper left side of the stomach are ligated with stout chromic catgut,

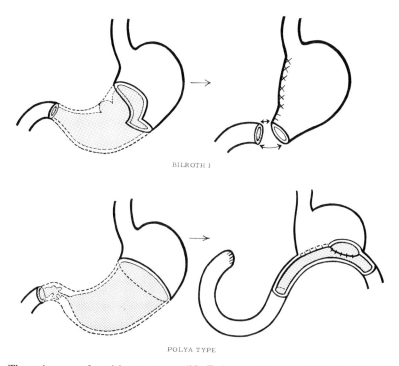

BILROTH I

POLYA TYPE

Fig. 15.33 The main types of partial gastrectomy. (MacFarlane and Thomas: *Textbook of Surgery*)

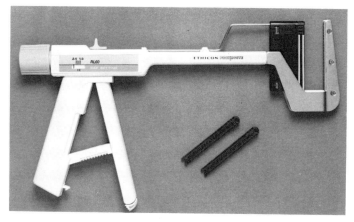

Fig. 15.34 Reloadable linear stapler. (Proximate™ RL60, Ethicon.)

synthetic absorbable or silk and then divided. An occlusion clamp is applied across the stomach at the desired level and the organ resected.

The cut end of the stomach is funnelled with two layers of sutures towards the greater curvature and the anastomosis made to the duodenum. The first posterior and second anterior seromuscular layers of the anastomosis consist of continuous 2.5 (2/0) chromic catgut or a synthetic absorbable suture or interrupted silk sutures. The second posterior and first anterior layers consist of a continuous 3 (0) chromic catgut or a synthetic absorbable suture placed through and through all layers of the stomach and bowel. Instruments used for the anastomosis are discarded before wound closure.

Billroth II Operation. In all the following variations of this operation, the duodenum is divided between crushing clamps and closed with a continuous chromic catgut or a synthetic absorbable suture followed by a second layer of catgut, synthetic absorbable, non-absorbable or silk sutures. Alternatively, an automatic stapling device such as Proximate^{TM} (Ethicon, Fig. 15.34) can be used to divide the duodenum. The row of staples on the duodenal stump is buried by a layer of interrupted seromuscular sutures of chromic catgut or a synthetic absorbable. The stomach is resected and anastomosed to a loop of jejunum. With the original Billroth II operation, now rarely performed, the cut end of the stomach is closed and the jejunum joined to a fresh opening in the stomach. Staples can be used also to close the gastric pouch (cut end of the stomach) and complete the anastomosis (Fig. 15.35). The Polya operation is perhaps the most common and consists of an end to side anastomosis between the entire cut end of the stomach and the jejunum, posterior to the transverse colon. An anterior Polya resection consists of an end to side anastomosis made in a similar manner but anterior to the transverse colon. The Hoffmeister resection consists of closing the cut end

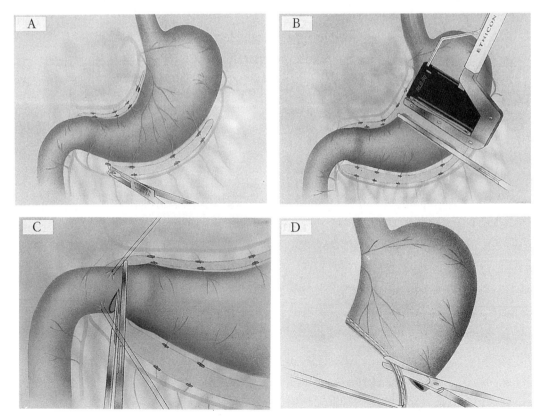

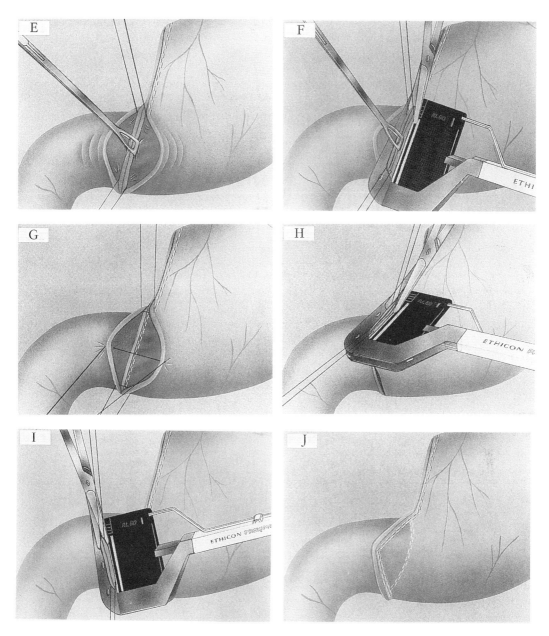

Fig. 15.35   Bilroth 1, resection and anastomosis with staples. (A) The greater and lesser curvatures of the stomach are mobilised and the omental vessels are ligated with clips. (Absolok★ absorbable.) (B) The stomach is closed with one application of the linear gastric stapler. A clamp is placed just below the stapler, and the stomach transected using the cutting guide on the edge of the stapler anvil as a guide. (C) The duodenum is transected between clamps on the resection side and stay sutures placed on the patient side to prevent retraction of the duodenal stump. (D) A portion of the gastric staple line, slightly smaller than the diameter of the transected duodenum, is excised. (E) The posterior edges of the duodenal and gastric openings are approximated, serosa to serosa, with two traction sutures; the tissue edges are approximated at the midpoint with a Babcock clamp. (F) The stapler jaws are positioned around the approximated tissue and the stapler fired. Extraneous tissue is excised. (G) A third everting traction suture is used to form a triangle with the posterior staple line as the base. (H and I) The remaining sides of the anastomosis are closed, mucosa to mucosa by two successive applications of the stapler. (J) The completed anastomosis with the anterior wall made transparent to show reconstruction. (*Surgical Stapling Techniques*, Ethicon.)

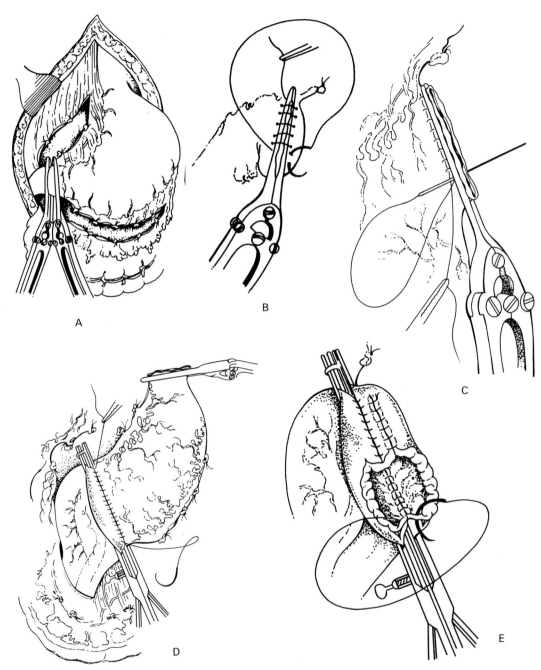

Fig. 15.36 Polya type of gastrectomy. Mobilisation of stomach; division and closure of duodenum (A) The stomach and first part of duodenum are mobilised, and the latter is divided between clamps. (B) The duodenal stump is first closed with an invaginating sero-muscular suture passed from side to side above the clamp, followed by a second invaginating suture. If this is impracticable the first suture line is covered with omentum or is buried by being sutured against the pancreas. (C) Sewing machine stitch, an alternative method of closing duodenal stump when the stump is short and may be difficult to invaginate. (D) The proximal loop of jejunum is brought through a window in the transverse meso-colon, and, with the aid of twin clamps, is anastomosed to the stomach at the selected level. The first layer of suture is shown. (E) The stomach has been transected and the distal segment removed; the upper part of the cut end is then closed, and the lower part only is used for the anastomosis. (Rintoul: *Farquharson's Textbook of Operative Surgery*.)

of the stomach, leaving a 51 mm (2 in) stoma on the greater curvature to which the jejunum is anastomosed. Alternatively, a central 51 mm (2 in) stoma may be formed by partially closing the cut end of the stomach from each side. The loop of jejunum is then anastomosed to the opening.

Total gastrectomy

This is occasionally performed for malignancy and the dissection approximates to that for partial gastrectomy but is more extensive. The instruments are for gastrectomy plus thoracotomy set (page 829). In most instances a thoraco-abdominal approach is employed. A Billroth I type of anastomosis may be used, joining the oesophagus to the duodenum, but more commonly an oesophagojejunostomy is established.

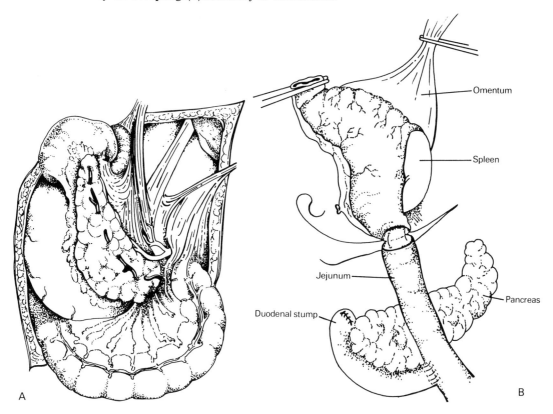

Fig. 15.37   Total gastrectomy by the abdominothoracic approach. A. The diaphragm has been incised from the rib margin into the oesophageal hiatus. The mobilized spleen and stomach have been turned forwards and to the right exposing the splenic and left gastric arteries at their origin from the coelic axis. B. The mobilized stomach and spleen have been reflected upwards and a Roux loop of jejunum has been brought up for anastomosis to the oesophagus. (Rintoul: *Farquharson's Textbook of Operative Surgery.*)

Vagotomy (adominal approach)

Definition

Division of the vagus nerves often in conjunction with gastro-jejunostomy in the treatment of peptic ulcer or pyloroplasty.

Position

Supine.

Instruments

> General set (Figs. 14.1–14.28)
> Laparotomy set (Figs. 15.1–15.7)
> Gastro-enterostomy set (page 426) if gastro-jejunostomy is to be carried out.
> Laparotomy ligatures and sutures.

Outline of procedure

The incision may be midline or paramedian. The left triangular ligament is divided to mobilize the left lobe of the liver, which is displaced to the right with a pack.

The transverse colon and small intestine are displaced downwards with a pack. Utilising deep retractors and traction, the stomach is drawn downward to expose the gastro-oesophageal junction. After incising the covering peritoneum, a finger is passed upwards to gently mobilize the oesophagus within the posterior peritoneum.

The lower 5 to 8 cm (2 to 3 inches) of the oesophagus is drawn into the abdomen and immobilised with a tape or tubing sling. One method adopted is when the anterior (left) vagus nerve, which may have two divisions is identified and sectioned between forceps. The upper end is ligated with non-absorbable ligatures, and the lower end withdrawn to expose other branches of the nerve. These are excised for a length of 3 to 5 cm (1½ to 2 inches). The posterior (right) vagus nerve lies behind the oesophagus. This is identified and excised in a similar manner to the anterior nerve. If a gastro-jejunostomy is to be carried out, this follows the vagotomy.

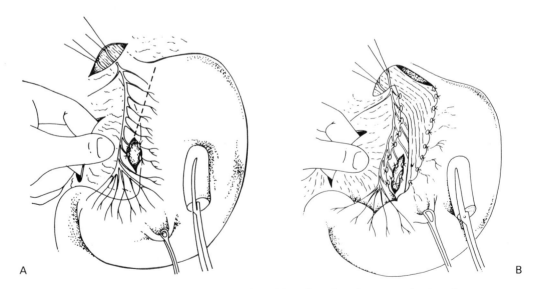

A   B

Fig. 15.38 Highly selective vagotomy in which individual branches of vagal nerve passing into the upper two-thirds of the stomach are divided, whilst sparing the vagal supply to the antrum and pylorus. A. Shows crow's foot fanning of anterior nerve of Latarget, and commencement of division of anterior leaf of lesser omentum. Dotted line indicates the line of separation to be used at a higher level. B. Showing separation of posterior leaf of lesser omentum and window created into lesser sac. (Rintoul: *Farquharson's Textbook of Operative Surgery.*)

Another method is highly selective vagotomy which is illustrated in Figures 15.38 and 15.39. In this procedure, only the individual branches of the vagus nerve passing into the upper two thirds of the stomach are divided. This spares the vagal supply to the antrum and pylorus, so obviating the need for drainage. The abdomen is closed as for laparotomy.

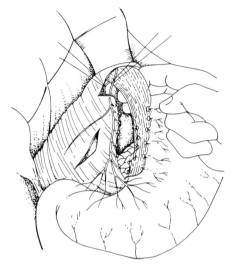

Fig. 15.39 Highly selective vagotomy: finished dissection showing extent of oesophageal clearance. (Rintoul: *Farquharson's Textbook of Operative Surgery.*)

Intussusception

Definition

Obstruction from invaginated bowel.

Position

Supine with Trendelenburg for colonic invagination.

Instruments

As for gastrectomy (p. 428) (resection of bowel may be necessary).
   Automatic bowel stapler

Outline of procedure

Through a paramedian or midline incision, the deformity is reduced by gentle pressure exerted on the head of the invaginated portion of the bowel. Warm packs are applied and if the bowel is non-viable, it is resected in the usual manner and the wound closed.

Resection of small bowel

Definition

Resection of a portion of the small intestine.

Position

Supine.

Instruments

As for gastrectomy (p. 428).
  Automatic bowel stapler

Outline of procedure

The incision may be paramedian or midline (an exception being when treating a strangulated hernia and in this case the bowel may be delivered via the hernial orifice).

  The mesenteric vessels supplying the loop of bowel are identified and ligated with chromic catgut, synthetic non-absorbable or silk. Crushing and occlusion clamps are applied at each side of the affected section of bowel which is then resected. The occlusion clamps are retained until an end to end anastomosis has been made, using two layers of continuous chromic catgut or a synthetic absorbable. Anastomosis instruments are discarded before wound closure in the usual manner.

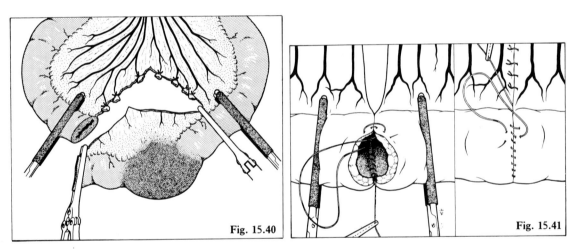

Fig. 15.40   Technique of resection in small bowel. (Rintoul: *Textbook of Operative Surgery.*)

Fig. 15.41   End-to-end anastomosis of small bowel by two layers of continuous suture. The *Connell* suture shown in the first drawing prevents eversion of the mucosa. (Rintoul: *Farquharson's Textbook of Operative Surgery.*)

Right hemicolectomy

Definition

Resection of the right half of the colon.

Position

Supine.

Instruments

As for gastrectomy (p. 428).
  Automatic bowel stapler

Outline of procedure

Through a right paramedian or midline incision, the ascending colon and distal part of the ileum are mobilised from the lateral peritoneal fold. The ureter and duodenum are ident-

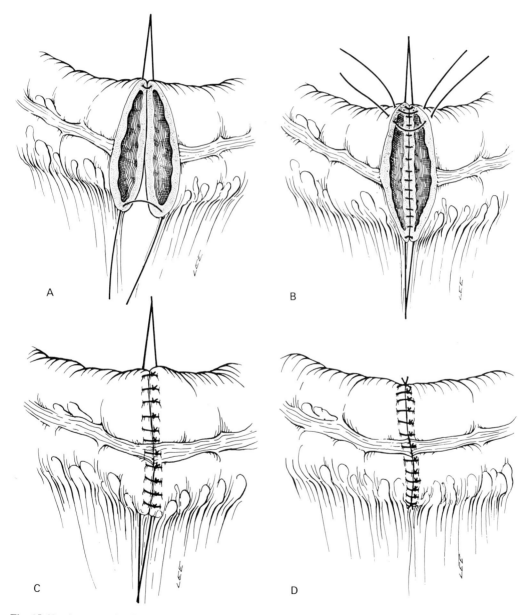

Fig. 15.42 Anastomosis of two cut ends of the colon. (A) Stay sutures are placed for a single layer anastomosis. (B) Principles of a single layer anastomosis. (C & D) Anastomosis completed. (Rintoul: *Farquharson's Textbook of Operative Surgery*.)

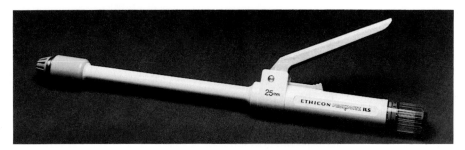

Fig. 15.43   Disposable intraliminal stapler system. (Proximate ILS, Ethicon.)

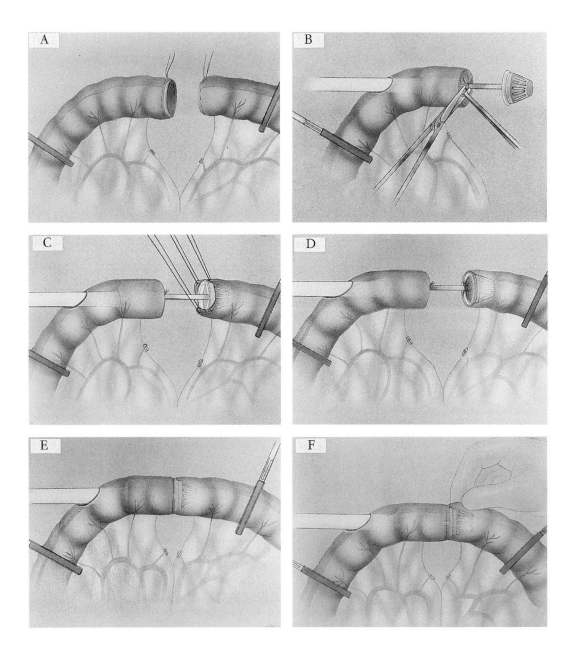

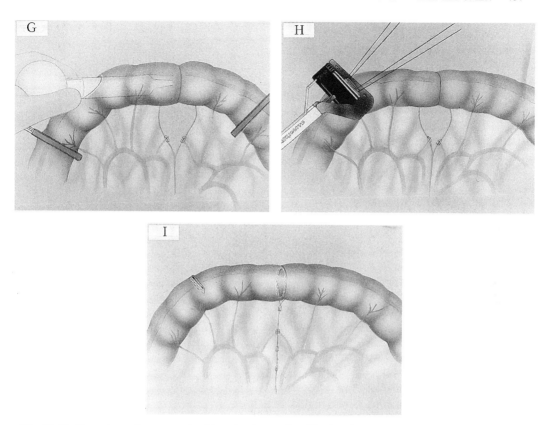

Fig. 15.44 Resection and anastomosis of bowel using staples. (*Surgical Stapling Techniques* — Ethicon.)
(A) After the appropriate segment of colon is mobilized and the mesentary dissected back at least 2 cm beyond the proximal and distal points of transection, the colon is resected in the usual manner. Purse string sutures are then placed on each end of the transected bowel. (B) After insertion into the bowel lumen through a colotomy, the intraluminal stapler is opened 4–6 cm. The instrument is advanced until the anvil protrudes through the open end of the bowel. At that time the purse string suture is tied down firmly around the centre rod, and excess suture and tissue trimmed to avoid bunching. (C) Traction sutures or Allis tissue forceps may be used to facilitate placement of the posterior wall of the bowel over the instrument anvil. (D) Once the anvil has been fully introduced into the bowel lumen, the purse string suture is tied down firmly around the centre rod. Excess suture and redundant tissue is carefully trimmed, making certain that the purse string remains intact. (E) After properly aligning the two bowel segments, the stapler is closed, and the staple height set by turning the adjusting knob clockwise. As the instrument is fired, staples are driven through the tissue and formed against the anvil; at the same time, a knife blade advances to cut a uniform stoma between the proximal and distal bowel segments. (F) Before attempting to remove the stapler, the instrument is opened slightly by turning the adjusting knob counterclockwise approximately 1/2 to 3/4 turn, rotating the stapler 180° in either direction to ensure tissue release. The anastomotic staple line is then gently lifted over the lip of the anvil by hand or with a traction suture. The instrument is then removed whilst slightly rotating or rocking it. (G) The integrity of the anastomosis is checked by introducing fluid via a syringe inserted through the colectomy. (H) The colotomy is closed with one application of a linear stapler. (I) The completed anastomosis with the anterior wall made transparent to show the lumen and staple lines.

ified, the mesentery incised, and the mesenteric vessels ligated with chromic catgut, a synthetic absorbable or silk before division. Two sets of clamps are applied across the bowel on either side of the area of resection. The bowel is divided between each of the sets and removed. The occlusion clamps are retained in position until the anastomosis is completed (Fig. 15.42). Anastomosis may be accomplished using staples; this technique is shown in Figures 15.43 and 15.44. The instruments used for the anastomosis are discarded, the defect

in the posterior peritoneum and mesentary sutured, and the wound closed in the usual manner. Crushing and occlusion clamps are applied transversely across the colon and obliquely across the ileum, the bowel is resected and the occlusion clamps retained until the anastomosis is completed with sutures in the usual manner. (Fig. 15.41). Alternatively a stapled anastomosis can be undertaken. The principle consists of bringing the two ends of the bowel together over an 'anvil', with a purse string suture (Fig. 15.45) and then inserting a row of staples through the wall of the colon, and at the same time cutting a central core with a circular knife (Fig. 15.42). The instruments used for the anastomosis are discarded, the defect in the posterior peritoneum and mesentery sutured and the wound closed.

Total colectomy

Definition

Resection of the ascending, transverse and descending colon.

Position

Supine with some degree of Trendelenburg.

Instruments

As for gastrectomy (p. 428).
   Automatic bowel stapler
   Intestinal occlusion clamps, right-angled (Finch), 2.

Outline of procedure

The incision may be midline or paramedian. The colon is mobilised from the distal end of the ileum to the sigmoid flexure, ligating and dividing the mesenteric and superior haemorrhoidal vessels with stout chromic catgut, a synthetic absorbable or silk. Resection of the colon between two sets of crushing and occlusion clamps is performed and anastomosis made between the ileum and the rectum (ileorectostomy) in the usual manner, or the rectum is closed with interrupted synthetic non-absorbable or silk sutures and an ileostomy performed. If the resection is low, the rectal anastomosis may be made with a series of interrupted mattress sutures of 3 (0) chromic catgut, a synthetic absorbable or silk which are left long and not tied until all have been placed in position.

Abdominoperineal resection of the rectum and part of the colon

Definition

Mobilisation of the diseased portion of the colon which is pushed into the hollow of the pelvis for removal via the perineal route, and the establishment of a terminal colostomy.

Position

Lithotomy and Trendelenburg with a sandbag or similar support under the buttocks.

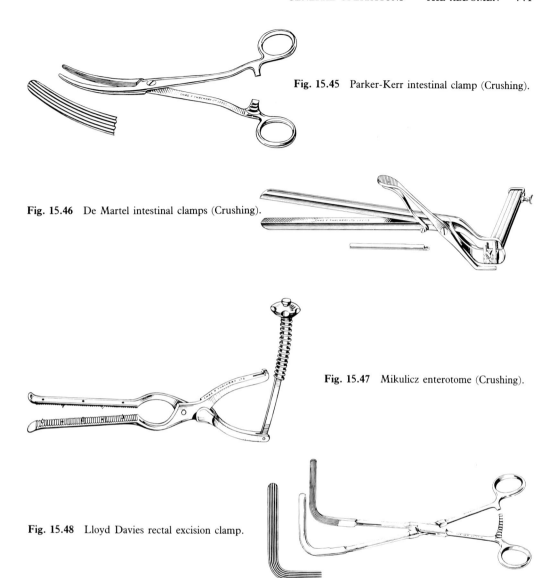

Fig. 15.45 Parker-Kerr intestinal clamp (Crushing).

Fig. 15.46 De Martel intestinal clamps (Crushing).

Fig. 15.47 Mikulicz enterotome (Crushing).

Fig. 15.48 Lloyd Davies rectal excision clamp.

Instruments

Anterior part of the operation
General set (Figs. 14.1–14.28)
Laparotomy set (Figs. 15.1–15.7)
Long scalpel handle No. 4L with No. 20 blade (Bard Parker)
Long dissecting forceps, toothed, 25 cm (10 in)
Long dissecting forceps, non-toothed, 25 cm (10 in)
Long scissors, curved on flat, 23 cm (9 in) (Nelson)
Scissors, straight, 20 cm (8 in) (Mayo)
Intestinal occlusion clamps, straight (Doyen), 2

Intestinal occlusion clamps, curved (Doyen), 2
Intestinal crushing clamps (Payr or Joll), 2
Intestinal crushing clamps (de Martel or Zachary Cope), set of 3
Suprapubic retractor (Doyen)
Suction tubing, nozzles and tube anchoring forceps
Diathermy leads, electrodes and lead anchoring forceps
Ligatures and sutures as for laparotomy
Long tissue forceps, 20 cm (8 in) (Lane's or Fagge's), 5

Posterior part of operation
General set (Figs. 14.1–14.28)
Extra towel clips, 5
Long scalpel handle No. 4L with No. 20 blade (Bard Parker)
Long tissue forceps, 20 cm (8 in) (Lane's or Fagge's), 5
Deep retractors, narrow blade (Paton), 2
Rugines curved and straight (Faraboeuf)
Bone nibbling or gouge forceps (single action)
Bone nibbling or gouge forceps (compound action)
Bone cutting forceps, curved (Liston)
Long scissors, straight, 20 cm (8 in) (Mayo)
Long scissors, curved on flat, 20 cm (8 in) (Mayo)

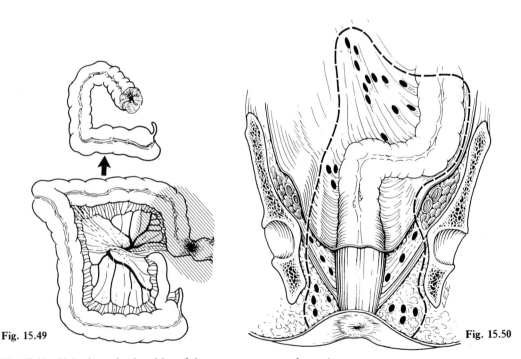

Fig. 15.49

Fig. 15.50

Fig. 15.49 Abdominoperineal excision of the rectum — extent of resection.

Fig. 15.50 Abdominoperineal excision of rectum — showing the tissues removed with the tumour in the distal rectum. (Rintoul: *Farquharson's Textbook of Operative Surgery.*)

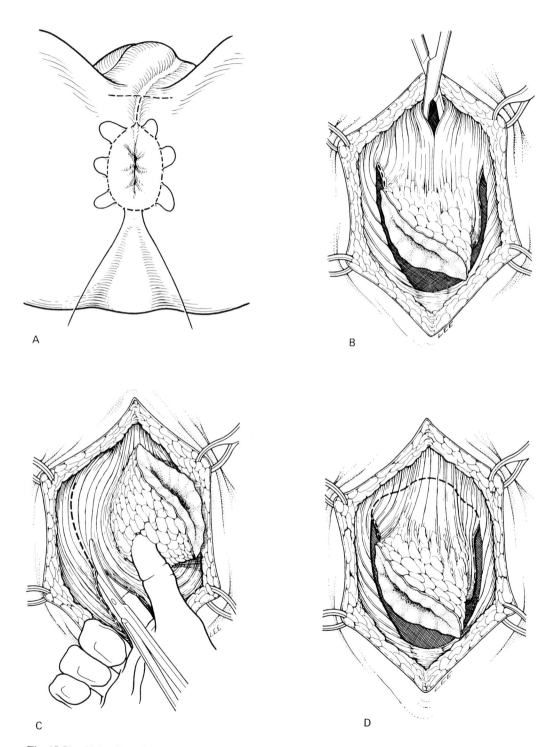

A

B

C

D

Fig. 15.51 Abdominoperineal excision of the rectum — perineal dissection. A. The anal purse string suture.
B. Dissecting the perineum. C & D Dividing the levators (Rintoul: *Farquharson's Textbook of Operative Surgery.*)

Urethral catheter, 18 to 20 Charrière gauge (Jacques, Nélaton, or Foley self-retaining) (If Foley catheter is used, a syringe containing 5 to 30 ml of sterile water to inflate the catheter cuff, and a ligature for the pilot tube will be required, unless this is self-sealing.)

Spigot

Large rubber or plastic drainage tube

3 and 4 (0 and 1) Chromic catgut or synthetic absorbable for ligatures

4 or 5 (1 or 2) Chromic catgut or a synthetic non-absorbable on a large half-circle cutting needle for deep sutures

5 (2) Synthetic non-absorbable or silk on a large half-circle cutting needle for anal purse-string sutures

2.5 (2/0) Synthetic non-absorbable or silk in large curved cutting needles for skin sutures.

Outline of procedure

Generally this operation is performed as a synchronous-combined procedure by two operation teams. In this case the instrument sets must be available on two trolleys for simultaneous use and it is very important that the swab count of each team is kept separate. To assist this, the instrument nurse assisting the surgeon performing the anterior part of the operation will ensure that only 'taped' swabs or packs are used in the vicinity of the pelvis and that instruments are not interchanged between the teams.

The anterior part of the operation. Through a lower midline incision the bowel is mobilised from the point of transection to the coccyx, ligating and dividing the inferior mesenteric vessels. Slender crushing clamps such as the de Martel's are applied across the colon, above the disease portion. The bowel is divided and the proximal end brought out through an incision at the selected site for the permanent colostomy. A rubber glove is secured over the distal clamp to prevent soiling of the peritoneum, and the diseased portion of the bowel and rectum is pushed into the hollow of the pelvis for removal by the surgeon performing the perineal part of the operation. The pelvic peritoneum is sutured with a continuous 2.5 (2/0) or 3 (0) chromic catgut or a synthetic absorbable before general wound closure.

The posterior part of the operation. A urethal catheter is inserted and the bladder emptied. The rectum is sealed by placing two purse-string sutures around the anus, and an elliptical incision made round the rectum exposing the levator ani muscles, which are divided. The urethra is identified and in co-operation with the surgeon performing the anterior part of the operation, the rectum is freed with scissors. The diseased bowel and rectum is removed through the posterior incision and the muscles approximated with chromic catgut. A long drainage tube (which will be attached to a suitable sterile bottle) is used to drain the pelvic space before skin closure with a synthetic non-absorbable or silk.

Anterior resection of the rectum and part of the colon

Definition

A sphincter-saving resection of the rectum and part of the colon with re-establishment of continuity by anastomosis.

Position

As for abdominoperineal resection.

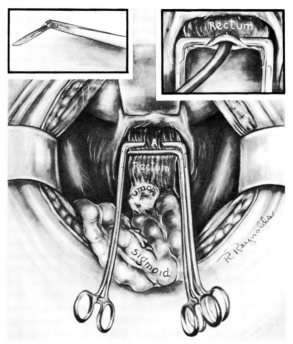

Fig. 15.52 Anterior (trans-abdominal) resection of the rectum — division of the bowel between clamps below the tumour. (Best, by kind permission.) (Farquharson and Rintoul: *Textbook of Operative Surgery, 6th Edn*)

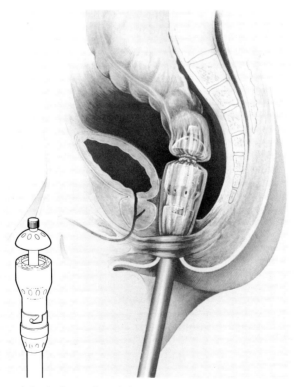

Fig. 15.53 Anterior (trans-abdominal) resection of the rectum — anastomosis of pelvic colon to stump of rectum — using AutoSuture® stapling technique. (AutoSuture Ltd.)

Instruments

As for abdominoperineal resection
  Minus de Martel clamps
  Plus automatic bowel stapler
  Plus Intestinal occlusion clamps, right-angled (Finch), 2
  Plus Proctoscope (Fig. 13.26).

Outline of procedure

Through a lower midline incision, the colon is mobilised from the point of transection to the ano-rectal junction, ligating and dividing the inferior mesenteric vessels. It is then divided between clamps, one a right-angled clamp (Finch) placed proximally to the two.

The mesorectum is separated from the back of the rectum at the level selected for division below the growth (not less than 6 cm from its inferior edge). The mesorectum is then clamped with two large artery forceps, divided and ligated leaving the rectum bared all round over a segment about 4 cm long.

The bowel is then clamped at the upper end of this bared segment with right-angled clamps, the rectum is transected, and the colon clamp brought into proximity to the open stump of the rectum. A row of seromuscular mattress Lembert sutures is inserted both laterally and medially and left untied. A further row of through and through mattress sutures is inserted and when all are placed the sutures are tied. This slides the colon down to the cut edge of the rectum, invaginates the suture line and completes the anastomosis. Finally the clamp is removed and the pelvic peritoneum sutured over the anastomosis to extraperitonealise the suture line. Stapling instruments are available which complete the anastomosis in one action, and enable resection to within about 2 cm ($\frac{3}{4}$ inch) segment of the rectal margin (Heald, 1980).

A drainage tube is inserted and the wound closed in layers in the normal manner.

Colostomy

Definition

The establishment of a temporary or permanent opening in the colon.

Position

Supine.

Instruments

  General set (Figs. 14.1–14.28)
  Laparotomy set (Figs. 15.1–15.7)
  Long scissors, curved on flat (McIndoe)
  Fine artery forceps, straight (mosquito)
  Fine tissue forceps (McIndoe), 6
  Glass or plastic colostomy rod and tubing
  Diathermy cable and electrodes
  Paraffin gauze dressing or colostomy bag (i.e. colostomy is to be opened immediately)
  Ligatures and sutures as for laparotomy.

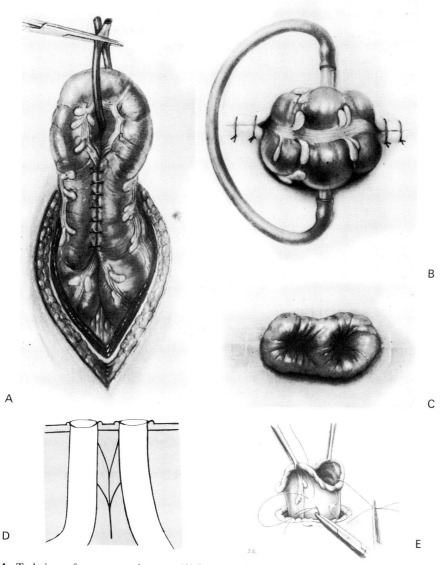

Fig. 15.54 Technique of transverse colostomy. (A) Loop of colon mobilised. (B) Colostomy rod in position. (C and D) Double barrel defunctioning type of colostomy. (E) Method of suturing colostomy to skin. Stitches are placed to pick up the mucosal edge, the bowel wall about 2 cm below (not penetrating the lumen), and finally the skin margin. (A, B, C and E: Farquharson and Rintoul: *A Textbook of Operative Surgery, 6th Edn.,* D: Macfarlane and Thomas: *Textbook of Surgery.*)

Outline of procedure

The incision can be paramedian, midline or in the iliac region as described for appendectomy. The colon is mobilised and a loop brought either through the original incision or through a separate stab wound (inguinal colostomy). An opening is made in the mesentery of this loop of bowel, and a glass or nylon rod (attached at one end to a short piece of tubing) is passed between the skin and bowel. The tubing is then attached to the other end of the

rod, forming a D-shaped loop which retains it in position. The wound is closed and petroleum jelly gauze placed around the exteriorised bowel. The colostomy is usually opened with a diathermy knife or cautery, but the apparatus should be available in case the surgeon decides to open the bowel in theatre. If the colostomy is opened immediately after operation, a self-adhesive colostomy bag may be applied. In this instance the cut edge of the bowel is sutured as shown in Figure 15.54.

Closure of colostomy

Definition

Re-establishment of intestinal continuity.

Position

Supine.

Instruments

> General set (Figs. 14.1–14.28)
> Deep retractors, narrow blade (Paton), 2
> Intestinal occlusion clamps, straight (Doyen), 2
> Fine tissue forceps (McIndoe), 5
> Fine artery forceps, curved on flat (mosquito), 10
> 2.5 (2/0) Chromic catgut, a synthetic absorbable or silk for ligatures
> 2.5 (2/0) Chromic catgut, a synthetic absorbable or silk on a small curved non-traumatic intestinal needle for closure of bowel
> 3 or 4 (0 or 1) Chromic catgut or a synthetic absorbable on a medium half-circle round-bodied or Mayo needle for peritoneum and muscle
> 2.5 (2/0) Synthetic non-absorbable or silk on a large curved or straight cutting needle for skin sutures.

Outline of procedure

An extraperitoneal or intraperitoneal closure may be performed. If an extraperitoneal closure is contemplated, the spur between the upper and lower portion of the colostomy will have been crushed previously by an enterotribe (see Fig. 15.47).

For extraperitoneal closure an elliptical incision is made around the colostomy and the skin and bowel freed down to the peritoneum. The segment of skin attached to the colostomy is excised and the opening in the colon closed with one layer of continuous chromic catgut or synthetic absorbable and one layer of interrupted a synthetic non-absorbable or silk sutures. The peritoneum and muscle are plicated over the sutured colon and the wound is closed.

For intraperitoneal closure the dissection is the same except that the peritoneum is opened at each side of the exteriorised colon. The bowel is sutured in the manner already described or is divided at each side of the colostomy, and an end to end anastomosis made. The wound is closed.

Ileostomy

Definition

The establishment of an opening into the ileum (generally permanent).

Position

Supine.

Instruments

As for colostomy
  Intestinal occlusion clamps, straight (Doyen), 2
  2.5 (2/0) Chromic catgut or a synthetic absorbable on a small curved non-traumatic
    intestinal needle for ileum closure. Ileostomy bag.

Outline of procedure

This operation is usually done for ulcerative colitis. Through a low paramedian or midline
incision, the ileum is mobilised and two occlusion clamps applied at the selected point for
ileostomy. The ileum is transected and the proximal end brought out through a small
circular wound made in the right side of the abdomen. The distal end of the ileum is closed
with 2.5 (2/0) chromic catgut or a synthetic absorbable and the wound is closed. The base
of the exteriorised ileum is sutured to the abdominal wall and the mucosa is then everted.
The cut edge of the mucosa is sutured to the skin with 2.5 (2/0) chromic catgut or a synthetic
absorbable. An ileostomy bag is usually applied immediately at the end of the operation.

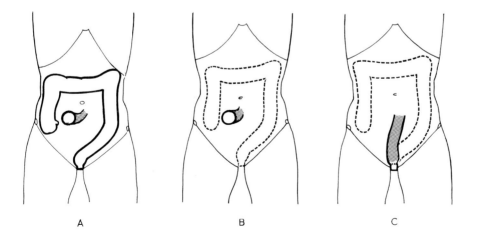

Fig. 15.55 The types of operation performed for ulcerative colitis. (A) Ileostomy. (B) Ileostomy with resection
of the colon and rectum. (C) Resection of colon with ileorectal anastomosis. (Macfarlane and Thomas: *Textbook
of Surgery*.)

Splenectomy

Definition

Removal of the spleen.

Position

Supine.

Instruments

As for laparotomy, including ligatures and sutures (p. 411).

Outline of procedure

A midline, left paramedian or transverse incision is made. The spleen is palpated, and if there are any adhesions these are clamped with forceps before dividing. The gastrosplenic ligament is first divided and then the lateral peritoneal fold of the lienorenal ligament is incised, allowing the spleen to be brought forward into the wound. The major splenic vessels are either clamped with sets of two strong artery forceps and divided, or are individually ligatured with double strong synthetic non-absorbable or silk and cut after the ligatures have been tied. The spleen is then free and may be removed. The wound is closed in layers.

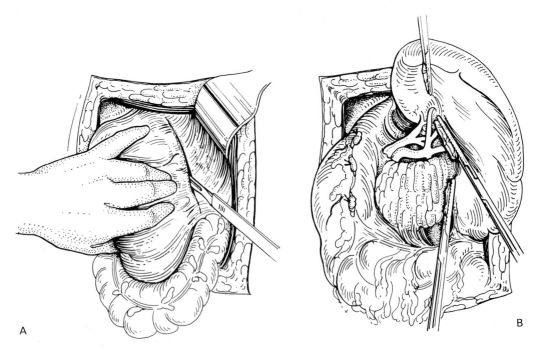

A   B

Fig. 15.56 Splenectomy (left). The spleen is lifted forwards and is mobilised by incision of the peritoneum passing from its lateral surface on to the posterior abdominal wall, *i.e.* the posterior layer of the lieno-renal ligament. (right) The gastro-splenic ligament is divided between clamps and ligatured. The thin anterior layer of the lieno-renal ligament is then incised to expose the splenic vessels and the tail of the pancreas. (Rintoul: *Farquharson's Textbook of Operative Surgery.*)

Inguinal or scrotal herniorrhaphy

Definition

The obliteration of a sac containing viscera, which have protruded from the abdomen, either as a direct hernia through Hesselbach's triangle, or as an indirect hernia through the internal ring.

Position

Supine.

Instruments

General set (Figs. 14.1–14.28)

2.5 and 3 (2/0 and 0) Chromic catgut or a synthetic absorbable for ligatures

3 or 4 (0 or 1) Chromic catgut or a synthetic absorbable on a small or medium half-circle round-bodied needle for the hernial sac, and on a half-circle cutting needle for the muscle tendon

Repair material of choice, e.g., polyamid monofilament or braided; polyester braided; polybutester; polypropylene; stainless steel wire; and mesh made from polyamid, braided silk or wire (Chapter 8); small or medium stout half-circle needles, such as Mayo needles, or special types such as fish-hook shape may be used to facilitate the suturing with the chosen material

2.5 (2/0) Synthetic non-absorbable or silk on medium or large curved or straight cutting needles for skin sutures

(Alternatively, Michel or Kifa clips or skin staples may be used.)

Gallie's repair, extra instruments

Fascia forceps, right and left, 2

Fasciatome or fascia stripper

Gallie's living suture needles — small, medium and large

2.5 and 3 (2/0 and 0) Synthetic non-absorbable or silk on small half-circle round-bodied needles for securing graft.

Outline of procedure

Through an incision overlying the inguinal canal, the spermatic cord is mobilised and retracted with a piece of ribbon gauze or tubing. By separating the coverings of the cord, the hernial sac is found and isolated. It is opened to make quite sure that it is empty, transfixed, ligated with 3 or 4 (0 or 1) chromic catgut or a synthetic absorbable at the internal ring, and is cut off. This is all that is necessary in infants who require no repair of the muscles at this stage.

There are many repair procedures, including the *Bassini operation* which consists of interrupted a synthetic non-absorbable or silk sutures from the border of the internal oblique and transversus abdominus muscles to the inguinal ligament deep to the spermatic cord. In *Gallie's repair* a strip of fascia lata is removed from the lateral aspect of the thigh either with a fasciatome or via a long incision extending from just above the knee to the great trochanter. This fascia is then sutured 'zigzag' fashion across the posterior inguinal wall to strengthen it. A *nylon darn* consists of a continuous monofilament or braided polyamid (nylon) suture, introduced forwards and backwards across the posterior inguinal wall, extending from the

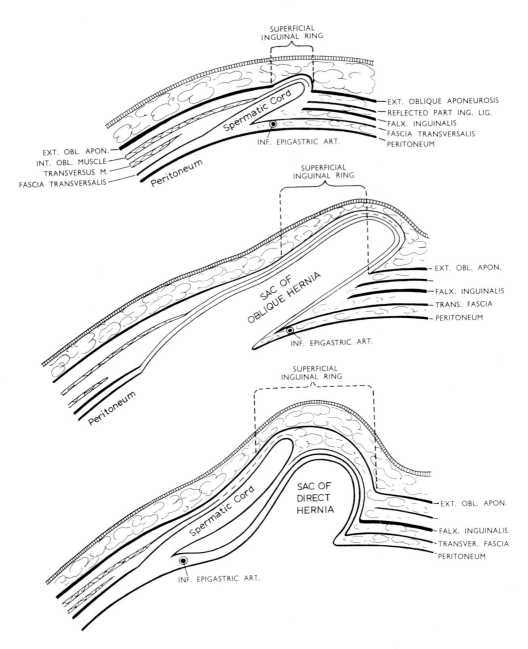

Fig. 15.57 Diagrammatic sections of the long axis of the inguinal canal. In all three diagrams the external spermatic fascia is shown to be continuous with the aponeurosis of the external oblique muscle.

(1) The upper diagram shows the normal spermatic cord and its coverings.

(2) The middle diagram shows an oblique inguinal hernia. Note the relationship of the hernial sac to the inferior epigastric artery. In an oblique hernia the sac descends within the coverings of the spermatic cord.

(3) The lowest diagram shows a direct inguinal hernia. Note the relationship of the neck of the hernial sac to the inferior epigastric artery. In a direct inguinal hernia the external spermatic fascia is the only covering which the hernia shares with the spermatic cord. (Bruce, Walmsley and Ross.)

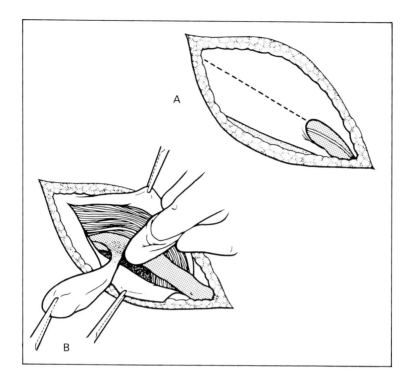

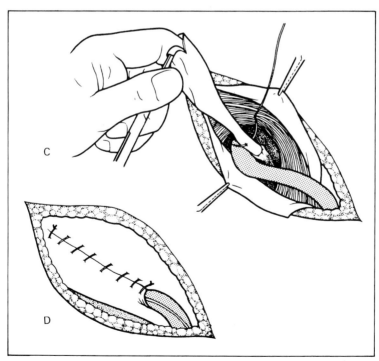

Fig. 15.58 Simple herniotomy for oblique inguinal hernia; (A) incision in external oblique aponeurosis, (B) separation of sac by gauze dissection, (C) transfixion ligature of the sac at its neck, and (D) repair of external oblique aponeurosis. (Rintoul: *Farquharson's Textbook of Operative Surgery*.)

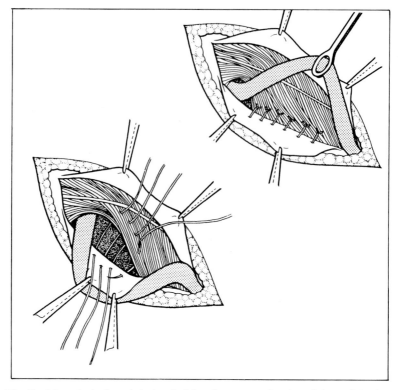

Fig. 15.59   The Bassini method of repair in inguinal hernia — approximation of the conjoined muscles and tendon to the inguinal ligament, behind the spermatic cord; this is held out of the way, under cover of the lower flap of external oblique. (Rintoul: *Farquharson's Textbook of Operative Surgery.*)

internal oblique and transversus abdominus muscles to the inguinal ligament without actually drawing them into approximation.

Stainless steel wire or braided polyamid silk mesh may be used to strengthen the posterior wall. A piece of suitable shape and size is sutured around its periphery to the muscles described above.

The hernia repair may be further strengthened by overlapping the external oblique, suturing the upper margin to the inguinal ligament and using the part below the incision for an overlap. This means that the anterior wall of the inguinal canal has a double instead of a single layer of external oblique. The wound is closed.

Femoral herniorrhaphy

Definition

This is similar to an inguinal hernia but the sac protrudes through the femoral ring into the femoral canal.

Position

As for inguinal hernia.

Instruments

As for inguinal hernia (p. 451).

Outline of procedure

The hernial sac is exposed below the inguinal ligament, freed, ligated and excised as previously described. The femoral canal is then usually closed from above by opening the inguinal canal and suturing the conjoined tendon to the pectineal ligament with interrupted silk or thread sutures. The operation then proceeds as for inguinal hernia.

Umbilical hernia

Definition

A protrusion of intestine through the umbilicus or muscle surrounding the umbilicus. (In congenital form, the loop of intestine can easily be seen through a thin transparent membrane and is not strictly speaking a true hernia, for the bowel has never been inside the abdomen. The acquired hernia in children is due to the scar of the umbilicus giving way because of some strain (e.g., coughing). In adults, usually the obese patient, the hernia occurs above or below the umbilical scar itself.

Position

Supine.

Instruments

As for inguinal hernia (p. 451).

Outline of procedure

A transverse elliptical incision is made above or below the umbilicus. The sac is isolated, opened, and the omentum contained either dissected free or clamped and resected. The redundant sac is excised, and the peritoneal opening closed with 4 or 5 (1 or 2) chromic catgut or a synthetic absorbable. Repair is accomplished by overlapping the aponeurosis transversely with interrupted a synthetic non-absorbable or silk mattress sutures (Mayo procedure). The skin wound is closed.

Ventral hernia

Definition

A protusion of abdominal viscera through an opening in the linea semilunaris, linea alba or through the scar of an abdominal incision.

Position

Supine.

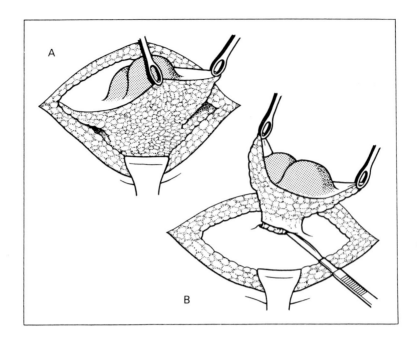

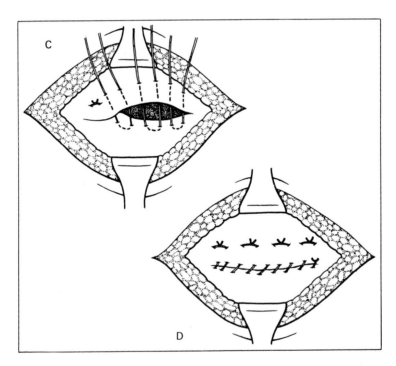

Fig. 15.60 Mayo's operation for umbilical hernia — repair by overlapping or fascial sutures. (A) Clearance of the aponeurosis centrally towards the neck of the sac. (B) Circular division of the neck of the sac and its fibrous covering. (C) Mattress sutures inserted to draw one flap under cover of the other. (D) Overlapping completed by suturing down free edge of superficial flap.

Instruments

As for inguinal hernia (p. 451).

Outline of procedure

Through the selected incision the sac is identified and obliterated. The abdominal wall is repaired either with a fascial strip or a non-absorbable suture material (see inguinal hernia) and the wound is then closed.

Strangulated hernia

Definition

Gangrene of an intestinal loop contained within a hernial sac, due to compression of its mesentery and blood-vessels.

Position

Supine.

Instruments

As for inguinal hernia (p. 451)
Fine tissue forceps (McIndoe), 5
Fine artery forceps, straight (mosquito), 5
Intestinal occlusion clamps, straight (Doyen), 2
Intestinal occlusion clamps, curved (Doyen), 2
Intestinal crushing clamps (Pyar, Joll or Schoemaker), 2
Artery forceps, straight, 20 cm (8 in) (Spencer Wells), 10
Long artery forceps, curved on flat (Moynihan gall-bladder), 5
Hernia director and bistoury
2.5 and 3 (2/0 and 0) Chromic catgut or a synthetic absorbable on small or medium non-traumatic intestinal needles for resection anastomosis
Ligatures and sutures as for inguinal hernia.

Outline of procedure

The approach and dissection follows that for inguinal hernia or umbilical hernia, etc. The sac is opened and the gangrenous contents prevented from slipping into the abdomen whilst the constricting area is divided, perhaps with a director and bistoury under direct vision. Warm, moist packs are applied to the bowel and if it does not appear viable after five minutes, a resection of the affected part is carried out in the usual manner. Repair is carried out in the usual manner.

Haemorrhoidectomy

Definition

The excision of internal piles.

Position

Lithotomy or jack-knife.

Instruments

Sponge-holding forceps (Rampley), 5
Towel clips, 5
Rectal speculum (Kelly, Gabrial, etc.)
Scalpel handle No. 3 with No. 10 blade (Bard Parker)
Dissecting forceps, toothed, 2
Scissors, straight, 15 cm (6 in) (Mayo)
Scissors, curved on flat, 15 cm (6 in) (Mayo)
Artery forceps, straight (Moynihan), 10
Dissectors (MacDonald and Durham), 2
Pile clamps (Kocher, curved), 6
Aneurysm needle
2.5 (2/0) Chromic catgut or a synthetic absorbable for fine ligatures
6 (3) Chromic catgut, a synthetic absorbable, or silk on a medium curved round-bodied
    needle for pile transfixion and ligation
Stout rubber or plastic drainage tube and safety-pin
(Three small packs made from petroleum jelly gauze, or ribbon gauze soaked in antiseptic,
    may be required to pack around the tube to control oozing from pile areas after
    operation.)

Outline of procedure

The three piles are each clamped with forceps and individually dissected upwards off the
muscular coat of the anal canal until a pedicle is formed. This pedicle is transfixed at the

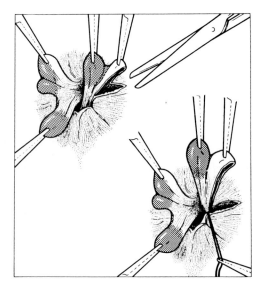

Fig. 15.61 Haemorrhoidectomy by the dissection-ligature technique. (Rintoul: *Farquharson's Textbook of Operative Surgery.*)

base, ligated and two-thirds of the pile cut off together with the tag of skin corresponding to the pile. A drainage tube may be inserted.

Anal fissure

Definition

A small vertical ulcer at the anal margin.

Position

Lithotomy or jack-knife.

Instruments

As for haemorrhoidectomy
    Malleable probe
    Small retractors, double hook, 2
    Sinus forceps
    Curetting spoon, double end (Volkmann)
    Petroleum jelly gauze roll.

Outline of procedure

The anal margins are retracted and a knife directed against the floor of the ulcer dividing the internal sphincter fibres. There is usually a small tag of skin (the so-called 'sentinel pile') in the region of the fissure, and this is cut away to provide free drainage. The wound is plugged with petroleum jelly gauze.

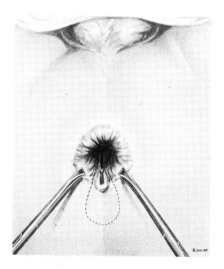 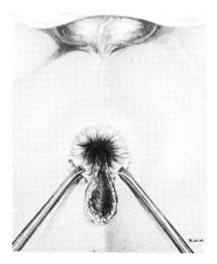

Fig. 15.62   Excision of an anal fissure. (Rintoul: *Farquharson's Textbook of Operative Surgery.*)

Fistula in ano

Definition

A sinus or sinuses between the anal canal and the skin in the region of the anus.

Position

Lithotomy or jack-knife.

Instruments

As for anal fissure.

Outline of procedure

The sinuses are opened to provide free drainage, care being taken to divide only the subcutaneous sphincter muscle, otherwise, incontinence may result. The surgeon may require a sterile dye to assist identification of the sinuses and indigo carmine or methylene blue together with a syringe and cannula should be available.

REFERENCES AND FURTHER READING

FARQUHARSON, E. L. AND RINTOUL, R. F. (1972) *Textbook of Operative Surgery.* Edinburgh: Churchill Livingstone.
RINTOUL, R. F. (1986) *Farquharson's Textbook of Operative Surgery*, 7 edn. Edited by R. F. Rintoul, Edinburgh: Churchill Livingstone
HEALD, R. (1980) *Nursing Mirror*, **150**, No. 1, 30.
MacFARLANE, D. A. AND THOMAS, L. P. (1972) *Textbook of Surgery.* Edinburgh: Churchill Livingstone.

16

Operations on the breast

Incision of breast abscess

Definition

The incision and drainage of an abscess due to acute mastitis.

Position

Supine.

Instruments

Sponge-holding forceps (Rampley), 2
Towel clips, 5
Scalpel handle No. 3 with No. 10 blade (Bard Parker)
Dissecting forceps,toothed, 2
Dissecting forceps, non-toothed, 2
Scissors, curved on flat, 13 cm (5 in) (Mayo)
Sinus forceps, 18 cm (7 in)
Probe, malleable silver
Artery forceps, straight (Moynihan), 5
20 ml syringe with wide-bore exploration needles
Sterile culture tube
Latex rubber or plastic drainage tubing and safety-pin or suction drain
2.5 (2/0) Synthetic non-absorbable or silk on a large curved cutting needle for securing
   drainage tubing.

Outline of procedure

An incision or incisions are made radiating from the nipple. If the abscess is loculated, care
is taken to drain each compartment. A split drainage tube is inserted and secured to the skin
with a suture. Alternatively a suction drainage tubing is inserted and secured by suturing
the skin around the tubing. A firm dressing is applied.

Excision of simple adenoma or amputation of the breast (simple mastectomy)

Definition

The removal or a simple adenoma; or amputation of the mammary gland, most commonly
for chronic mastitis.

Position

Supine, with arms extended on narrow arm boards (Fig. 5.17).

Instruments

General set (Figs. 14.1–14.28)
Local infiltration set (Fig. 10.35) with adrenaline 1:400,000 (optional)
Artery forceps, curved on flat (Kelly Fraser, Dunhill, etc.), 25
Large tissue forceps (Lane or Fagge), 5
Diathermy leads, electrodes and lead anchoring forceps
Short rubber or plastic drainage tube and safety-pin for adenoma; or long drainage tube and Redi-vac or Activac for mastectomy
2.5 and 3 (2/0 and 0) Chromic catgut or a synthetic absorbable for ligatures
2.5 (2/0) Synthetic non-absorbable or silk on a large curved or straight cutting needle for skin sutures.

Outline of procedure

A simple adenoma is removed through an incision placed over the swelling, but extending radially from the nipple to conserve the secreting ducts. The wound is closed with or without drainage.

For simple mastectomy, the skin and subcutaneous tissues over the incision line may be infiltrated with 100 to 300 ml of a 1:400,000 adrenaline solution to minimise bleeding. An elliptical, vertical incision is then made extending from the axilla to the sternum, enclosing the nipple in the centre of the ellipse. The skin is dissected from the breast until the surgeon has reached the limits of the gland in all directions. The breast is peeled off the deep fascia (without cutting into it) towards the axilla, using light strokes of the knife, until the axillary tail of the gland is reached. The blood vessels at this point are ligated before freeing the breast, which is then removed. A drain is placed in the lower end of the wound which is closed in the usual manner. A negative pressure may be applied to this drainage tube in the manner described on page 467.

Modified radial mastectomy

Definition

Removal of the mammary gland, together with the pectoralis minor muscle, and the axillary glands. The operation is performed for malignant tumours of the breast.

Position

Supine with arms extended on narrow arm boards, or only one secured and the other (operation side) held by a seated assistant. The arm is more easily supported in a flexed position, holding the elbow in one hand and the wrist in the other. The elbow must not be allowed to drop below the plane of the operation table or abducted more than a right angle to the body, for the nerves may be stretched over the humeral head and cause paralysis.

Figs. 16.1–16.4 (Rintoul: *Farquharson's* Textbook of Operative Surgery).

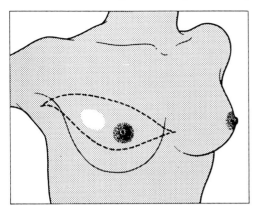

Fig. 16.1 Elliptical incision including the nipple and skin overlying the tumour.

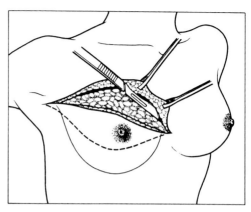

Fig. 16.2 The upper skin flap is dissected free.

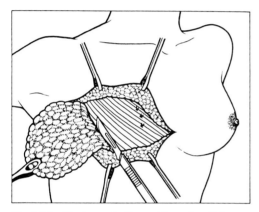

Fig. 16.3 The breast is dissected laterally off the pectoralis major.

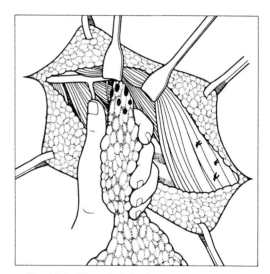

Fig. 16.4 The apical glands and axillary tail is mobilised using the breast for traction. It is not always necessary to sacrifice the pectoralis minor muscle as in this case.

Instruments

General set (Figs. 14.1–14.28)

Local infiltration set (Fig. 11.60) with adrenaline 1:400,000 (optional)

Artery forceps, curved on flat (Kelly Fraser, two-thirds serrated jaws), 25

Artery forceps, curved on flat (Dunhill, fully serrated jaws), 25

Large tissue forceps (Lane or Fagge), 6

Diathermy leads, electrodes and lead anchoring forceps

Long plastic drainage tube and Redi-vac, Portovac or Activac

2.5 *and* 3 (2/0 and 0) Chromic catgut or a synthetic absorbable and silk or thread for ligatures

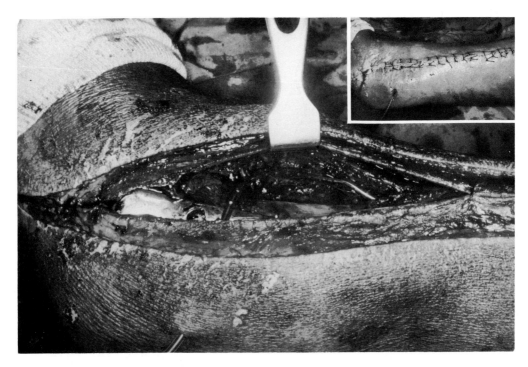

Fig. 16.5 Perforated suction catheter in position prior to wound closure (inset shows catheter protruding from separate stab incision). Operation depicted is that on a limb although a similar technique is used for draining a mastectomy wound. (Biomet Ltd.)

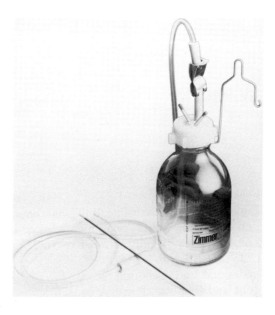

Fig. 16.6 The Redi-vac suction device showing vacuum bottle, suction catheter and insertion trocar. (Zimmer Biomet Ltd.)

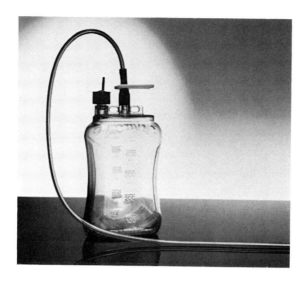

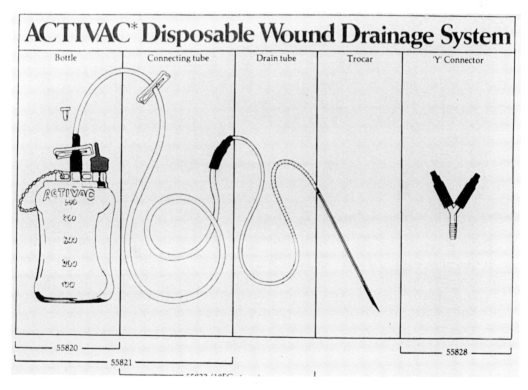

Fig. 16.7   Activac disposable drainage system. (Johnson & Johnson Ltd.)

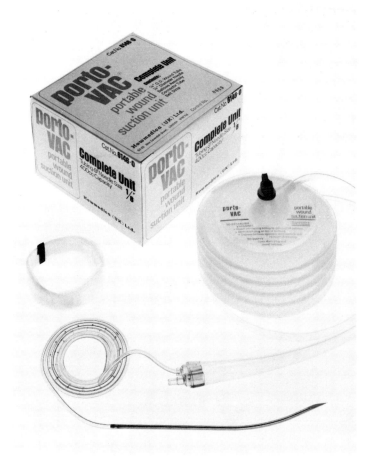

Fig. 16.8   Portovac portable wound suction unit. (Howmedica (U.K.) Ltd.)

3 (0) Chromic catgut or Dexon on a medium half-circle round-bodied needle for axillary sutures

2.5 (2/0) Synthetic non-absorbable or silk on a large curved or straight cutting needle for skin sutures (Skin graft instruments may be required, page 745).

Outline of procedure

The skin and subcutaneous tissues over the incision line may be infiltrated with 100 to 300 ml of 1:400,000 adrenaline solution to minimise bleeding. An elliptical incision is then made, above and below the nipple to include the skin overlying the tumour which is in the centre of the ellipse. Fig. 16.1. The skin flaps over the axilla are reflected to expose the pectoralis major and minor muscles which are severed from their insertions. The fat and glands contained in the axilla are cleared by dissection, carefully avoiding damage to the major blood vessels, subscapularis nerve and the nerve of Bell. The skin flaps overlying the breast are reflected and the breast removed, if necessary together with the pectoralis muscles underneath, extending from the sternum medially to the border of the latissimus dorsi

muscle. A long drainage tube is inserted into the axilla through a separate stab incision, the skin flaps are approximated with tissue forceps and the wound is closed.

The long drainage tube is either coupled to an under-water collection bottle (Chapter 25), or preferably a slight negative pressure is applied by connecting a Redi-vac bottle to the open end of the tube.

FURTHER READING

RINTOUL, R. F. (1986) *Farquharson's Textbook of Operative Surgery*, 7th edn. Edinburgh: Churchill Livingstone.

17

Dental operations

Dental extraction

Definition

The removal of a tooth or root either under local or general anaesthesia.

Position

Supine, or sitting with the head and neck extended slightly.

Instruments

Mouth gag (Mason or Doyen)
Dental props, set
Tongue forceps
Angled tongue depressor
Dental conveying forceps, stout and fine, 2
Dental extraction forceps, set

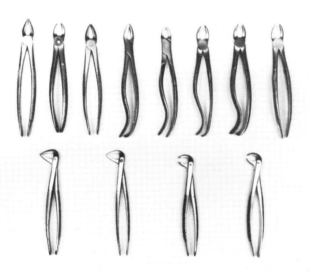

Fig. 17.1 Examples of upper and lower dental extraction forceps. (Birmingham Dental Hospital.)

Dental elevators and probes, set
Mouth mirror
Local anaesthetic, e.g., 2 per cent lignocaine (Xylocaine) and dental syringe may be
  required
Mouth wash.

Outline of procedure

If general anaesthesia is to be administered, mouth props are inserted to prevent the patient
from closing his jaw. Following the administration of a local anaesthetic, five minutes are
allowed to elapse before the operation is commenced. The teeth are extracted and the patient
is allowed a gentle mouth wash before leaving the dental chair.

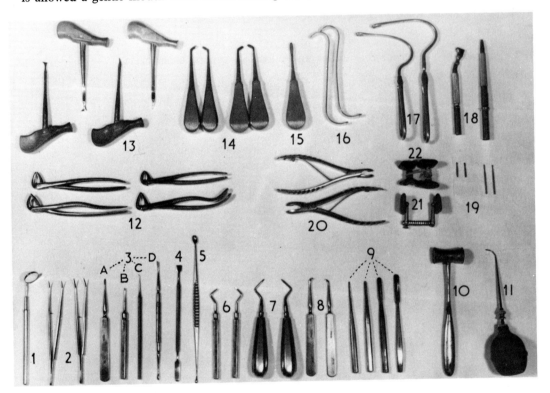

Fig. 17.2 Removal of impacted wisdom tooth.
1. Dental mirror.
2. Dental conveying forceps, fine and stout, 2.
3. (A) Root elevator straight.
   (B) Probe.
   (C) Probe and scaler.
   (D) Specula and spoon.
4. Spatula.
5. Curette (Volkmann).
6. Apical elevators, left and right, 2.
7. Apical elevators, left and right, 2.
8. Small gouges (Jenkins), 3 mm, 4 mm, 6 mm, and
   8 mm, 4.
9. Small mallet (Rowland).
10. Small mallet (Rowland).
11. Dental cavity syringe.
12. Dental extraction forceps, appropriate shape.
13. Root elevators (Winter), 4.
14. Root elevators (Hospital), right and left, 4.
15. Root elevator (Read).
16. Retractors, cheek, 2.
17. Retractors, cheek, 2.
18. Dental drill handpieces, straight and angled, 2.
19. Dental burrs, fissure and rose-end type.
20. Bone-nibbling or gouge forceps, 2 sizes.
21. Gag (Brunton).
22. Mouth prop (Hewitt).

Not illustrated:
Suction tubing, fine nozzles and tube anchoring
forceps.

Removal of impacted wisdom tooth

Definition

The removal of the third molar tooth, the eruption of which is partially or completely prevented by its contact against the second molar tooth.

Position

Supine, with some reverse Trendelenburg.

Instruments

As Figure 17.2.

Outline of procedure

An incision is made in the gum overlying the impacted tooth. The cortex of the bone which

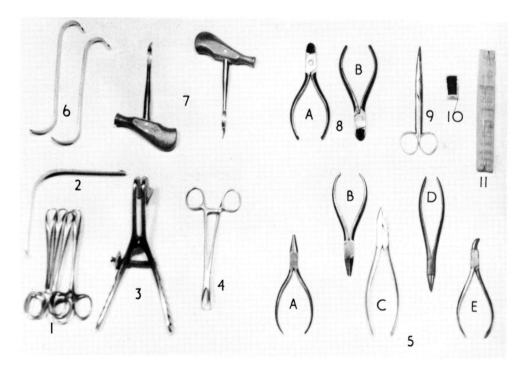

Fig. 17.3 Wiring of mandible, utilising teeth.

1. Towel clips, 4.
2. Right-angled tongue depressor.
3. Mouth gag (Mason).
4. Tongue forceps (Mayo).
5. (A) Collar pliers.
   (B) Collar pliers.
   (C) Collar pliers.
   (D) Snipe nose pliers.
   (E) Contouring pliers.

6. Cheek retractors, 2.
7. Root elevators (Winter), right and left, 2.
8. (A) Wire-cutting forceps, straight. Wire-cutting forceps, angled on flat.
9. Scissors, curved on flat, 13 cm (5 in) (Mayo).
10. Silk or thread, stout.
11. Stainless-steel wire.

covers the tooth is drilled or gouged away. The tooth is removed and the incision closed either with 2 (3/0) chromic catgut, a synthetic absorbable, or silk.

Treatment of a fractured mandible

Definition

Reduction of a fractured mandible, followed by immobilisation, in this case by wiring the upper and lower teeth together.

Position

Supine, with some reverse Trendelenburg

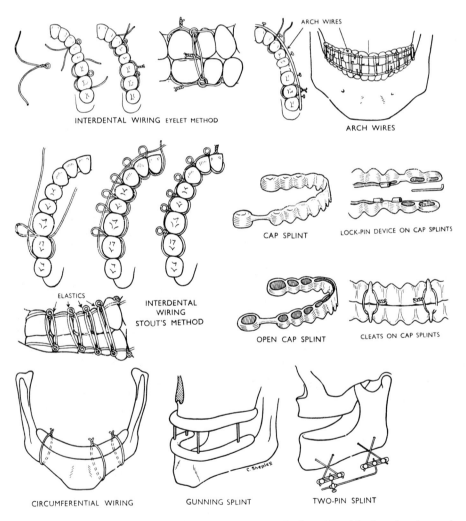

Fig. 17.4 When there are teeth in both fragments, a fracture may be immobilised by interdental or arch wiring, or by cap splints. When the jaw is edentulous, a Gunning splint (or preferably the patient's dentures), circumferential wiring or the two-pin splint is used. (J. N. Wilson and Watson Jones.)

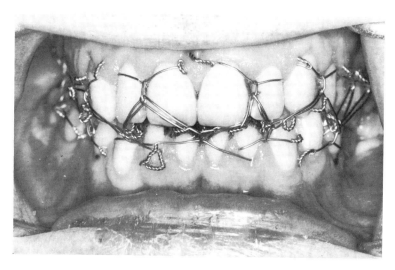

Fig. 17.5   Interdental eyelet wiring. (Photo, courtesy Mr N. L. Rowe, F.D.S.R.C.S., M.R.C.S., L.R.C.P. Consultant in Oral Surgery, Queen Mary's Hospital, Roehampton.)

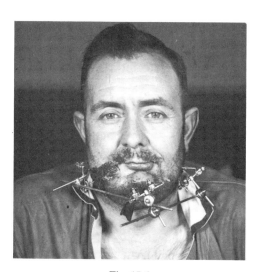

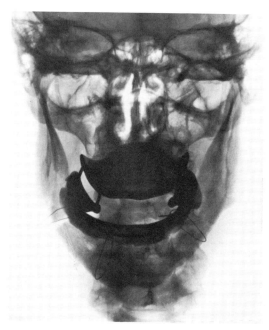

Fig. 17.6   Fig. 17.7

Figs. 17.6 and 17.7   Double fracture of the mandible immobilised by two-pin splints, one on each side of the jaw. Fracture of an edentulous mandible immobilised by a Gunning Splint with circumferential wiring. (Courtesy R. Watson-Jones.)

Instruments

As Figure 17.3.

Outline of procedure

With a pharyngeal pack in position; wires with loops are wound around the necks of two adjacent teeth of one side of the lower jaw. The wires are twisted together so that the loops or eyelets protrude at gum level from the space between the two teeth.

This procedure is repeated on the other side of the lower jaw and at correspondingly opposite positions around the teeth in the upper jaw. This results in protruding eyelets spaced evenly around the jaw.

The wires are now passed through eyelets on opposing jaws. The pharyngeal pack is removed, the tie wires tightened and the lower teeth secured in normal occlusion with the upper teeth; this immobilises the fracture.

Alternative methods of jaw immobilisation are shown in Figures 17.4, 17.6 and 17.7.

FURTHER READING

WILSON, J. N. (1982) *Watson-Jones' Fractures and Joint Injuries*, 6th edn. Edinburgh: Churchill Livingstone.

18

Ear, nose and throat operations

SURGICAL APPROACHES TO THE MIDDLE EAR AND MASTOID

There are several methods of approach to the middle ear space and mastoid; these include permeatal, endaural, postaural, posterior tympanotomy and middle fossa approaches. Each of these is suited to specific surgical procedures, although the selection of any particular one will depend on clinical assessment of the possible range and extent of the proposed procedure.

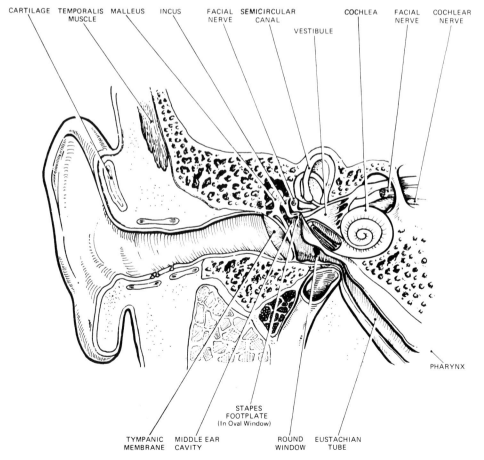

Fig. 18.1 Anatomical cross section of the ear. (Down's Surgical Ltd.)

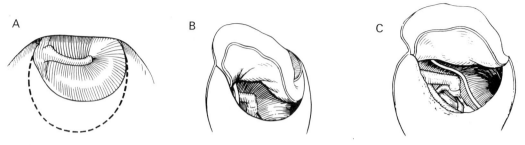

Fig. 18.2 Permeatal surgical approach. (A) The incision. (B) Reflection of the tympanomeatal flap. (C) Exposure of the middle ear cavity. (Ballantyne).

Permeatal approach

This approach is often used for stapedectomy, ossicular chain reconstruction or examination, destruction of the membranous labyrinth in uncontrolled unilateral Ménière's disease associated with severe sensorineural deafness, tympanic neurectomy and removal of some glomus — jugulare tumours. A curved incision is made in the posterior canal skin which is then reflected forwards from the bone beneath by blunt dissection to expose the posterior part of the mesotympanum (Fig. 18.2A).

Exposure of the posterior half of the middle ear cavity reveals the chorda tympani nerve situated just deep to the tympanic membrane (Fig. 18.2C). Gentle reflection of the nerve reveals the long process of incus, incudostapedial joint and the oval window region.

The posterosuperior part of the middle ear cavity is exposed fully by curetting the bony meatal wall and this reveals the stapedius tendon, pyramidal process, stapes and oval window. The tympanic meatal flap is replaced at the conclusion of the operation.

Endaural approach

The endaural approach is used mainly for removal of cholesteatoma in the epitympanum, correction of acquired mental stenosis and occasionally modified radical mastoidectomy or fenestration.

The incision is commenced in the cartilage-free gap between the anterior end of the helix posteriorly and the tragus anteriorly, and continued in a circular fashion between the cartilaginous and bony meatus (Fig. 18.3A). The periosteum in the lower meatal part of the incision is reflected off the bone to expose the supramental spine (of Henle), the supramental triangle (of Macewen) and the bony cortex of the mastoid process (Fig. 18.3B).

The temporalis muscle is reflected upwards, the meatal skin mobilised from the bone down to the tympanic ring to expose the epitympanum (Fig. 18.3C). The mastoid antrum and air cells are exposed with a power driven cutting burr, the attic is visualised by drilling forwards from the antrum (Fig. 18.3D). The short process of the incus and malleoincudal joint are identified. The horizontal semi-circular canal is exposed by removal of the incus.

Postaural approach

This approach is often used as it provides goods visualisation of the entire mastoid bowl, the epitympanum and the anterior recess of the deep meatus. The operations most

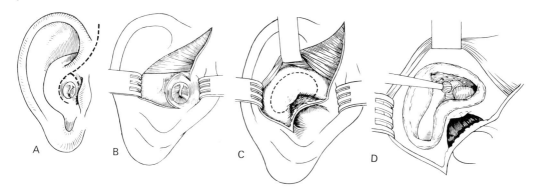

Fig. 18.3 *Endaural approach.* (A) Incision. (B) Exposure of the mastoid and temporalis fascia. (C) Reflection of meatal skin. (D) Exposure of mastoid antrum.

frequently carried out via this approach include: simple, modified radical and radical mastoidectomy, combined approach tympanoplasty, in Menière's disease, facial nerve surgery, tumours in the middle ear cavity, extensive glomus-jugulare tumours and some cases of congenital atresia.

A curved incision is made behind the ear and division of subcutaneous tissues and muscle carried out by diathermy. The overlying periosteum is divided, the flaps separated to expose the mastoid cortex, suprameatal triangle and bony posterior meatal margin (Figs. 18.5A and B).

The temporalis muscle is displaced upwards exposing the zygoma root. The posterior canal skin is reflected from the bone as far as the tympanic margin (Fig. 18.5B). The mastoid antrum is exposed as in the endaural approach (Figs. 18.3C and D).

Posterior tympanotomy

This is an extension of the postaural approach used for patients with cholesteatoma of the mastoid bowl, attic and mesotympanum and is often combined with tympanoplasty (p. 490). It may also be used for patients with generalised and irreversible active mucosal disease of the mastoid bowl and tympanic cleft.

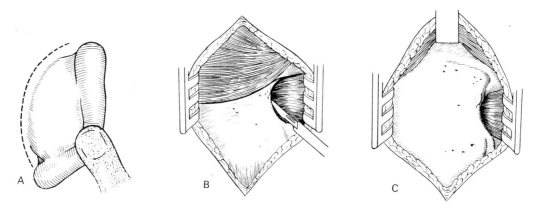

Fig. 18.4 *Postaural approach.* (A) Incision. (B) Reflection of periosteum. (C) Reflection of meatal flap.

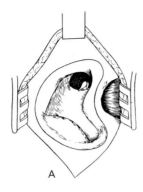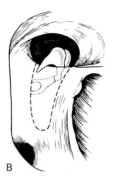

Fig. 18.5 *Posterior tympanotomy.* (A) Reflection of meatal flap. (B) Posterior tympanotomy. (Ballantyne.)

The incision and reflection of periosteum are as for the postaural approach (Figs. 18.4A and B). The posterior canal skin is reflected forwards from the bone, and the tympanic membrane reflected from the sulcus to determine the extent of the middle ear disease. The meatal flap may be reflected forwards after mobilisation if attic or posterior marginal perforation is present. The mastoid antrum is exposed as for the endaural approach.

A simple mastoidectomy is carried out, exentering the entire mastoid bowl. The bony dissection is continued into the root of the zygoma to expose the epitympanum, short process of the incus and malleo-incudal joint (Fig. 18.4C).

A posterio tympanotomy is performed, by gradually thinning down the posterior meatal bony wall, thereby connecting the mastoid cavity and the posterior mesotympanum. The slot is lateral to the facial nerve and medial to the tympanic annulus.

Middle fossa or transtemporal supralabyrinth approach

This approach to the internal auditory meatus is one of several used for procedures such as vestibular and cochleovestibular neurectomy, the removal of acoustic neuromas, the excision of cholesteatoma and tumours of the facial nerve in the supralabyrinth region and selective resection of the meatal segment of the vestibular nerve.

The skin incision is carried along the anterior attachment of the pinna and in a superior-anterior direction from the root of the zygoma to the superior margin of the temporalis region (Fig. 18.6A). Five muscle flaps are created from the temporalis muscle and fixed to the surrounding surgical drapes with traction sutures (Fig. 18.6B).

In conjunction with suction-irrigation, a craniotomy opening is made using a power cutting drill (Fig. 18.6C). The craniotomy opening is extended with rongeurs to give a good view of the petrosquamous attachment of the dura and veins between the dura and cranium (Fig. 18.6D). A incision is made in the dura to drain cerebral spinal fluid, and it is then elevated from the floor of the middle cranial fossa in a posterior-anterior direction. The petrosquamous attachment of the dura and veins encountered are diathermised (Fig. 18.6E).

The dura is elevated from the base of the middle cranial fossa and continued over the meatal plane to expose the facial hiatus (Fig. 18.6F). A self-retaining dura retractor is inserted followed by a Cushing retractor which rests over the petrosal sulcus. Visualising through the operating microscope, the bone over the arcuate eminence is removed with a diamond burr (Fig. 18.G). The meatal fundus (Fig. 18.1) is exposed by removing bone in the 60° sector indicated in Figure 18.6H. The meatal dural sac is then exposed by removing

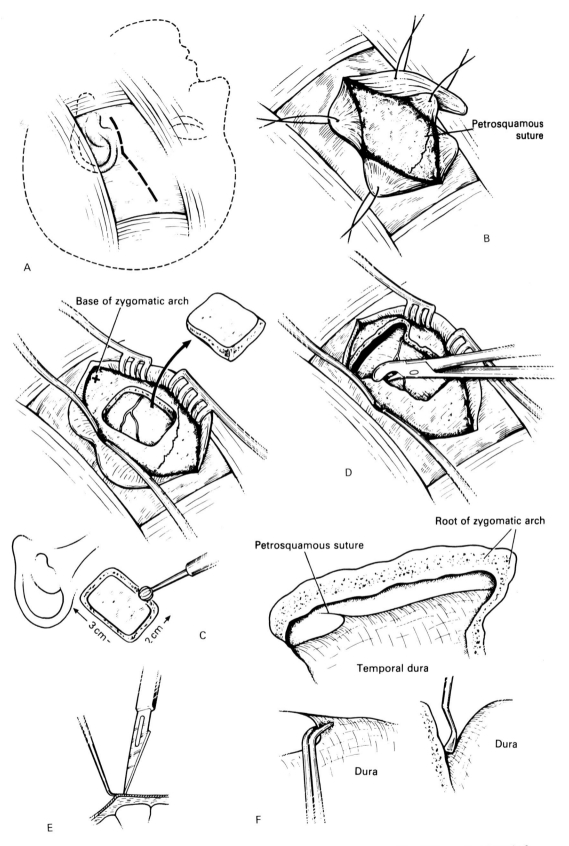

Base of zygomatic arch

Petrosquamous suture

Root of zygomatic arch

Petrosquamous suture

Temporal dura

Dura

Dura

A

B

C

3 cm

2 cm

D

E

F

Fig. 18.6 (continued overleaf)

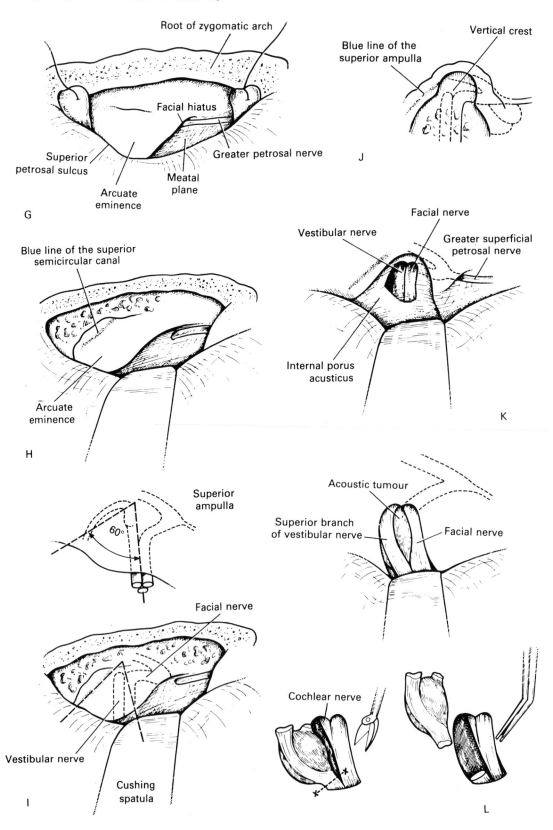

G

Root of zygomatic arch

Facial hiatus

Superior petrosal sulcus

Greater petrosal nerve

Meatal plane

Arcuate eminence

J

Blue line of the superior ampulla

Vertical crest

H

Blue line of the superior semicircular canal

Arcuate eminence

K

Facial nerve

Vestibular nerve

Greater superficial petrosal nerve

Internal porus acusticus

I

Superior ampulla

60°

Facial nerve

Vestibular nerve

Cushing spatula

Acoustic tumour

Superior branch of vestibular nerve

Facial nerve

Cochlear nerve

L

Fig. 18.6 Middle fossa approach to the internal auditory meatus. (A) The skin incision is made along the anterior attachment of the pinna, and continued in a superior-anterior direction from the root of the zygoma to the superior margin of the temporalis muscle. (B) Five temporalis muscle flaps are cut and fixed to the surrounding surgical drapes with non-absorbable sutures. (C) Craniotomy opening centred over the base of the zygomatic arch. (D) Extension of the craniotomy opening to give good view of the petrosquamous attachment of the dura. (E) Dura raised with a hook and incised to drain cerebral spinal fluid over the temporal lobe. This facilitates traction of the temporal lobe to expose the floor of the middle cranial fossa. (F) The dura is elevated from the floor of the middle cranial fossa. The petrosquamous attachment of the dura, and veins found along the base of the middle cranial fossa, are bipolarly diathermized. (G) Elevation of the dura is stopped after exposing the meatal plane for 2 cm anteriorly to the arcuate eminence. Exposure of the middle meningeal artery is not necessary. (H) The bone over the arcuate eminence is removed with a diamond burr. The contours of the bony semicircular canal are delineated. Note the position of the 'blue line' of the membranous canal. (I) The internal auditory canal is identified by removing bone in a sector of 60° anterior to the superior semicircular canal. This exposes the blue area of the meatal fundus without risk to the facial nerve and the basal turn of the cochlear. (J) Exposure of the meatal fundus, including the vertical crest (Bill's bar), for the identification of the facial and superior vestibular nerves. (K) Bone is removed over the meatal sac; the vestibular and facial nerves usually become visible through the thin dura. (L) An example of a surgical procedure through the middle fossa approach — removal of an accoustic tumour. *Top*: The superior and inferior vestibular branches are sectioned as distally as possible, allowing the tumour to be eased out from the canal without damage to the cochlear nerve. *Left*: The vestibular nerve is transected proximal to the tumour at the entrance to the internal auditory canal. *Right*: The tumour removed; divided vessels diathermized bipolarly. (Fisch in *Rob and Smith's Operative Surgery* 4th edn, edited by Ballantyne and Morrison.)

Figs. 18.8 to 18.10   Instruments for myringotomy. (Down's Surgical Ltd.)

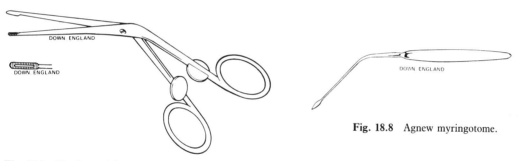

Fig. 18.8   Agnew myringotome.

Fig. 18.7   Heath aural forceps.

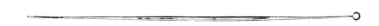

Fig. 18.9   Jobson Horne probe.

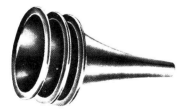

Fig. 18.10   Yearsley aural specula.

Figs. 18.11 to 18.16   Aural instruments. (Down's Surgical Ltd.)

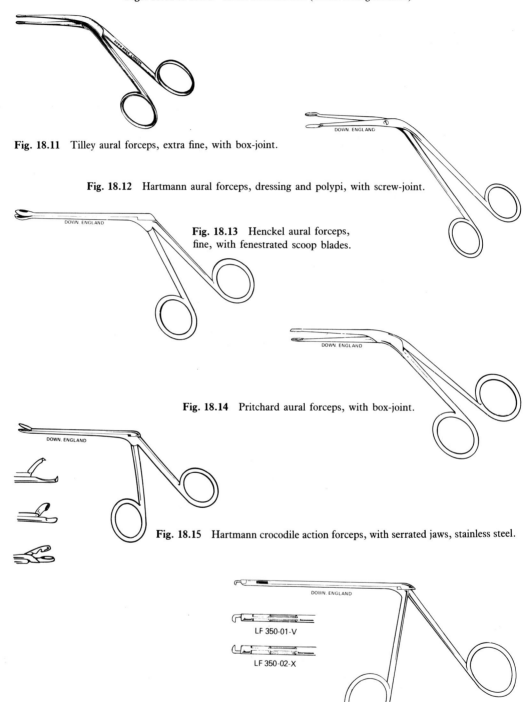

Fig. 18.11   Tilley aural forceps, extra fine, with box-joint.

Fig. 18.12   Hartmann aural forceps, dressing and polypi, with screw-joint.

Fig. 18.13   Henckel aural forceps, fine, with fenestrated scoop blades.

Fig. 18.14   Pritchard aural forceps, with box-joint.

Fig. 18.15   Hartmann crocodile action forceps, with serrated jaws, stainless steel.

LF 350-01-V

LF 350-02-X

Fig. 18.16   Wishart guillotine forceps, for head of malleus, right.

Figs. 18.17 to 18.23   Aural instruments. (Down's Surgical Ltd.)

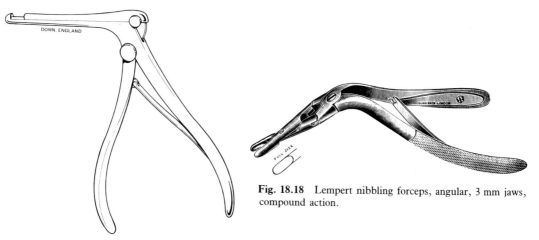

Fig. 18.18   Lempert nibbling forceps, angular, 3 mm jaws, compound action.

Fig. 18.17   Kerrison ronqeurs, upward cutting, four widths.

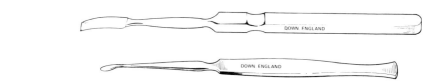

Fig. 18.19   Lempert rugines, broad and narrow.

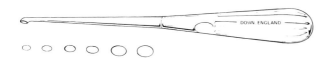

Fig. 18.20   Lempert scoops, oval, 6 sizes, 3.5 to 6 mm.

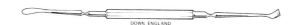

Fig. 18.21   Freer separator and elevator, fine.

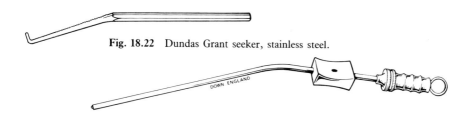

Fig. 18.22   Dundas Grant seeker, stainless steel.

Fig. 18.23   Lempert suction and irrigation tube, with Tucker valve plate, with stilette to clean out after use, 6 F.G., 2 mm diam., electro-plated.

the bone over it with a diamond burr. This visualises the vestibular and facial nerves through the thin dura (Fig. 18.6J).

The removal of an acoustic neuroma via this route is illustrated in Figure 18.6K–L.

OPERATIONS ON THE EAR

Myringotomy

Definition

Incision of the tympanic membrane.

Position

Supine, with the head inclined away from the affected ear.

Instruments

> Sponge holding forceps, small (Rampley)
> Aural speculae (Yearsley or Pritchard) 3 sizes
> Jobson Horne probe
> Myringotome (Agnew)
> Dressing forceps (Heath)
> Suction tubing, fine nozzles and tube anchoring forceps
> Operating microscope.

Outline of procedure

The operation is almost always carried out with the aid of an operating microscope. A speculum is placed into the outer ear and a myringotome used to make an incision in the tympanic membrane. The discharge which wells forth is gently aspirated by suction.

In secretory otitis media (blue drum, or 'glue' ear) a Shephard's teflon grommet drain tube may be inserted in the ear drum to ventilate the middle ear. This is usually left in position until it comes away by itself (Fig. 18.24).

Mastoidectomy

Definition

The removal of diseased mastoid air cells.

Position

Supine, with some reversed Trendelenburg and the head inclined away from the affected side.

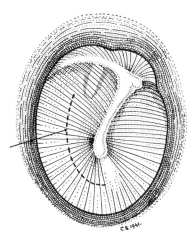

Fig. 18.24 Myringotomy. In acute suppurative otitis media the incision is as shown. For a diagnostic paracentesis a small stab is usually made anteriorly in a radial direction. (Hall and Colman.)

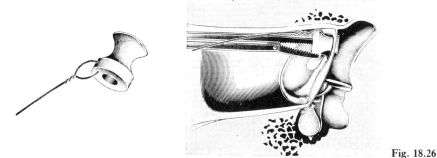

Fig. 18.25

Fig. 18.26

Figs. 18.25 to 18.26   Shepard grommet drain tube, Teflon (Down's Surgical Ltd.)

Instruments

Sponge-holding forceps (Rampley), 5
Towel clips, 5
Scalpel handles No. 3 with No. 10 and No. 15 blades (Bard Parker), 2
Dissecting forceps fine toothed (Lane and Gillies), 2
Dissecting forceps fine non-toothed (McIndoe), 2
Artery forceps, curved on flat (Kilner), 10
Aural forceps (Hartmann)
Aural forceps (Heath)
Dressing forceps (Pritchard)
Hook aural (Hartmann)
Probe aural (Jobson Horne)
Needle holder (Kilner multiple joint or Gillies)
Raspatory (Lempert)
Raspatory (Freer)

Medium retractors (Czerny), 2
Retractors, self-retaining (Mayo angled, and West straight), 2
Fine scissors, curved, 10 cm (4 in) (Kilner)
Stitch scissors, 13 cm (5 in)
Power drill, range of cutting burrs, connecting tubing or drive cable
Cartridge syringe for 2 ml adrenaline cartridges (1 : 250,000)
Fine exploring needles, sizes 18 and 14
Gelatine sponge, ribbon gauze, adrenaline, bone wax, B.I.P.P. paste in gallipot
2 (3/0) Plain catgut or synthetic absorbable for ligatures
2 (3/0) Plain catgut or synthetic absorbable on a small half-circle cutting needle for
  subcutaneous sutures
2 (3/0) Synthetic non-absorbable or silk on a small curved cutting needle for skin sutures
Operating microscope

Outline of procedure

If the operation is for acute mastoiditis, a conservative mastoidectomy is performed. The skin over the incision line is infiltrated with a 1 in 250,000 adrenaline solution to minimise bleeding. A curved incision is made behind the junction of the auricle with the scalp, and a periosteal elevator used to reflect this skin flap and ear to expose the underlying bone above and behind the external auditory meatus.

The bone over the mastoid antrum is drilled away till the antrum is opened, the diseased cells removed, but the middle ear is not opened. Either the mastoid cavity is packed with ribbon gauze impregnated with B.I.P.P., etc., and a portion of the gauze left protruding from the wound, or a post-auricular drain consisting of rubber or plastic drainage tubing is inserted. The wound is closed with catgut or a synthetic absorbable and silk or nylon skin sutures. The surgeon may also pack the external auditory canal with suitably impregnated ribbon gauze.

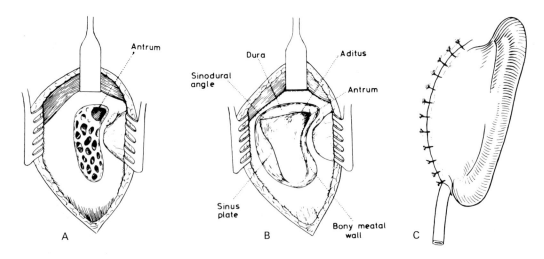

Fig. 18.27 Mastoidectomy. A post auricular incision is made, the periosteum and meatal flap reflected and the mastoid antrum exposed (Fig. 18.4A to C). (A) Antrum exposed. (B) Air cells removed, extenteration complete, bony cavity formed with antrum as its deepest point, bounded above by the dural plate, posteriorly by the sinus plate, and anteriorly by the bony meatal wall and aditus. (C) Wound closed with drainage. (Ballantyne.)

Modified radical mastoidectomy

In a radical mastoidectomy the middle ear and mastoid are turned into one cavity, drained permanently to the outside through an enlarged external auditory meatus. It is now customary to complete the operation with the creation of a new ear drum with a graft of temporal fascia.

The bone of the posterior wall of the external auditory meatus is removed and any middle ear pathology dealt with. Care is taken to avoid damage to the facial nerve which runs along the inner wall of the middle ear. The mastoid cavity and the middle ear are packed as previously described and the wound closed.

Mastoidectomy may also be performed through an endaural incision. This is known as Lempert's approach.

Microtia and meatal atresia of the external auditory canal

Definition

Correction of maldevelopment of the external auditory meatus which is often associated with maldevelopment of the middle ear. Depending on the degree of congenital abnormality the operation usually consists of repositioning the pinna and refashioning of the middle ear.

Position

As for mastoidectomy.

Instruments

As for mastoidectomy (p. 485).
Skin grafting set.

Outline of procedure

Microtia. This abnormality may be due to maternal rubella or the taking of thalidomide during pregnancy. The new pinna may have to be reconstructed in stages with a skin tube pedicle (Chapter 24). Cartilage taken from the patient's rib, from the mother, or from another person may be used. A new ear drum is constructed, often from cialit-preserved homologous dura mater, or temporal fascia. The newly constructed external auditory canal is skin grafted. The operation may be carried out in several stages.

Meatal atresia. There are various degrees of abnormality but the pinna is always situated away from its normal position forwards and downwards towards the angle of the jaw. A 'Z' plasty is carried out behind the ear to eventually move the external auditory meatus to a normal position (Fig. 18.28A).

The mastoid process is generally exposed via a postaural incision (Figs. 18.4A and B, p. 477), and exenteration of the antrum completed. The ossicles are exposed and where the meatus is present, the meatal skin is elevated, followed by enlargement of the underlying bony meatus with a cutting burr (Figs. 18.28B and C). The meatal skin tube is then refashioned and packed into position with a B.I.P.P. pack; the 'Z' plasty is closed (Fig. 18.28F) and a week later the defect in front of the pinna is skin grafted. Where the meatus is not present there are often abnormalities of the ossicles. This necessitates refashioning of the ossicles and tympanoplasty; the combined approach may be used (p. 491).

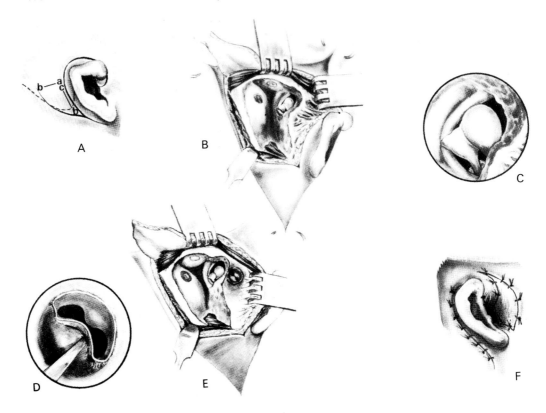

Fig. 18.28 Surgery of meatal atresia. (A) Z plasty incision, the more normal the pinna the shorter the distances a-b and b-c are made. (B and C) Exposure of the ossicles. (D and E) Elevation of the meatal skin and enlargement of the underlying bony meatus. (F) Closure of the Z plasty leaving a bare area in front of the pinna which is skin grafted in a second stage operation. (Ballantyne.)

Otoplasty (See Chapter 24)

Osteoma of the external auditory canal

Definition

Removal of a simple bony tumour of the external auditory canal.

Position

As for mastoidectomy

Instruments

As for mastoidectomy, p. 485.

Outline of procedure

The exposure is similar to that for mastoidectomy. The skin is elevated off the tumour which is drilled away, often using diamond paste burrs.

OPERATIONS TO IMPROVE AURAL FUNCTION

Stapedectomy

Definition

Removal of stapes in cases of conductive or mixed deafness due to otosclerosis in which there is a good bone-air gap, and insertion of a prosthesis in order to re-establish sound conduction to the inner ear.

Position

As for mastoidectomy.

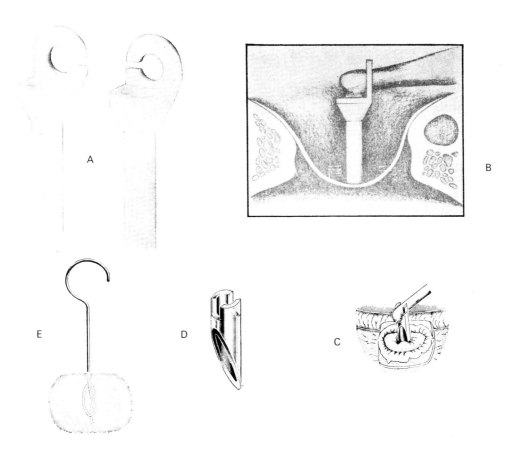

Fig. 18.29 (A and B). Shea Teflon piston attached to tip of the incus with the lenticular process seated in a cup at the prosthesis head. By fitting on to the tip of the incus where the stapes was formerly attached, the prosthesis closely approximates the original angle to the oval window and provides a more normal reconstruction. (C and D) Shea slotted prosthesis. (E) Prefabricated wire loop with gelatine sponge. (Down's Surgical Ltd.)

Instruments

As for mastoidectomy (p. 485).
   Stapedectomy set etc. (Fig. 18.31).
   Saline irrigation set.

Outline of procedure

Previously mobilisation of stapes was carried out but this seldom gave permanent results as the stapes usually became fixed again. Stapedectomy is carried out via a permeatal approach (Fig. 18.30); the favoured procedure being to remove the stapes, seal off the oval window with a piece of temporal fascia, vein or gelatin sponge and to replace the stapes with a prosthesis such as a specially shaped polyethylene tube of suitable length, or a teflon piston, or a piece of stainless steel hooked over the incus. This is to connect the incus to the oval window, thereby restoring the function of the ossicular chain.

Tympanoplasty

Definition

Repair of the ear drum by myringoplasty (a graft of temporal fascia, vein or Cialit-preserved homograft (dura mater) and if necessary reconstruction of the ossicular chain with polyethylene, teflon, or stainless steel, or grafts of cartilage taken from the nasal septum, or bone chips, or sterile preserved ossicles taken from cadavers or other patients and preserved in the deep freeze, or patient's own refashioned ossicles.

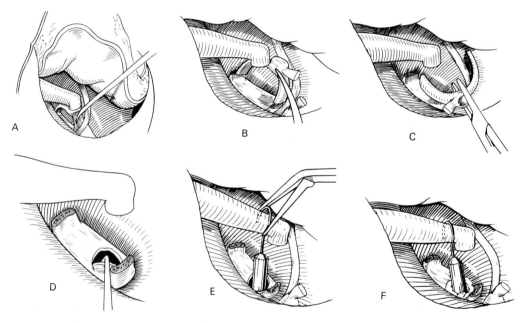

Fig. 18.30 Stapedectomy, approach by permeatal incision (Fig. 18.2). (A) The stapedius tendon is cut with a curved sickle knife. (B) Fracture of the stapedial cura. (C) Removal of the stapes superstructure. (D) Removal of the footplate to accommodate the prosthesis (in Ménière's disease, the whole of the stapes footplate would be removed if the labyrinth is to be destroyed). (E) Insertion of stainless steel piston. (F) Sealing the gap between the piston and oval window with gelatin sponge. (Ballantyne.)

Position

As for stapedectomy.

Instruments

As for stapedectomy.
  Tympanoplasty instruments (Fig. 18.31).
  Biological adhesive (non-toxic fibrinogen glue)

Outline of procedure

Tympanoplasty is a delicate operation to reconstruct the sound conducting mechanism in cases of diseases such as chronic otitis media, or trauma, which has resulted in disruption of the mechanism thereby causing hearing loss. It may be combined with procedures for the eradication of chronic disease — such as generalised cholesteatosis and intractable catarrhal otis media.

There is a wide variety of operative procedures which can be adopted. These include partial myringoplasty, total myringoplasty and combined approach tympanoplasty (posterior tympanotomy). The posterior, or less frequently the transmeatal approach, may be used for partial myringoplasty or simple myringoplasty.

Partial myringoplasty — partial restoration of the tympanic membrane — consists in some instances of inserting a piece of preserved tympanic membrane between the elevated squamous epithelium of the drum and its pars fibrosa (Fig. 18.32A). Other defects may be repaired by using a fragment of fibrous annulus and meatal skin attached to a tympanic membrane fragment (Fig. 18.32B).

Total myringoplasty — complete restoration of the tympanic membrane — is carried out after removing all scar tissue around the whole circumference of the perforation (Fig. 18.33A–C). This may be termed a simple myringoplasty. An appropriate allograft is inserted, correctly aligned, and glued into position with biological glue applied to the meatal cuff. Correct packing to ensure subsequent healing is essential (Fig. 18.33D–F and Fig. 18.34A–C).

Simple myringoplasty is used when pathology appears safe and either the osicular chain is intact following the dissection of all tympanic and annular remnents, or simple ossiculoplasty has been performed.

A tympanic membrane graft with its periosteal cuff attached is placed donor manibrium to host manibrium, thereby ensuring correct anatomical resetting of the drum. A biological glue is used to attach the manibrium to the drum, meatal cuff to the bony edges, and fibrous annulus into the sulcus.

Combined approach — posterior tympanotomy — aims to remove all pathology in such a way as to allow preservation or restoration of the posterior bony wall and bony sulcus to provide support for an allograft tympanic membrane.

A postaural incision is made and a posterior tympanotomy carried out (Figs. 18.4 and 18.5). All drum remnants including the fibrous annulus, diseased tissue, and unsafe ossicles with the exception of the stapes footplate are removed (Fig. 18.35A–D). When all diseased tissue has been removed from the middle ear cavity attention is given to anatomical restoration.

A suitable tympano-ossicular allograft is manoeuvred into an anatomically normal position, and then secured where necessary with biological glue (Fig. 18.35E–F). The

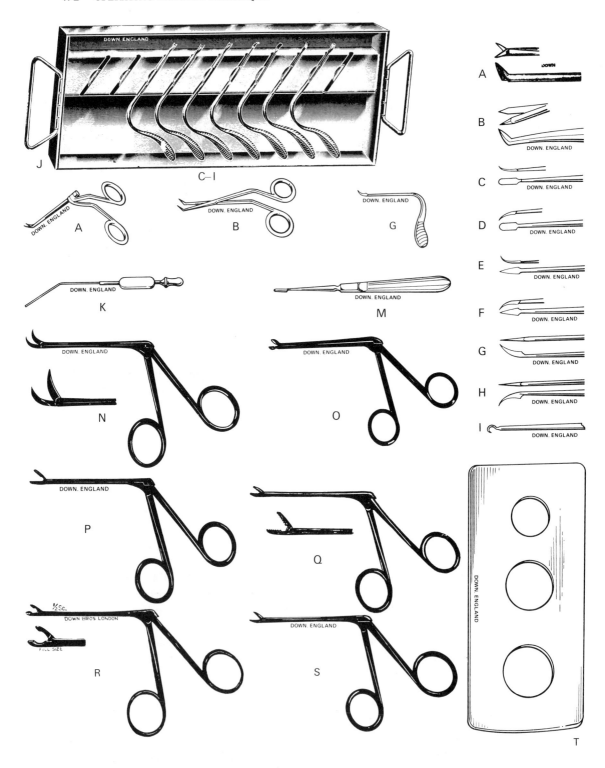

Fig. 18.31 Zoellner's tympanoplasty instruments. As used at the Royal National Throat, Nose and Ear Hospital, London. (Down's Surgical Ltd.)

Key:
A. Zoellner's scissors, bayonet shaped, tubular model, with upward cut, lateral action.
B. Zoellner's scissors, angular, with upward cut, lateral action, screw joint.
C. Zoellner's fine raspatory, curved to right, with thumb grip, matt finish.
D. Ditto, curved to left, with thumb grip, matt finish.
E. Zoellner's fine spear-pointed needle, curved to right, with thumb grip, matt finish.
F. Ditto, curved to left, with thumb grip, matt finish.
G. Zoellner's knife, upward cutting, with thumb grip, matt finish.
H. Ditto, downward cutting, with thumb grip, matt finish.
I. Zoellner's small hook, with thumb grip, matt finish.
J. Zoellner's rack to hold instruments above, figs. C to I with three space clips for additional similar instruments; arranged to protect the knives, etc. during sterilisation and afterwards to make the different instruments easily discernible.

K. Zoellner's suction tube, nickle plated with fine detachable end, 5 sizes 18, 20, 22, 24 and 26 s.w.g. × 19 mm ($\frac{3}{4}$ in) long.
M. Zoellner's raspatory, curved on flat, narrow bladed on metal handle.
N. Ormerod's aural scissors, extra fine, curved upwards crocodile action, black finished.
O. Ormerod's aural forceps with extra fine circular cup crocodile action jaws, black finished.
P. Ormerod's aural forceps with extra fine elongated cup crocodile jaws, black finished.
Q. Hartmann's aural forceps with extra fine serrated crocodile action jaws, black finished.
R. Aural forceps extra fine, double cup oval jaws 1.75 mm × 0.75 mm crocodile action, black finished.
S. Scissors, extra fine, crocodile action jaws, black finished.
T. Zoellner's Skin Graft Plate, 152 × 76 mm (6 × 3 in) with three holes 22, 28, 32 mm ($\frac{7}{8}$, $1\frac{1}{8}$ and $1\frac{1}{4}$ in) diameter.

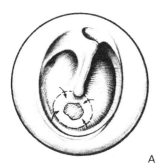 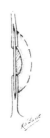 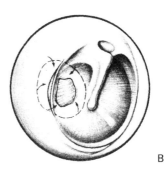 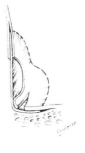

Fig. 18.32 Partial myringoplasty — allograft. (A) Small defect requiring a piece of preserved tympanic membrane to be inserted between the elevated squamous epithelium of the drum and its pars fibrosa. (B) Another defect which required the insertion of a fragment of fibrous annulus and meatal skin attached to a fragment of tympanic membrane. (Marquet in *Rob and Smith's Operative Surgery* 4th edn, edited by Ballantyne and Morrison.)

incudo-stapedial joint may be restored in a number of ways (Fig. 18.36A–E). Alternatively a prosthesis may be inserted in the manner described under stapedectomy (page 489), and a total typanoplasty carried out. The mastoid cavity is drained before wound closure to prevent increase in air pressure in the middle ear and possible displacement of the drum graft (Fig. 18.37A–B).

Surgical treatment of Ménière's disease

Definition

Surgical relief of Ménière's disease (attacks of rotational vertigo, tinnitus and deafness) after failure of conservative treatment. There are many specialised operations for this condition, which include transmeatal and translabyrinth cochleovestibular neurectomy. This procedure consists of exposing the internal auditory canal and dividing both the inferior and superior vestibular nerves and the cochlear nerve (Fig. 18.38A–B).

Other operative procedures include the destruction of the vestibular end-organs without causing further damage to the organ of Corti or the facial nerve.

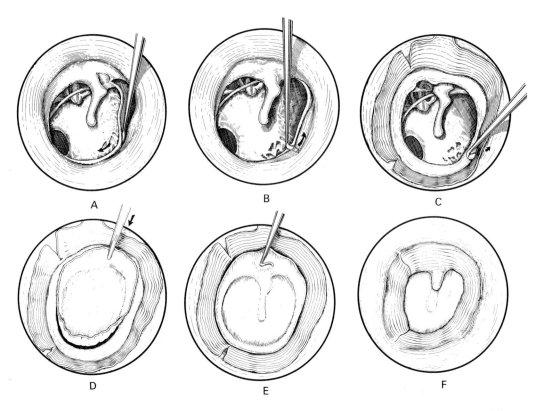

Fig. 18.33 Total myringoplasty — allograft. (A–C) Removal of scar tissue around whole circumfrence of the perforation and dissection of the outer epithelial layer from the fibrous layer towards the periphery. The integrity of the ossicular chain is checked and if necessary restoration carried out. Care is taken to ensure that all epithelial remnants are removed. (D) Allograft of correct size and shape placed in position. (E) Sheath of allograft material which corresponds with the donor's handle of the malleus is aligned with the denuded handle of the host's malleus. Biological glue may be used to secure the graft in position. (F) The host's epithelial remnants of the drum and skin of the auditory canal are replaced on the surface of the periosteal cuff. (Marquet in *Rob and Smith's Operative Surgery* 4th edn, edited by Ballantyne and Morrison.)

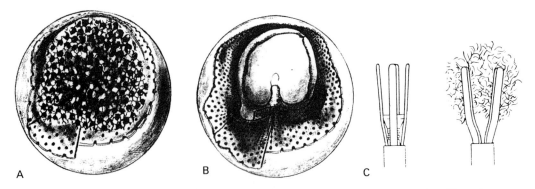

Fig. 18.34 Packing, following middle ear surgery. (A) A piece of perforated silastic, rolled up like a cigarette paper, is inserted into the auditory canal and pushed gently against the wall covered by the new stretched epithelium. (B) Three or four artificial sponges soaked in an antibiotic steroid ointment are gently inserted into the canal using sponge forceps (C). (Marquet in *Rob and Smith's Operative Surgery* 4th edn, edited by Ballantyne and Morrison.)

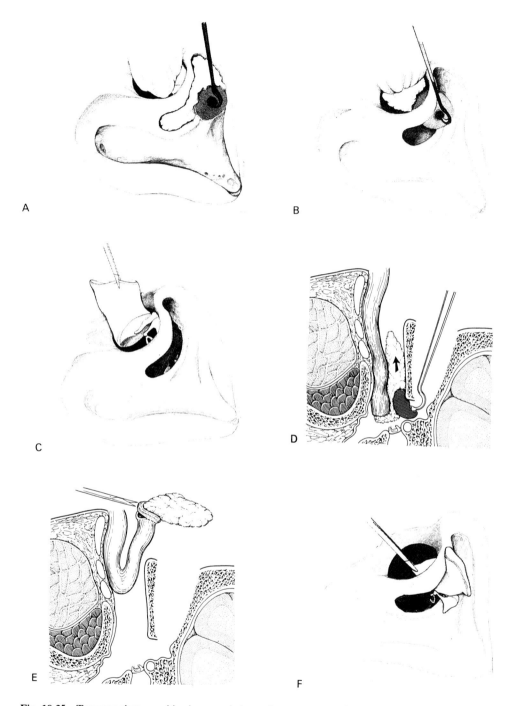

Fig. 18.35 Tympanoplasty combined approach (posterior tympanotomy).
(A–E) Removal of all drum remnants, including the fibrous annulus, and any diseased tissue (e.g.
cholesteatoma). This is accomplished with artificial sponges and a specially designed sponge elevator.
Ossicle remnants are also excised, but a normal mobile stapes is retained and the host's tensor tympani is
cleaned and preserved.
(F) Introduction of suitable tympano-ossicular chain allograft into the middle ear.
(Marquet in *Rob and Smith's Operative Surgery* 4th edn, edited by Ballantyne and Morrison)

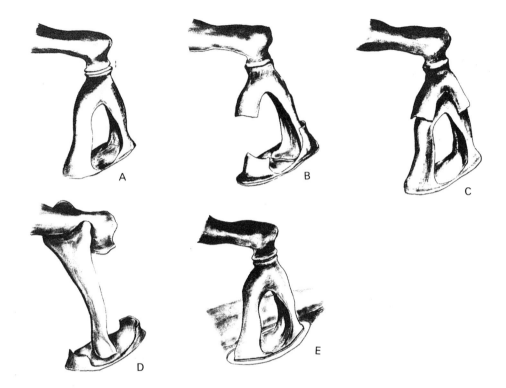

Fig. 18.36 Restoration of the incudo-stapedial joint.

A. Repositioning of lenticular process on top of a normal mobile stapes.

B. Using a partial stapes, with the anterior crus on top of a normal mobile footplate without superstructure.

C. Positioning the head of an allograft stapes on top of the original one.

D. Implanting an alloplastic or autogenic modelled ossicle.

E. In exceptional cases, when the footplate is non-existent, the normally attached stapes allograft may be placed on the oval window. The cuff and ossicles are then glued to the bony wall of the host.

(Marquet in *Rob and Smith's Operative Surgery* 4th edn, edited by Ballantyne and Morrison)

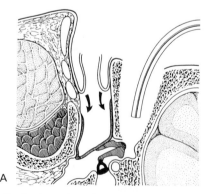
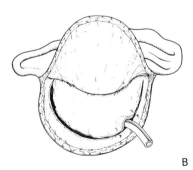

Fig. 18.37 Drainage following tympanoplasty. A–B. Drainage tube is positioned in mastoid cavity before closure to prevent any increase in air pressure which could displace the drum graft. (Marquet in *Rob and Smith's Operative Surgery* 4th edn, edited by Ballantyne and Morrison)

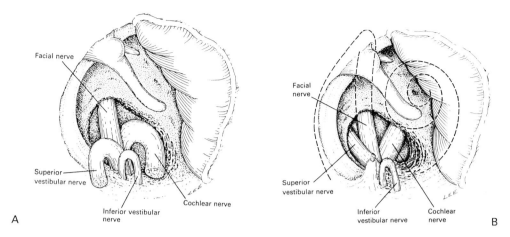

Fig. 18.38 Transmeatal cochleovestibular neurectomy.
A. Exposure of the nerves lying in the internal auditory canal.
B. Sectioning of both vestibular nerves and the cochlear nerve; a small segment of each is removed.
(Garcia-Ibanez and Alvarez de Cozar in *Rob and Smith's Operative Surgery* 4th edn, edited by Ballantyne and Morrison)

OPERATIONS ON THE NOSE AND ACCESSORY SINUSES

Pre-operative nasal packing

Definition

Packing of the nasal cavity before operation either to effect local anaesthesia (e.g., lignocaine (Xylocaine) 4 per cent) or to provide vasoconstriction and haemostasis for the surgeon (e.g., 5 to 10 per cent cocaine solution with 1 in 10,000 adrenaline added. Too much adrenaline may cause ventricular fibrilation if halothane or trilene general anaesthesia is used).

Position

Supine.

Instruments

> Speculae Nasal (Thudichum), set
> Dressing forceps, nasal (Tilley or Wilde)
> Roll of 25 mm (1 in) ribbon gauze
> Lignocaine 4 per cent
> Adrenaline 1 in 10,000
> Graduated measure, 15 ml ($\frac{1}{2}$ oz)
> Head light, or head mirror and lamp
> Towel or swab to protect the patient's lips.

Outline of procedure

The ribbon gauze is impregnated with solution, and one or both nasal cavities are packed

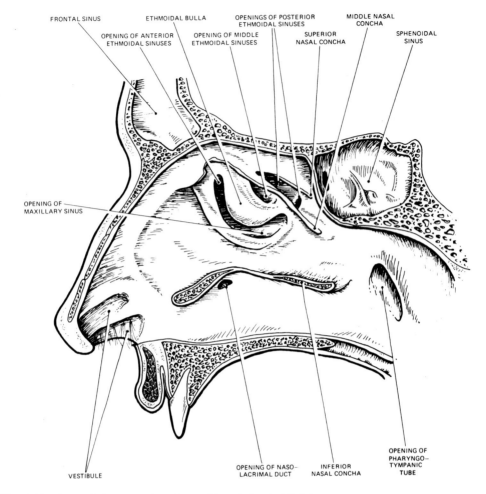

FRONTAL SINUS ETHMOIDAL BULLA OPENINGS OF POSTERIOR ETHMOIDAL SINUSES MIDDLE NASAL CONCHA

OPENING OF ANTERIOR ETHMOIDAL SINUSES OPENING OF MIDDLE ETHMOIDAL SINUSES SUPERIOR NASAL CONCHA SPHENOIDAL SINUS

OPENING OF MAXILLARY SINUS

VESTIBULE OPENING OF NASO-LACRIMAL DUCT INFERIOR NASAL CONCHA OPENING OF PHARYNGO-TYMPANIC TUBE

Fig. 18.39 Anatomical cross-section of nose. (Down's Surgical Ltd.)

using a nasal speculum and dressing forceps. The ribbon gauze is first passed along the floor of the cavity, and successive layers are built up until it is filled. The pack is left in place for at least 15 minutes before operation, and is removed gently to avoid trauma of the nasal mucosa. Spraying the nose with 5 per cent cocaine first makes packing with ribbon gauze less unpleasant if the patient is conscious.

Reduction of a nasal fracture

Definition

Anatomical re-alignment of a fractured nasal bone.

Position

Supine.

Figs. 18.40 to 18.43   Nasal instruments. (Down's Surgical Ltd.)

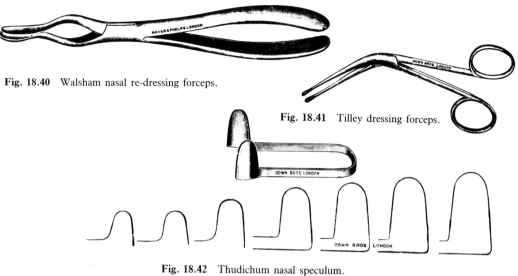

Fig. 18.40   Walsham nasal re-dressing forceps.

Fig. 18.41   Tilley dressing forceps.

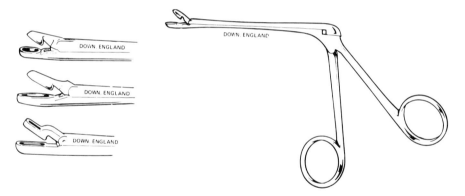

Fig. 18.42   Thudichum nasal speculum.

Fig. 18.43   Grunwald nasal turbinate forceps, with narrow punch jaws, 3 patterns.

Instruments

Dressing forceps nasal (Tilley)
Re-dressing or re-fracture nasal forceps (Walsham)
Mallet small (Rowland), optional
Specula nasal (Thudichum)
25 mm (1 in) ribbon gauze which may be impregnated with petroleum jelly
Scissors, dressing
Suction tubing, fine nozzles and tube anchoring forceps
Plaster of Paris strips 50 mm (2 in) × 150 mm (6 in) or Stent material, and hot water in
  a small bowl
Adhesive strapping and a few small swabs

Figs. 18.44 to 18.50 Nasal instruments. (Down's Surgical Ltd.)

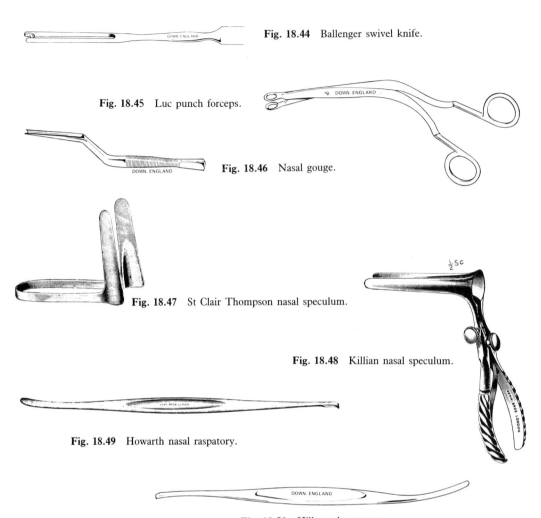

Fig. 18.44 Ballenger swivel knife.

Fig. 18.45 Luc punch forceps.

Fig. 18.46 Nasal gouge.

Fig. 18.47 St Clair Thompson nasal speculum.

Fig. 18.48 Killian nasal speculum.

Fig. 18.49 Howarth nasal raspatory.

Fig. 18.50 Hill nasal raspatory.

Outline of procedure

If the injury is old the nasal bone may be re-fractured with a small mallet, utilising a swab to protect the skin.

One jaw of the Walsham's forceps is introduced into the nose and pressed against the nasal bone on the selected side. The other jaw provides counter-pressure against a swab placed on the outside of the nose.

The fragments of the nasal bone are manipulated into anatomical position and the nose packed with ribbon gauze. If the fracture fragments are stable no further procedure is carried out. If unstable, the fracture is immobilised either with three strips of plaster of Paris (two diagonally across the bridge of the nose extending from forehead to cheek, one across the forehead) or Stent. A Stent splint is fashioned by softening the material in hot water and moulding it into shape. The splints are retained in position with adhesive plaster.

Figs. 18.51 to 18.53 Nasal instruments (cont'd). (Down's Surgical Ltd.)

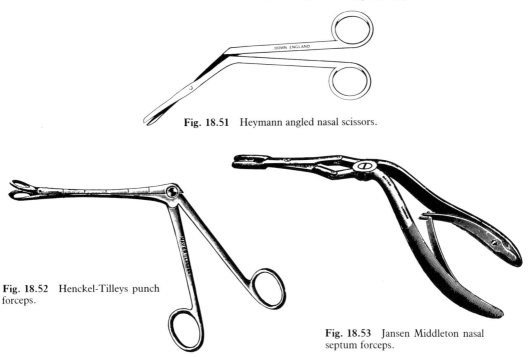

Fig. 18.51 Heymann angled nasal scissors.

Fig. 18.52 Henckel-Tilleys punch forceps.

Fig. 18.53 Jansen Middleton nasal septum forceps.

Nasal polypectomy

Definition

Removal of nasal polypi, under general or local anaesthesia.

Position

Supine.

Instruments

    Nasal speculae (Thudichum) set
    Nasal speculae (St Clair Thompson), set
    Nasal dressing forceps (Henckel-Tilley)
    Nasal snare, wire
    Punch forceps, small and large (Weil), 2
    25 mm (1 in) ribbon impregnated with petroleum jelly
    Suction tubing and fine nozzles and tube anchoring forceps.

Outline of procedure

Using a nasal speculum, the wire loop of the snare is manoeuvred around each polyp in turn and withdrawn, bringing the excised polyp with it; the Weil's forceps are used to grasp and

remove tags, avulsing them with a twisting action. Packing the nasal cavity or cavities completes the operation.

Turbinotomy or turbinectomy

Definition

The removal part of hypertrophied nasal turbinate.

Instruments

    Nasal specula (Thudichum), set
    Nasal specula (St Clair Thompson), set
    Nasal dressing forceps (Tilley or Wilde)
    Nasal snare, wire
    Punch forceps, small and medium (Weil or Luc), 2
    Nasal scissors, angled (Heymann)
    25 mm (1 in) ribbon gauze impregnated with petroleum jelly
    Suction tubing, fine nozzles and Robin tube anchoring forceps.

Outline of procedure

Using a nasal speculum, the surgeon inserts the angled scissors and divides the turbinate bone along its base for a short distance. The wire snare is inserted and the loop passed over the turbinal with the barrel of the snare lying along the cut made. The snare is withdrawn and the enlarged portion of the turbinal removed with forceps.

The nasal cavity or cavities are packed with ribbon gauze in the usual manner.

Submucous resection of the nasal septum

Definition

The removal of the deflected bony and cartilaginous parts of a nasal septum to rectify an obstructed airway.

Position

Supine.

Instruments

    Sponge-holding forceps (Rampley), 5
    Scalpel handles No. 3 with No. 10 and No. 15 blades (Bard Parker), 2
    Towel clips, 5
    Fine dissecting forceps, toothed (Gillies)
    Dressing forceps, angled (Tilley)
    Dressing forceps, angled (Wilde)
    Gauges nasal, angled (Tilley and Killian)
    Knife nasal (Dundas Grant)
    Knife swivel (Ballenger)

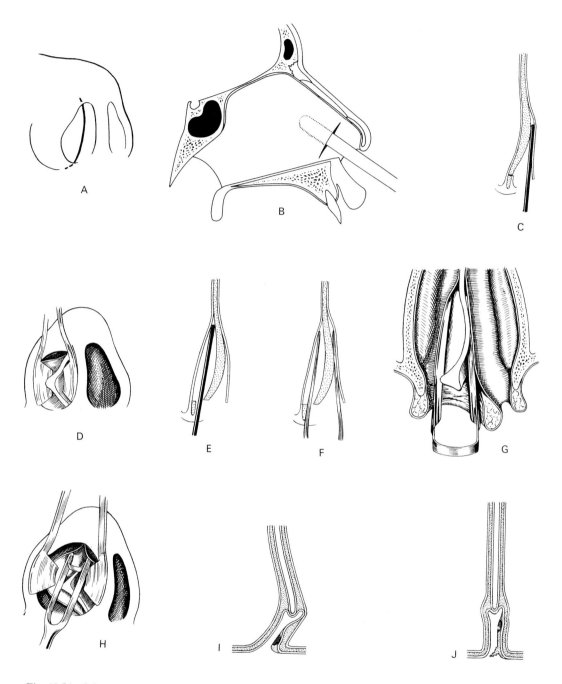

Fig. 18.54 Submucous resection of the nasal septum. (A) Incision of one side of nasal septum. (B) and (C) Plane of cleavage between cartilage and perichondrium opened by blunt dissection. (D) to (G) Cartilage incised, opening second plane of cleavage between cartilage and perichondrium on other side. (H) Removal of cartilage with Ballenger's swivel knife. (I and J) Groove of perichondrium lying on crest of maxilla and vomer. The crest of the bone is freed from soft tissue, fractured in the mid-line, and then removed with a hammer and gouge or bone forceps. (Ballantyne.)

Mallet (Heath)
Mouth gag (Mason)
Probe, malleable silver
Punch forceps (Luc) medium and small
Punch forceps (Weil)
Raspatory, nasal (Hill)
Raspatory, nasal (Howarth)
Retractors, small single hook, 3
Scissors, nasal angled (Heymann)
Septum forceps, nasal (Jansen Middleton)
Speculum, nasal, self-retaining (Killian)
Speculae, nasal, long (St Clair Thompson) set of 3
Speculae, nasal, short (Thudichum) set of 4
Tongue depressor, angled
Tongue forceps (Mayo)
Suction tubing, fine nozzles and tube anchoring forceps
Needle holder (Kilner multiple joint)
2 (3/0) Chromic catgut or synthetic absorbable on a small half-circle cutting needle for
    mucosa sutures
B.I.P.P. (optional)
Lubricant in galli-pot e.g., liquid paraffin
Rubber glove fingers for nasal pack (distended with ribbon gauze) optional
Plaster of Paris strips or Stent impression material for nasal splint (optional).

Outline of procedure

A small incision is made behind the junction of the skin and mucous membrane on one side
of the nasal septum. A Thudichum's nasal speculum is inserted, and using a long raspatory
through this incision, the mucoperichondrium is dissected free from the septum along one
side.

An incision is then made through the cartilage along the line of the original incision and
the raspatory introduced to strip off the mucoperichondrium on the other side of the
septum. Care is taken not to puncture the mucosa on this side. The small nasal speculum
is changed for a longer one (St Clair Thompson's), which is inserted so that the blades pass
between the nasal septum and mucosa on each side. This separates the mucosa away from
the septum and the cut edge of the septal cartilage lies in the centre of the speculum.

As much as necessary of the cartilage is removed with a Ballenger's swivel knife, which
is first passed backwards and then downwards, and finally forwards. Pieces of the vomer
and vertical plate of the ethmoid are removed with punch forceps and the irregular spur
which is usually present along the lower edge of the septum is removed with an angled
gouge. The long speculum is removed and the tubinates are examined using a Thudichum's
speculum. If these are hypertrophied, a turbinotomy or turbinectomy may be performed.

Some surgeons suture the mucosal incision before inserting two rubber glove fingers (one
in each nostril) which have been packed with petroleum jelly gauze.

Antrostomy (intranasal operation)

Definition

An intransal opening into the maxillary antrum usually performed for chronic suppuration.

Position

Supine.

Instruments

Sponge-holding forceps (Rampley), 5
Scalpel handle No. 3 with No. 15 blade (Bard Parker)
Towel clips, 5
Curetting spoon (Volkmann)

Figs. 18.55 to 18.59   Antrum instruments. (Down's Surgical Ltd.)

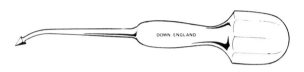

Fig. 18.55   Tilley antrum trocar.

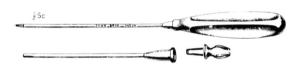

Fig. 18.56   Tilley Lichwitz antrum trocar and cannula.

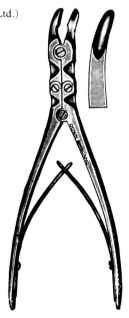

Fig. 18.57   Luer Jansen gouge or punch forceps.

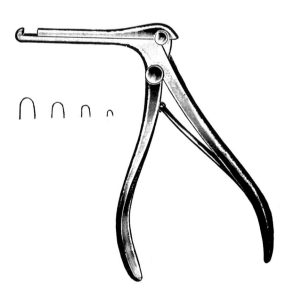

Fig. 18.58   Kerrison's rongeur, upward cutting.

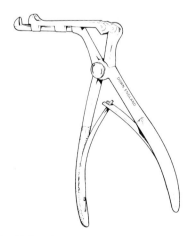

Fig. 18.59   Citelli gouge or punch forceps.

Dissector (Hill)
Dressing forceps nasal (Tilley or Wilde)
Small gouges 4 mm, 6 mm, 8 mm, (Jenkins)
Harpoon antrum (Tilley)
Irrigation syringe and warm saline
Power drill, cutting burrs, connecting tubing or drive cable
Punch forceps (Citelli)
Punch forceps, small and medium (Luc)
Punch forceps, small and medium (Weil)
Probe, malleable silver
Scissors, nasal, angled (Heymann)
Snare nasal wire
Speculae nasal (Thudichum) set
Speculae nasal (St Clair Thompson) set
Trocar antrum and cannula
Suction tubing, nozzles and tube anchoring forceps
(Two rubber glove fingers distended with petroleum jelly ribbon gauze may be required).

Outline of procedure

An intra nasal antrostomy consists of performing a turbinectomy or turbinotomy (removing the anterior end of the inferior turbinate) followed by the insertion of an antrum harpoon, or using burrs to make an opening through the lateral nasal wall into the antrum. This opening is then enlarged with a burr or punch forceps, followed by irrigation of the antrum with warm water. The nasal cavity may be packed using two rubber glove fingers as previously described.

Radical antrostomy or Caldwell Luc operation

Definition

An opening into the antrum approached via the mouth through the anterior wall of the maxilla, leaving a large antrostomy into the nose.

Position

Semi-sitting head and neck flexed
or Supine.

Instruments

Sponge-holding forceps (Rampley), 5
Scalpel handle No. 3 with Nos. 10 and 15 blades (Bard Parker)
Towel clips, 5
Curetting spoon (Volkmann)
Dissecting forceps, toothed (Lane), 2
Dissecting forceps, non-toothed, 13 cm (5 in), 2

Dressing forceps, angled (Tilley)
Dressing forceps, angled (Wilde)
Gouge forceps (Jansen)
Gouge or punch forceps (Citelli)
Harpoon antrum (Tilley)
Irrigation syringe and warm saline
Mouth gag (Mason)
Needle holder (Kilner multiple joint)
Punch forceps nasal (Grunwald)
Punch forceps (Luc) large and medium
Punch forceps (Weil)
Raspatory nasal (Hill)
Raspatory nasal (Howarth)
Power drill, burrs, connecting tubing or drive cable
Retractors, malleable, medium
Rugine (Faraboeuf)
Scissors, curved on flat, 13 cm (5 in) (Mayo)
Scissors, stitch, 13 cm (5 in)
Scissors, nasal angled (Heymann)
Speculum nasal self-retaining (Killian)
Speculae, nasal, long (St Clair Thompson), set of 3
Speculae, nasal small (Thudichum), set of 4
Tongue depressor, angled
Tongue forceps (Mayo)
Trocar, antrum and cannula
Cartridge syringe for 2 ml adrenaline cartridge 1: 250,000
Fine exploring needles, sizes 18 and 14
Suction tubing and tube anchoring forceps
3 or 2.5 (0 or 2/0) Chromic catgut, synthetic absorbable or silk on a small half-circle round-bodied needle for mucosa suture
Lubricant in galli-pot e.g., Liquid paraffin
2 Rubber glove fingers for nasal pack (distended with ribbon gauze).

Outline of procedure

The upper lip on the affected side is retracted upwards and the tissues just above the gingivolabial reflection infiltrated with adrenaline 1: 250,000 solution. An incision is made in the mucosa lying over the anterior wall of the maxilla. The mucous membrane is reflected from the surface of the bone, and an opening fashioned in the wall of the antrum, using a power driven burr followed by punch forceps.

Any diseased mucosa in the antrum is scraped away, and the cavity is irrigated with warm saline. An opening is made into the nasal cavity through the lateral bulge at the interior meatus using a burr. The opening is enlarged with punch forceps to about 1.5 cm long by 1 cm wide, and an incision made through the mucosa which is then incised to create an opening which matches the bony opening. The cavity may then be packed with B.I.P.P. ribbon gauze, the end of which is brought out via the antrostomy opening and taped to the cheek. The gum is then closed with catgut or a synthetic absorbable suture.

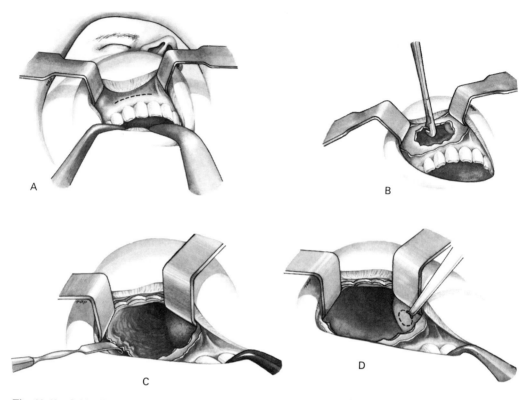

Fig. 18.60   Caldwell–Luc operation. (A) Incision. (B) Soft tissue elevated from bone, antrum opened, enlargement of bony opening with punch forceps. (C) Removal of antral lining. (D) Site of antrostomy opening into nose. (Ballantyne.)

Ethmoidectomy (intranasal operation)

Definition

Removal of the anterior wall of the ethmoidal labyrinth and ethmoidal cells for chronic allergic inflammatory conditions.

Position

Supine.

Instruments

As for submucous resection (p. 502)
Frontal sinus probe
Frontal sinus curette.

Outline of procedure

A submucous resection of the nasal septum may be performed to provide better access to the ethmoidal labyrinth.

Basically, the operation consists of removing the ethmoid cells which lie around the passage leading from the frontal sinus to the nasal cavity. The operation is performed almost entirely with a long nasal speculum, frontal sinus probe, punch forceps, such as Luc's and the frontal sinus curette.

Fronto-ethmoidectomy

Definition

Removal of diseased ethmoid cells and the creation of a drainage channel through that area from the frontal sinus.

Position

Supine.

Instruments

Sponge-holding forceps (Rampley), 5
Towel clips, 5
Scalpel handles No. 3 with Nos. 10 and 15 blades (Bard Parker), 2
Bone nibbling forceps, curved on flat
Artery forceps fine curved on flat, mosquito, 10
Dressing nasal forceps (Tilley)
Curette frontal sinus
Dissecting forceps, toothed (Gillies and Lane), 2
Dissecting forceps non-toothed 13 cm (5 in), 2
Needle holder (Kilner multiple joint, or Gillies)
Power drill, burrs, connecting tubing or drive cable
Punch forceps frontal sinus (Citelli)
Punch forceps, small and medium (Luc)
Rasps frontal sinus (Watson-Jones), set of 3
Retractors small double hook
Retractors, self-retaining (Mayo hinged and West straight or Ferris Smith), 2
Rugines, small, curved and straight (Farabacue), 2
Scissors, curved on flat 13 cm (5 in) (Mayo)
Scissors, fine curved, 10 cm (4 in) (Kilner)
Scissors, stitch, 13 cm (5 in)
Skin hooks (Gillies), 2
Speculae, nasal (St Clair Thompson), set of 2
Tissue forceps, fine (McIndoe), 5
Suction tubing, fine nozzles and tube anchoring forceps
2 (3/0) Plain catgut or synthetic absorbable for ligatures
2 and 2.5 (3/0 and 2/0) Chromic catgut or synthetic absorbable on small half-circle round-bodied needles for subcutaneous sutures
1.5 (4/0) synthetic non-absorbable or silk on a small curved cutting needle for skin sutures. sutures.

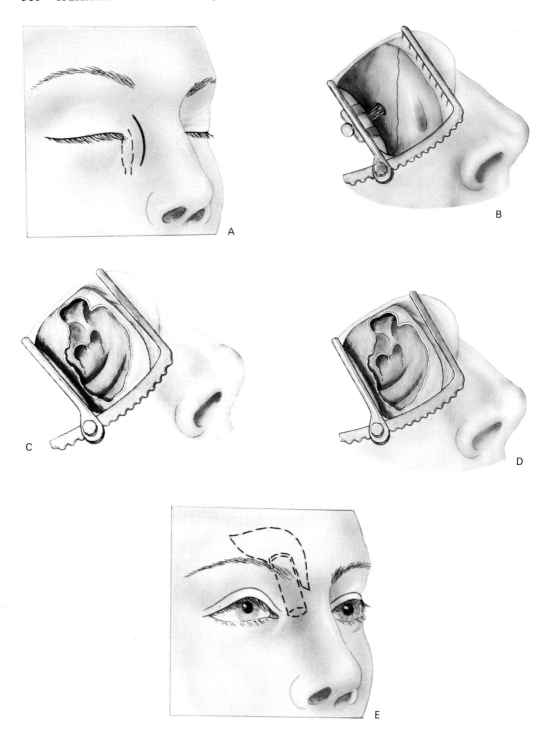

Fig. 18.61 Exposure of the frontal, ethmoidal and sphenoidal sinuses. (A) The incision. (B) Ligation of the ethmoidal vessels either with ligatures or clips. (C) Exposure of the ethmoidal sinuses. (D) Exposure of the frontal sinus. (E) Maintenance of frontal sinus drainage. (Ballantyne.)

Outline of procedure

A curved incision is made medial to the medial canthus of the eye. The periosteum is reflected off the maxilla, and frontal bone and medial orbital wall. The lacrymal sac is displaced laterally and the ethmoidal vessels exposed, and ligated.

The thin ethmoidal bone medial to the orbit is penetrated and ethmoid cells exenterated to expose the anterior wall of the ethmoid sinus which is then removed. Exenteration of the anterior ethmoid cells, working in an upwards direction exposes the frontal sinus. The bony wall of the frontal sinus floor is removed and the diseased contents evacuated.

A plastic or rubber tube may be inserted between the cavity and the nose, being left to protrude at one end of the nostril, where it is secured with a suture. Haemostasis is secured and the subcutaneous tissues approximated before closing the skin with fine silk or synthetic non-absorbable sutures.

OPERATIONS ON THE THROAT AND MOUTH

Direct laryngoscopy

Definition

Direct examination of the larynx with an endoscope which places the mouth, pharynx and larynx in a straight line (the Boyce position).

Position

Supine.

Instruments

    Laryngoscope with appropriate size of blade (Mackintosh Magill or Chevalier Jackson, etc.) (Chapter 11, p. 346)
    Tongue forceps (Mayo)
    Angled tongue depressor
    Laryngeal swab holders and small mops
    Laryngeal biopsy forceps
    Adrenaline 1 in 1,000
    Graduated measure
    Suction tubing, nozzles and tube anchoring forceps
    Diathermy leads, electrodes and lead anchoring forceps.

Outline of procedure

The patient is anaesthetised and with his neck flexed and head extended the laryngoscope is inserted. A biopsy may be taken with the biopsy forceps and the area swabbed with small mops soaked in adrenaline solution, or diathermised.

For bronchoscopy and oesophagoscopy, see Chapter 27 Thoracic operations.

Peritonsillar abscess or quinsy

Definition

An abscess between the surgical capsule of the tonsil and the superior constrictor muscle and fascia of the adjacent lateral pharyngeal wall.

Position

Sitting, facing the surgeon, or lateral position with the table in slight Trendelenburg.

Instruments

Scalpel handle No. 3 with No. 15 blade (Bard Parker) wrapped with adhesive plaster, tip only exposed.
Sponge-holding forceps (Rampley) and small sponges or swabs, 5
Mouth gag (Mason or Doyen)
Tongue forceps (Mayo)
Angled tongue depressor
Scissors, straight with sharp outer edges.
Sinus forceps
Pharyngeal spray and 4 per cent lignocaine
Sterile throat swab
Mouth washes (used with great caution and with patient bending forwards).

Outline of procedure

A little topical anaesthesia is generally employed. An incision is made with the guarded knife through the maximum bulge in the soft palate, parallel with the posterior margin and extending approximately about 2 cm inwards from the anterior pillar of the fauces. Sinus forceps are introduced quickly into the incision and separated.

Tonsillectomy and adenoidectomy

Definition

Enucleation of the tonsils either by dissection or guillotine, and curetting of the adenoids.

Position

Dissection. Supine, with the head and neck in extension. A 'jack' may be used to support the mouth gag during operation. One of the best gag supporters is two Draffin poles, one on each side, resting on the operating table, thus leaving the patient's chest unobstructed. Adenoidectomy as below.
Guillotine: First supine with the head to one side, and then lateral for adenoidectomy.

Instruments

Sponge holding forceps (Rampley), 5
Towel clips, 5

Figs. 18.62 to 18.68   Tonsil instruments. (Down's Surgical Ltd.)

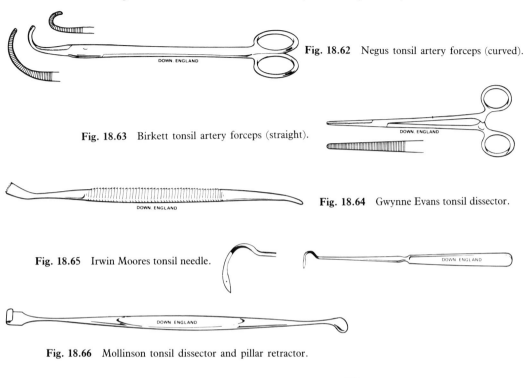

Fig. 18.62   Negus tonsil artery forceps (curved).

Fig. 18.63   Birkett tonsil artery forceps (straight).

Fig. 18.64   Gwynne Evans tonsil dissector.

Fig. 18.65   Irwin Moores tonsil needle.

Fig. 18.66   Mollinson tonsil dissector and pillar retractor.

Fig. 18.67   Eves tonsil snare.

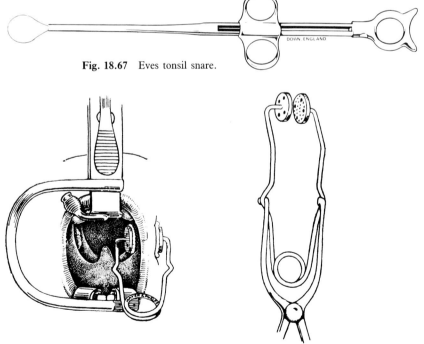

Fig. 18.68   Beneys tonsil compressor.

Figs. 18.69 to 18.73   Tonsil and adenoidal instruments. (Down's Surgical Ltd.)

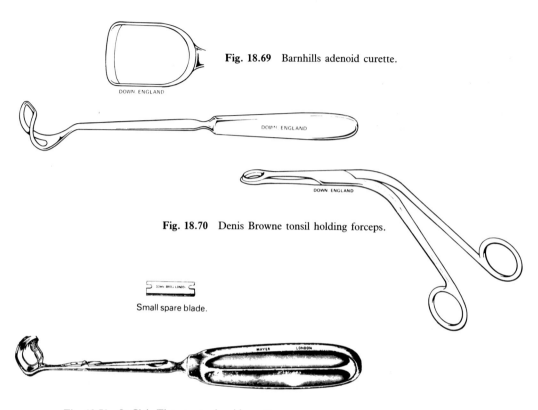

Fig. 18.69   Barnhills adenoid curette.

Fig. 18.70   Denis Browne tonsil holding forceps.

Small spare blade.

Fig. 18.71   St Clair Thompson adenoid curette.

Fig. 18.72   Woods curved tonsil scissors.

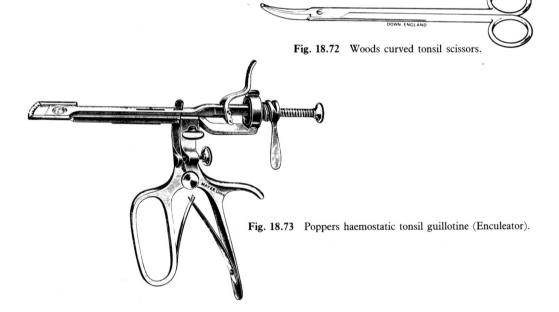

Fig. 18.73   Poppers haemostatic tonsil guillotine (Enculeator).

Dissector (Hill)
Dissector tonsil and pillar retractor (Beavis)
Artery forceps, tonsil, curved and straight (Negus, Birkett)
Compression clamps, tonsil (Beneys)
Curette, adenoid (St Clair Thompson)
Dissecting forceps, long fine, toothed and non-toothed (Waugh)
Guillotine, tonsil, haemostatic
Holding forceps, tonsil (Denis Browne)
Ligature needle, tonsil (Irwin Moores)
Mouth gag and blades (Boyle-Davis)
Mouth gag (Mason)
Scissors, tonsil, curved and straight (Wilson)
Snare, tonsil (Eve)
Tongue forceps (Mayo)
Angled tongue depressor
Suction tubing, nozzles and tube anchoring forceps
2 (3/0) Synthetic absorbable or non-absorbable, catgut or silk for ligatures
Adrenaline 1 in 1,000 (optional)
Graduated measure
Iced water.

Outline of procedure

Dissection operation: A Boyle-Davis mouth gag is inserted, and if an endotracheal tube has not been placed in position, the anaesthetic gases are conveyed to the back of the pharynx through a tube attached to the side of the tongue blade.

The tonsil is grasped with holding forceps and drawn inwards, exposing the anterior pillar of the fauces. Using curved scissors, or a dissector, and incision is made through the mucous membrane at the junction between the tonsil and the anterior pillar. The tonsil is freed by blunt dissection, first at the upper part and then the lower. After the tonsil has been removed, bleeding vessels are clamped and tied, or under-run and tied with silk or linen thread. The other tonsil is removed in a similar manner and both tonsil beds are inspected for complete haemostasis before gag is removed.

Guillotine operation: A mouth gag is inserted and the tongue grasped with tongue forceps. The guillotine is passed into the mouth and the right tonsil positioned in the ring. With the haemostatic type instrument (tonsil enucleator), the clamp mechanism is closed to crush the tonsil 'pedicle' for about 20 seconds before depressing the knife blade to separate the tonsil from its bed. With the simple type instrument, when the tonsil has been pressed well into the ring, the knife blade is depressed and the tonsil removed by a slight twist of the guillotine. The second tonsil is removed, and compression clamps applied to a taped swab in each tonsil fossa. The child is immediately turned on its side for the removal of the adenoids. The guillotine operation is less common than dissection.

Adenoidectomy. The adenoids are removed with a curette which is passed behind the soft palate, pressed hard against the posterior pharyngeal wall, and moved in a downwards sweeping action. Care is taken to avoid damage to the mucosa of the posterior pharyngeal space.

The patient's face and neck are bathed with ice-cold water, and if haemorrhage persists a Boyle-Davis gag may be inserted for further inspection of the tonsil fossae.

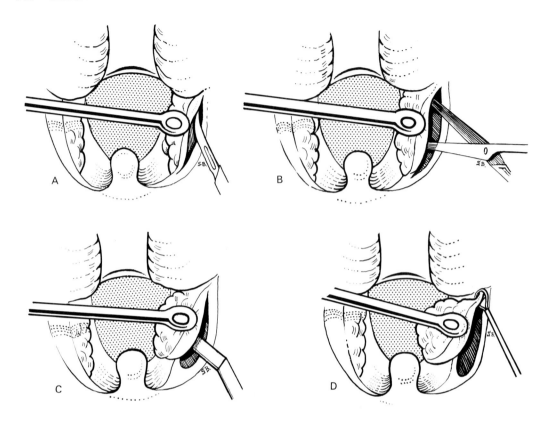

Fig. 18.74 (A) Shows incision of anterior pillar. Tonsil is drawn out with forceps putting pillar on the stretch to define the attachment to tonsil. (B) Blunt dissection of tonsil by scissors inserted through incision in anterior pillar. Dissection is done by forceps, dissector or scissors. (C) Shows tonsil dissected out of its bed, leaving pedicle below the lower pole. (D) Snare placed round the pedicle. (Hall and Colman).

Tracheostomy

Definition

The establishment of an opening into the trachea below the larynx, and the insertion of a tube for the purpose of providing an airway.

Position

Supine, with a sandbag under the shoulder blades, neck extended, with the head thrown well back and the chin in the midline. (Fig. 5.18, p. 126).

Instruments

As for tracheostomy (Fig. 18.76)
Sponge-holding forceps (Rampley), 5
Towel clips, 5

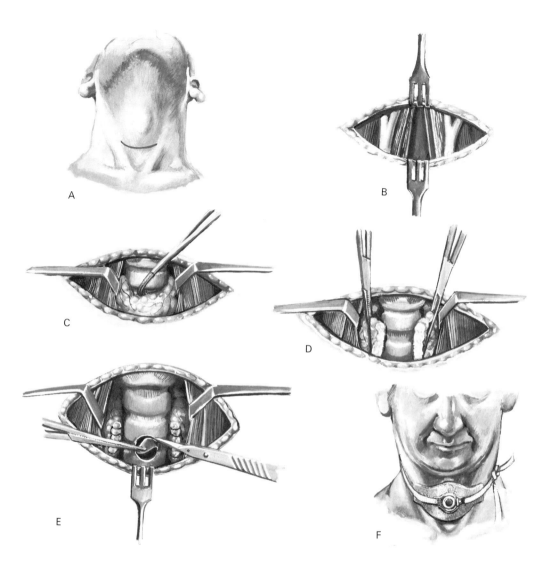

Fig. 18.75 Elective tracheostomy (transverse incision). (A) Incision. (B) Separation of sternothyroid and hyoid muscles. (C) Identification of thyroid isthmus, incision through pretracheal fascia, separation of thyroid isthmus. (D) Division of thyroid isthmus between haemostats. (E) Incision of trachea, creation of circular opening. (F) Tracheostomy tube inserted, retained by tapes passed around the neck and secured with a reef knot. (Ballantyne.)

Needle holder (Kilner)

Suction tubing, nozzles and tube anchoring forceps

2.5 and 3 (2/0 and 0) Chromic catgut or synthetic absorbable for ligatures

3 (0) Chromic catgut or synthetic absorbable on a small half-circle round-bodied needle for muscle sutures.

2 (3/0) Synthetic non-absorbable or silk on a small curved cutting needle for skin sutures

(Local anaesthesia requisites (Fig. 11.60) may be required).

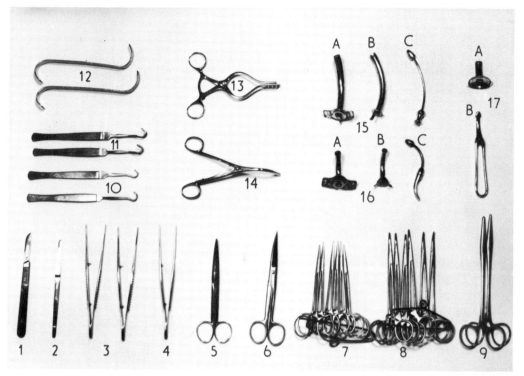

Fig. 18.76 Tracheostomy or laryngostomy.

1. Scalpel handle No. 3 with No. 10 blade (Bard Parker).
2. Scalpel handle No. 9 with No. 15 blade (Bard Parker).
3. Fine dissecting forceps, toothed (Gillies), 2.
4. Fine dissecting forceps, non-toothed (McIndoe), 1.
5. Scissors, curved on flat, 13 cm (5 in) (Mayo).
6. Scissors, stitch.
7. Fine artery forceps, straight, mosquito, 6.
8. Fine artery forceps, curved on flat, mosquito, 6.
9. Artery forceps, straight, 18 cm (7 in) (Spencer Wells), 2.
10. Small retractors, sharp and blunt, single hook, 2.
11. Small retractors, double hook, 2.
12. Medium retractors, malleable copper.
13. Retractor, self-retaining (West).
14. Tracheal dilating forceps (Bowlby or Trouseau).
15. Long tracheostomy tubes (Chevalier Jackson), assorted sizes. A, outer tube; B, inner tube; C, pilot or introducer.
16. Medium tracheostomy tubes (Parker), assorted sizes. A, outer tube; B, inner tube; C, pilot or introducer.
17. Laryngotomy tube (Butlin), 3 sizes. A, tube; B, pilot or introducer.

Outline of procedure

Emergency tracheostomy is carried out less frequently nowadays. Endotracheal intubation is usually carried out first for respiratory obstruction. Where this is impracticable, or for prolonged pulmonary mechanical ventilation, elective tracheostomy may be undertaken and an appropriate plastic or rubber cuffed tube inserted. Silver tracheostomy tubes are still used for maintaining an airway either before or after operations on the larynx.

A tracheostomy set of tubes and instruments arranged in the correct order of use should be kept sterile and ready in all operating theatres. It is important that the tapes are already attached to the outer tubes, as many valuable minutes may be lost placing these in position during operation.

It is important that the head and neck are maintained perfectly in the midline during the whole operation. A transverse or vertical midline incision is made over the upper part of

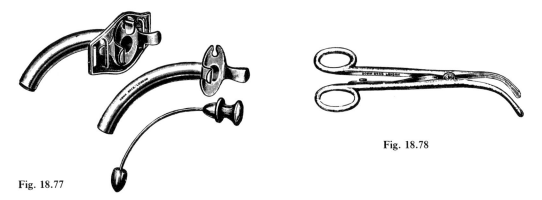

Fig. 18.77

Fig. 18.78

Fig. 18.77   Chevalier Jackson tracheostomy tubes. (Down's Bros Ltd.)

Fig. 18.78   Trouseau tracheal dilating forceps. Sizes available 16–34 Charrière gauge.

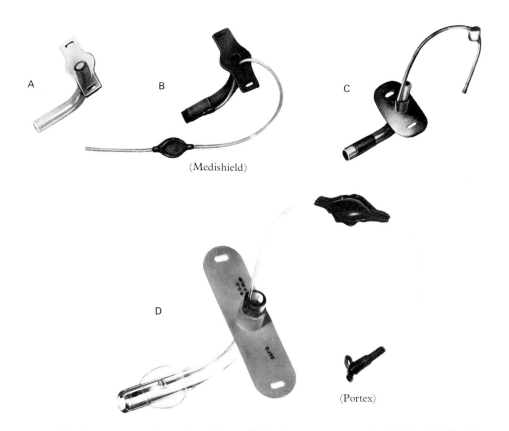

A

B

(Medishield)

C

D

(Portex)

Fig. 18.79   Tracheostomy cannulae or tubes. Sizes available: A, B and C, 27, 30, 33, 36, 39 and 42 Charrière gauge or 3 to 12 Magill tube scale.

A. Morrant Baker plastic tracheostomy cannula, with fixed plastic flange slotted for retaining tape.

B. Morrant Baker rubber tracheostomy cannula, with fixed rubber flange slotted for retaining tape and detachable inflatable rubber cuff.

C. James Rubber tracheostomy cannula, with detachable rubber flange slotted for retaining tape and fixed inflatable rubber cuff.

D. Portex cuffed plastic tracheostomy tube.

the trachea just below the cricoid cartilage. The incision is extended through the deep fascia, and the sternothyroid and hyoid muscles retracted laterally.

The isthmus of the thyroid gland is either clamped across, divided and ligated, or displaced. Another layer of the fascia is incised, the cricoid cartilage steadied with a single sharp hook, and the trachea is opened through a vertical stab wound which divides about two rings of cartilage. The trachea dilators are inserted into this incision, separated, and a tracheal tube inserted. Some surgeons cut a small flap of cartilage when making their incision in order to accommodate the circumference of the tube better, especially the cuffed, rubber variety (which may be used as an alternative to those illustrated, see Fig. 18.79). This cartilage flap is sutured to the skin to prevent it slipping back accidentally into the trachea should the tube become displaced, and to help in changing the tube.

The skin is closed in the usual manner. The tapes secured round the neck and a dressing of tulle gras applied under the tube flange.

Laryngofissure

Definition

An opening through the thyroid cartilage into the larynx to remove a tumour or tumours.

Position

As for tracheostomy.

Instruments

> General set (Figs. 14.1–14.28)
> Laryngofissure and laryngectomy set (Fig. 18.80)
> Tongue forceps (Mayo)
> Angled tongue depressor
> Mouth gag (Mason)
> Suction tubing, nozzles and tube anchoring forceps
> Diathermy leads, electrodes and lead anchoring forceps
> Connection and tubing for anaesthetic machine
> Corrugated rubber or plastic drainage tubing
> 2.5, 3 and 4 (2/0, 0 and 1) Chromic catgut or synthetic absorbable for ligatures
> 2.5 and 4 (2/0 and 1) Chromic catgut or synthetic absorbable (or stainless-steel wire) on medium half-circle cutting and round-bodied needles for larynx and muscle sutures.
> 2.5 or 2 (2/0 or 3/0) Synthetic non-absorbable or silk on a medium curved cutting needle for skin sutures.

Outline of procedure

A preliminary tracheostomy may have been performed. A midline incision is made from the hyoid bone to the cricoid cartilage. Soft tissues are retracted and the thyroid cartilage divided with shears or a cartilage saw, care being taken to divide the mucous membrane of the larynx in the midline. (This is to avoid damage to the vocal cords.) The cut edges of the cartilage are retracted to expose the interior of the larynx. The tumour is excised, haemostasis secured with diathermy, and the wound closed in layers, with drainage. Stainless-steel wire or chromic catgut is used to close the larynx.

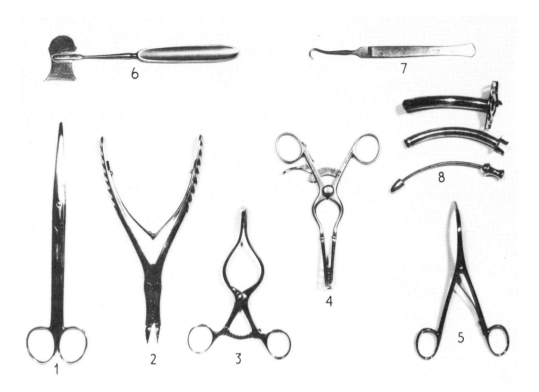

Fig. 18.80   Laryngofissure or laryngectomy.
1. Scissors, straight 20 cm (8 in) (Mayo).
2. McIndoe bone cutting forceps.
3. Retractor, self-retaining (West).
4. Retractor, self-retaining (Mayo, angled).
5. Tracheal dilators (Bowlby or Trousseau).
6. Cartilage saw.
7. Small retractor, sharp single hook.
8. Long tracheostomy tube (Chevalier Jackson, large size).

Laryngectomy

Definition

Removal of the entire larynx, and establishment of a permanent tracheostomy.

Position

As for laryngofissure.

Instruments

As for laryngofissure.
Synthetic non-absorbable or silk may be used in preference to catgut sutures for the deep closure.

Outline of procedure

A midline incision is made from the hyoid bone to the cricoid cartilage. The body of the hyoid bone may be divided in the midline and the ends retracted.

The muscle attachments at the sides of the larynx are freed and the trachea is severed. The endotracheal tube is withdrawn, and a wide tracheostomy tube (wrapped with tulle gras) is inserted into the severed end and connected to the anaesthesia machine.

The larynx is elevated and freed, clamping the vessels as dissection proceeds. The pharynx is then opened and the larynx removed. When haemostasis is complete, the pharynx is closed with interrupted chromic catgut, synthetic absorbable or silk sutures.

The incision is closed, with drainage, and the skin margins in the lower part of the wound are sutured around the tracheal opening.

There are a variety of post-laryngectomy tubes (e.g., Lombard's which is metallic), but a very satisfactory tube can be fashioned from the lower 6 cm (2.5 in) or so of a size 10 Magill endotracheal tube with a safety pin put across it. If the rubber produces skin irritation, a plastic tube can be used. In laryngectomy and pharyngo-laryngectomy a feeding tube is passed either beforehand in the ward, or towards the end of the operation in the theatre.

Partial amputation of the tongue

Definition

Removal of varying amounts of the tongue for carcinoma, but usually not less than half when the growth is limited to one side. Radical dissection of the cervical glands (Chapter 22) may also be performed, either before, during, or after this operation.

Position

Supine.

Instruments

As for tracheostomy
General set (Figs. 14.1–14.28)
Mouth gag (Doyen or Mason)
Tongue forceps (Mayo)
Angled tongue depressor
Fine artery forceps, curved on flat mosquito, 10
Fine artery forceps, straight, mosquito, 10
Fine tissue forceps (McIndoe), 5
Suction tubing, nozzles and tube anchoring forceps
Diathermy leads, electrodes and lead anchoring forceps.
2 and 2.5 (3/0 and 2/9) Chromic catgut or synthetic absorbable for ligatures
2.5 and 3 (2/0 and 0) Chromic catgut or synthetic absorbable on small half-circle round-bodied needles for sutures
3 (0) Synthetic non-absorbable or silk on a medium half-circle round-bodies needle for stay sutures.

Outline of procedure

A preliminary tracheostomy is performed and the pharynx packed with ribbon gauze. Three

stay sutures are inserted into the tongue and left long. One of the sutures is placed behind the growth and the other two at each of the tip of the tongue.

The mucous membrane on the floor of the mouth is freed and the tongue split longitudinally down the centre. The tongue is freed from the hyoid bone and the posterior position divided across well behind growth. Any blood-vessels seen during dissection are picked up with artery forceps and ligated or under-run, if possible before they are divided. Haemostasis may be achieved also with diathermy.

The cut edge of the tongue is sutured and the mucous membrane approximated also if possible.

Partial excision of the jaw

Definition

Partial removal of the mandible for malignancy. This operation is usually combined with radical dissection of the cervical glands (Chapter 22).

Position

Supine, with sandbag under the shoulder blades, neck extended and head thrown well back, with the chin central and in the midline.

Instruments

As for partial amputation of the tongue
Wire saw and handles (Gigli or Olivercrona)
Saw guide (de Martel)
Jaw saw (Wood)
Bone awls, set
Bone-nibbling forceps, small and medium, 2
Bone-cutting forceps (Liston)
Bone-cutting forceps (Horsley compound action)
Small rugines, curved and straight (Faraboeuf), 2
Bone-holding forceps (St Thomas)
Ligatures as for partial amputation of the tongue, plus 2/0 and 0 synthetic non-absorbable or silk.

Outline of procedure

An L-shaped or T-shaped incision is made over the neck and lower mandible. Radical dissection of the cervical glands is carried out and the muscles attached to the mandible are freed. The tongue and the parotid gland are retracted and the portion of the jaw to be removed is divided with a saw. The bone is disarticulated from the joint and resected.

The wound is closed in layers with drainage in the usual manner. If the mucosa cannot be approximated, the wound will be partially packed and an intra-oral or buccal skin graft will be performed at a later date by the plastic surgeon. In order to restore the facial contours after such an extensive excision, the dental surgeon may co-operate with the otolaryngologist

and plastic surgeon to provide a prosthesis, which will also help to maintain the graft in position during healing.

REFERENCES AND FURTHER READING

BALLANTYNE, J. (1976) *Operative Surgery: The Ear*. London: Butterworth.
BALLANTYNE, J. (1976) *Operative Surgery: Nose and Throat*. London: Butterworth.
HALL, I. S. AND COLMAN, B. H. (1976) *Diseases of the Nose, Throat and Ear*. Edinburgh: Churchill Livingstone.

19

Operations on the face

Excision of superficial ulcer of the face

Definition

The removal of a superficial dermal ulcer.

Position

Supine.

Instruments

Sponge-holding forceps (Rampley), 2
Towel clips, 4
Scalpel handles Nos. 3 and 9 with Nos. 10 and 15 blades (Bard Parker)
Fine dissecting forceps, toothed (Gillies), 2
Fine dissecting forceps, non-toothed (McIndoe), 2
Scissors, curved 10 cm (4 in) (Kilner or strabismus)
Fine pointed scissors, curved (iris)
Fine double-hook retractors, 2
Skin hooks (Gillies or Kilner), 2
Fine tissue forceps (McIndoe), 4
Artery forceps, straight, mosquito, 5 to 10
Artery forceps, curved on flat, mosquito, 5 to 10
Fine needle holder (Gillies, Kilner, etc.)
2 and 1.5 (3/0 and 4/0) Plain catgut or a synthetic absorbable for ligatures
2 (3/0) Plain catgut or a synthetic absorbable on a small curved round-bodied needle for fat sutures
1.5 or 1 (4/0 or 5/0) Synthetic non-absorbable or silk on a small curved non-traumatic cutting needle for skin sutures
(Skin graft instruments may be required (Fig. 24.15)).

Outline of procedure

An elliptical incision is made following the facial lines and with the ulcer in the centre of the ellipse. The ulcerated skin is dissected free and the surrounding skin flaps undermined. If the skin can be approximated, it is closed wih fine interrupted sutures; if it cannot, a skin flap is rotated or a split-skin graft performed, using a soft textured graft such as that which can be obtained from the inner aspect of the upper arm.

Removal of sebaceous or dermoid cysts, naevi, etc.

This is similar to the operation above but with the addition of the following instruments:
  Dissector (MacDonald or Durham)
  Double-end curetting spoon (Volkmann)
  Medium retractors, double hook, 2.

20

Gynaecological and obstetric operations

Marsupialisation of Bartholinian cyst

Definition

The removal of a cyst due to blockage of the duct of the Bartholin gland which is in the lateral vaginal wall on either side.

Position

Lithotomy, Figure 5.15.

Instruments

Sponge-holding forceps (Rampley), 5
Towel clips, 5
Scalpel handle No. 3 with No. 10 blade (Bard Parker)
Dissecting forceps, toothed (Lane), 2
Dissecting forceps, non-toothed, 15 cm (6 in)
Scissors, curved on flat, 13 cm (5 in) (Mayo)
Tissue forceps (Allis), 5
Dissector (MacDonald or Durham)
Fine artery forceps, straight, mosquito, 10
Needle holder (Mayo)
Corrugated drain
2.5 (2/0) Chromic catgut or a synthetic absorbable for ligatures
3 (0) Chromic catgut or a synthetic absorbable on a small half-circle round-bodied needle for deep sutures.

Outline of procedure

An incision is made over the swelling in the long axis of the labium majora, and deepened down to the cyst wall. The cyst (or abscess) is grasped with tissue forceps and a large cruciate incision made right through to the shiny internal surface of the cyst. After removal of the cyst any divided blood-vessels encountered are picked up and ligated. The wound edges are avulsed with chromic catgut or synthetic absorbable sutures leaving a cavity which is usually drained with a corrugated drain.

Excision of the vulva (vulvectomy)

Definition

Removal of the vulva.

Position

Lithotomy.

Instruments

General set (Figs. 14.1 to 14.28).
Urethral catheter, self-retaining (Foley size 18 Charrière gauge)
20 ml syringe and sterile water for inflating catheter balloon
Proflavine emulsion or similar gauze pack
2.5 and 3 (2/0 and 0) Chromic catgut or a synthetic absorbable for ligatures
4 or 5 (1 or 2) Chromic catgut or a synthetic absorbable on a medium half-circle Mayo's
  needle with a trocar point for sutures.

Outline of procedure

An outer, oval incision is made, surrounding both labia majora if necessary. An inner, oval incision is also made and this lies just within the mucocutaneous junction, to include the urethral orifice, passing around the vaginal orifice. The incisions are extended down to the urethra. Just above the urethra the cut edges are joined together, but the cut edge of the vagina below is approximated to the cut edge of the skin all around. A self- retaining catheter is inserted and the vagina packed with a length of X-ray detectable gauze to control bleeding.

Perineorrhaphy

Definition

Repair of a complete or incomplete rupture of the perineum.

Position

Lithotomy.

Instruments

As vulvectomy
Ligatures and sutures as vulvectomy
3 (0) Chromic catgut or a synthetic absorbable on a small half-circle round-bodied needle
  for plication of rectum
3 (0) Chromic catgut or a synthetic absorbable on a curved non-traumatic intestinal needle
  for rectal closure (complete rupture only).

Outline of procedure

Incomplete rupture (where a segment of perineum remains, with the rectum and anal sphincter intact; there is no potential rectovaginal fistula). Tissue forceps are applied to the estimated edge of the original vaginal opening. Traction on these forceps stretches the torn edge of the perineum which is cut away between the forceps to expose an edge of mucosa and skin. The edge of the mucosa is dissected up and the posterior vaginal wall freed from the rectum. A triangular-shaped piece of vaginal wall (with its base at the perineum) is excised, and the levator ani muscles identified and drawn together with mattress sutures of chromic catgut or a synthetic absorbable. The triangular gap is approximated longitudinally with a continuous chromic catgut or a synthetic absorbable suture, and the vagina is packed in the usual manner. The procedure is completed by inserting a self-retaining catheter into the bladder.

Complete rupture. This operation is similar to that just described, but in addition it is necessary to reconstruct the rectum and the anal sphincter; there is a very real risk of rectovaginal fistula formation.

The septum separating the rectum and vagina is cut away, so exposing the mucous membrane of both. The rectum is freed and the torn ends of the sphincter identified. The rectum is sutured and the sphincter brought together with strong chromic catgut or a synthetic absorbable. The operation then resembles incomplete rupture with repair of the levator ani muscles and closure of the triangular gap formed by partial excision of the posterior vaginal wall. Finally, a catheter and vaginal X-ray detectable gauze pack are inserted.

Anterior colporrhaphy, amputation of cervix and posterior colpoperineorrhaphy (Manchester or Fothergill repair)

Definition

Repair of a cystocele (prolapse of the bladder into the vagina) and repair of a rectocele (prolapse of the rectum into the vagina).

Position

Lithotomy.

Instruments

    General set (Figs. 14.1 to 14.28)
    Dilation and curettage set (Fig. 20.2)
    Artery forceps, straight (Moynihan), 24
    Urethral catheter, self-retaining (Foley size 18 Charrière gauge)
    20 ml syringe and sterile water for inflating catheter balloon
    2.5 and 3 (2/0 and 0) Chromic catgut or a synthetic absorbable for ligatures
    3 (0) Chromic catgut or a synthetic absorbable on a small half-circle round-bodied needle for plication of the bladder
    4 or 5 (1 or 2) Chromic catgut or a synthetic absorbable on a small half-circle Mayo needle with a trocar point for sutures
    X- ray detectable gauze pack for the vagina.

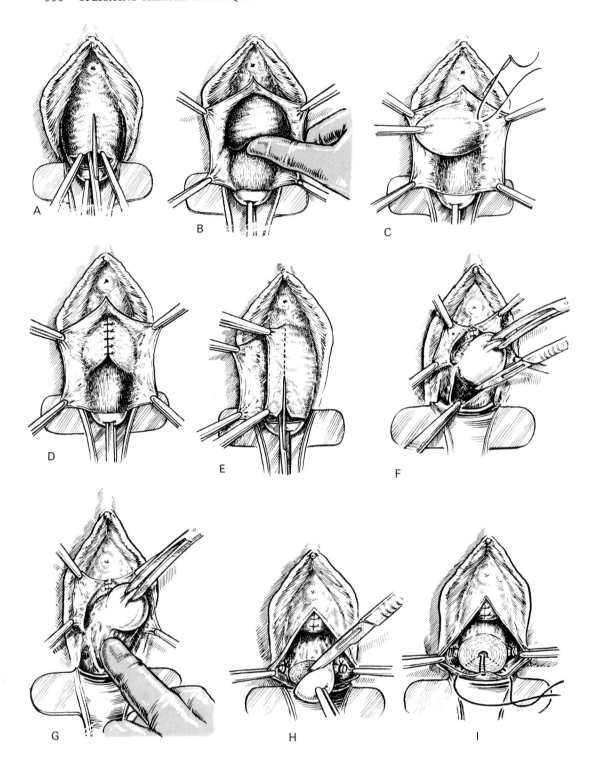

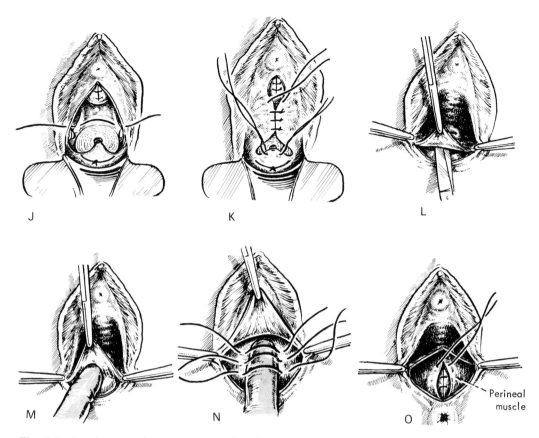

Fig. 20.1 Anterior colporrhapy, amputation of cervix and posterior colpoperineorrhaphy. (A) Opening up the anterior vaginal wall. (B) Mobilising cystocele from cervix. (C) Placing the tightening suture as far laterally as possible. (D) Obliteration of the cystocele completed. (E) Removing redundant vaginal wall. This is followed by closure with a continuous catgut suture. (F) The cystocele has been repaired. The cervix is being stripped of vaginal wall. (G) Posterior vaginal wall being stripped back. Elongated transverse cervical and uterosacral ligaments have been sutured and divided. (H) Amputation of cervical stump. (I) Covering the posterior stump with vaginal wall. (Note: amputation of the cervix may not be performed.) (J) Tying the transverse cervical ligaments in front of the cervix and so shortening them and raising the uterus. (This is the so-called Fothergill suture: sometimes two are put in). (K) Covering cervical stump and closing the vaginal wall. On release of the cervical stump the uterus returns to the pelvis. (L) Mobilisation of the posterior vaginal wall. (M) Separating rectocele from posterior vaginal wall. (N) Obliterating the rectocele by tightening the fascial layer. (O) Excess vaginal skin is removed. The perineal muscles are sutured over the obliterated rectocele. The skin and vagina are closed as in perineorrhaphy. (Garrey, Govan, Hodge and Callander: *Gynaecology Illustrated.*)

Outline of procedure

Anterior colporrhaphy. An Auvard's speculum is inserted and the cervix grasped with vulsellum forceps. The surgeon may then perform a dilation and curettage of the uterus if the patient is post menopausal and has cervical bleeding.

Traction is placed on the vulsellum forceps, pulling the cervix down and thereby stretching the anterior vaginal wall. An incision is made just above the junction of the cervix with the vaginal wall and blunt pointed scissors are inserted to separate the bladder from the vagina. A bladder sound is inserted, and the dissection continued up to a point just

below the urethra, care being taken to avoid opening the bladder, and the vaginal wall is then split up the midline along the extent of the separated portion. These skin flaps are retracted laterally and the bladder mobilised from the cervix and up and away from view. The cystocele is repaired by plicating the pubocervical fascia with 3 (0) chromic catgut or a synthetic absorbable, thereby making a buttress between the bladder and vagina.

Amputation of the cervix. If there is a vault prolapse, then a partial amputation of the cervix may be performed. This is done after dissecting up two flaps of mucous membrane from the cervix, one in front and one behind. The partial amputation of the cervix is performed and the two flaps of mucous membrane sutured so that the mucosa is invaginated towards the lining of the cervix to form a reconstructed cervical os.

The anterior incision is closed with several mattress sutures which are placed lateral to the cut edge of the vaginal wall on each side. These sutures are tied and the redundant vaginal wall excised, so narrowing the vagina. The procedure is completed with a row of interrupted chromic catgut or synthetic absorbable sutures.

Posterior colpoperineorrhaphy. The Auvard's speculum is removed and an elliptical transverse section of skin excised with scissors, care being taken to avoid opening the rectum, as it may be stuck down in the Pouch of Douglas. The rectum is freed with dissecting scissors and the posterior vaginal wall is slit up the midline. The rectocele is repaired by approximating the levator ani muscles with mattress sutures of chromic catgut or a synthetic absorbable. The redundant vaginal mucosa is excised and the edges brought together with continuous chromic catgut or synthetic absorbable sutures.

The transverse incision in the posterior vaginal wall is sutured longitudinally, which again tightens the vagina. The operation is completed by inserting a self-retaining catheter into the bladder and packing the vagina with an X-ray detectable gauze pack.

Dilation of the cervix and curettage of the uterus

Definition

Dilation of the cervix and scraping away the uterine mucosa.

Position

Lithotomy.

Instruments

Sponge-holding forceps (Rampley), 2
Vaginal speculum (Auvard)
Vaginal speculum (Sim)
Uterine dilators (Hegar)
Uterine curette (Sims)
Bladder/urethral sound
Uterine sound (Simpson)
Endometrial biopsy curette (Sharman)
Uterine dressing forceps (Bozeman)
Female catheter, metal
Towel clips (4).

(**Figs. 20.2–20.12**   Chas. F. Thackray Ltd.)

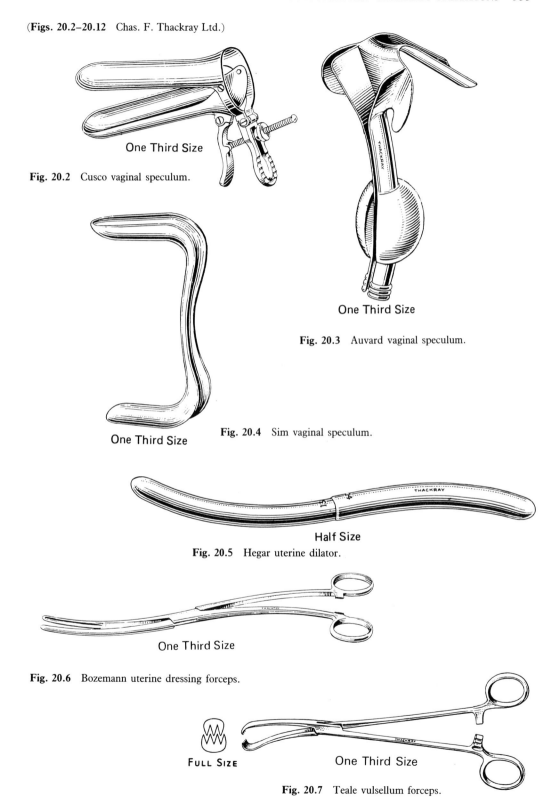

One Third Size

Fig. 20.2   Cusco vaginal speculum.

One Third Size

Fig. 20.3   Auvard vaginal speculum.

One Third Size

Fig. 20.4   Sim vaginal speculum.

Half Size

Fig. 20.5   Hegar uterine dilator.

One Third Size

Fig. 20.6   Bozemann uterine dressing forceps.

Full Size   One Third Size

Fig. 20.7   Teale vulsellum forceps.

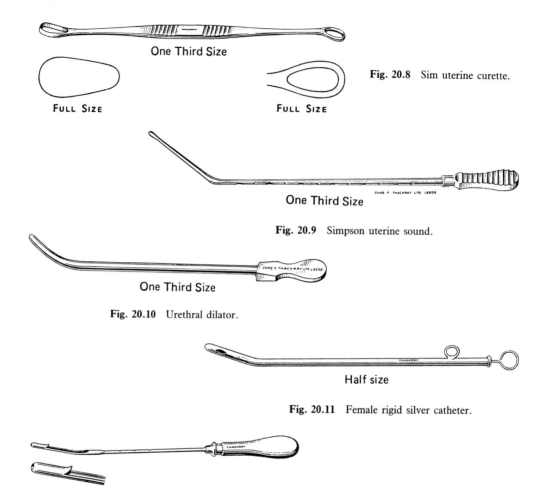

One Third Size

Fig. 20.8   Sim uterine curette.

FULL SIZE

FULL SIZE

One Third Size

Fig. 20.9   Simpson uterine sound.

One Third Size

Fig. 20.10   Urethral dilator.

Half size

Fig. 20.11   Female rigid silver catheter.

Fig. 20.12   Sharman endometrial biopsy curette.

Outline of procedure

An Auvard's speculum is inserted and the cervix drawn down and steadied with one or two vulsellum forceps. The position and length of the uterus are gauged with a uterine sound and progressively larger sizes of uterine dilators are inserted until the os is large enough to introduce the curette. The surgeon always holds each dilator between his thumb and forefinger, with the other fingers extended at the side, so that should the dilator slip, these extended fingers will come into contact with the buttocks and prevent the dilator penetrating too deeply and perforating the uterus. A uterine curette is inserted and the mucosa scraped gently and systematically. The curetted mucosa is sent for histological examination.

If the procedure is being carried out for retained products of conception, the initial stages follow that described above, but in this case the retained products are removed preferably with ovum or sponge-holding forceps instead of a curette, and the uterine sound is not used. An X-ray detectable gauze pack may then be inserted into the vagina.

Instruments for immediate laparotomy should be available in case of accidental perforation of the uterus and inadvertent damage to intra-abdominal structures.

Hysterosalpingography and fallopian insufflation

Definition

An injection of a radio-opaque medium for X-ray examination of the interior of the uterus and Fallopian tubes; and insufflation of the Fallopian tubes with CO_2 to test their patency.

Position

Lithotomy.

Instruments

D and C set
For hysterosalpingography add:
Leech Wilkinson cannula or Sprockman
Bivalve vaginal speculum.

Outline of procedure

For hysterosalpingography , a Sim's speculum is inserted and the radio-opaque medium (Urografin 76 per cent) injected into the uterine cavity with a special syringe. An X-ray is taken immediately.

A bi-valve speculum is inserted and the cervix drawn down and steadied with one or two pairs of vulsellum forceps. The position and length of the uterus are gauged with a uterine sound and progressively larger sizes of uterine dilators are inserted up to the outside diameter of the insufflation nozzle. The insufflation nozzle is inserted into the cervical canal and CO_2 under pressure is injected into the uterus up to 180 mmHg. Patency of the Fallopian tubes is determined either by applying a stethoscope to the abdominal wall and listening to the gas escaping into the peritoneal cavity from each tube as the pressure is applied, or observing a direct reading Kymograph which records pressure variations as the CO_2 is injected. (The dilation may then be continued followed by endrometrial biopsy.)

Cervical and uterine polypus, biopsy and cauterisation of the cervix

Definition

Removal of a polypus from the cervix or interior of the uterus; biopsy of the cervix for histological examination; cauterisation for cervical erosion and chronic cervicitis.

Position

Lithotomy.

Instruments

Dilation and curettage (Fig. 20.2–12)
Scalpel handle No. 3 with No. 10 blade (Bard Parker)
Dissecting forceps, toothed (Lane), 2
Dissecting forceps, non-toothed, 18 cm (7 in), 2

Scissors, curved on flat, 18 cm (7 in) (Mayo)
Needle holder (Mayo)
Diathermy or cautery apparatus, leads and electrodes for cervical cauterisation
3 or 4 (0 or 1) Chromic catgut or a synthetic absorbable on a small half-circle Mayo needle
    with a trocar point for sutures.

Outline of procedure

Cervical polypus. A Sim's speculum is inserted and the polyp grasped with ring forceps or artery forceps. The polypus is twisted until it comes away, and the cervical canal is gently scraped with a small curette.

    Uterine polypus. A Sim's speculum is inserted and the cervical os dilated until the opening is large enough to grasp the polyp with forceps which are then twisted as described above. If bleeding is persistent, the surgeon will pack the uterine cavity with a length of X-ray detectable gauze.

    Cervical biopsy. This operation is generally performed in conjunction with dilatation and curettage of the uterus, sometimes following a Papanicolaou cervical smear in which suspicious cells have been found. A small wedge or cone of cervix is excised and sent for histological examination, and the incision is approximated with chromic catgut or a synthetic absorbable. The vagina may be packed with an X-ray detectable gauze pack.

    Cervical cauterisation. A bi-valve or Sim's speculum is inserted and heat applied to the ulcerated area by means of a cautery or diathermy electrode. If diathermy is being used, the indifferent electrode is applied to the patient's thigh with the usual precautions (Chapter 3). The vagina will be packed with an X-ray detectable gauze pack. Spiritous antiseptics must not be used for skin preparation due to the danger of explosion with diathermy or cautery. (Cauterisation may be undertaken using a laser beam or cryoprobe.)

Laparoscopy (peritoneoscopy)

Definition

Inspection of the peritoneal cavity by means of a laparoscope introduced through the abdominal wall.

Position

Steep Trendelenburg with legs in lithotomy.

Instruments

Laparoscopy
    Sponge-holding forceps (Rampley), 2
    Towel clips, 5
    Scalpel handle No. 3 with No. 11, 15 or 12 blade (Bard Parker)
    Dissecting forceps, toothed (Lane), 2
    Dissecting forceps, non-toothed, 15 cm (6 in)
    Scissors, curved on flat, 13 cm (5 in) (Mayo), 1
    Needle holder (Mayo), 1
    Laparoscope, such as the Frangeheim (as Fig. 20.13) or Olympus double puncture

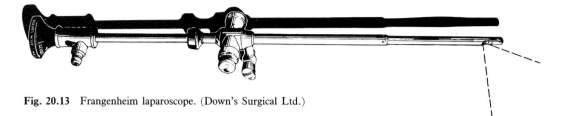

Fig. 20.13 Frangenheim laparoscope. (Down's Surgical Ltd.)

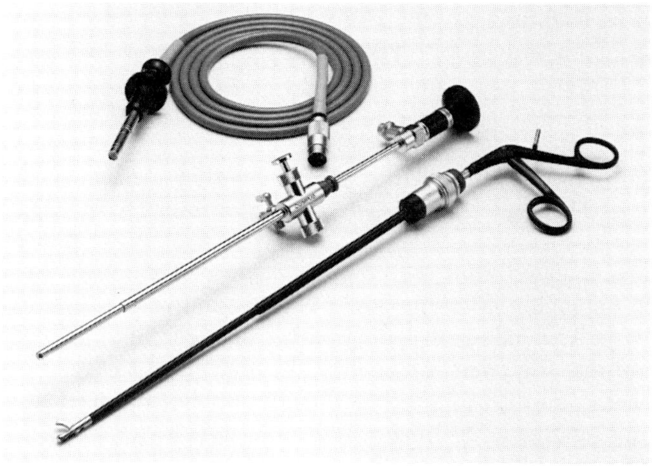

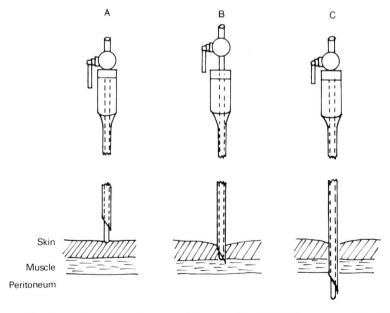

Fig. 20.14 Therapeutic double puncture laparoscope 5 mm diameter. (Olympus, Key Med.)

Fig. 20.15 (A) Needle at skin surface, inner core fully extended. (B) Needle in abdominal wall, inner core fully retracted at point, air intake raised above shoulder. (C) Needle point through abdominal wall, inner core descends rounded end now prevents point of outer sheath from damaging bowel, etc. Air intake sits down on shoulder as point enters peritoneal cavity.

Palmer biopsy drill forceps
Verres trocar and cannula
Diathermy leads and electrodes
Fibre light lead and projector
2.5 or 3 (2/0 or 0) chromic catgut or a synthetic absorbable for ligatures and on small
    half-circle cutting needle for subcutaneous sutures if required
2.0 (2/0) synthetic non-absorbable or silk on straight or curved cutting needle for skin
    sutures.
Vaginal examination
Instruments as for D and C may be required
Gentian violet solution and 10 ml syringe with cannula.

Outline of procedure

The Verres needle is inserted through a small 2 cm skin incision made transversely just
below the umbilicus. The same incision is used later for inserting the laparoscope trocar and
cannula.

The needle is manipulated until the point is felt to pass through the outer layer of the
rectus sheath then impinging upon the posterior layer and with a little more pressure enter
the abdominal cavity. The sudden dropping of the inner core into the needle (Fig. 20.15) is
a further indication that the point has entered the abdominal cavity.

The needle is then connected to a carbon dioxide supply controlled through an apparatus
such as the Semm's automatic insufflator and some three litres of gas are allowed to pass
into the abdominal cavity. This takes three to four minutes and care is taken not to raise
the intra-abdominal pressure by more than 20 mmHg as this could seriously interfere with
the return of blood to the heart by stopping the flow in the inferior vena cava which could
lead to acute hypotension.

Verres needle is removed and the laparoscope trocar and cannula are now inserted slightly
diagonally through the puncture hole used for the Verres needle, through the rectus sheath
and into the abdominal cavity. The trocar is removed and the telescope with its
accompanying light carrier is passed through the cannula into the abdominal cavity.

Procedures carried out with the laparoscope (Fisher, 1970)

1. *Infertility.* Tubal patency can be demonstrated by methylene blue installation through
a cervical cannula by a second operator. A solution of gentian violet, is instilled into the
uterus; with the laparoscope the surgeon by visualising dye transit can confirm tubal
patency. Similarly the restriction of dye dispersal by fine adhesions is easily demonstrated.
At the same time ovarian biopsy can be taken to establish the presence of primordial follicles
or functioning corpora lutea or graffian follicles.

2. *Ectopic pregnancy.* When there are doubts in cases of early tubal abortion laparoscopy
can reveal the presence of the tubal gestation and the surgeon can then proceed to laparotomy and definitive surgery. Conversely, a ruptured retention cyst which is settling can
be left alone and thus laparotomy avoided.

3. *Unexplained abdominal pain.* Much of the gynaecologist's practice concerns pain in the
pelvis. In these instances laparoscopy provides a means of obtaining a correct diagnosis in
cases of unsuspected endometriosis and other causes of pelvic inflammatory response. Thus
definitive treatment is possible and the patient's pain relieved.

4. *Amenorrhoea.* The investigation of amenorrhoea today will include a laparoscopy,

visualising the ovaries and enabling a biopsy to be taken. This step can be most useful in establishing the likelihood of the ovaries responding to treatment. In the absence of primordial follicles there is little evidence that stimulation by gonadotrophins will be of value. Similarly, the presence of multiple micro-cysts in the ovary indicate the need for extreme caution in the management of gonadotrophin stimulation therapy.

5. *Sterilization.* It is possible by introducing suitably insulated bipolar diathermy forceps through a special trocar/cannula second small incision to divide the Fallopian tubes by diathermy coagulation in one or more places and thus effect sterilization by interrupting tubal continuity.

At the close of the operation the carbon dioxide is first expelled from the abdominal cavity via the cannula which is then removed. The skin incision is closed with synthetic absorbable or silk. Alternatively subcutaneous sutures of catgut or synthetic absorbable may be used.

Abdominal hysterectomy

Definition

Partial or entire removal of the uterus through an abdominal incision.

Position

Trendelenburg.

Instruments

General set (Figs. 14.1 to 14.28)
Laparotomy set (Figs. 15.1 to 15.7)
Self-retaining retractor Balfour, with Doyen blade.
Supra pubic retractor (Doyen)
Long heavy scissors, curved on flat 25 cm (10 in)
Vulsellum forceps (Teale), 2
Uterine dressing forceps
Artery forceps, curved on flat, 20 cm (8 in) (Mayo Oschner or Kocher), 10
Artery forceps, curved on flat, 24 cm ($9\frac{1}{2}$ in) (Mayo Oschner or Kocher), 6
An X-ray detectable gauze pack for the vagina
2.5 and 3 (2/0 and 0) Chromic catgut or a synthetic absorbable for ligatures, fine and medium
5 (2) Chromic catgut or a synthetic absorbable on large half-circle Mayo needles with trocar points for transfixion sutures and uterine, vaginal vault, peritoneum and muscle sutures
3 (0) Chromic catgut or a synthetic absorbable on a medium half-circle round-bodied needle for reconstruction of pelvic floor
2.5 (2/0) Synthetic absorbable or silk on a large straight or curved cutting needle for skin sutures (Kifa and Michel clips or skin staples may be required.)

Outline of procedure

The vagina is swabbed with antiseptic solution and plugged with a length of X-ray detectable gauze, which is left protruding for subsequent removal during operation. Removal and safety

(**Figs. 20.16–20.18**   Chas. F. Thackray Ltd.)

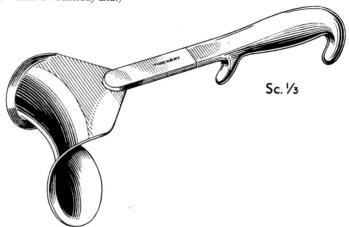

Fig. 20.16   Doyen supra-pubic retractor.

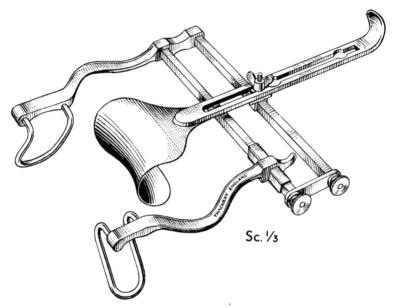

Fig. 20.17   Balfour self-retaining retractor with Doyen blade.

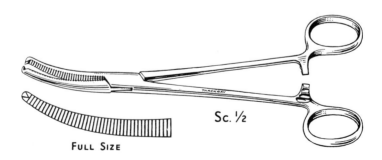

Fig. 20.18   Mayo Oschner artery forceps, curved on flat.

ensuring removal will be easier if a pair of sponge-holding forceps is attached to this pack and left lying between the patient's legs.

The abdomen is opened through a Pfannenstiel or lower midline incision which passes through the skin, linea alba and peritoneum (page 414). The bowel which may protrude is displaced towards the diaphragm with two or three large gauze packs. The uterus is drawn out of the pelvis and two pairs of Kocher's or Mayo-Oschner forceps are applied across the broad ligament either inside or outside the ovaries, depending on whether they are to be removed or not. It is usual to try to leave at least one ovary for endocrine function. The broad ligament is opened on each side between these forceps and a flap of peritoneum is cut from the front of the uterus. The bladder is separated from the front of the cervix by blunt dissection and is pushed well below the point of transection. Pairs of clamps are placed across the cardinal ligaments and uterine arteries on each side, carefully avoiding the ureters and ureteric arteries by feeling through the peritoneum if necessary, and the uterine vessels are divided between the clamps.

The pack is removed from the vagina, the fornix of the vagina is cut into, the cervix seized with a pair of vulsellum forceps and drawn upwards, and the uterus is removed by dividing the vagina from the cervix all round.

Transfixion sutures are placed and tied around the clamped stumps of the ovarian vessels, round ligament and uterine arteries. The cut edge of the vagina is closed with interrupted or continuous chromic catgut or synthetic absorbable sutures. The flap of peritoneum is sutured over the cut edge of the posterior peritoneum, covering the cervical or vaginal stump and the transfixed round ligaments. The surgeon may suture the round ligaments to the vault of the vagina before reconstructing the pelvic floor with 4 (0) chromic catgut or synthetic absorbable sutures. The abdominal wound is closed in layers.

Wertheim's hysterectomy

Definition

Total hysterectomy, bilateral salpingo-oöphorectomy, with removal of the upper part of the vagina and lymphatic glands which drain the pelvis.

Position

Trendelenburg, Figure 5.12.

Instruments

As for abdominal hysterectomy
Hysterectomy clamps, right-angled (Wertheim), 2
Diathermy leads, electrodes and lead anchoring forceps
Urethral catheter, self-retaining (Foley size 18 Charrière gauge)
20 ml syringe, and sterile water to inflate catheter balloon
An X-ray detectable gauze pack for vagina
Ligatures and sutures as for hysterectomy.

Outline of procedure·

This follows the procedure of total hysterectomy but with the following additions.

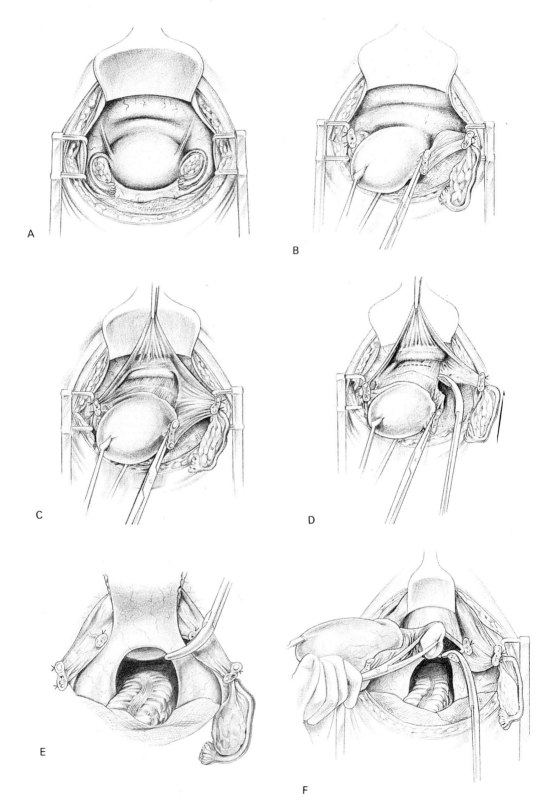

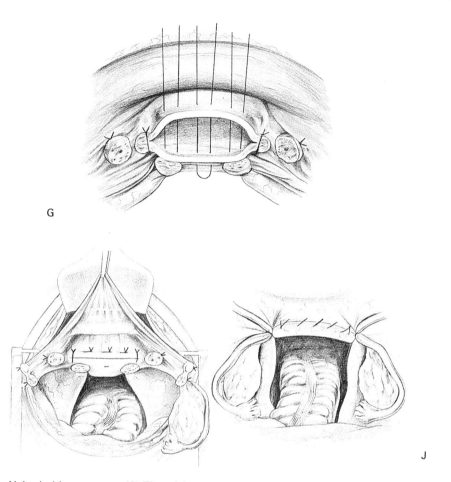

Fig. 20.19 Abdominal hysterectomy. (A) The pelvic organs are exposed through a Pfannenstiel or lower midline incision. (B) Division of broad ligaments; the pedicles contain round ligament, Fallopian tube, and ovarian branches of the uterine artery. (C & D) The utero-vesical peritoneal fold is divided, and the bladder mobilised from the front of the cervix. (E) The uterine vessels are divided after placing curved Mayo Oschner or Kocher's forceps across the base of the broad ligament. The vagina is opened anteriorly with a scalpel. (F) Removal of the uterus with the help of vulsellum forceps. (G) The vaginal angles are secured with single sutures and the vagina is closed with mattress sutures. The utero-sacral ligaments are included in the lateral mattress sutures. (H) The vagina having been closed, the field is ready for peritonealisation. (I) Closure of the pelvic peritoneum. (*A Digest of Obstetrical and Gynaecological Procedures*, Ethicon Ltd.)

The rectum is freed from the vagina which is divided across well beyond the cervix, after applying strong right-angled clamps (Wertheim's). In this way, when the uterus is removed, the growth on the cervix is covered by a section of the vagina clamped over it, thereby preventing soiling of the peritoneal cavity. After the vagina has been closed and the vessels ligatured, the connective tissue on the side walls of the pelvis and around the vessels is carefully dissected free, together with the iliac and obturator glands. In order to properly clear the pelvis the ureters and vessels *must* be visualised. There is danger that clearing the tissues from around the ureters will interfere with their blood supply.

The pelvic floor is reconstructed as before and the wound closed in layers. As the bladder has been extensively separated, it is usual to leave a catheter *in situ* for a few days postoperatively.

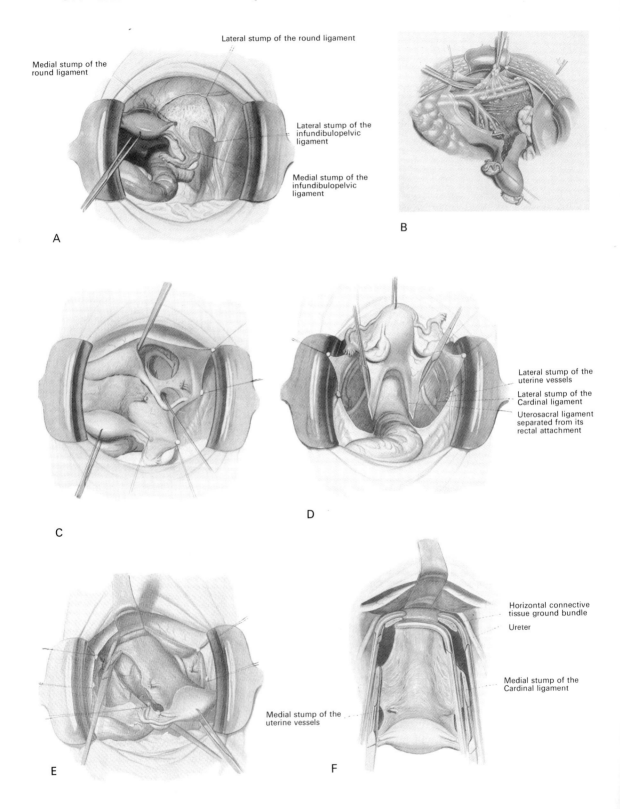

Medial stump of the round ligament

Lateral stump of the round ligament

Lateral stump of the infundibulopelvic ligament

Medial stump of the infundibulopelvic ligament

A

B

C

D

Lateral stump of the uterine vessels

Lateral stump of the Cardinal ligament

Uterosacral ligament separated from its rectal attachment

E

F

Horizontal connective tissue ground bundle

Ureter

Medial stump of the Cardinal ligament

Medial stump of the uterine vessels

Fig. 20.20   Wertheim's hysterectomy for carcinoma of cervix — extent of excision. (A) The abdomen has been opened and the round ligaments have been divided. The infundibulopelvic ligament has also been divided between ligatures. The ligatures are left long and act as retractors. The peritoneum in front of the uterus has been cut through so that the broad ligament has been opened up. (B) The right external iliac vessels and their lymph nodes have been exposed by the division of the peritoneum between the right ovariopelvic ligament and the right round ligament. A taped swab has been placed in the right paravesical fossa to arrest bleeding. The glands and cellular tissue are being cleared from the left external iliac vessels. The uterus is drawn well over to the opposite side so that the obturator fossa is exposed. The obturator nerve, artery and vein are well seen and the left ureter can be seen passing under the uterine artery. (C) The uterine artery has been divided between ligatures and the roof of the ureteric canal cut through. The cardinal ligament can be seen in the diagram with the aneurysm needle placed below it. In front of the cardinal ligament lies the paravesical space while behind the ligament lies the pararectal space. (D) The cardinal ligament has been divided on each side. The uterus has been drawn forwards, the peritoneum of the pouch of Douglas has been cut through transversely and the bowel has been separated from the posterior vaginal wall. (E) The uterosacral ligament on the left side has been clamped and divided. A clamp has been placed across the left cardinal ligament, and the tissues distal to the clamp have been cut through. (F) The uterus and appendages have been separated from their attachments, the cardinal ligaments and the uterosacral ligaments having been divided. A large Wertheim clamp has been placed over the vagina. On each side of the vagina below this level the paravaginal tissues which form the horizontal part of the ground bundle have been clamped and divided. (Howkins and Bourne: *Shaw's Textbook of Gynaecology*.)

Vaginal hysterectomy

Definition

Removal of the uterus through the vagina, usually done when a prolapse is also present.

Position

Lithotomy.

Instruments

General set (Figs. 14.1 to 14.28)
Artery forceps, straight, 20 cm (8 in) (Spencer Wells), 10
Deep retractors, narrow blade (Deaver or Paton), 2
Artery forceps, heavy curved on flat (Mayo-Oschner or Kocher), 6
Vulsellum forceps (Teale), 2
Scissors, heavy curved on flat, 20 cm (8 in) (Mayo)
Vaginal speculum (Auvard)
Urethral catheter, self-retaining (Foley size 18 Charrière gauge)
20 ml syringe, and sterile water to inflate catheter balloon
4 and 5 (1 and 2) Chromic catgut or a synthetic absorbable for all ligatures, transfixion
   sutures and closure sutures on large half-circle Mayo needles with trocar points
An X-ray detectable gauze pack for vagina.

Outline of procedure

An Auvard's speculum is inserted, and the cervix grasped with vulsellum forceps, pulled down and steadied. An incision is made below the urinary orifice and round the cervix. The bladder is freed from the uterus in front, and the rectum from the uterus posteriorly. The anterior and posterior peritoneum is opened and traction applied to the cervix so that clamps

can be applied to the cardinal ligament and uterine arteries. The fundus of the uterus is delivered from the abdomen and clamps applied to each round ligament. The round ligament is severed between the clamps and the uterus is removed. The vessels and ligaments are transfixed and ligated with chromic catgut or a synthetic absorbable. The anterior and posterior peritoneum are sutured together, exteriorising the round ligaments and uterine vessels which are sutured over by closing the vaginal wall.

A catheter is inserted and the vagina plugged with a proflavine emulsion gauze or similar pack.

Oöphorectomy, salpingectomy, myomectomy

Definition

Removal of an ovary; Fallopian tube; or one or more uterine fibroids.

Position

Trendelenburg. (Supine for ectopic gestation.)

Instruments

As for abdominal hysterectomy (p. 539).
Suction tubing, nozzles and tube anchoring forceps for ectopic gestation.

Outline of procedure

The uterus is exposed through a Pfannenstiel or subumbilical midline incision. For *oöphorectomy* for the removal of ovarian cyst, the pedicle of the ovary or tumour is transfixed with strong chromic catgut or a synthetic absorbable, clamping with Mayo-Oschner forceps before division. The tumour is removed and the raw edges of the tied pedicle are covered with peritoneum secured with fine chromic catgut or synthetic absorbable sutures. Alternatively, for cysts, an ovarian cystectomy may be performed, whereby an incision is made through the ovarian cortex around the base of the cyst, which is then shelled out by sharp dissection. The incision in the ovary is then sutured, care being taken to obliterate the dead space (Fig. 20.22).

In *salpingectomy*, the inflamed tubes are usually adherent behind the uterus. They are carefully freed by blunt dissection and clamped across with double clamps before dividing. A catgut or synthetic absorbable transfixion ligature is now passed around the cut tube and vessels at each side of the division. This operation is performed also for ruptured ectopic gestation and in this case suction is used to remove blood from the peritoneal cavity.

For sterilization the Fallopian tube is drawn up with dissecting forceps in a position where the broad ligament is relatively bloodless and curved clamps are placed in position on each side. The tissue enclosed by the two clamps is then excised with a scalpel. Subsequently the tissues enclosed in the clamps are ligatured. No effort is made to bury the cut ends of the Fallopian tube. Although the operation is simple, it gives excellent results and subsequent adhesions have been shown to cause no trouble. Sterilization is often performed nowadays through a laparoscope using diathermy or occlusion clips.

In *myomectomy*, the uterus is incised and the fibroids shelled out. The uterine incision is closed with two layers of chromic catgut or a synthetic absorbable and the abdominal incision closed in the usual manner. The common complications are haemorrhage and sepsis.

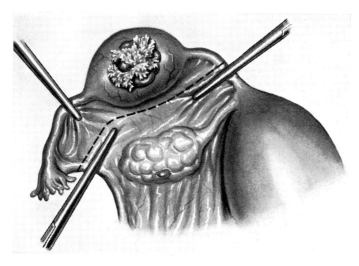

Fig. 20.21 Removal of the Fallopian tube for ectopic gestation. Further clamps are placed across the broad ligament so that no part escapes ligation. (Farquharson and Rintoul: *Textbook of Operative Surgery, 6th edn.*)

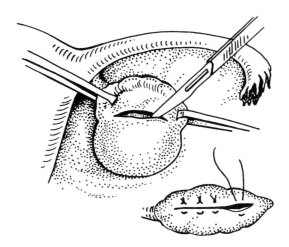

Fig. 20.22 Ovarian cystectomy, the cyst being shelled out through an incision in the ovarian cortex around its base. The ovary is then repaired by suture (Rintoul: *Farquharson's Textbook of Operative Surgery*).

Hysteropexy

Definition

A plastic operation on the uterus, performed for retroversion.

Position

Trendelenburg.

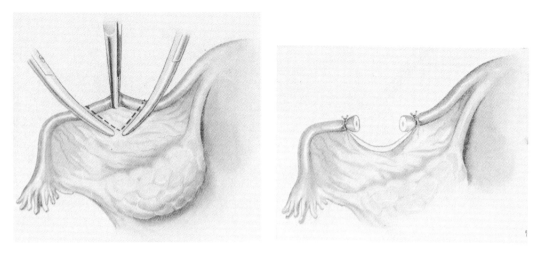

Fig. 20.23   Operation for sterilization. The method of the Viennese school.

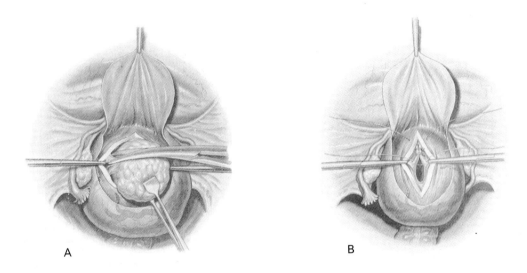

A

B

Fig. 20.24   Myomectomy (A) Enucleation of the tumour from the uterus. The myoma is drawn out with a vulsellum forceps, and adhesions separated with the help of Mayo's scissors. (B) In this case the cavity of the uterus has been opened and the mucous membrane is being closed with interrupted catgut sutures. The peritoneal flap is then sutured back in position. (Howkins and Bourne: *Shaw's Textbook of Gynaecology.*)

Instruments

As for laparotomy (Figs. 14.1 to 14.28 and 15.1 to 15.7)
    Artery forceps, curved (Mayo-Oschner or Kocher), 2.

Outline of procedure

There are several operations for this condition, but only one, that of ventrosuspension or shortening of the round ligaments (Gilliam's operation), will be described here.

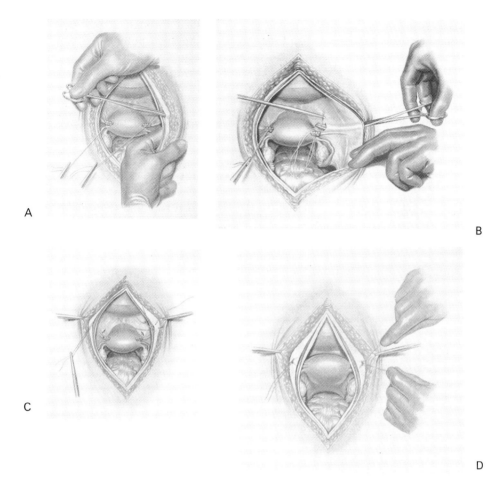

Fig. 20.25 Ventrosuspension of the uterus (Gilliam's operation) (A) Forceps, preferably curved, being introduced between the anterior rectus sheath and the rectus muscle. (B) The surgeon has passed the forceps round the outer border of the rectus and manoeuvred the points inwards to the internal abdominal ring. The peritoneum has been nicked over the points which are slightly opened to receive the ends of the suture used to plicate the round ligament. (C) The round ligament suture is now withdrawn along the track of the forceps and its ends are secured by threading them on a needle which anchors them to the anterior rectus sheath. (D) When tied this suture firmly draws the uterine cornu against the peritoneal surface of the posterior aspect of the rectus muscle and holds the uterus in a position of anteversion. (Howkins and Bourne: *Shaw's Textbook of Gynaecology.*)

A transverse, curved incision is made just above the pubis. This incision is carried down to the rectus sheath only, which is then incised in a vertical direction and the peritoneum is opened. The uterus is raised and a transfixion ligature placed on each round ligament about 1 cm (half an inch) from where it joins the uterus. The two ends of this ligature are left about 25 cm (10 in) long.

The skin is separated from the anterior rectus sheath for a small area on each side of the incision. Using scissors, the anterior rectus sheath is separated from the rectus muscle in a downward and outward direction towards the internal abdominal ring. Curved artery forceps are manoeuvred along this so-formed track on each side of the incision to the internal ring. They pass through the internal abdominal ring and are manoeuvred along the round

ligament to the point of ligature, where they are pushed through a stab incision in the peritoneum. The ligature is grasped and the forceps withdrawn, pulling the round ligament through the internal abdominal ring to appear between the anterior rectus sheath and muscle. The round ligaments are secured to the anterior rectus sheath with sutures of strong silk and the ligatures are used as an additional suture to make fixation doubly sure.

This procedure shortens the round ligaments by doubling them over and the suspension of the uterus is tightened, thereby correcting retroversion. The wound is closed in layers.

Caesarean section

Definition

Removal of the fetus through an incision in the abdominal wall and the uterus.

Position

Supine, with lateral tilt away from the surgeon followed by Trendelenburg. 10°–20°.

Instruments

As for hysterectomy
    Supra pubic retractor (Doyen)
    Uterine forceps (Green-Armytage), 5
    Obstetric forceps
    Suction tubing, nozzles and tube anchoring forceps
    2 ml syringe and needles with ergometrine 0.5 mg
    Mucus extractors and general apparatus for resuscitation of the child (cord clamps, scissors, etc.).

Outline of procedure

The patient comes to theatre with a catheter *in situ* which is released but not removed during the operation. A vertical lower midline or Pfannenstiel incision is made extending from the umbilicus to the pubis. The bowel is displaced towards the diaphragm with packs and a 10 cm (4 in) incision made in the uterus. For lower segment operations (the majority of procedures), the incision is made horizontally in the uterus (after separating the bladder from the uterus) just where the peritoneum is reflected off the bladder, and for upper segment operations, the incision is in the midline vertically. This requires a clean scalpel.

Fig. 20.26   Lower segment Caesarian section.
A. Exposure of the lower uterine segment through a Pfannenstiel or lower mid-line incision; Doyens supra-pubic retractor in situ. The peritoneal fold is incised with scissors, and the lower uterine segment opened with a scalpel.
B. The incision is completed by stretching with index fingers, extending it laterally.
C. The baby's head is delivered after rupturing the membranes.
D. Folowing an intravenous dose of oxytocic drug, the placenta is dellvered by gentle traction.
E. The incision angles are secured with single sutures. The first layer of the lower uterine segment is closed with a continuous suture involving half a thickness of the incision . .
F. Closure is completed by suturing the second layer with a continuous suture.
    Closure of the peritoneum with continuous sutures.
    (*A Digest of Obstetrical and Gynaecological Procedures, Ethicon Ltd.*)

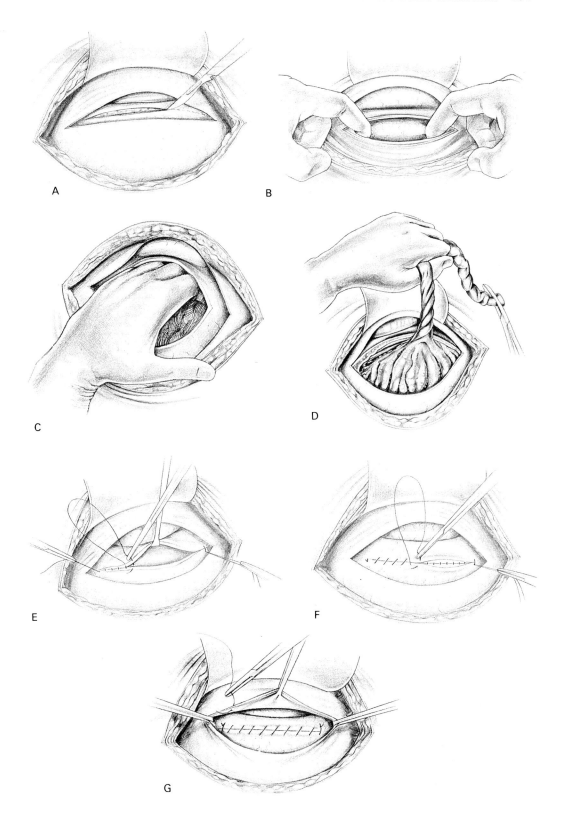

The incision is completed with scissors and by manual stretching. The fetus is delivered and the umbilical cord clamped with forceps and divided. Whilst the midwife or paediatrician resuscitates the child, the placenta is delivered and the cut edges of the uterus grasped with Green-Armytage forceps. Suction is used to remove amniotic fluid.

Ergometrine is injected intravenously to cause contraction of the uterine muscles and thereby arrest haemorrhage. The incision in the uterus is closed with two layers of chromic catgut or synthetic absorbable sutures, the first layer passing through the muscle coat but not the mucosa, and the second layer is inserted to invert the first layer. The uterovesical peritoneum is sutured and the wound closed in the usual manner.

Clots are expressed from the vagina by pressure on the abdomen and a pad applied to the vulva.

REFERENCES AND FURTHER READING

ETHICON (1980) *A Digest of Obstetrical and Gynaecological Procedures*. Edinburgh: Ethicon Ltd.
GARREY, M. M., GOVAN, A. D. T., HODGE, C. H. AND CALLANDER, R. (1972) *Gynaecology Illustrated*. Edinburgh: Churchill Livingstone.
HOWKINS, J. AND BOURNE, G. (1971) *Shaw's Textbook of Gynaecology*. Edinburgh: Churchill Livingstone.
MACLEOD, D. AND HOWKINS, J. (1966) *Bonney's Gynaecological Surgery*. London: Baillière Tindall.
MOVAIR, T. J. (1972) *Hamilton Bailey's Emergency Surgery*. Bristol: Wright.
RINTOUL, R. F. (1986) *Farquharsons Textbook of Operative Surgery*. Edinburgh: Churchill Livingstone.

21

Neurosurgical operations

Angiography

Definition

Serial X-ray examination of the cerebral vascular tree following the injection of a water soluble radio-opaque medium into a main artery in the neck, (the needle being introduced percutaneously) or via a femoral catheter.

Position

Supine, with the head extended, preferably on a Lysholm skull table.

Instruments

Sponge-holding forceps, (Rampley), 5
Towel clips, 5
Scalpel handle (Bard Parker) with No. 11 blade
20 ml syringes, 3
Sterile normal saline, pyrogen-free, 60 ml
Arterial puncture needles, i.e., Lindgren arterial needles; carotid or vertebral type
    needles, adult and child size; or femoral arterial catheters, trocar and cannula
Adaptors and silicone tubing, 15 cm in length
Local anaesthesia requisites (Fig. 11.60)
Water soluble radio-opaque contrast medium, e.g., Iopamidol, Omnipaque.

Outline of procedure

After cleansing the skin and draping, a bleb of local anaesthetic is raised anterior to the sternomastoid, and then the carotid sheath or region of the vertebral artery is infiltrated. The needle is mounted on a syringe filled with saline and is inserted into the appropriate artery through a nick in the skin. After ensuring that there is a good backflow of blood from the selected vessel, the assembly is kept patent by slow injection of saline.

After positioning the patient for radiography, the saline-filled syringe is exchanged for a syringe containing contrast medium which is then rapidly injected intra-arterially whilst X-rays are taken. Normally these consist of three views, antero-posterior, lateral and oblique,

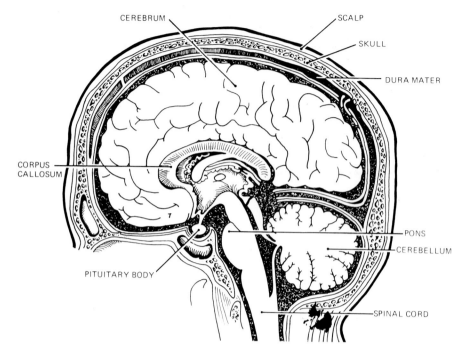

Fig. 21.1 Cross section of skull showing brain. (Down's Surgical Ltd.)

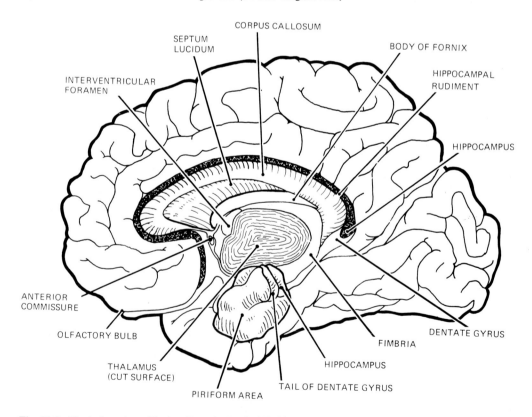

Fig. 21.2 Vertical section of brain. (Down's Surgical Ltd.)

taken serially. Each time, 8 to 10 ml of contrast medium is injected. Alternatively, if vertebral or multiple aneurysms are suspected, 4-vessel angiography is carried out via a femoral catheter. The groin is cleansed and draped in the usual manner, and the trocar and cannula inserted through the palpated external iliac artery. The trocar is withdrawn, and the cannula is pulled back until its presence within the vessel is indicated by a flow of arterial blood. The catheter guide wire is threaded through the cannula until it reaches the selected level in the aorta. The catheter is then passed over the guide wire for the predetermined distance, and after confirmatory radiographs to check its position, the guide and cannula are withdrawn, leaving the catheter in place. The injection of radio-opaque medium follows in a similar manner to that for carotid angiography.

Encephalography

Definition

X-ray examination of the ventricular system and subarachnoid spaces surrounding the brain by fractional replacement of cerebrospinal fluid with water soluble radio-opaque contrast medium.

Position

Sitting, with head flexed 20°, usually in an encephalography chair.

Instruments

Spinal set (Fig. 11.61).
Water soluble radio-opaque contrast medium e.g. Iopamidol, Omnipaque.

Outline of procedure

Local anaesthesia and lumbar puncture is performed, omitting manometry. Using 5 ml quantities, c.s.f. is gradually replaced with a water soluble radio-opaque contrast medium, an X-ray being taken after 10 ml replacement to check that contrast medium is entering the brain ventricles. After the required amount of contrast medium is injected, the lumbar puncture needle is removed, the patient placed supine and further X-rays are taken. A sample of the aspirated c.s.f. is sent for analysis.

Myelography

Definition

X-ray examination of the spinal canal after the injection of a water soluble radio-opaque medium into the subdural space.

Position

Lateral with knees and neck moderately flexed, or sitting.

Instruments

Spinal set (Fig. 11.61)
Water soluble radio-opaque contrast medium, e.g. Iopamidol, Omnipaque.

Outline of procedure

Local anaesthesia and lumbar puncture is performed in the third or fourth lumbar inter-space. Pressure readings without, and then with jugular compression are taken and 5 to 6 ml of c.s.f. withdrawn for analysis. The contrast medium is then injected and the patient X-rayed supine and prone on a tilting table. The contrast medium is left *in situ*.

Cysternal puncture

Definition

The subarachnoid injection of a water soluble radio-opaque contrast medium for myelography in cases of 'failed lumbar puncture' due to 'dry tap' secondary to total spinal block. The contrast medium is injected into the cysterna magna.

Position

Sitting with the neck flexed.

Instruments

Spinal set (Fig.11.61)
Cysternal puncture (short bevel) needle
Needle guard
Steel rule, 15 cm (6 in).
Water soluble, radio-opaque contrast medium, e.g. Iopamidol, Omnipaque.

Outline of procedure

A skin bleb of local anaesthetic is raised in the mid-line of the neck, halfway between the external occipital protuberance and the sixth cervical spinous process. After infiltration of the neck musculature, the cysternal puncture needle (with the guard set at 55 mm) is then slowly inserted in the mid-line to traverse the posterior atlanto-occipital membrane and enter the cysterna magna at the base of the brain. After withdrawing 5 to 6 ml of c.s.f. for analysis, contrast medium is injected, the needle withdrawn and X-rays taken as in myelography.

Ventriculography

Definition

An X-ray examination of the ventricular system of the brain after partial replacement of the ventricular c.s.f. with a water soluble, radio-opaque contrast medium.

Figs. 21.3 to 21.7 Neurosurgical instruments — craniotomy/burr hole. (Down's Surgical Ltd.)

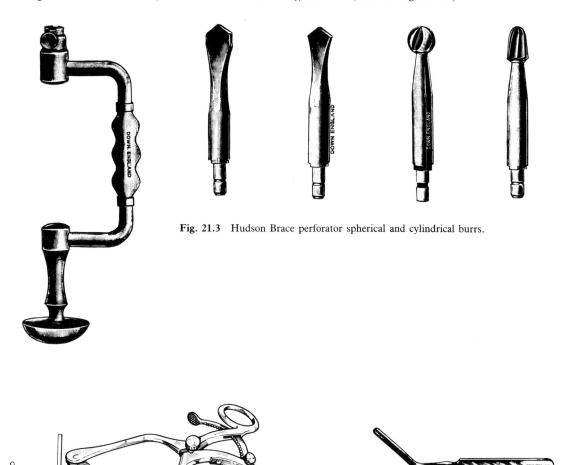

Fig. 21.3 Hudson Brace perforator spherical and cylindrical burrs.

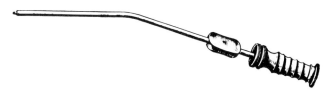

Fig. 21.4 Schnitker scalp retractor, curved, self-retaining with blunt swivel blades.

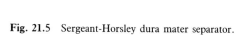

Fig. 21.5 Sergeant-Horsley dura mater separator.

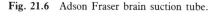

Fig. 21.6 Adson Fraser brain suction tube.

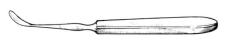

Fig. 21.7 Adson curved periosteal elevator.

Position

Supine or sitting in the neurosurgical chair.

Instruments

Sponge-holding forceps (Rampley), 5
Scalpel handle No. 4 with No. 22 blade (Bard Parker)
Scalpel handle No. 5 with No. 15 or 11 blade (Bard Parker)
Fine dissecting forceps, non-toothed (McIndoe)
Fine dissecting forceps, toothed (Gillies)
Medium dissecting forceps, non-toothed
Medium dissecting forceps, toothed (Lane's)
Artery forceps, straight (Moynihan), 5
Scissors, stitch
Scissors curved (Metzenbaum)
Scissors curved (strabismus)
Scissors straight (iris)
Dura hooks, sharp and blunt
Periosteal elevator (Adson)
Dissector (McDonald)
Trephine seeker/small aneurysm needle
Dura separator (Sergeant's)
Dressing forceps (Tilley or Olivecrona)
Bone nibblers, curved on flat and angled on side 2
Skull perforators and burrs (Hudson)
Skull brace (Hudson)
Retractors, self-retaining (Shnitkers)
Fine needle holder (West)
Diathermy leads, electrodes, scabbard and lead anchoring forceps
Spinal manometer
CSF specimen bottles
10 ml syringe
Bonney's Blue
Steel rule and skin pen
Ventricular cannula
Towel clips 5
Irrigation syringe
Pint measure with warm saline
Local anaesthesia requisites (Fig. 11.60)
Suction tubing, fine nozzles and tube anchoring forceps
Fine Nélaton catheters, polyvinyl or latex rubber with spigots, 5
250 ml conical flask fitted with a two-holed rubber stopper, glass air-vent and 100 cm of silicone tubing and fine metal concentric connector
Horsley's bone wax gelatine sponge, patties
2 or 1.5 (3/0 or 4/0) Synthetic non-absorbable on small curved round-bodied needles for dura
2 (3/0) Synthetic non-absorbable on small curved cutting or straight cutting needles for skin.

Figs. 21.8 to 21.14 Neurosurgical instruments — craniotomy/burr hole (*cont'd.*) (Down's Surgical Ltd.)

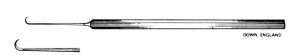

Fig. 21.8 Cairns dural hook, fine, sharp.

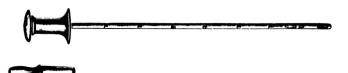

Fig. 21.9 Jefferson ventricular cannula and tubing connection.

Fig. 21.10 Dandys ventricular drainage cannula. (Full size approx.)

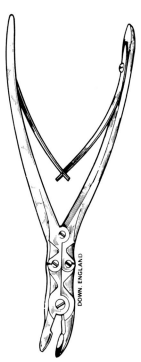

Fig. 21.11 Luer-Jansen rongeur, double action, slightly curved on flat.

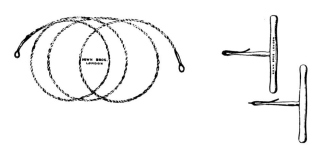

Fig. 21.12 Gigli Wire saw and handle. (Used in pairs.)

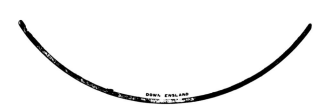

Fig. 21.13 Cairn-De Martel wire saw guide.

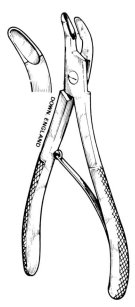

Fig. 21.14 Cairns rongeur with fine angled on flat jaws, curved handles.

Outline of procedure

Local anaesthetic is infiltrated into the areas selected for ventricular puncture. A 5 cm straight incision is made 3.5 cm from the midline, either on the frontal or parietal eminences. Two artery forceps are clipped on to the deepest galeal layer as retractors and after clearing back the periosteum, artery forceps are replaced with a self-retaining retractor which by virtue of pressure from the blades creates haemostasis.

The hole is drilled first by using the perforator and then the appropriate matching burr. The dura is elevated with a dural hook, incised in a cruciate fashion and the lifted edges diathermised. The underlying brain is diathermised and incised at the entry point for insertion of the cannula. The lateral ventricles are cannulated on either side and c.s.f. pressure measured if required. Samples of c.s.f. are taken separately from each side for analysis.

The cannulae may be exchanged for fine catheters through which c.s.f. is fractionally replaced with a water soluble radio-opaque contrast medium in 5 ml increments to give a total replacement of 5 to 6 ml with normal size ventricles.

The catheters are spigoted and the scalp closed in two layers after haemostasis has been secured. Following radiography, the catheters (which project through the suture line) are either removed, or in cases of chronic raised intracranial pressure, one is left coupled to the drainage flask for 24 to 48 hours to minimise the risk of brain compression or 'coning'.

Burr hole and biopsy abscess drainage

Definition

Diagnostic needle biopsy of pathological intracerebral tissue or cyst drainage via a burr hole.

Position

Supine, lateral or prone depending on selected site for biopsy.

Instruments

As for ventriculography
  Glass microscope slides, 7.6 cm × 2.5 cm (3 in × 1 in)
  In cases of brain abscess a selection of short rubber tubing of medium bore, 5 cm long
    will be required: also antibiotic solution.

Outline of procedure

Up to and including the dural incision the procedure approximates that for ventriculography. The burr hole is sited so that on 'needling' the brain a relatively 'silent' area is traversed.

The brain substance is explored with a fine brain needle passed in radiate fashion, to discover pathological tissue or cysts. When a possibly pathological area of brain is entered, a gentle aspiration biopsy is taken through the needle and pressure-smeared between two microscope slides which are placed in formol saline and sent for pathological examination.

Cysts and abscess cavities are drained through medium-bore tube drains. Antibiotics are instilled and abscess cavities are assessed thereafter by computerised axial tomography. The scalp is closed in two layers.

Craniotomy and craniectomy

Definition

Craniotomy is incision through the scalp and underlying muscle, with fashioning of a muscle-hinged osteoplastic flap of the skull in order to gain access to the brain. *Craniectomy* denotes removal of a bone from the skull vault, either by enlargement of burr holes or removal of osteoplastic bone flap, again to afford access to the brain. Included under this heading is reduction of a depressed fracture of the skull vault.

Craniotomy

Position

Supine for frontal, temporal or parietal exposures; prone for occipital and posterior fossa exposures; sitting for posterior fossa exposures or lateral for temporo-parietal flaps (Mayfield frame may be used, Fig. 21.32).

Instruments

Use of the Oxford instrument table facilitates instrumentation (Figs. 21.33 or 21.34).
    General set (Figs. 14.1 to 14.28), except large retractors
    As for ventriculography (p. 556)
    Artery forceps, curved on side, 24
    Dissector, double end (Durham)
    Aneurysm needles small and medium
    Scissors, dura mater (Schmeiden)
    Micro instruments, various
    Brain retractors, malleable, various sizes
    Punch forceps (Hajecks, DeVilbiss)
    Wire saw and handles (Gigli or Olivecronas)
    Saw guard (Cairn-de-Martel)
    Haemostasis clips and insertion/removal forceps (Raney)
    Dissecting forceps (Adson)
    Rongeur, pituitary, straight and angled (Cushing).
    Retractors, self-retaining (West, Mayo hinged, etc.), 2
    Fine needle holders (West or Kilner), 2
    20 ml syringe
    Elastic rubber bands for securing forceps in groups
    Plastic drainage tubing and wound suction apparatus (Redivac, Activac or Portovac)
    Diathermy leads, forceps electrodes, scabbard and lead anchoring forceps
    (Bone awl or micro hand drill with twist drills and drill guard may be needed, plus
        stainless steel wire)
    2 or 1.5 (3/0 or 4/0) Synthetic non-absorbable or silk on small curved round bodied
        needles for dura
    2 (3/0) Synthetic non-absorbable or silk on small curved cutting or straight cutting needles
        for skin.

Figs. 21.15 to 21.20 Neurosurgical instruments — craniotomy/burr hole (*cont'd.*). (Down's Surgical Ltd.)

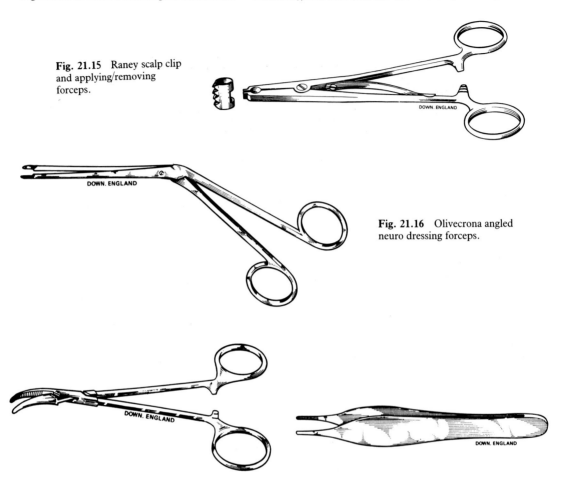

Fig. 21.15 Raney scalp clip and applying/removing forceps.

Fig. 21.16 Olivecrona angled neuro dressing forceps.

Fig. 21.17 Cairns artery forceps, curved-to-side, box-joint.

Fig. 21.18 Adson dressing forceps, serrated points.

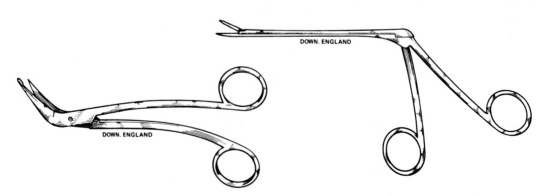

Fig. 21.19 Schmeiden (or Taylor) dural scissors, angular with probe-pointed under blade, screw-joint.

Fig. 21.20 Selverstone micro alligator forceps, light smooth jaws.

Figs. 21.21 to 21.25 Neurosurgical instruments — craniotomy/burr hole (*cont'd.*). (Down's Surgical Ltd.)

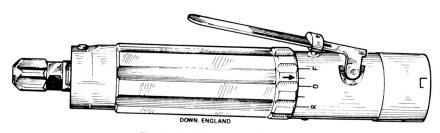

Fig. 21.21 Air powered driver.

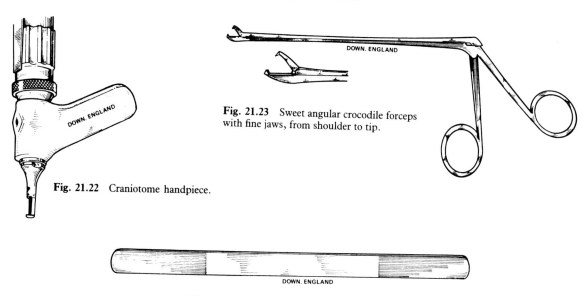

Fig. 21.23 Sweet angular crocodile forceps with fine jaws, from shoulder to tip.

Fig. 21.22 Craniotome handpiece.

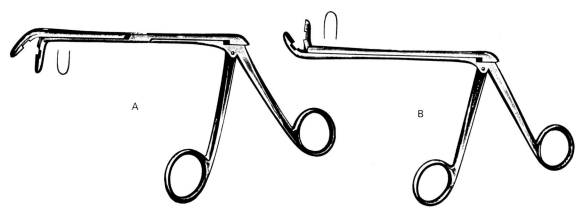

Fig. 21.24 Cairns malleable strip retractors.

Fig. 21.25 Cushing rongeur. For pituitary body. Maybe straight (not illustrated), angled forwards (A) or angled backwards (B).

Figs. 21.26 to 21.31   Examples of neurosurgical micro instruments. (Down's Surgical Ltd.)

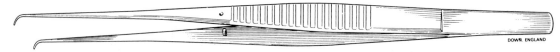

Fig. 21.26   Dissecting forceps, straight.

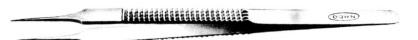

Fig. 21.27   Micro forceps, taper jaws, with smooth tungsten carbide inserts.

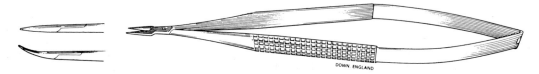

Fig. 21.28   Micro needleholder, straight, spring handles, tungsten carbide faced smooth jaws.

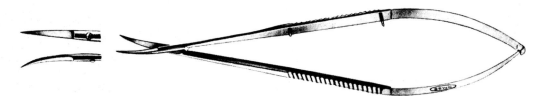

Fig. 21.29   Jacobson micro scissors, straight, spring handle.

Fig. 21.30   Yasargil micro forceps.

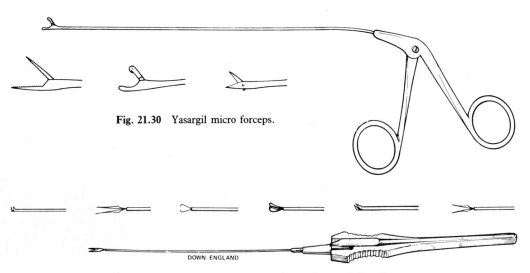

Fig. 21.31   Micro instruments, squeeze action, angled shaft.

Outline of procedure

Depending on the site and extent of brain exposure required, either a solitary burr hole will be made which is enlarged as necessary to form a limited craniectomy (e.g., for access to the Gasserian ganglion, certain temporal haematoma, subtemporal decompressions or emergency intracranial vascular surgery); or alternatively several burr holes are made in rhombic form and linked with a wire saw to form a bony 'trapdoor' hinged on the temporal muscle. This is the classical osteoplastic flap.

Elevation of a depressed fracture of the skull vault. To gain access to the fracture margins, a skin incision is made which possibly will include existing scalp wounds if the fracture be compound. The galeal bleeding is arrested with artery forceps which are grouped conveniently with rubber bands and clipped to the drapes.

The periosteum is reflected from the fracture lines for 5 to 10 mm each side and a burr hole made on sound bone to one side of the depression in order to afford access to the

Figs. 21.32 to 21.35 Radcliffe Infirmary, Oxford.

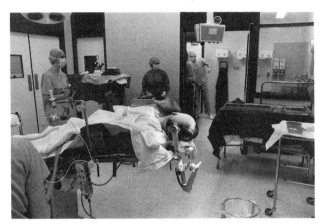

Fig. 21.32 Mayfield frame used to immobilise head for craniectomy.

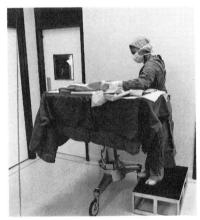

Fig. 21.33 Oxford instrument table, outer pack covers opened.

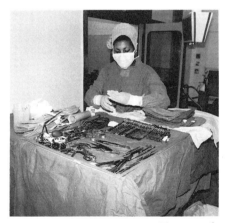

Fig. 21.34 Oxford instrument table prepared for craniectomy.

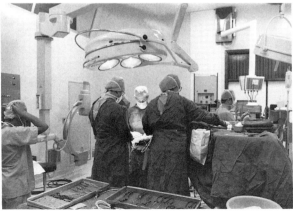

Fig. 21.35 Oxford instrument table in use during a neurosurgical procedure. Alternative method of draping to that depicted in Chapter 10.

extradural space. Alternatively small comminuted fragments of bone often found impacting the fracture in the depressed position are nibbled away, any extradural haematoma being removed by suction. The dura is freed from the skull and an Adson elevator or bone spike inserted into the burr hole or bony defect. Using intact bone as the fulcrum, the depressed fragments are gently elevated into anatomical position and haemostasis is secured.

If the dura is penetrated resulting in a c.s.f. leak, the rent must be exposed and explored. Minimal pulped brain is gently irrigated, removed with suction and finally haemostasis secured with bipolar diathermy or Cushing clips. The dural rent is closed with fine silk interrupted sutures or a fascial patch, the donor site being conveniently temporal fascia or even fascia lata.

The scalp is closed (after inserting a drain) as for venticulography.

Evacuation of extradural haematoma. (This may only require instruments as for ventriculography providing the additional cranial instrument set is kept sterile for immediate use.)

A limited temporal craniectomy is made as previously described. The bleeding point is exposed — usually where the middle meningeal vessels emerge from the bony tunnel in the temporal bone to cross to the dura. Bleeding is arrested by coagulation or by under-running the vessels with a fine suture. The dura is then secured with dural 'hitch' stitches to the pericranium thereby occluding dead space and preventing extradural ooze under the bone edges, which can predispose towards extradural clot reaccumulation. After haemostasis is

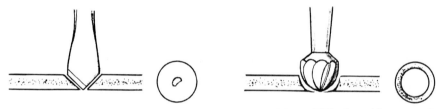

Fig. 21.36 Cutting a burrhole utilising skull perforator and spherical burr. (Gillingham: *Neurosurgery.*)

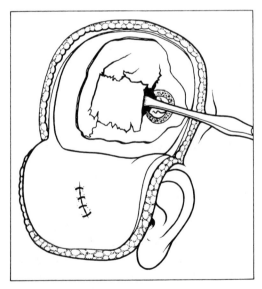

Fig. 21.37 Method of elevating a depressed fracture of the skull through on opening made with burr or trephine in *undamaged* bone adjoining the defect. In compound fractures all bone fragments should be removed. (Rintoul: *Farquharsons' Textbook of Operative Surgery.*)

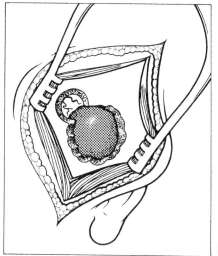

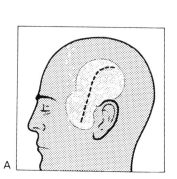

Fig. 21.38 Operation for extra-dural haemorrhage. The initial opening in the skull is made with a burr or trephine, and is then enlarged with Rongeur forceps to allow adequate access to the clot. *Inset* shows area to be infiltrated with local anaesthetic and the incision employed. (Rintoul: *Farquharsons' Textbook of Operative Surgery.*)

secured and a suction drain inserted the scalp is closed routinely with two layers of synthetic non-absorbable or silk sutures to both muscles and scalp.

Subdural haematoma. (This may only require instruments as for ventriculography as above.) These are removed normally by making two burr holes at suitable sites and then after dural incision the fluid or clot is aspirated by suction. Any remaining clot is flushed out by gentle irrigation utilising a fine catheter, the saline being introduced at one burr hole and the clot expelled via the other. If the clot be solid and too firm to evacuate, an osteo-plastic flap must be turned and the clot removed under direct vision.

In chronic subdural haematoma the brain shrinks and there is often some difficulty in expanding it to refill the space left by the evacuated haematoma. In this case saline is injected either via a lumbar puncture, or the lateral ventricle is cannulated and filled directly with saline via a Cushing brain needle.

Raising an osteoplastic flap. This is a preliminary procedure for all extensive intracranial procedures. The initial stages follow those previously described but a larger planned scalp incision is made. After scalp reflexion to the base of the planned incision, bleeding points are diathermised and the scalp flap covered with a saline soaked pack.

Two radial diathermy incisions are made down to bone in the temporal muscle, so that a fan-shaped section over the site of the osteoplastic bone flap will remain attached to temple and also to the reflected bone. This soft-tissue bridge is responsible for revascularisation of the bone flap after replacement when the operation is completed.

Five or six trephine holes are made at intervals on the circumference of the proposed bone flap. After deflecting the underlying dura from beneath the margins of the burr holes, first the bone base of the flap beneath the temporalis muscle is divided or narrowed enough to fracture through when the flap is reflected. The remaining burr holes are then linked one after the other with a de Martel saw guide and wire saw, or craniotome chamfering the bone edges to prevent the replaced bone flap from sinking inward.

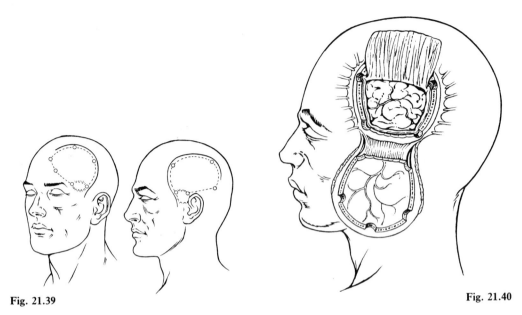

Fig. 21.39

Fig. 21.40

Fig. 21.39 The position of osteoplastic flaps for exposure in the frontoparietal and parietal areas. Dotted lines are shown between burr holes.

Fig. 21.40 Method of turning down a flap based on the temporalis muscle. The skin flap has been reflected along with the skull flap and the dura opened as a U-shaped flap.

The bone is then rapidly prised up and reflected, followed by removal of any bone spikes at the base. It is then wrapped with a saline soaked pack, which is secured to the drapes with rubber bands and towel clips. Occasionally the bone flap may be totally removed at this stage when a large decompression is needed rapidly. Bone haemostasis is secured with diathermy or bone wax and the edges are then covered with moist lintine strips followed by a fresh towel to cover all instruments *in situ* to that moment.

The dura is always reflected toward the vertex of the skull. A point near to the bone margins toward the base of the skull and free from blood vessels is selected and picked up with a sharp hook. It is then nicked with a scalpel and the nick enlarged with a director and scalpel sufficiently to introduce a small patty. The brain being protected by the patty, the dura is opened with dural scissors. Vessels to be traversed are bipolarly diathermised or under-run. The dural flap is reflected and covered with a moist patty. The dura is kept moist throughout the operation.

Tumours are gently separated out with brain retractors, scissors, diathermy and suction tube, or removed 'piecemeal' with a diathermy loop as in the case of large meningiomata. Alternatively, there is increasing use of ultrasonic aspirators which remove tumour tissue with minimal disturbance to adjacent normal tissue. A description of the Cusa Cavitron ultrasonic aspirator is included in Chapter 3, page 100. The cavity left by infiltrative tumours is gently irrigated until haemostasis is complete. Oozing is controlled with gelatin sponge, Oxycel or Surgicel covered with a moist cotton-wool pack which is sucked dry. This pack is later removed with the aid of irrigation.

For closure the dura is first 'hitch stitched' to the pericranium as described previously, then closed with interrupted synthetic non-absorbable or silk sutures. The bone flap is replaced *in situ* and sutured in place with periosteal synthetic non-absorbable or silk sutures.

In some cases the flap is fixed with twisted loops of stainless steel wire inserted in holes drilled in the flap and surrounding intact vault bones. Whilst drilling, the brain is guarded to avoid accidental deep penetration. The scalp may be drained using a subgaleal suction drain.

Posterior fossa exploration. A midline, 'crossbow' or lateral linear incision is made through previously infiltrated neck musculature. Artery forceps on each side of the incision are grouped together with rubber bands. The neck musculature is incised with diathermy down to bone and the occipital bone bared widely, stripping the muscles back with a periosteal elevator and large self-retaining retractors.

Two burr holes are made one on either side of the midline over the cerebellum. Using nibblers, a large craniectomy is made bilaterally and the crest of midline bone between these removed. The posterior aspect of the foramen magnum rim is removed, as is usually the posterior arch of the atlas and even the axis together with the axis' spinous process.

The dura is opened widely and held back with 'hitch stitches'. The brain is explored by 'needling' and retraction, pathological tissue being dealt with as previously described. The dura is left open and the muscles closed in layers to effect a watertight closure. Skin is then closed in two layers.

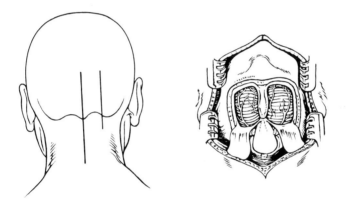

Fig. 21.41   Posterior fossa approach, midline and lateral incision.

Cranioplasty

Definition

Repair of skull defects with bone, acrylic resin or Vitallium prostheses.

Position

As for the appropriate craniotomy. If iliac bone or rib is to be used for a bony cranioplasty, the patient is placed in the lateral or half-lateral position.

Instruments

As for craniotomy
    Bone graft set (Fig. 23.94)
    Pistol grip hand drill, twist drills and drill guard

Stainless steel wire
Prosthesis; acrylic polymer and monomer, acrylic plate or Vitallium plate.

Outline of procedure

The cranial defect is exposed by reflexion of the scalp flap and careful sharp dissection to leave freshened bone margins and intact dura underlying the defect. The bone edges are 'stepped or chamfered' until the prepared prosthesis sits snugly in position. Holes are drilled in the surrounding bone at suitable intervals and the prosthesis is firmly wired into place with stainless steel wire. After twisting the wire ends these are cut and buried in the drill holes. The scalp is closed in two layers often with a suction drain in place for 24 hours post-operatively.

If an autogenous bone graft is used to repair the defect, the bone is removed from the appropriate donor site. A plate of cortical and cancellous bone can be removed *en bloc* from the inner aspect of the ileum, alternatively two or three sections of rib of sufficient length to bridge the skull defect may be used. A rib is split lengthwise and wired *in situ* in parallel strips to roof over the defect. Any cancellous chippings are lightly packed in the interspaces and the scalp closed routinely.

Stereotactic surgery

Definition

Deep ablative surgery of the white matter, basal ganglia or brain stem projection fibres by means of a special probe utilising electro-coagulation or extreme cold (cryoprobe) as the destructive agent. Accuracy of siting is accomplished by means of a stereotactic frame applied to the skull coupled with contrast radiography demonstrating fixed intracerebral landmarks as points of reference.

Position

Sitting (Leksell and cryoprobe); or prone (Guiot) depending on which stereotactic frame is used.

Instruments

As for ventriculography (p. 556)
    Micro hand drill, twist drills and drill guard
    Lead shot
    Cryoprobe or electro-coagulation unit
    Stereotactic frame (Leksell, Cooper, Guiot Gillingham, etc.).

Outline of procedure

One stage procedure. The ventricles are outlined by contrast radiography and the stereotactic frame applied to the skull. By reference to a standard sterotactic atlas, the probe is inserted and localised into the required position and a lesion performed in increments until the desired effect is obtained in the conscious patient. There are a number of different operations which can be carried out. The following is an example which illustrates the principles.

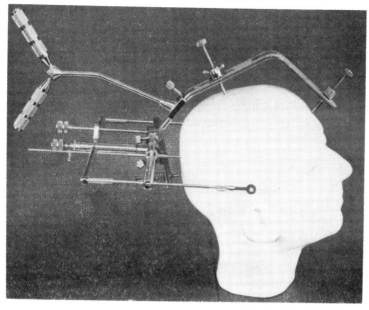

Fig. 21.42 Guiot Gillingham stereotactic frame. (Eschmann Bros and Walsh Ltd.)

Two stage procedure. The preliminary stage is performed, followed two days later by the main operation. An example is stereotactic thalamopallidotomy, designed to relieve the tremor and rigidity of Parkinsonism.

Stage one consists of inserting lead shot landmarks on the surface of the skull. Using the stereotactic frame bar as a guide, three incisions are made through the scalp: one traverse frontally as low as possible towards the nasion; another longitudinally over the coronal suture and a third longitudinal or transverse incision low on the occipital bone towards the external occipital protuberance. All the incisions are placed in the midline. Using a guarded drill, several holes are drilled in the outer table of the skull so that five or six lead shot can be inserted and secured with bone wax, arranged in a W fashion to give a 'spread' of shot across the skull midline at the three sites.

The scalp is closed routinely and an air encephalogram taken with several radiographic views to include the lines of shot and the septum pellucidum as well as the third ventricle. By computation, by consideration of the position of lead shot and various other intracranial landmarks, accurate co-ordinates of the globus pallidus and ventro-later nucleus of the thalamus are worked out. From this, the position of the parietal burr hole required in a direct line behind these targets is also worked out.

Stage two, the patient is conscious, placed in the prone position, with the head resting in a neurosurgical horseshoe and the limbs exposed. The original incisions are re-opened and the lines of lead shot exposed. The shot selected for siting an anchor point for the Guiot frame is removed and after enlarging the socket left behind, a special screw is driven home into the outer skull table. The procedure is repeated at the other incisions and after removing all surplus lead shot markers, the bar of the Guiot frame is secured to the anchor points and the wounds closed around the screws.

Two burr holes are then made and the dura incised to expose brain. The first is sited over the frontal horn of the lateral ventricle which is then catheterised. The second burr hole is

made over the parietal eminence on the side for the lesion, a pre-determined site, usually about 3 to 3.5 cm above the external occipital protuberance and centred 16 mm from the midline.

The Guiot frame is secured to the central bar with the depth electrode touching the brain surface. A water soluble radio-opaque contrast medium 3 ml is instilled into the ventricle and by manipulating the head is manoeuvred into the third ventricle to outline the anterior and posterior commissure. The sights of the Guiot frame are then aligned on the globus pallidus by using these points of reference and an image intensifier.

The contrast medium is aspirated and the frontal burr hole closed. The electrode is slowly inserted into the brain 16 mm from the midline until the ventro-lateral nucleus of the thalamus is entered. This usually results in a dramatic cessation or diminuation of tremor. A radiofrequency current of known strength and duration is then passed through the electrode to make a small spherical lesion in the thalamus. Alternatively the cryoprobe tip is cooled to -30 to $-100°C$ and after a predetermined time, warmed up again (Chapter 3).

After an acceptable result is achieved, the electrode is pushed further anteriorly, traversing the internal capsule to enter the globus pallidus. A second lesion is then made, which usually dramatically improves dexterity and alleviates the increased rigidity. The apparatus is then removed and the incisions closed.

By similar techniques, electrodes and probes can produce lesions in the frontal association to cause a controlled, more exact leucotomy; suprafellar cysts can be approached and ascending pain fibres in cases of intractable pain can be destroyed in the brain stem, with minimal interference to brain function.

Insertion of ventriculo-atrial or ventriculo-petritoneal shunt

Definition

The establishment of artificial c.s.f. drainage to heart or peritoneal cavity in cases of primary or secondary hydrocephalus.

Position

Supine, with head rotated to the left, sandbag under the shoulders and an X-ray film cassette beneath the patient's chest.

Instruments

As for ventriculography (p. 556)
  Fine arterial bulldog clamps, 3
  Small gauges, 3 mm, 4 mm, 6 mm (Hahn or Jenkins), 3
  Suitable valve (Pudenz or Spitz-Holter)
  Fine bore silicone tubing assorted sizes
  Eynard connectors, 2.

Outline of procedure

Ventriculo-atrial shunt, (Pudenz ventricular access device insertion). A preliminary chest radiograph confirms the level of the right atrium. A right sub-mandibular incision is made and

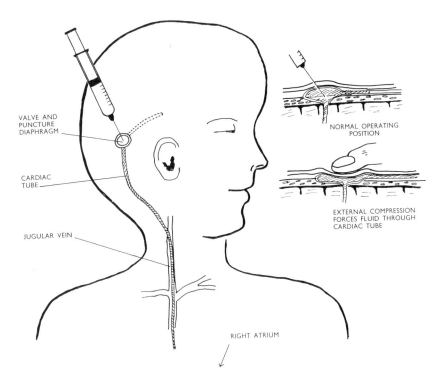

VALVE AND
PUNCTURE
DIAPHRAGM

CARDIAC
TUBE

JUGULAR VEIN

NORMAL OPERATING
POSITION

EXTERNAL COMPRESSION
FORCES FLUID THROUGH
CARDIAC TUBE

RIGHT ATRIUM

Fig. 21.43 Pudenz valve for ventriculo-atrial shunt.

the posterior branch of the common facial vein or the right internal jugular vein is exposed and freed from surrounding tissues.

A supramastoid occipital scalp incision 5 cm (2 in) long is made well above the line of the lateral sinus, and using a small gouge a hole is drilled in the attenuated skull. The dura is incised and the enlarged occipital horn of the lateral ventricle is catheterised with the top-half of the Pudenz catheter. This is then occluded with the bulldog clip to prevent leakage of c.s.f.

(*It is always necessary to insert the reservoir in the shunt circuit. As this is required, the gouge-hole must be enlarged to fit the rim of the disc snugly and bone haemostasis secured with bone wax. The radio-opaque Tantalum impregnated silicone plug is then cut off from the end of the outlet tube and distal catheter or catheter and valve fitted and tied to the centre of the outlet of the flushing disc which is then tied with fine synthetic non-absorbable or silk. The disc is then inserted and sutured to the periosteum margins of the bone defect.*)

Two synthetic non-absorbable or silk ligatures are passed around the right internal jugular vein, or the posterior branch of the common facial vein if the latter is of sufficiently large calibre to admit the Pudenz tube valve. The top ligature is tied to occlude the vessel. The Pudenz atrial catheter is checked for correct functioning of the four slit valves at the atrial end. The vessel is nicked and the catheter inserted toward the superior vena cava until it is estimated to be within the right atrium.

A few millilitres of a water soluble radio-opaque medium is injected via an Eynard connector whilst a radiograph of the chest is taken to verify correct positioning of the valve. Alternatively the catheter can be inserted under ECG control using hypertonic saline instilled. After any necessary adjustment, so that the valve tip is well within the right atrium,

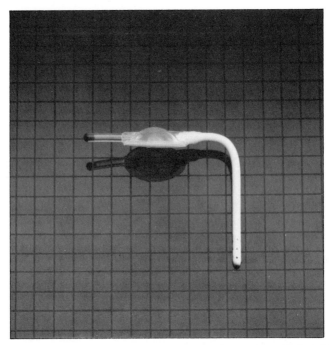

Fig. 21.44 Ventricular assist device 12 mm convertible, designed for neonates. (Pudenz-Schulte Medical (USA), Forth Medical Ltd (UK).)

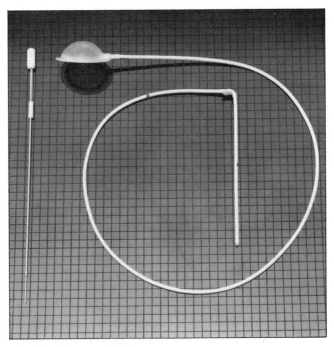

Fig. 21.45 Ventricular assist device with catheter. (Pudenz-Schulte Medical (USA), Forth Medical Ltd (UK).)

the Pudenz tube is secured in the neck with the lower ligature. The tubing of the lower end of the valve is then tracked from the neck incision to the scalp incision, using large artery forceps forced along the subcutaneous tissues. After trimming to a suitable length, the top and bottom tubes are linked over a fine connector supplied with the valve (or to the flushing disc) with synthetic non-absorbable ties. After checking fontanelle tension and the flusher if fitted, for correct function, both wounds are closed in two layers.

Ventriculo-peritoneal shunt. Ventricular catheterisation is performed as above with a single length of fine silicone tubing with several side holes cut near the top end. The tubing is then tunnelled subcutaneously, if necessary with supplementary small incisions down the neck and across the right anterior chest wall to a secondary incision sited just below the right costal margin.

The peritoneal cavity is opened at this site and after trimming to length and cutting several side holes in the silicone tubing, the latter is inserted into the suprahepatic space and sutured to peritoneum with watertight closure. The wounds are closed in layers.

Trans-sphenoidal hypophysectomy

Definition

Surgical excision of the normal pituitary or pituitary tumours with only limited intra cranial extension, via a transethmoidal — sphenoidal approach.

Position

Supine, in reversed Trendelenburg.

Instruments

As for fronto-ethmoidectomy (p. 509)
  Bi-valve speculum (Hardy modified Cushing)
  Dissector (Angell James) set
  Rongeurs, upward and downward cutting (Love Kerrison)
  Pituitary forceps (Bateman)
  Nasal septum instruments may be required (p. 502)
  Diathermy needle, leads and lead anchoring forceps
  Curved suction tube (insulated)
  Ligatures and sutures as for Fronto-ethmoidectomy (p. 509)
  B.I.P.P. and ribbon gauze
  Operating microscope.

Outline of procedure

This approach is used more frequently now as an alternative to transcranial removal of the pituitary. The normal pituitary gland may be removed for the hormonally-dependent tumour, as in metastatic spread of carcinoma of the breast or prostate, and cases of uncontrolled complications of diabetis such as retinopathy. Tumours of the pituitary requiring excision are usually associated either with Cushing's disease, acromegaly, or pressure on the optic chiasma which may cause blindness.

Figs. 21.46 to 21.51 Instruments for Trans-sphenoidal Hypophysectomy. (Down's Surgical Ltd.)

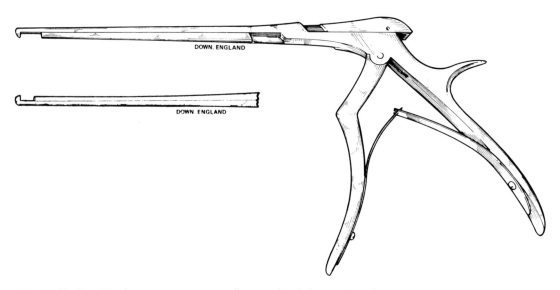

Fig. 21.46 Love Kerrison rongeurs, extra small, upward and downward cutting.

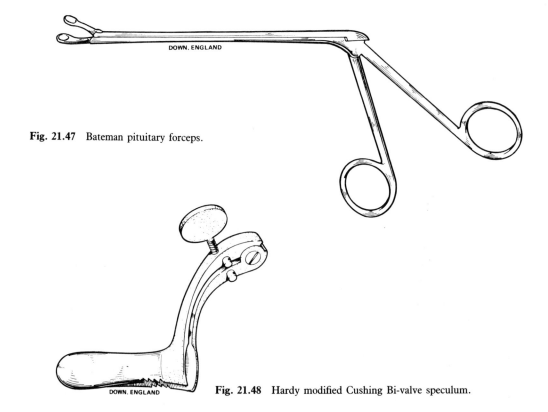

Fig. 21.47 Bateman pituitary forceps.

Fig. 21.48 Hardy modified Cushing Bi-valve speculum.

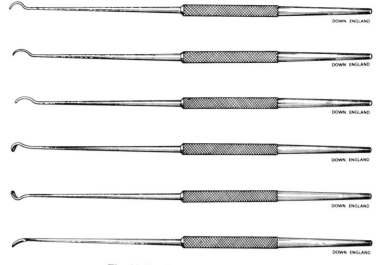

Fig. 21.49   Angell James dissectors.

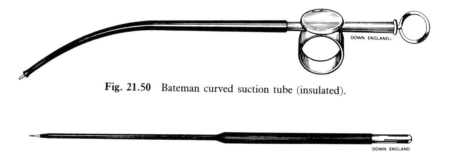

Fig. 21.50   Bateman curved suction tube (insulated).

Fig. 21.51   Angell James diathermy needle.

Ethmoidosphenoidal exenteration is carried out either by the Patterson approach (infra-orbital — Fig. 21.52A), or by the Howarth approach — Fig. 21.52B. The intersphenoidal septum is perforated and removed after exposure of the right sphenoidal sinus, and the operating microscope is brought into use.

A long-handled power driven burr is used to remove the central section of the anterior wall of the pituitary fossa. The burr hole is enlarged with punch forceps.

The pituitary gland is exposed through a cruciate incision in both layers of the dura, the extent being dependent on the size of the extent of the intercavernous venous system. Pituitary dissectors are used to separate the gland which is removed from the fossa with forceps, care being taken to excise all remnants.

The fossa is plugged with a graft of muscle, usually excised from the lateral aspect of the patient's thigh; this is to control oozing of blood or cerebro-spinal fluid. The nose is packed with B.I.P.P. gauze and the incision sutured as for fronto-ethmoidectomy.

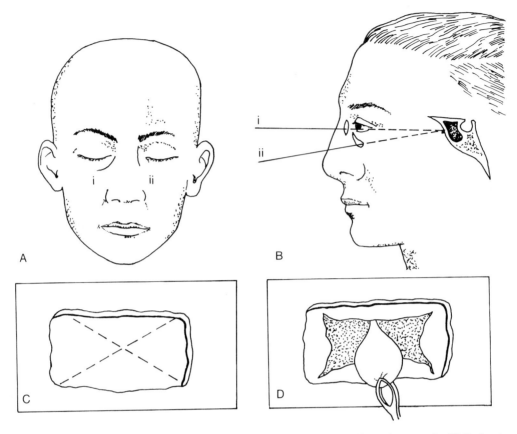

Fig. 21.52 Trans-sphenoidal hypophysectomy. (A) i-Patterson approach, ii-Howarth approach. (B) Perforation of the intersphenoidal septum. (C) Anterior wall of pituitary fossa perforated with burr and aperture enlarged with punch; cruciate incision in dura. (D) Removal of pituitary. (Gillingham: *Neurosurgery*.)

Repair of spina bifida and meningocoele

Definition

The repair of a congenital defect in the vertebral column which allows herniation of the malformed meninges and the spinal cord or caudu equina.

Position

Prone.

Instruments

General set (Figs. 14.1 to 14.28)
Fine artery forceps, curved on flat, mosquito, 25
Fine dissecting forceps, toothed (Gillies), 2
Fine dissecting forceps, non-toothed (McIndoe), 2

Fine tissue forceps (McIndoe), 12
Fine scissors, curved on flat, iris, 2
Long scissors, curved on flat (McIndoe)
Suction tubing, fine nozzles and tube anchoring forceps
Diathermy leads, electrodes, scabbard and lead anchoring forceps
2 (3/0) Plain catgut or synthetic absorbable on small curved round-bodied needles
2 (3/0) synthetic non-absorbable or silk on small curved cutting needles.

Outline of procedure

The margins of the herniated sac or exposed neural disc are feed from the overlying skin which is then retracted gently. The underlying neural tissue is gradually freed from the surrounding fascia on the margins of the lamina defect with preservation of all possible neural tissue. Haemostasis must be meticulous. The edges of the neural disc are then sunk beneath a flap of reflected fascia tailored from the paravertebral tissues. This layer is closed with fine synthetic non-absorbable or silk, plain catgut or synthetic absorbable to secure a watertight closure.

In the case of meningocoele when no neural disc is exposed, after freeing adherent nerve roots from the sac of the meningocoele, the sac is excised, the roots returned to the spinal canal and the sac edges resutured together.

The skin is closed, if necessary with the formation of rotation flaps and extensive undermining, in two layers to give a tensionless three layer closure in all.

Laminectomy

Definition

Removal of laminae, usually to provide access to a prolapsed intervertebral disc which may be pressing on a nerve root.

Position

Knee/elbow, as Fig. 5.23, or lateral, or prone position of flexion with Wilson frame.

Instruments

General set (Figs. 14.1 to 14.28)
Laminectomy set (Fig. 21.53)
Diathermy leads, electrodes and lead anchoring forceps
Suction tubing, nozzles and tube anchoring forceps
Corrugated drainage tubing
2.5 (2/0) Plain catgut or synthetic absorbable for ligatures
1 (5/0) Synthetic non-absorbable or silk on a small curved round-bodied non-traumatic needle for dural tears
4 or 5 (1 or 2) Chromic catgut or synthetic absorbable, etc., on a large half-circle cutting needle for muscle sutures
3 (0) Synthetic non-absorbable or silk on a large curved cutting needle for skin sutures.

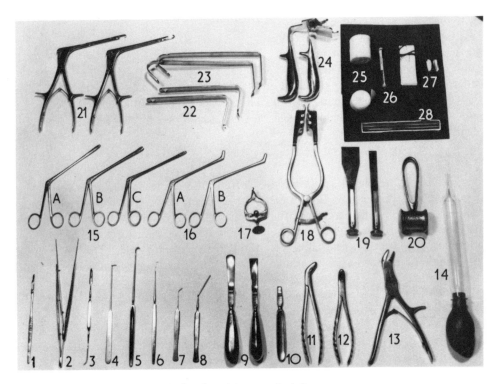

Fig. 21.53 Laminectomy — removal of prolapsed intravertebral disc.

1. Scalpel handle No. 5 with No. 15; blade (Bard Parker).
2. Long fine dissecting forceps, toothed and non-toothed (Waugh), 2 of each.
3. Dissector (Macdonald).
4. Nerve hook, medium (Adson), 2.
5. Nerve hook, large (Love).
6. Nerve hook, small (Adson).
7. Seeker (Horsley).
8. Dura mater separator (Sergeant-Horsley).
9. Rugines, large (Mitchell), straight and round end.
10. Rugine, small (Faraboeuf).
11. Gouge or bone-nibbling forceps, angled on side.
12. Gouge or bone-nibbling forceps, angled on flat.
13. Gouge forceps, angled on side, compound action.
14. Irrigation syringe.
15. Pituitary forceps (Cairn Cushing).
    A. Straight, small.
    B. Straight, medium.
    C. Straight, large.
16. Pituitary forceps (Cairn Cushing).
    A. Angled, small.
    B. Angled, medium.
17. Retractor, self-retaining (Little).
18. Retractor, self-retaining (Adson).
19. Broad osteotomes, 38 mm (1½ in) and 25 mm (1 in).
20. Mallet (Heath).
21. Punch forceps (Duggan), forward and backward cutting.
22. Retractors, laminectomy (Charnley), 2.
23. Retractors, laminectomy (Hibb), 2.
24. Retractors, laminectomy (Penrose), 2.
25. Ribbon gauze 25 mm (1 in) and 50 mm (2 in).
26. Bone wax (Horsley).
27. Patties made from cottonoid, large and small.
28. Plastic corrugated drain.

Outline of procedure

A midline incision is made over the spines of the vertebrae from which the lamine are to be removed. This incision is deepened and the erector spinae muscles are reflected from the vertebrae with a rugine of broad osteotome (Fig. 21.56A).

The dura is exposed by excising the ligamentum flavum with a scalpel and the overlying lamina with bone-nibbling forceps. Retraction on the nerve root exposes the intervertebral disc which, if bulging, is incised with a fine scalpel and extracted with pituitary forceps.

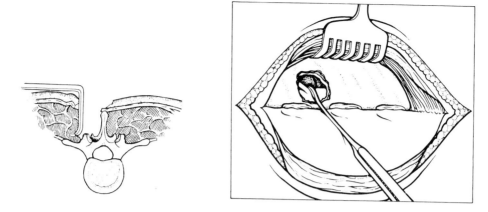

Fig. 21.54 (*Left*) Laminectomy for intervertebral disc protrusion. Stripping of soft tissues from the spinous processes and laminae.

Fig. 21.55 (*Right*) The fenestration operation for intervertebral disc protusion. The ligamentum flavum and the contiguous margins of two laminae have been removed on the affected side. The nerve root and the main theca have been retracted to expose the protrusion of the disc.

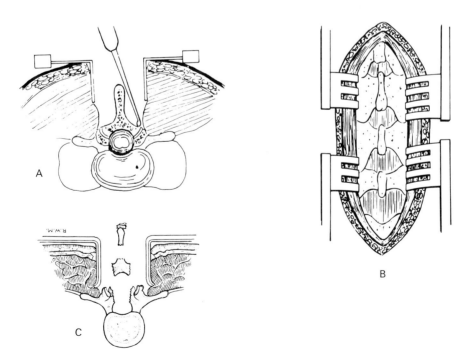

Fig. 21.56 (A) Reflection of the erector spinae muscles from vertebrae. (B) Self-retaining retractors inserted. (Gillingham.) (C) Removal of spinous processes. (Farquharson and Rintoul: *A Textbook of Operative Surgery*.)

It may be necessary to expose a disc space above or below that selected if the findings are inconclusive in the first instance.

The wound is closed with or without drainage.

Excision of spinal cord tumour

Definition

The removal of a spinal cord tumour following cervical, dorsal or lumbar laminectomy.

Position

Prone neurosurgical position with some flexion of the spine; lateral flexed position or laminectomy position (Fig. 5.23).

Instruments

As for laminectomy
Dura scissors (Schmeiden)
Micro instruments (p. 586)
Ligatures and sutures as for laminectomy.

Outline of procedure

A midline incision is made over the spines of the vertebrae. This incision is deepened and the erector spinae muscles reflected from the vertebrae with a rugine or broad osteotome (Fig. 21.56A). Self-retaining retractors are inserted. Sufficient spinous processes and interspinous ligaments, are removed to expose the area of exploration. The laminae are removed initially without disturbing ligamentum flavum.

Further operative stages will depend upon the type and extent of the tumour, but generally the exposed ligamentum and extra dural fat is excised for intra dural tumours by incision of the dura with scalpel and scissors. Stay sutures are placed in the edges of the cut dura to act as retractors and these lie over moist lintine strips arranged along each side of the wound.

The tumour is freed by sharp and blunt dissection together with adherent meninges, and haemostasis is secured with diathermy, gelatine sponge, Oxycel or Surgical. The dura is closed with interrupted synthetic non-absorbable or silk sutures, and if excision of the tumour has left a defect this is covered with gelatine sponge or film. The wound is closed as for laminectomy, with or without drainage.

Lumbar sympathectomy

Definition

Removal of the lower three lumbar sympathetic ganglia and intervening trunk for vasospastic disturbances.

Position

Supine.

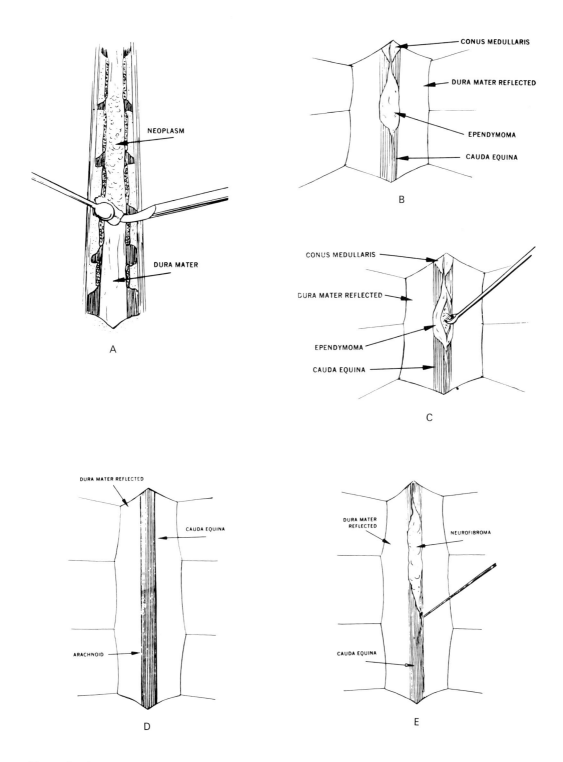

Fig. 21.57 Spinal cord tumours. (A) Extra-dural neoplasm. (B and C) Ependymoma. (D and E) Neurofibroma, the tumour may be submerged under portions of the cauda equina. (Gillingham: *Neurosurgery.*)

Instruments

As for laparotomy (Figs. 15.1 to 15.7)
  Illuminated retractor (Coldlight)
  Long dissecting forceps, non-toothed, 25 cm (10 in), 2
  Long dissecting forceps, toothed, 25 cm (10 in)
  Long scissors, curved on flat, 23 cm (9 in) (Nelson)
  Silver clips and galley (McKenzie)
  Insertion forceps for silver clips
  Ligatures and sutures as for laparotomy (p. 411).

Outline of procedure

The chain of ganglia may be approached by either of two incisions. If the sympathectomy is unilateral, an incision, rather like a kidney incision is made, but rather further forward. This incision extends from the margin of the twelfth rib towards the umbilicus, splitting the external oblique and transversus muscles in line with their fibres in the manner described for appendectomy in Chapter 15. The ganglia are approached by retracting the peritoneum which is not opened.

If the sympathectomy is bilateral, the approach *may* be midline or paramedian, opening the peritoneum anteriorly, retracting the viscera and opening the posterior peritoneum to expose the ganglia situated on each side of the abdominal aorta.

The second, third and fourth lumbar ganglia and the intervening trunk are dissected free and removed after ligating the proximal and distal points with silver clips. The wound is closed in the usual manner for laparotomy.

Division of the sensory root of the trigeminal nerve (Dandy's operation)

Definition

Intracranial fractional division of the sensory root of the trigeminal nerve for the relief of intractable trigeminal neuralgia.

Position

Sitting with the head in a frontal support to afford access to the temporal region and face on affected side (Fig. 5.20).

Instruments

As for ventriculography (p. 558)
  Trigeminal retractor, large self-retaining (Dandy's)
  Brain retractors, malleable
  Headlight
  Blunt meningeal hooks, 2
  Silver clips and galley (Cushing's)
  Insertion forceps for silver clips
  Bone-cutting forceps (de Vilbiss)
  Dural scissors (Dott)
  Ligatures and sutures as for ventriculography (p. 558).

Outline of procedure

A moderate sized temporal craniectomy is made extending well downward to the floor of the middle cranial fossa. The middle meningeal vessels are clipped or diathermised and divided. An extradural subtemporal dissection is made toward the midline until the dural fold overlying the trigeminal ganglion is exposed.

The dura is incised and by blunt dissection with meningeal hooks the sensory root of the trigeminal nerve is isolated and the motor root identified. The appropriate sensory division of the trigeminal nerve is then divided and the temporalis muscle is sutured in two layers after haemostasis has been secured. The scalp is sutured routinely in two layers without drainage.

Peripheral nerve anastomosis

Definition

Secondary repair of an injured peripheral nerve by anastomosis.

Position

Musculospiral (radial), ulnar or medium nerves; supine, with the arm extended on an arm table. Sciatic or popliteal; prone.

Instruments

General set
Fine dissecting forceps, toothed (Gillies), 2
Fine dissecting forceps, non-toothed (McIndoe), 2
Micro dissecting forceps (Figs. 21.26, 21.27 and 21.62)
Micro scissors (Figs. 21.29 and 21.59)
Micro artery forceps (Fig. 21.60)
Fine artery forceps, curved on flat (Mosquito), 6
Fine artery forceps, sharp points
Iris scissors, curved on flat, sharp points
Razor blade breaker and holder (Fig. 21.58)
Razor blades
Plastic tubing or tape for nerve traction
Retractor, self-retaining (Mayo)
Plaster of Paris back slab, or similar splint
Nerve sutures for both operation areas
1 or 0.75 (5/0 or 6/0) synthetic non-absorbable on a small curved round-bodied non-traumatic needle
19 Micron metallised synthetic non-absorbable suture
Ligatures and sutures for an arm operation
2 and 2.5 (3/0 and 2/0) Plain catgut or synthetic absorbable for ligatures
3 (0) Chromic catgut or synthetic absorbable on a medium half-circle cutting needle for muscle sutures
2.5 (2/0) synthetic non-absorbable or silk on a medium curved cutting needle for skin sutures.

Figs. 21.58 to 21.62   Micro nerve instruments. (Down's Surgical Ltd.)

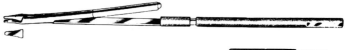
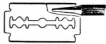

Fig. 21.58   Razor blade breaker and holder.

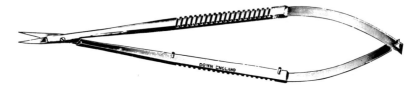

Fig. 21.59   Jacobson micro scissors, straight, spring handle.

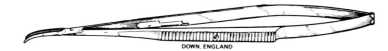

Fig. 21.60   Yasargil artery forceps, serrated jaws, spring handles with catch.

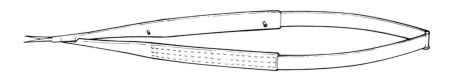

Fig. 21.61   Micro needleholder, straight, spring handles, Tungsten Carbide faced smooth jaws.

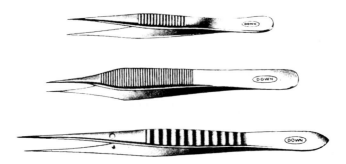

Fig. 21.62   Jacobson dissecting forceps, fine, smooth, straight jaws.

Ligatures and sutures for a leg operation

2.5 and 3 (2/0 and 0) Plain catgut or synthetic absorbable for ligatures

4 or 5 (1 or 2) Chromic catgut or synthetic absorbable on a medium or large half-circle cutting needle for muscle sutures

2.5 or 0 (2/0 or 0) Synthetic non-absorbable or silk on a large or medium curved cutting needle for skin sutures.

Outline of procedure

The incision is made and the muscles split or retracted to expose the nerve. The proximal and distal portions of the divided nerve are mobilised so that they can be brought together without tension. This usually means that the skin incision must be extended and the nerve mobilised for a considerable distance proximal to the division.

The bulbous fibrous neuroma is excised with the razor blade, and 'stay' sutures are placed in the nerve sheath. These 'stay' sutures are used as temporary retractors and to approximate the nerve ends, which are anastomosed with interrupted synthetic non-absorbable or metalised polyamid sutures placed through the nerve sheath only. Care is taken to complete the anastomosis without rotation of the nerve ends. A piece of Millipore or silastic material may be wrapped around the anastomosis to form a protective tunnel.

If the nerve is partially divided, after careful dissection a loop suture is carried out (Fig. 21.66). A large defect between the cut ends of the nerve may require a nerve graft. Figure 21.67 shows a cable grafting technique.

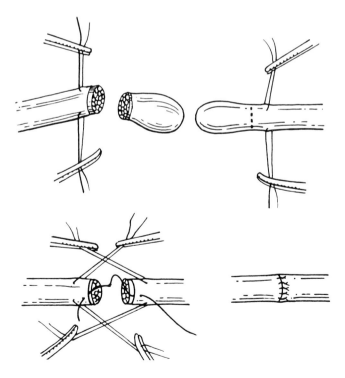

Fig. 21.63 Nerve suture. Note the guide suture inserted into the epineurium at corresponding points on the circumference and held with dissimilar pair of forceps. These help to maintain correct orientation of the nerve ends throughout the repair. (Rintoul: *Farquharsons' Textbook of Operative Surgery*.)

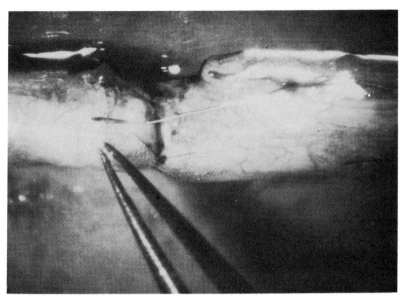

Fig. 21.64 Funicular repair of a digital nerve inserting a metallized polyamid microsuture through the nerve sheath.

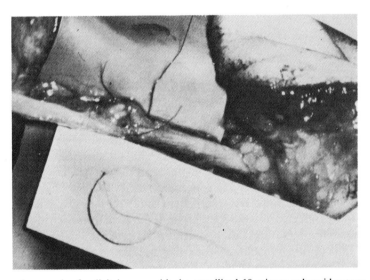

Fig. 21.65 Secondary repair of a digital nerve with the metallized 19 micron polyamid suture. (O'Brien: *Microvascular Reconstructive Surgery.*)

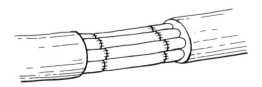

Fig. 21.66 Loop suture used to repair partial division of a nerve. The intact and damaged fascicles are carefully separated and the damaged portion resected and repaired as shown.

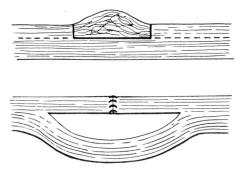

Fig. 21.67 Cable grafting. Multiple lengths of a smaller expendable nerve may be used to bridge the gap in a larger nerve. Shows sutures between epineurium of the graft and perineurium of the fascicles (by microsurgical techniques).

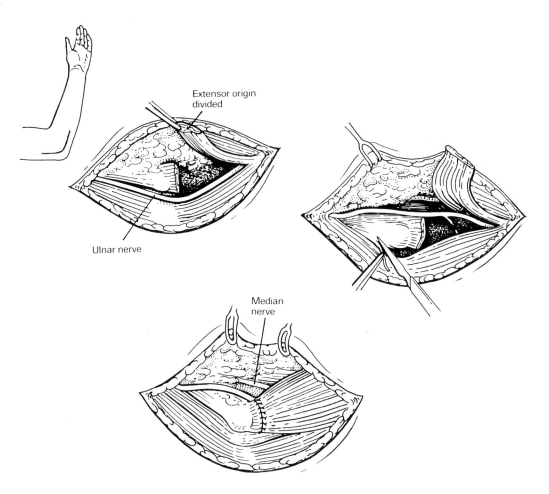

Fig. 21.68 Anterior transposition of the ulnar nerve. The nerve is brought to lie in front of the elbow deep to the extensor muscles and in the same plane as the median nerve.

The muscle is sutured over the nerve and the skin is closed. The limb is immobilised with a splint and bandages in a position which affords the least tension on the nerve suture line.

Transposition of ulnar nerve

Definition

Anterior translocation of the ulnar nerve from its normal position behind the medial epicondyle to a soft tissue channel made medially in the flexor carpi ulnaris, thereby alleviating recurrence of symptoms due to stretching of the nerve.

Position

Supine, with the arm extended on an arm table and small sandbag.

Instruments

As for peripheral nerve suture.

Outline of procedure

A curved incision is made, extending above and below the elbow, with its centre lying over the medial epicondyle. The skin flaps are reflected and the nerve dissected free from behind the epicondyle. Loops of rubber tubing or tape are placed around the nerve which is retracted medially. The flexor carpi ulnaris is partially detached from the epicondyle, and reflected to form a channel into which the nerve is laid.

The muscle can be sutured over the nerve with interrupted chromic catgut, synthetic absorbable or left unsutured and the skin closed with interrupted synthetic non-absorbable silk or nylon.

FURTHER READING

RINTOUL, R. F. (1986) *Farquharson's textbook of Operative Surgery*. Edinburgh: Churchill Livingstone.
GILLINGHAM, F. J. (1970) *Neurosurgery*. London: Butterworth.
O'BRIEN, B. McC. (1977) *Microvascular Reconstructive Surgery*. Edinburgh: Churchill Livingstone.

22

Ophthalmic operations

A very large proportion of ophthalmic operations are performed under local anaesthesia if the patient is co-operative. In small children, restless adults and also major procedures such as retinal detachment general anaesthesia is usually administered. The operating microscope is used extensively (see Chapter 12).

Local anaesthesia consists of installation of cocaine proxymetacaine (Ophthaine), or amethocaine 4 per cent at intervals before operation. In addition, for operations on the eyelids a 1 or 2 per cent lignocaine (Xylocaine) 0.5 per cent bupivacaine (Marcain) is injected

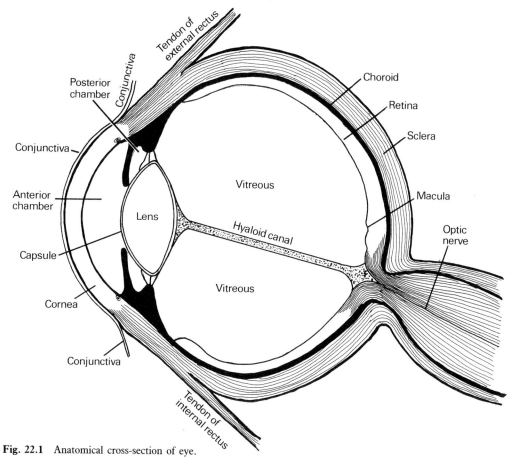

Fig. 22.1 Anatomical cross-section of eye.

subcutaneously. For operations on the eyeball itself and ocular muscles, a retrobulbar injection of lignocaine (Xylocaine), 0.5 per cent bupivacaine (Marcain) is made. The lignocaine (Xylocaine) solution may be combined with 1 in 100,000 adrenaline which acts as a haemostic agent. Local anaesthesia is often used in conjunction with sedatives such as diazamuls, pethidine and phenergan or basal anaesthetics.

Excision of chalazion

Definition

The removal of a cystic degenerated Meibomian gland in the eyelid.

Position

Sitting or supine with head elevated.

Instruments

Sponge holding forceps (Rampley), 2
Scalpel handle, No 3 with No 15 blade (Bard Parker)
Fine dissecting forceps, toothed and non-toothed, fixation
Iris scissors, curved on flat, sharp points
Iris scissors, straight, sharp points
Tarsal cyst forceps (Greene)
Meibomian cyst curettes, 3 sizes
Fine needle holder (Barraquer)
Towel clips (Backhaus), 4
Hand cautery and points
0.7 (6/0) Synthetic non-absorbable or black silk on small cutting needle for skin closure.

Outline of procedure

The cyst is usually removed via the conjunctiva but occasionally through the skin. In either case, the skin overlying the lesion is infiltrated with local anaesthetic, and if the cyst is to be removed through the conjunctiva, this may be ballooned out with local anaesthetic.

A chalazion clamp is applied with the cyst projecting into the ring of the forceps. Approach to the cyst through the conjunctiva is made through an incision vertical to the lid margin, for this type of wound closes readily without sutures. The cyst is curetted unless it is large, or has recurred in which case it is dissected out with sharp scissors or a scalpel.

If the cyst is approached through the skin, the incision is made parallel with the lid margin and is closed afterwards with a few interrupted synthetic non-absorbable or silk sutures.

Ectropion correction

Definition

The correction of an eyelid deformity (usually the lower lid), where relaxation of the skin and muscles of the eyelid cause permanent exposure of the conjunctiva.

Figs. 22.2–22.7 Examples of fixation and suture forceps. (John Weiss and Son Ltd, and Down's Surgical Ltd.)

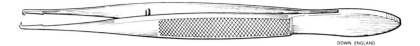

Fig. 22.2 Moorfields non-toothed fixation forceps.

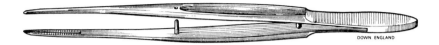

Fig. 22.3. Jayles toothed fixation forceps.

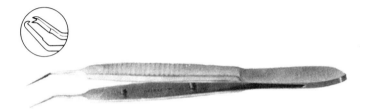

Fig. 22.4 MacPherson suture tying, angled, toothed forceps.

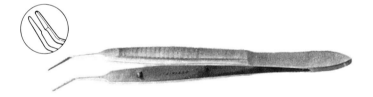

Fig. 22.5 MacPherson suture tying, angled, non-toothed forceps.

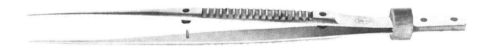

Fig. 22.6 Bipolar diathermy forceps, straight, fine tips.

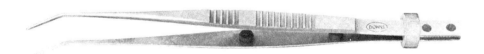

Fig. 22.7 Bipolar diathermy forceps, angled fine tips.

Figs. 22.8 to 22.15 Examples of instruments for eyelid operations. (Chas. F. Thackray Ltd and Down's Surgical Ltd.)

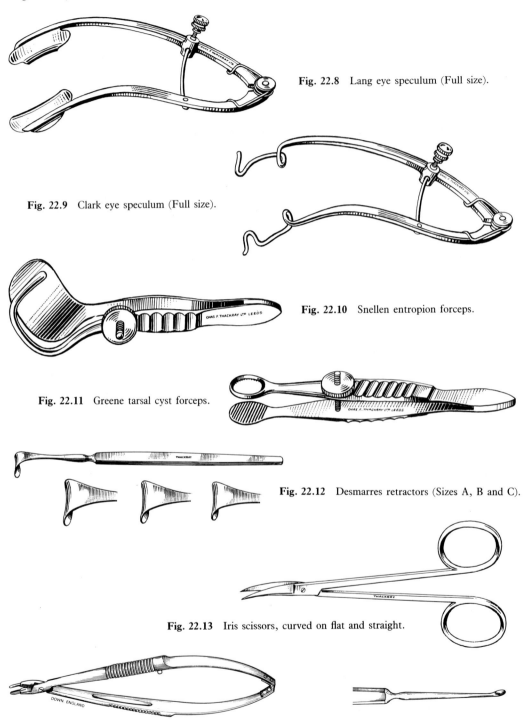

Fig. 22.8 Lang eye speculum (Full size).

Fig. 22.9 Clark eye speculum (Full size).

Fig. 22.10 Snellen entropion forceps.

Fig. 22.11 Greene tarsal cyst forceps.

Fig. 22.12 Desmarres retractors (Sizes A, B and C).

Fig. 22.13 Iris scissors, curved on flat and straight.

Fig. 22.14 Barraquer needle holder.

Fig. 22.15 McHardy meibomian curette.

Position

Supine.

Instruments

As above, plus
  Eyelid retractors, left and right (Clark or Lang), 2
  Fine skin hooks (Kilner), 2
  Mapping pen and gentian violet
  1 (6/0) Synthetic absorbable on small cutting needle for orbicularis.

Outline of procedure

There are several operations for this condition, including skin grafting procedures. Basically the operation consists of tightening the lower lid to correct the abnormal position. One such operation is the V–Y procedure.

Kilners hooks are used to bring together the eyelid skin to a point where the ectropion is corrected. A mapping pen, dipped in gentian violet may be used to mark the redundant fold. An incision is made along the marked line and an arrow headed area excised (Fig. 22.16A).

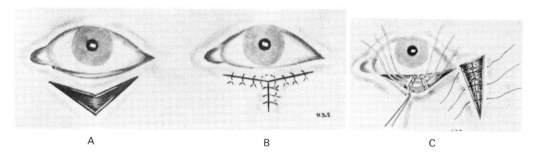

A   B   C

Fig. 22.16 Ectropion and entropion correction, (A and B) V-Y operation for ectropion excision of arrow-headed area of skin which is sutured as a Y. (C) Fox's operation for entropion of lower lid, resection of tarsus, skin and muscle. (Stallard.)

Entropion correction

Definition

The correction of an eyelid deformity where inward rotation or inversion of the eyelid may cause trauma by the rubbing of the lashes on the cornea.

Position

Supine.

Instruments

As Ectropion.

Outline of procedure

There are several plastic operations for atonic (senile) entropion. The objective is to space the atrophic tarsus and atonic orbicularis muscle which have allowed the lid to become too long from side to side. A lid clamp is used to evert the lower lid and a triangular segment of conjunctiva and tarsus excised at the lid margin, and just lateral to the centre of the eyelid.

Fox's operation is an additional procedure in which a triangle of skin, base up and just temporal to the lateral canthus is excised and also an ellipse of orbicularis muscle is resected.

Synthetic absorbable sutures are used to unite the resected tarsus and conjunctiva. The orbicularis muscle is also sutured with synthetic absorbable and the skin incision is closed with interrupted sutures of 0.7 (6/0) synthetic non-absorbable or black silk.

Dacrocystorhinostomy

Definition

The establishment of a permanent opening between the lacrimal sac and the nasal cavity.

Position

Supine.

Instruments

Sponge holding forceps (Rampley), 2
Scalpel handles No. 3 with No. 15 blade (Bard Parker)
Fine dissecting forceps, toothed (Jayles), 2
Fine dissecting forceps, toothed (St Martins'), 2
Fine dissecting forceps, non-toothed (Moorfields), 2
Spring scissors (Wescott)
Fine artery forceps, curved on flat, mosquito, 10
Rougine (Rolletts)
Elevator, muco-periosteal (Traquair)
Hooks (Kilner), 2
Dilator, canaliculus (Nettleship)
Lacrimal probes, set
Punch forceps (Citellis and Duggan or Ferris-Smith), 3
Power driven diamond burrs, connecting tubing or cable
or
Small chisels or osteotomes, 4 mm, 6 mm, 10 mm
Small mallet (Rowland)
Needle holders (Castroviejo and Barraquer), 2
Syringe and lacrimal cannula
pp 10 polythene tubing to cannalicolae, mounted on retrobulbar needle 26 g × 50 mm
Sac Knife
Fine suction nozzles, tubing and tube anchoring forceps
Diathermy forceps electrodes, cable and cable forceps.
Towel clips (Backhaus), 4

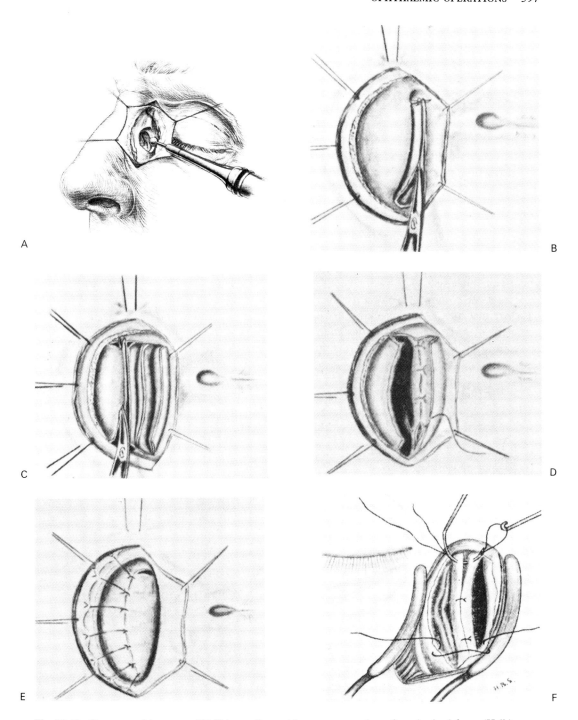

Fig. 22.17 Dacrocystorhinostomy. (A) Using a diamond burr to remove bone from lacrimal fossa. (Hall.) (B) Left lacrimal sac cut transversely at entrance to naso-lacrimal duct. (C) T incisions in nasal mucosa. (D) Suture of posterior panels of lacrimal sac. (E) Suture of anterior panels. (F) Suture of posterior panels of nasal mucosa. (Stallard: *Eye Surgery*.)

1 (6/0) Synthetic absorbable on $\frac{1}{2}$ circle spatulated needle for lacrimal sac and deep sutures
2 (4/0) Synthetic non-absorbable or silk on small $\frac{1}{2}$ circle cutting needle for traction sutures
1 (6/0) Synthetic non-absorbable or silk on small curved cutting needle for skin sutures.

Outline of procedure

A curved incision is made to expose the whole of the anterior lacrimal crest. Traction sutures are inserted to facilitate reflection of the orbicularis muscle, with an elevator, from the frontal process of the maxilla medial to the lacrimal crest. Haemostasis is achieved by the use of traction sutures or haemostasis by diathermy.

The lacrimal fascia is incised and the lacrimal sac separated by blunt dissection from the lacrimal fossa down to the opening of the naso-lacrimal duct. The sac is retracted and 2 to 3 mm of bone removed from the anterior lacrimal crest and lower part of the lacrimal fossa using a power driven diamond burr, or punch forceps. The thin parchment — like bone of the posterior part of the lacrimal fossa is fractured with a blunt dissector, and using punch forceps or a power burr the opening is enlarged, care being taken to avoid damage to the underlying mucosa.

A sac knife is used to make a transverse cut across the end of the sac where it enters the naso-lacrimal duct. After checking the patency of the sac lumen, the medial wall is opened vertically with the blade of the sac knife almost down to the fundus where a T-cut is made (Fig. 22.17B). The nasal mucosa is incised to match the opening in the lacrimal sac (Fig. 22.17C) and the patency and position of each canaliculus checked with a lacrimal probe.

The anastomosis between the sac and nasal mucosa is carried out as illustrated in Figures 22.17D to 22.17F. The orbicularis incision is closed with interrupted synthetic absorbable sutures and the skin sutured with synthetic non-absorbable or silk.

Strabismus operations

Definition

Advancement or recession of the ocular muscles in the treatment of squint.

Position

Supine.

Instruments

Eye speculum, guarded (Lang)
Strabismus hooks (Graefe or Chavasse), 2
Fine artery forceps, curved on flat (Mosquito), 4
Fine dissecting forceps, toothed (Jayles or Fixation)
Fine dissecting forceps, non-toothed (Moorfields)
Scissors straight sharp points
Scissors, straight blunt points
Scissors, spring (Wescott)
Muscle forceps (Prince)
Needle holder (Barraquer)

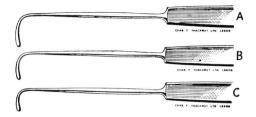

Fig. 22.18   Graefe strabismus hooks. (A) Large;
(B) Medium; (C) Small.

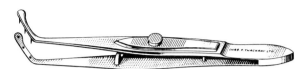

Fig. 22.19   Prince strabismus forceps.

Screw callipers
Rule, stainless steel 15 cm (6 in)
Diathermy forceps, electrodes, cable and cable forceps
Towel clips (Backhaus), 4
2 (4/0) Synthetic non-absorbable or silk on small curved cutting needle for traction
1.5 (5/0) Synthetic absorbable *or* 0.5 (8/0) synthetic non-absorbable or virgin silk on small
   curved cutting needle for conjunctiva.

Outline of procedure

These operations are usually performed under general anaesthesia. Eye muscle action is
weakened by recession and strengthened by resection.
   An eye speculum is inserted, traction sutures are placed just into the sclera, and a cres-
centic incision made in the conjunctiva, parallel with, or at the limbus of the eye. The
conjunctiva is freed from the underlying fascia and insertion of the ocular muscle on the
sclera, to a point well in the capsule tenons on one side, and a strabismus hook inserted
under the muscle. The capsule on the other side of the muscle, where the hook presents
its point, is incised and a second hook introduced from this side. Sutures may be inserted
at the point chosen for division of the muscle to replace it into the new insertion.
   The two hooks are separated, the muscle is divided across at a point near to its insertion
in the sclera, and for recession is sutured to a new scleral insertion usually in the same
meridian as the original insertion, and just behind (Fig. 22.20).
   Where resection is being carried out, the amount of muscle selected for resection is
removed and the shortened stump of muscle sutured to the sclera at the muscle insertion.
   The conjunctiva is closed with continuous synthetic non-absorbable or virgin silk sutures.

Corneal transplants

Definition

Transplantation of a corneal graft from an enucleated eye of another human being in the
treatment of suitable corneal opacities, or irregularities such as keratoconus and keratectasis.

Position

Supine.

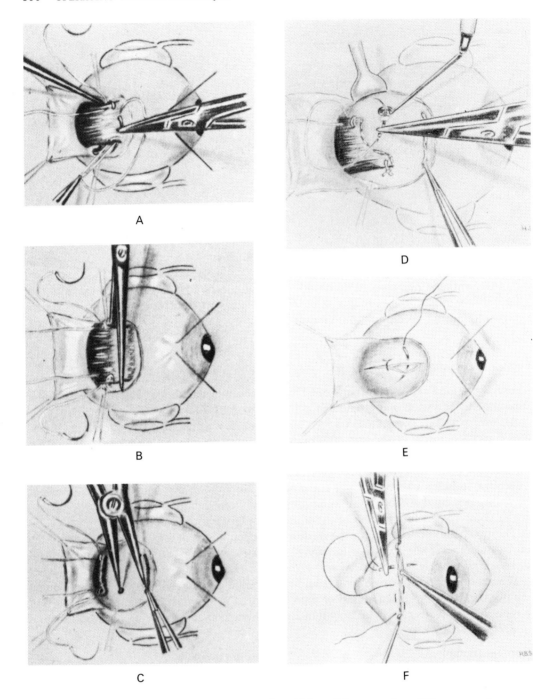

Fig. 22.20 Recession operation for squint. (A) Recession of left medial rectus, edges of Tenons capsule retracted, muscle elevated with strabismus hook, traction sutures being inserted. (B) Division of muscle at its insertion. (C) Marking position of recession with calipers. (D) Suturing muscle to new scleral insertion. (E) Closure of Tenons capsule. (F) Closure of conjunctiva. (Stallard: *Eye surgery*.)

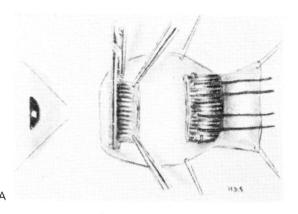
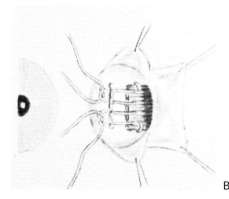

A

B

Fig. 22.21 Resection of left lateral rectus. (A) Muscle for resection held with two pairs of forceps, resection completed with sutures. (B) Suturing of rectus to new scleral insertion. (Stallard: *Eye Surgery.*)

Instruments

(These are the essential instruments required, as there are many individual instruments which may only be of use to a particular surgeon.)

Eye speculum

Lid clamps (Castroviejo)

Scalpel handle with No. 15 blade

Fine artery forceps, curved on flat (Mosquito), 6

Fine dissecting forceps, toothed (Jayles), 2

Fine dissecting forceps, non-toothed, (Moorfields) 2

Fine dissecting forceps (Micro)

Support for donor eye (Tudor Thomas)

Scissors, right and left (Troutman)

Diamond knife or razor fragment in holder

Needle knife (Bowman)

Double-bladed knife or corneal trephines of various sizes

Fine needle holder (Micro)

Ultra fine needle holder (Troutman)

Syringe and Ryecroft cannula

Towel clips (Backhaus), 4

1 (4) Synthetic non-absorbable or silk on small, half circle, reverse cutting needle for traction sutures of rectus muscles

0.7 (7/0) Synthetic non-absorbable or silk on small curved needle with cutting edge on concavity of needle point, for cross-over suture to hold graft in place whilst final sutures are being inserted

0.2 (10/0) Synthetic non-absorbable on small curved needle with cutting edge on convexity of needle point for sutures to secure graft in position.

Outline of procedure

There are many corneal transplant operations, but basically each consists of grafting a circular piece of healthy corneal tissue on to a prepared central area of the recipient's cornea.

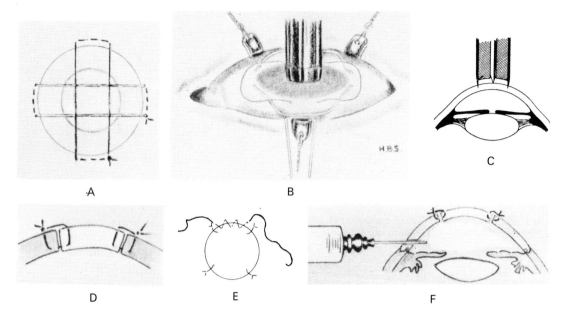

Fig. 22.22   Corneal graft. (A) Temporary limbal indirect graft retention sutures. (B) and (C) Application of trephine to cornea; rectus traction sutures and graft retention sutures in position. (D) and (E) Method of suturing graft. (F) Injection of sterile air into anterior chamber. (Stallard: *Eye Surgery*.)

The operation outlined is that for a full thickness corneal graft. The donor eye is held in a suitable stand, and a graft cut from the cornea using a trephine of appropriate size; the cornea disc remains in the trephine. The trephine is then held over the site from which the graft was taken and the central plunger screwed down to eject the graft, so that it lies with its endothelial surface bathed in the intra-occular fluid of the donor eye.

After insertion of an eye speculum, traction sutures of synthetic non-absorbable or white silk passed transversely through the insertions of the superior and inferior rectus muscles, are used to immobilise the eye with the centre of the cornea vertical to the ceiling.

A fine needle knife is passed into the anterior chamber at the limbus in the upper temporal quadrant, and is quickly withdrawn to avoid loss of aqueous. Sterile air or healonid is injected into the anterior chamber to reduce the risk of endothelial damage from the trephine. Transverse and vertical indirect limbal mattress sutures are inserted as Figure 22.22A to assist in the retention of the graft during its fixation by direct sutures. The epithelium of the donor cornea is normally scraped away with a scalpel blade to eliminate rejection by the recipient.

A disc of opaque cornea, corresponding with the size of the graft is cut with a trephine, gentle and even pressure being applied until the anterior chamber is entered. The trephine is gradually lifted from the circular incision, and any remaining incompletely severed tissue is cut with a diamond knife or razor fragment in a holder or scissors. If scissors are used, these are inclined so that the posterior blade severs Descemets membrane a little wider than the circumference of the graft.

A circular spatula is manoeuvred between the cornea and the iris through the trephine hole and any remaining tags of the Descemets membrane trimmed with scissors.

The graft is gently manipulated into its position in the trephine opening, care being taken

to avoid damage to the endothelium; the surface of the graft is flush with the surrounding cornea. The loops of the indirect limbal mattress sutures are positioned over the graft and drawn sufficiently taut to steady the graft. Interrupted or continuous 0.2 (10/0) synthetic non-absorbable sutures are inserted to unite the corneal graft to the host; these remain in position for two weeks. Air is injected into the anterior chamber, and the suture line is completed with a continuous suture of synthetic absorbable, which is removed after six months.

The temporary graft retention sutures are removed. The upper lid is drawn over the eye and retained in position with tullegras, an eye pad dressing and eye shield.

Iridectomy

Definition

Excision of a segment of iris. This is performed for many conditions, including cysts or tumours of the iris, anti-glaucoma operations, iris prolapse, as part of intra-capsular cataract extraction, etc.

Position

Supine.

Instruments

(Essential instruments only are listed as there are many kinds of forceps, etc., which are personal and only of interest to a particular surgeon.)

Eye speculuae (Clarkson-Lang and Barraquer)
Diamond knife or razor fragment in holder
Fine artery forceps, curved on flat (Mosquito), 4
Fine dissecting forceps, toothed fixation (Jayles)
Micro forceps to suit a particular surgeon
Eye scissors (De Wecker)
Iris scissors, sharp points, curved and straight
Iris hook
Iris repositor (Bowman)
Fine needle holder (Barraquer)
Lacrimal cannula with 2 ml syringe for irrigation (balanced sodium chloride solution)
Towel clips (Backhaus), 4
1 (4) Synthetic non-absorbable or silk on small half circle round bodied needle for traction sutures
0.5 (8/0) Synthetic non-absorbable or virgin silk on small curved cutting needle for conjunctival sutures.

Outline of procedure

After insertion of an eye speculum, traction sutures of synthetic non-absorbable or white silk passed transversely through the insertions of the superior and inferior rectus muscles are used to immobilise the eye in the desired position. A conjunctival flap is made to protect the incision afterwards.

Figs. 22.23–22.30   Examples of iris and lens instruments. (Downs Surgical Ltd and John Weiss and Son Ltd.)

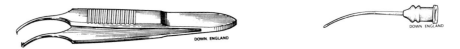

Fig. 22.23   Graft iris forceps.   **Fig. 22.24**   Morrison-Butler lacrimal cannula.

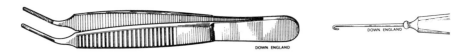

Fig. 22.25   Arruga iris forceps.   **Fig. 22.26**   Bowman iris hook.

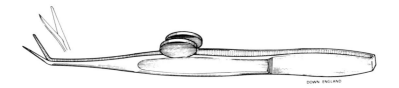

Fig. 22.27   de Wecker iris forceps.

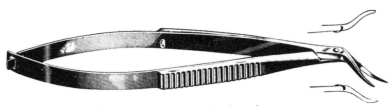

Fig. 22.28   Troutman enlarging scissors.

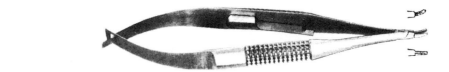

Fig. 22.29   Catford micro needle holder.

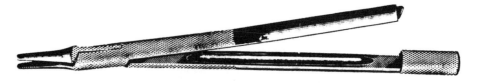

Fig. 22.30   Razor blade fragmenter and holder.

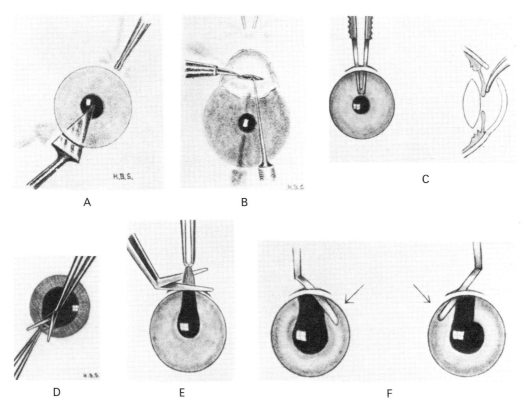

Fig. 22.31 Iridectomy. (A) Insertion of diamond knife or razor fragment. (B) Limbal incision. (C) Iris forceps inserted into anterior chamber in closed position. (D) Narrow iridectomy using de Wecker scissors. (E) Broad iridectomy. (F) Deposition of iris pillars. (Stallard: *Eye Surgery*.)

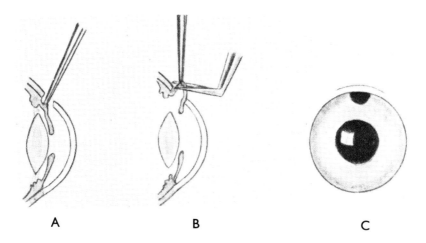

Fig. 22.32 Peripheral iridectomy. (A) The iris root is grasped with von Graefe's straight iris forceps. (B) The iris is withdrawn into the incision and peripheral iridectomy is performed with de Wecker's scissors. (C) Peripheral coloboma after replacement of the iris. (Stallard: *Eye Surgery*.)

Fixation forceps are placed at a point close to the limbus and opposite the site for the limbal incision. A conjunctival flap is raised and a diamond knife or razor fragment is inserted about 0.5 mm behind the limbus and passed slightly obliquely through the cornea. The knife is then withdrawn to avoid loss of aqueous. An incision is made in the limbus and the anterior chamber entered. The closed tip of an iris forceps is introduced into the anterior chamber just beneath the cornea. When the iris sphincter is reached, the forceps are opened and a tiny fold of iris grasped as close to the sphincter as possible. This fold of iris is withdrawn and cut off with de Wecker's scissors held at the lips of the wound. The iridectomy may be narrow or broad (Figs. 22.31A to 22.31F); any blood from the cut iris is soaked up with a small cellulose sponge held over the incision. Reposition of the iris pillars are accomplished with a repositor (Fig. 22.31F).

Any blood remaining in the anterior chamber is washed out with balanced sodium chloride solution and the incisions are closed with virgin silk. Balanced sodium chloride solution is injected into the anterior chamber, the eyelids closed and normal dressing applied.

Trabeculectomy

Definition

Excision of a short length of the canal of Schlemm leaving the two cut ends of the canal open directly into aqueous humour, with no trabecular tissue intervening. Carried out for glaucoma to relieve the outflow obstruction of aqueous humour.

Position

Supine.

Instruments

As for iridectomy plus
    Scleral hook (Cruise)
    Corneal splitter (Tooke)
    Syringe 2 ml
    Diathermy forceps, electrodes, cable and cable forceps
    0.7 (7/0) Synthetic absorbable on small curved cutting needle.

Outline of procedure

After insertion of an eye speculum, a traction suture is inserted through the belly of the superior rectus muscle.

A concentric conjunctival incision is made and a flap reflected over the cornea, to expose the limbus. Episcleral tissue is scraped forwards with an angled cornea splitter. A 5 mm incision is made in the limbus and further radial incisions are made from the ends of this, posteriorly through half of the sclera.

Under high power magnification of the operating microscope, a 4 mm incision is made over the scleral spur to enter the anterior chamber. Using fine forceps to hold the deep corneo-scleral flap, 4 mm are excised with fine scissors.

A peripheral iridectomy is carried out. The scleral flap is replaced and secured by tightening the synthetic absorbable loops before tying. The conjunctival flap is closed with virgin silk and saline injected into the anterior chamber before applying dressings as for iridectomy.

Cataract extraction

Definition

The removal of an 'opaque' crystalline lens.

Position

Supine.

Instruments

Eye speculum (Clark or Lang)
Diamond knife or razor fragment in holder
Eyelid retractors (Desmarre), 2
Fine dissecting forceps, toothed and non-toothed, fixation
Iris scissors, curved on flat, sharp points
Iris scissors, straight, sharp points
Capsule forceps (Arruga or MacPherson)
Eye scissors (de Wecker)
Iris repositor (Bowman)
Razor fragment in holder
Angled corneal splitter (Tooke)
Corneal scissors (Troutmans)
Vectis (Snellen)
Fine needle holder (Barraquer)
Fine needle holder (Castroviejo)
Anterior chamber cannula (Ryecroft) with irrigator (Southampton) for irrigation (Sodium chloride 0.9%)
Chymar, Trypsin, Zonulysin (to digest suspensory ligaments)
Cryo-probe and cryo machine
1 (4) Synthetic non-absorbable or white silk on small half-circle cutting needle for traction sutures
0.5 (8/0) Synthetic non-absorbable or virgin silk on small curved cutting needle for corneo-scleral and conjunctival sutures
0.2 (10/0) Synthetic non-absorbable on small micro point needle for implant fixation.

Outline of procedure (intra-capsular)

This operation may be performed under local anaesthesia, consisting of 4 per cent cocaine conjunctival instillation, retrobulbar injection of 2 per cent lignocaine (Xylocaine) and facial nerve injection of 2 per cent lignocaine (Xylocaine) or 0.5 per cent bupivacaine (Marcain) to prevent the patient from closing his eyelids.

After insertion of an eye speculum, a traction suture is inserted through the belly of the superior rectus muscle. (Fig. 22.33A) The conjunctiva is incised above the limbus, under-mined, and curved incisions are made on each side. A flap of conjunctiva is reflected over the limbus. Half thickness incisions are made in the limbus and pre-section corneo-scleral sutures inserted (Fig. 22.33B).

The episcleral tissue just posterior to the limbus is held with forceps and an incision made with the diamond knife or razor fragment 2 mm posterior to the corneo-scleral junction.

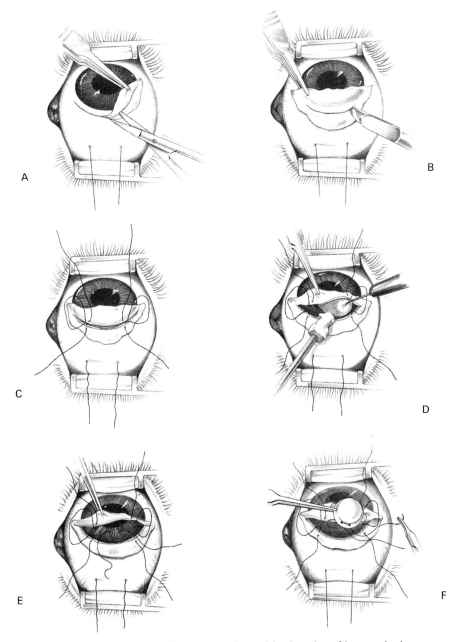

Fig. 22.33 Cataract operation — intra capsular cryoextraction and implantation of intra ocular lens.
(A) Preparation of the limbal-based flap; superior rectus traction suture in place. (B) Ab-externo incision; anterior chamber is not penetrated with knife until several sutures are pre-placed. (C) Pre-extraction sutures in place prior to completion of incision with knife or scissors. (D) The superior rectus traction suture is released and intracapsular cryoextraction performed; pre-placed sutures facilitate prompt accurate wound closure. (E and F) A 0.2 (10/0) synthetic non-absorbable suture (Prolene) is placed through the iris and attached to haptic rim of intra ocular lens. (G) A peripheral iridectomy is performed to permit draining of aqueous from the posterior chamber. (H) Intra ocular lens is sutured into position. (I) Interrupted sutures are placed at intervals to assure a watertight closure. Pressure in the anterior chamber is maintained with air bubbles until suturing is completed. (J) Air is replaced with balanced sodium chloride solution to re-pressurise the anterior chamber. (K) The conjunctiva is closed using a continuous 1 (6/0) synthetic absorbable suture. (*A Digest of Ophthalmic Procedures*, Ethicon Ltd.)

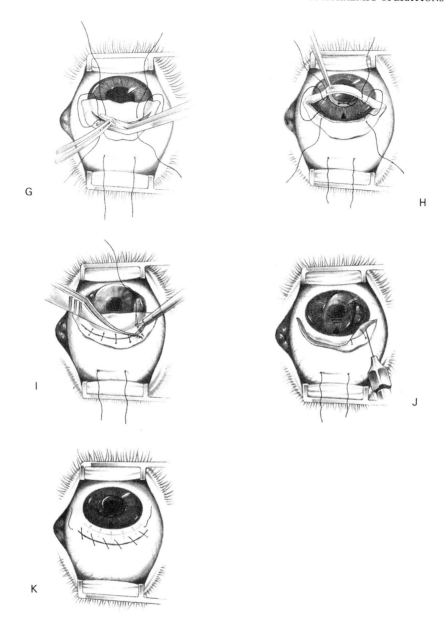

Three synthetic absorbable stay-sutures are inserted to facilitate closure of the corneal flap after the lens has been removed. The corneo-scleral incision is completed with a diamond knife; alternatively corneal scissors are used. A peripheral iridectomy may be performed (Fig. 22.33D).

A fine anterior chamber cannula is used to inject a drop of Zonulysin in the vicinity of the nasal and temporal suspensory ligaments; this is left to digest the ligaments for a period between 1 minute and $3\frac{1}{2}$ minutes. The anterior chamber is then irrigated with saline to remove traces of enzymes.

Because of the greater tensile strength which can be applied, cryo-extraction of the lens (Fig. 22.33D) is the method of choice in preference to capsule forceps. This equipment is described in Chapter 3, page 98.

After the lens has been extracted the iris usually falls into position. The stay sutures are drawn together, and 0.5 per cent isotonic pilocarpine injected into the anterior chamber through a lacrimal cannula to constrict the pupil and prevent forward movement at the vitreous. The corneo-scleral incision is closed with synthetic absorbable, and balanced sodium chloride solution is injected into the anterior chamber (Fig. 22.33J).

The conjunctival incision is closed with virgin silk and the normal dressing applied.

Although intra capsule extraction has been described the procedure can be undertaken by an extra capsular extraction operation. Extra capsular extraction is usually indicated when the lens capsule is fragile as in elderly patients. The initial operative procedure is similar to that for intra capsular extraction. The piece of capsule to be removed is sectioned with a cystotome and then removed with forceps (Figs. 22.34). The lens is delivered with a lens expressor and, the corneo-scleral stay sutures drawn tight. The anterior chamber may be irrigated with saline if any lens tissue or flecks of blood remain.

Aspiration of the lens is accomplished, first by carrying out a capsulotomy through the anterior capsule followed by aspiration with an infusion aspiration machine or co-axial cannula.

Frequently, after cataract operations the surgeon may insert a plastic lens implant into the posterior chamber. One such operation is illustrated in Figure 22.33.

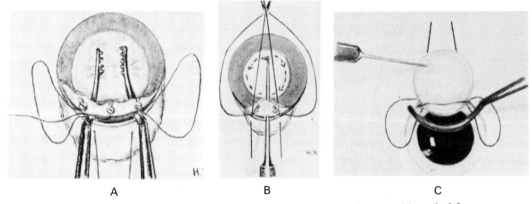

| A | B | C |

Fig. 22.34 Extra capsular extraction. (A) Cataract extraction. Anterior capsulectomy with toothed forceps. (B) Anterior capsulectomy with cystotome. Preliminary to extracapsular cataract extraction. (C) Right cataract extraction. Delivery of the lens by expressor and a cystotome, after which the corneo-scleral sutures are drawn tight. (Stallard: *Eye Surgery*.)

Retinal detachment

Definition

Loss of continuity between the internal and external limiting membranes i.e., detachment of the retina from the choroid.

Position

Supine.

Instruments

Eye speculae (Clark and Lang), 2
Fine artery forceps, curved on flat, mosquito, 10
Fine dissecting forceps, 2/3 teeth, fixation (St Martins')
Fine dissecting forceps, 1/2 teeth, fixation (Jayles), 2
Fine dissecting forceps, non-toothed, fixation (Moorfields), 2
Fine scissors, straight, blunt points (Strabismus)
Iris scissors, straight, sharp points
Spring scissors (Wescott)
Strabismus hooks (Grafe or Chevasse), 2
Eyelid retractors (Desmarre), 2
Eyelid retractor (Fergusson)
Dilator canaliculus (Nettleship)
Caliper
Fine needle holder (Castroviejo)
Bulldog clips, 4
Diathermy forceps, electrodes, cables and cable forceps
Towel clips (Backhaus), 4
Cryotherapy, retinal cryoprobe
Gass indentor, appropriate explant
Fine pen and methylene blue (Optional)
4 (1) and 2 (4/0) synthetic non-absorbable or black silk on small half-circle round bodied needle for traction sutures
1.5 (5/0) Synthetic non-absorbable on small curved cutting needle
0.5 (8/0) Synthetic non-absorbable or silk on small cutting needle for conjunctiva
0.7 (6/0) Synthetic non-absorbable or silk on small curved cutting needle for marker suture.

Outline of procedure

There are many operations for retinal detachment but the principle is to seal the retinal break or breaks. This may be accomplished by cryotherapy, scleral indentation; scleral encircling; or photocoagulation.

Cryotherapy: After insertion of a speculum, a marker suture of silk is inserted to identify the horizontal meridian. The conjunctiva episcleral tissues and tenons capsule are incised to expose the sclera (Fig. 22.35A) and the meridian of the retinal break is marked with a traction suture of synthetic non-absorbable inserted through the episcleral tissue.

Lengths of 2(4/0) synthetic non-absorbable or black silk are passed under the rectus muscles to facilitate control of the eye rotation. It may be necessary to divide a rectus muscle to gain access to a retinal break in the macular region or behind the equator of the globe, especially the upper quadrant.

Utilising an indirect ophthalmoscope the operator visualises the site of the retinal break. A cryoprobe is applied until the tissues around the retinal break are treated satisfactorily (Fig. 22.35C).

After satisfactory treatment it is usual to drain away inter-retinal fluid by scleral incision. This is a very delicate procedure. The scleral incision is closed with synthetic absorbable, and synthetic non-absorbable or silk sutures are used for the conjunctiva.

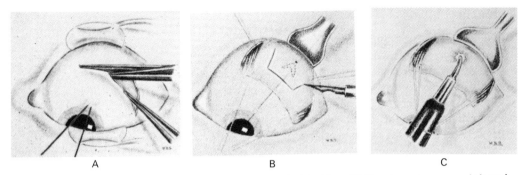

Fig. 22.35 Cryotherapy for retinal detachment. (A) Conjunctival incision. (B) Traction sutures passed through superior and lateral rectus muscles; arms of limbal suture separated position of retinal break and lamellar scleral flap marked with methylene blue. (C) Application of cryoprobe to sclera. (Stallard: *Eye Surgery.*)

Scleral indentation. This consists of an explant which is fixed to the sclera over the site of the retinal break (Fig. 22.36). The principle behind this is the fact that when the sclera is buckled and the retinal break lies against the choroid at the hump of the indentation, traffic of fluid from the vitreous is stopped and any sub-retinal fluid is absorbed through the choroid without the need for a drainage operation.

Scleral encircling. Usually undertaken in conjunction with cryotherapy. The purpose is to create an indent and achieve mechanical block of retinal breaks, and to maintain adequate intra-ocular pressure without risk of hypotony.

A silicone strap is passed under the four recti muscles. The strap is overlapped and secured in a silicone sleeve with synthetic non-absorbable sutures as illustrated in Figure 22.37.

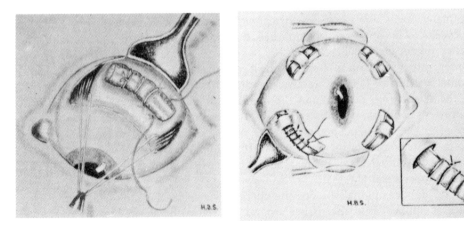

Fig. 22.36 (*Left*) Scleral indentation. Explant is fixed to sclera by two synthetic non-absorbable mattress sutures over site of retinal break. (Stallard.)

Fig. 22.37 (*Right*) Scleral encircling. Encircling silicone band passed through lamellar scleral tunnels in the four quadrants and secured by overlapping and two synthetic non-absorbable mattress sutures in the lower temporal quadrant. (Stallard: *Eye Surgery.*)

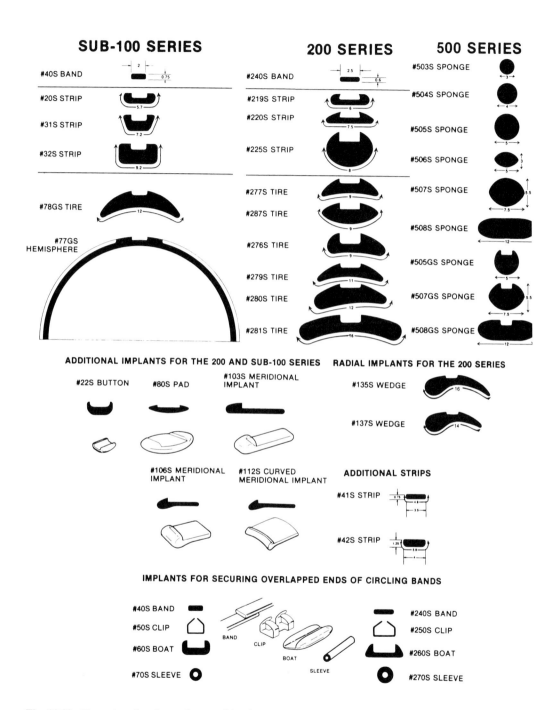

Fig. 22.38 Examples of ocular explants and implants. (John Weiss and Son Ltd.)

Simple enucleation

Definition

Removal of the entire eyeball for disease or injury.

Position

Supine.

Instruments

    Eye speculum
    Fine dissecting forceps, toothed, fixation
    Fine dissecting forceps, non-toothed, fixation
    Scissors (Westcotts)
    Iris scissors, sharp points, curved and straight, 2
    Scissors, enucleation
    Muscle hook
    Snare, enucleation
    Fine artery forceps, curved on flat mosquito, 5
    Fine needle holder (Barraquer)
    0.7 (6/0) Synthetic non-absorbable may be required for muscle sutures
    1.5 (5/0) Synthetic absorbable on a small curved cutting needle for conjunctival suture.

Outline of procedure

General anaesthesia usually administered for this operation.

    The conjunctiva is incised close to the limbus and into the internal and external commissures and into the superior and inferior fornices. The medial rectus, superior rectus, inferior rectus and lateral rectus muscles are divided in that order, utilising a muscle hook and Westcott's scissors. The external rectus is usually cut, leaving a small tab of muscle adherent to the sclera so that a scleral clamp or mosquito artery forceps can be applied to control the eyeball for subsequent enucleation.

    The eyeball is prolapsed from the orbit utilising this clamp, and the enucleation completed either by threading a tonsil snare over the eyeball and optic nerve, or dividing the nerve with enucleation scissors. A snare is never used if the eyeball is perforated.

    The superior, inferior, medial and lateral recti are sutured together in a cross. Haemorrhage is controlled by pressure or synthetic non-absorbable ligatures and the conjunctiva is closed with a running suture of silk.

    Orbital implants such as the Castro Viego plastic implant are now widely used following enucleation.

FURTHER READING

ETHICON (1981) *A Digest of Ophthalmic Procedures*, Livingston: Ethicon.
STALLARD, H. B. (1973) *Eye Surgery*. Bristol: Wright.

23

Orthopaedic operations

Tourniquets

Many orthopaedic operations are carried out in a bloodless field under pneumatic tourniquet. Pneumatic tourniquet cuffs are of two distinct types: those inflated with air directly by a hand pump, and those inflated by a flow of air/gas through an automatic controller (DHSS, 1985).

A correctly applied tourniquet cuff should compress the vessels just sufficiently to stop arterial blood flow, and no more. This entails using a cuff of adequate size; a wider cuff spreads the compression more evenly over a wider area of tissue. If a cuff rolls when inflated it is likely that it is of insufficient width (Spacy, 1985). The use of excessive pressure is not only unnecessary but carries with it the danger of irreversible ischaemia in the muscles and damage to nerve fibres. In most instances this means applying a pressure to the artery of about 50 mmHg (6.9 kPa, 0.5 p.s.i.) above systolic pressure. However, to compensate for the padding effect of muscle and fat, pressures above this level may be required to achieve arterial occlusion. It is important to ascertain the correct pressure which should be used with a particular design of cuff.

A tourniquet on the lower limb should be applied to mid-thigh, well clear of the knee joint; and for the upper limb, it should be placed at mid-biceps level well above the elbow joint. If a tourniquet is applied near to a joint or over a bony prominence, there is little padding effect of muscle and fat, therefore the pressure exerted may damage vessels or nerves by compressing them directly against the bone.

In almost every situation the limb is exsanguinated before inflating the tourniquet cuff. This may be accomplished with an Esmarch's rubber bandage which, after elevating the limb, is applied over a towel from extremity to the level of the tourniquet cuff. To minimise 'tourniquet time', this may be done after the patient has been draped; in which case a sterile Esmarch's bandage is required, which is prepared by being loosely rolled before sterilization in a pack (Spacy, 1985).

An alternative method of exsanguination is to use a pressurised device such as the Rhys-Davies exsanguinator (Fig. 23.1) (Camp Therapy Ltd). This is an inflated rubber sleeve which forms a cylinder, and when rolled onto a limb, produces exsanguination without subjecting the limb to high pressures. The sleeve is permanently inflated to a circumference of 46–47 cm (18–18½ in), corresponding to a pressure of approximately 60 mmHg (8.3 kPa, 0.6 p.s.i.). This is done with a hand pump connected to a hollow needle which is inserted into a concealed valve in the sleeve marked with an arrow. With time, slow air loss occurs, and the elastomer of which the sleeve is made may gradually stretch with prolonged use. In either case, pumping the sleeve up with more air is all that is required. The pressure of the cylinder can be directly checked by attaching the tubing of the inflation pump and needle

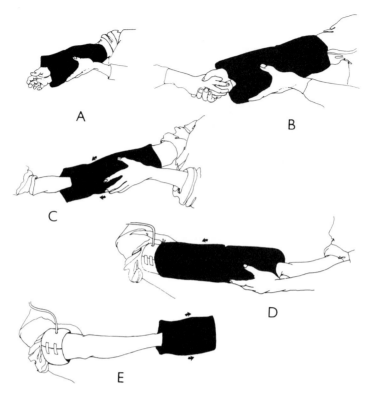

Fig. 23.1 Rhys-Davies exsanguinator (Camp Therapy Ltd.) (A) The patient's limb is elevated for one minute and then the sleeve is rolled onto the operator's arm until his hand comes out of the other end. (B) He then grasps the patient's hand or foot. (C) While pulling gently on the limb, the cylinder is rolled onto it. (D) The cyclinder is rolled up to the level of a padded pneumatic tourniquet cuff (for adult legs, assistance may be required to roll the sleeve onto the wider part of the thigh). (E) The tourniquet cuff is then inflated and the exsanguinator rolled off the limb.

to a sphygmomanometer via a T-connection. In an old cylinder which has stretched slightly, a somewhat larger circumference will be needed to achieve the optimal pressure. The method of application is shown in Figure 23.1.

Manually operated tourniquets are pumped up to the required pressure indicated on a pressure gauge. An example of these is the *Conn pneumatic tourniquet* (Fig. 23.2) (Biomet Ltd). The Conn tourniquet, which should be in direct contact with the skin and *not* applied over a towel, is inflated with the hand pump following exsanguination of the limb. The exsanguinator or Esmarch's bandage is then removed. The pressure applied to an arm should not exceed 275 mmHg (34 kPa, 5 p.s.i.), and to a leg, 550 mmHg (69 kPa, 10 p.s.i.). These pressures take into account the broad design of the cuff, and compensation for the padding effect of muscle and fat overlying the vessel wall.

Automatic tourniquet controllers generally incorporate a mechanism which enables the cuff inflation pressure to be pre-set by rotation of a pre-set pressure control knob. The intended cuff pressure is displayed on a pressure gauge, and at this stage the cuff control knob or switch is at the 'DEFLATE' position. When the cuff control knob is moved to the 'INFLATE' position, the pressure gauge displays the actual tourniquet cuff pressure. Any drop in cuff pressure during use, caused for example by leakage, should result in a drop in gauge pressure. Some automatic controllers compensate for small air leakages or increased pressure resulting from manipulation of the limb.

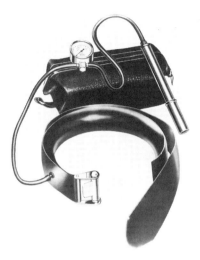

Fig. 23.2   The Conn tourniquet. (Biomet Ltd.)

Automatic tourniquets are available for use with either one or two cuffs, each cuff generally being controlled by a separate gas supply channel. This avoids affecting both cuffs should the gas supply to one cuff be disrupted. Two examples of automatic controllers are as follows:

1. Biomet Control Unit Model 885/A MK2 (Biomet Ltd) is a single cuff controller which is operated either from an external compressed air pipeline/cylinder supply, or charged using a cartridge of Dichlorodifluoromethane (Freon). The integral reservoir, when fully charged, holds 7.2 litres which is sufficient to enable disconnection from the supply line, and hence become portable and self-contained.

There are two pressure gauges fitted in the sloping front face. One gauge indicating the RESERVOIR PRESSURE is graduated from 0–100 p.s.i. (0–696 kPa, 0–5170 mmHg), which gives an approximate guide to reservoir tank content. The pressure relief valve connected to the reservoir tank is set to 'blow' at this pressure. The outer gauge labelled CUFF PRESSURE is graduated in 0–15 p.s.i. (0–104 kPa, 0–775 mmHg).

The tourniquet cuff tubing is connected to the controller by a male 'push on' fit connector. One female connector is provided, for inserting the Freon gas cartridge. Another male 'quick-lock' connector is for fitting a compressed air pipeline hose.

Instructions for use are as follows:

The cuff control switch should be in the DEFLATE position, and the PRESSURE CONTROL rotated fully anticlockwise. If a pipeline or cylinder air supply is being used, the hose is connected until the pressure relief valve operates. The reservoir pressure is allowed to settle at 80 p.s.i. (557 kPa, 4133 mmHg).

If a gas cartridge is being used to charge the reservoir, this is inserted until the reservoir pressure settles between 50–60 p.s.i. (348–418 kPa, 2583–3100 mmHg).

The tourniquet cuff is applied and connected to the control unit. The CUFF CONTROL switch is turned to INFLATE, and the cuff pressure adjusted until required pressure is indicated on CUFF PRESSURE GAUGE. When this is reached, the CUFF CONTROL switch is turned to 'HOLD'; an indicator shows GREEN when the tourniquet cuff is in use. The cuff is deflated by turning the CUFF CONTROL switch to 'DEFLATE'.

2. Braun self-compensating Tourniquet Model SCT (Braun and Co Ltd) is a twin cuff

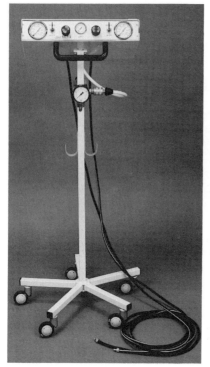

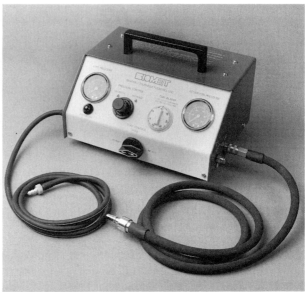

Fig. 23.3   **Fig. 23.4**

Fig. 23.3   Single cuff pneumatic tourniquet control unit operated from a Freon gas cartridge or pipeline/cylinder compressed air supply. (Model 855A, Mk 2, Biomet Ltd.)

Fig. 23.4   Double cuff pneumatic tourniquet control unit operated from a pipeline/cylinder compressed air supply. (Model SCT, Braun and Co Ltd.)

controller which is operated from an external compressed air pipeline/cylinder supply. The unit is mounted on a mobile stand with four anti-static castors.

The front panel has a supply gauge to indicate the air supply pressure. The two cuff control circuits are mounted on either side of the panel and each comprises a rotary knob marked REGULATOR, a switch labelled INFLATE/DEFLATE and a CUFF PRESSURE gauge graduated in mmHg over a range of 0–760 mmHg.

The tourniquet cuff tubing is connected to the controller by push-on tubing mounts. The single high pressure air inlet comprises a threaded male connection on the rear of the unit.

Instructions for use are displayed on top of the controller. For each cuff control circuit, with the switch in the DEFLATE position, the required pressure can be pre-set with the REGULATOR knob. This pre-set pressure is indicated on the CUFF PRESSURE gauge. The tourniquet cuff can be inflated by moving the switch to INFLATE; the CUFF PRESSURE gauge then shows the actual cuff pressure. The controller maintains a stable selected pressure until the cuff is deflated by moving the switch to deflate. Each cuff control circuit can be operated independently of the other.

Generally, surgeons do not leave a tourniquet in position for too long a time. If the limb has been exsanguinated, 1 hour is within safe limits, but for operations lasting much longer than this, the surgeon may release and re-inflate the tourniquet at hourly intervals.

An efficient system of recording the application and removal of tourniquets must be in operation. A tourniquet forgotten and left in position when the patient returns to the ward can be disastrous and result in the loss of a limb.

Skeletal traction (long bones)

Definition

The insertion of pins or wires through a bone in order to apply traction as an alternative to skin traction.

Position

Usually supine, but varies with the site for insertion.

Instruments

As Figure 23.5.
   Splints, weights, pulleys, traction frame, etc.

Outline of procedure

Skeletal traction may be used as a temporary procedure for the manipulation of a fracture during operation, or as a permanent means of maintaining this reduction after operation until the fracture heals. It is used either as fixed traction, or as sliding traction with weights and pulleys, etc., in combination with a splint.

For average adults with a traction of up to 9 kg (20 lb) a Steinmann pin size 4 mm ($\frac{5}{32}$ in) diameter is usually adequate, although for larger patients and a greater degree of traction it may be necessary to increase this diameter to 4.8 mm ($\frac{3}{16}$ in). If the pin is to be inserted with a hand or power drill, it should have a diamond-shaped point; but if a hand chuck and mallet are used, the point needs to be of a trocar shape.

When inserting a Steinmann pin, a small skin incision is first made at the entrance and then the exit of the pin. Each end is then attached to a Bohler's stirrup and the limb is immobilised on a splint in the usual manner.

Kirschner wires are very thin in comparison with Steinmann pins. However, when these wires are maintained under tension in a special stirrup (in a manner similar to a piano wire) the degree of traction obtainable is quite considerable and as a very small hole is made, bone damage is minimal. There are three sizes of wires, 0.9 mm (0.035 in), 1.15 mm (0.045 in), 1.6 mm (0.062 in) in diameter, the larger size being the most popular. Kirschner wires are inserted with a special hand or power drill, having a telescopic attachment which is extended to support the wire. This attachment collapses as the wire is inserted, the wire is stretched taut in the special Kirschner stirrup and splints applied as before. In both cases the point at which the pin or wire enters and leaves the skin is sealed with a piece of cotton-wool and plastic skin or collodion.

For fractures of the femoral shaft, a pin or wire is passed through the upper part of the tibia; and for fractures of the tibial shaft, the pin or wire is passed through the lower end of the tibia or os calcis.

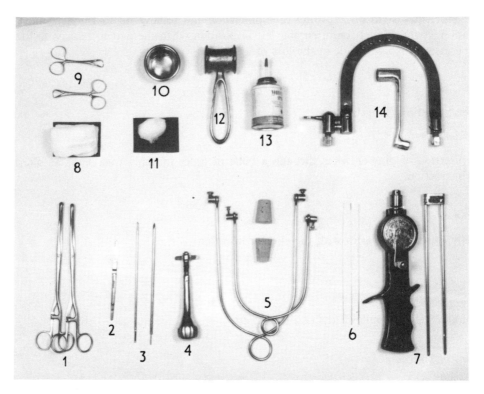

Fig. 23.5   Skeletal traction, Steinmann pin and Kirschner wire

1. Sponge-holding forceps (Rampley), 2.
2. Scalpel handle No. 9 with No. 15 blade (Bard Parker).
3. Traction pins (Steinmann) of appropriate diameter; diamond and trocar points illustrated.
4. Hand chuck for Steinmann pins.
5. Traction pin stirrups (Bohler), and corks for points of pins.
6. Traction wires (Kirschner), 3 sizes.
7. Drill with telescopic guide for insertion of Kirschner wires. (Chuck keys may be required.)
8. Swabs.
9. Towel clips, 2.
10. Gallipot containing skin antiseptic.
11. Cotton-wool for sealing around the protruding pins.
12. Mallet (Heath).
13. Nobecutane for sealing puncture wounds.
14. Traction wire stirrup (Kirschner) and key.

Skeletal traction (skull)

Definition

Traction applied to the skull in the treatment of cervical lesions, e.g., cervical dislocations, by means of a caliper.

Position

Supine, with no pillow.

Instruments

Batchelor's Zygoma hooks
Sponge-holding forceps (Rampley), 2

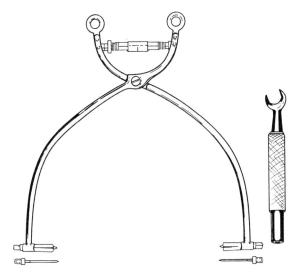

Fig. 23.6   Stratford (Cone) ice tongs caliper. Includes two sets of screw shouldered pins, adult and child; combined spanner/wrench for inserting pins and turning extending nut to accommodate inter-tip distance from 10 cm to 20 cm (Downs Surgical Ltd).

Scalpel handle No. 3 with No. 15 blade (Bard Parker)
Stratford (Cone) Ice Tongs caliper, with screw shouldered pins, and combined
    spanner/wrench (Fig. 23.6)
Local anaesthesia requisites (Fig. 11.60)
Traction cord, weights and pulleys, etc.

Outline of procedure

The ice tongs caliper is regarded as the most satisfactory form of skull traction, for they have little tendency to slip out after insertion.

Under local anaesthesia the penetrating pins are applied about 6 cm above each ear, just in front of the parietal eminence. This is done by adjusting the span of the caliper so that it just clears the skull on each side, and then screwing in the pins until they penetrate the skin. The extending nut is then turned with the spanner/wrench, thereby closing the caliper and driving the pins into the skull to the depth desired. Traction is applied by joining the caliper by cord to weights and pulleys attached to the patient's bed.

The bone and fracture set of instruments

The basic set consists of suitable instruments for the average bone operation. The very small or large bone instruments are added as required, and do not form part of the basic set unless they are in constant use.

Bone levers, hooks and holding forceps are generally used in pairs, especially for the manipulation of fractures. Bone-cutting and nibbling or gouge forceps may have single joints; or multiple joints (compound action), which allows considerable force to be applied with the minimum of effort, and are of great value when the bone is very hard.

Figs. 23.7 to 23.11   Bone cutting/gouge forceps. (Biomet Ltd.)

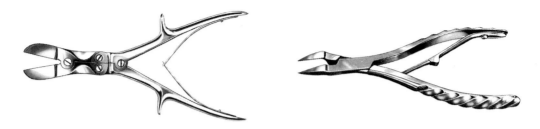

Fig. 23.7   Horsley bone cutting forceps (compound action).

Fig. 23.8   Stamms bone cutting forceps.

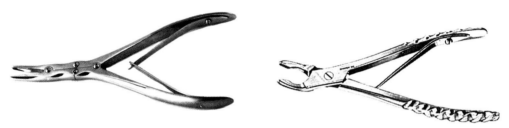

Fig. 23.9   Jansen-Zaufel bone rongeur (compound action).

Fig. 23.10   Wilms gouge forceps.

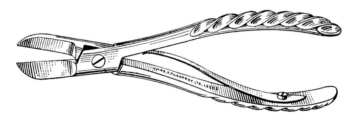

Fig. 23.11   Liston bone cutting forceps. (Chas. F. Thackray Ltd.)

Figs. 23.12 to 23.18   Bone levers, rugines, hook, and curetting spoon.

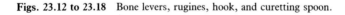

Fig. 23.12   Volkmann curetting spoon.
(Double end. Four sizes A, B, C and D.)

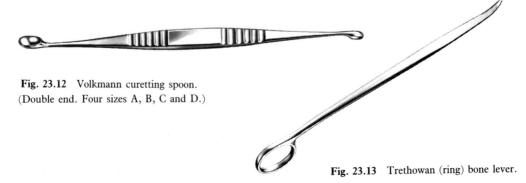

Fig. 23.13   Trethowan (ring) bone lever.

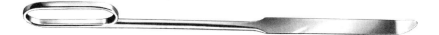

Fig. 23.14   Lane bone lever.

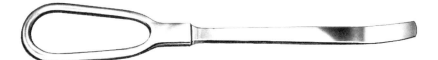

Fig. 23.15   Bristow bone lever.

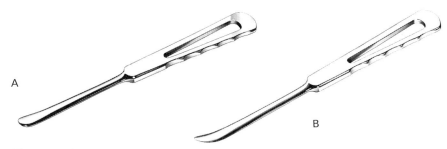

A

B

Fig. 23.16   St Thomas' bone levers.

Fig. 23.17   Faraboeuf rugine.

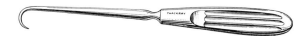

Fig. 23.18   Bone hook. (Chas. F. Thackray Ltd.)

Figs. 23.19 to 23.21   Bone holding forceps. (Biomet Ltd.)

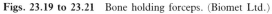

Fig. 23.19   Lane bone holding forceps.

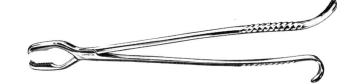

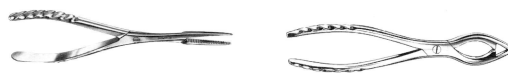

Fig. 23.20   Necrosis forceps (straight).

Fig. 23.21   Fergusson Lion bone holding forceps.

Figs. 23.22 and 23.23 Orthopaedic mallets. (Biomet Ltd.)

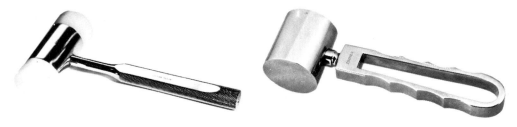

Fig. 23.22 Nylon faced mallet.

Fig. 23.23 Heath mallet.

Open reduction of a fracture

Definition

Reduction of a fracture by open operation.

Position

Dependent upon the location of the fracture.

Instruments

General set (Figs. 14.1 to 14.28)
Cutting forceps, compound action (Horsley)
Cutting forceps, straight (Liston)
Cutting forceps, angled on flat (Liston)
Elevators or levers (Bristow)
Elevators or levers, medium size (Lane), minimum of 2
Gouge or nibbling forceps, angled on side
Gouge or nibbling forceps, angled on flat
Gouge or nibbling forceps, compound action
Holding forceps (St Thomas' Hospital)
Holding forceps (Fergusson lion), 2
Hooks (Lane)
Mallet (Heath)
Mallet (Rowland)
Necrosis or sequestrum forceps, straight
Necrosis or sequestrum forceps, angled on flat
Periosteal elevators or rugines (large), (Mitchell), straight and round end
Periosteal elevator or rugine (small), (Faraboeuf).
(If internal fixation is contemplated, instruments for this are added. See appropriate section, e.g., plating and screwing.)
2.5 or 3 (2/0 or 0) Synthetic absorbable or plain catgut for ligatures
3, 4 or 5 (0, 1 or 2) Plain or chromic catgut or synthetic absorbable sutures on appropriate needle for that area of the body
2.5 or 3 (2/0 or 0) Synthetic non-absorbable or silk on a curved or straight cutting needle for skin sutures.

Outline of procedure

The open reduction of a fracture is performed when adequate reduction by closed methods has been unsuccessful or is impossible; when displacement, angulation or deformity are likely following closed reduction, e.g., fractures of the patella; to promote union and reduce stay in hospital, e.g., internal fixation of fractures of the middle and upper femoral shaft; to reduce mortality, e.g., internal fixation of femoral neck fractures and intertrochanteric fractures.

The fracture is exposed through a skin incision which is sufficiently long to provide adequate exposure with minimal retraction of soft tissues. This incision is generally not placed directly over bony prominences, and the fracture is approached through intermuscular planes rather than through muscle bellies.

The bone is exposed by minimal periosteal stripping and reduction is accomplished with bone levers, hooks or bone-holding forceps. If internal fixation is contemplated, the reduction may be maintained with ordinary bone-holding forceps or the self-retaining kind.

If the fracture has not been fixed internally some type of external splintage will be needed (Chapter 31). Occasionally internal fixation may be combined with external splintage as a temporary measure.

Drills, plates and screws

Internal fixation for bone surgery can take the form of a plate screwed into position on the surface of a bone; a screw passing through the bone to transfix the fracture; or an intramedullary nail or pin inside the bone.

There are very few metals which can be left inside the body without causing at least a severe reaction, if not complete corrosion. The 'noble' metals including gold and silver may be used, but are very expensive and often mechanically weak. It must be mentioned that tantalum is another metal which has been used for implants, but it has been shown that this metal can cause severe tissue reaction (not corrosion) and its use is now rather limited.

There are three metals which have been found suitable for surgical implants, although none of these is regarded as perfect. The three implant metals are: special wrought austenitic stainless-steel, Vitallium and Titanium.

The wrought austenitic stainless steel is manufactured from raw material made in accordance with BS3531: Part 2. It contains 10 to 14 per cent nickel, and 2 to 3.5 per cent molybdenum, in addition to iron residue and traces of other elements. The composition is shown in Table 23.1.

Table 23.1 Composition of wrought austenitic stainless steel manufactured to BS3531: Part 2.

Constituent element	Composition A	Composition B
Carbon	0.080% max.	0.030% max.
Silicon	1.00% max.	
Manganese	2.00% max.	
Nickel	10.0% to 14.0%	
Chromium	16.0% to 19.0%	
Molybdenum	2.0% to 3.5%	
Sulphur	0.010% max.	
Phosphorus	0.025% max.	
Copper	0.25% max.	
Iron	Balance	

There are two kinds of BS3531: Part 2 austenitic stainless steel. Composition A, having higher carbon content than composition B, is used for implants such as compression plates and screws which require a high tensile strength. Composition B is used for permanent implants such as hip prostheses. The main stipulation regarding the raw material is that all deliveries from the foundry are accompanied with a certificate of chemical analysis. This enables the batch to be traced at a later date if required, for example if a defect occurs in the manufactured implant. The material has excellent corrosion resistant properties, great toughness and can readily be worked by machine.

A similar austenitic stainless steel is the AO/ASIF* 316L, which is also a chromium-nickel-molybdenum material. This is prepared to strict tolerances with a special re-melting process, and specific processes for annealing and re-modelling the metal for optimum strength.

Austenitic stainless-steel is non-magnetic, but may become slightly magnetic as a result of cold working such as the drawing process used to manufacture Kirschner wires, Kuntscher nails and Steinmann pins. It cannot be hardened much more than a Rockwell C35 (a degree of hardness determined with a special testing machine) and is therefore not suitable for osteotomes which require a lasting sharp edge.

The resistance of austenitic stainless-steel to corrosion lies in its 2 to 3.5 per cent addition of molybdenum, but equally important are the highly polished surface finish, careful cleansing process, the creation of an oxide surface layer and removal of debris left in the implant during the polishing operations by 'passivating' the implant in a chemical bath, and adequate inspection after manufacture to detect flaws. It is interesting to note that the most satisfactory method of polishing implants is by reverse plating. In this method, which is the exact opposite of electrolytic plating (e.g., chromium plating), debris is 'thrown' off the implant even from the most inaccessible areas such as the threads of screws and cannulations of pins.

Under normal circumstances the protective oxide layer is self-sealing if the surface of an implant becomes slightly scratched. In spite of this, care must be taken to avoid scratching any implant during handling, as a point of corrosion may be set up which could cause severe reaction in the tissues.

It is appropriate here to mention the martensitic stainless-steels which are used in the manufacture of most surgical instruments. These stainless-steels are magnetic and can be hardened to a Rockwell C56 to C60 which is adequate for osteotomes and chisels, etc. Ordinary plated carbon steel can be hardened to a Rockwell C55 to C65 and for this reason some surgeons contend that carbon steel osteotomes retain a better edge than stainless-steel osteotomes. However, with improved manufacturing techniques, stainless-steel is fast approaching carbon steel in quality from this point of view.

Martensitic stainless-steel is rust resistant but it corrodes if left in the tissues and is therefore entirely unsuitable for internal use. A surgeon will take steps to remove a fragment of martensitic stainless-steel which has 'flaked off' from a surgical instrument and become embedded in the tissues.

Chrome/Cobalt/Molybdenum alloy (Vitallium) is a non-ferrous alloy (it does not rust) containing 57 to 63 per cent cobalt, 26.5 to 30 per cent chromium and 4.5 to 7 per cent molybdenum, with traces of other elements. (Table 23.2). The metal is virtually inert in the body tissues and is very strong but very difficult to work by machine. Most implants, even screws, are cast from molten metal because of this difficulty. The tensile strength is in the order of 63 to 66 kgf per mm^2 (40 to 42 tons per in^2).

---

* Arbeitsgemein fur Osteosynthesefragen (Association for the study of Problems of Internal Fixation — AO/ASIF)

Table 23.2 Composition of Chrome/Cobalt/Molybdenum alloy manufactured to BS3531

Constituent element	%
Chromium	26.5% to 30.0%
Molybdenum	4.5% to 7.0%
Iron	1.0% max.
Carbon	0.35% max.
Nickel	2.5% max.
Silicon	1.0 max.
Manganese	1.0 max.
Aluminium	0.14% max.
Titanium	0.14% max.
Cobalt	Balance

Non-ferrous alloys do not rely upon a high surface polish for part of their corrosion resistance, and slight damage to the surface is not quite so important as with the stainless-steels. But this does not mean that any less care should be taken during handling, for a highly polished smooth surface of an implant may be essential, e.g., for arthroplasty of joints.

Titanium alloy used for surgical implants contains about 90 per cent pure Titanium, the remaining elements varying in proportion according to the type of implant. The alloy contains also aluminium and vanaxium, and traces of oxygen, iron, and hydrogen. Commercially pure *titanium* is available as a series of oxygen alloys with a range of malleability (Table 23.3). Grade 5 has the greatest malleability, Grade 1 the lowest. Grade 5 is used for the manufacture of implants which require contouring during operation, e.g. mandibular implants. Grade 1 is employed for small bone plates.

Unlike austenitic stainless-steels, Titanium cannot be 'work hardened' by machining or cold drawing, so that the high tensile strength achieved in cold drawn stainless-steel wire as used for staples, Kirschner wires, Steinmann pins, Rush type pins cannot be reproduced in Titanium. However those implants usually made from the annealed material of stainless-steel, have less tensile strength and yield point (or ductility) as compared with Titanium before permanent deformation of the implant occurs under stress.

Table 23.3 Composition of Titanium and Titanium alloy manufactured to BS3531

Constituent element	Grades T1,T2,T3,T4,T5	Grade TA1
Oxygen	0.50% max.	0.20% max.
Iron	0.20% max.	0.30% max.
Aluminium	–	5.5–6.75%
Vanaxium	–	3.5–4.5%
Titanium	Balance	Balance
Carbon	Raw materials used for the production of an ingot shall contain not more than 0.08% Carbon	
Hydrogen	Plate, sheet, strip, bar and section for machining, wire forging stock forgings	0.0125% max. 0.010% max. 0.015% max.

Implants suitable for manufacture in Titanium include, hip prostheses, hip nails, bone plates and screws. For its strength the metal is exceptionally light, being about half the weight of the equivalent size in stainless-steel. It is extremely inert and resistant to corrosion by body tissue and fluids. Its ultimate tensile strength can be as high as 95 kgf per mm^2 (60 tons per in^2) but on average is in the region of 70 kgf to 79 kgf per mm^2 (44 to 50 tons per in^2). Titanium has been used clinically since 1957 and as a result of many papers on its successful use it is for some purposes replacing the other metallic implant materials.

Different metals should not be used in contact with one another in the body. Although all three metals described are relatively inert when used alone, severe reactions can occur if, for instance, a stainless-steel screw is used in contact with a chrome/cobalt/molybdenum (Vitallium) plate. This reaction is said to be partially an electrolytic and partially a chemical process. Whatever the cause, the end result is corrosion of the implant, and often non-union of the fracture or a discharging wound. *The scrub nurse must ensure that she does not give the surgeon implants made from different metals and which are to be used in contact with one another in the tissues.* Similarly, implants from different manufacturers should not be combined, e.g. screws from one source, plates from another. Even though the metals of each may be similar, different manufacturing processes could result in incompatibility.

It is possible for small fragments of metal to 'flake off' from instruments used for the insertion of implants. For this reason, it is desirable that all instruments used for handling implants are made from or tipped with the same metal as the implant; otherwise small fragments of metal may be transferred from the insertion instruments and set up local points of corrosion in the tissues. This is especially so with screwdrivers, which may slip off the screw during insertion.

Drills

Bone drills are made from three materials, martensitic stainless-steel, Vitallium and plated carbon steel. The first two types of drills are sterilized by steam, but the carbon steel drills must be dry-heat sterilized.

Drill points must be kept sharp and at slightly less than the 45 degrees angle point of the conventional industrial drills. If the drill shaft is not straight, or has been incorrectly aligned in the drill chuck, the result will be an oval hole in the bone. Correct alignment is checked by looking along the drill shaft as the chuck is rotated. A drill end (up to 6.4 mm ($\frac{1}{4}$ in) in diameter) should appear as a point about the size of a full stop on this page. A blunt drill appears as a larger point, and a wobbling drill as an oval-shaped point. In this case the drill must be re-aligned in the chuck, or discarded for straightening and re-sharpening before further use.

Vitallium drills appear to have several advantages over the other two types. They are rustless, have lasting sharpness and a safety feature — the ability to bend considerably without breaking.

Screws

Bone screws have threads which either extend for the full length of the screw or for only three-quarters of the length. Sherman 'self-tapping' screws have a fine pitch thread requiring a relatively large hole to be predrilled for the screw. Only the tips of the threads engage the bone. AO screws feature an asymmetric thread which ensures an improved hold (Figs. 23.30 and 23.33). This type of thread has been chosen for the AO system because the strength of bone is about ten times less than that of metal. Using an asymmetric thread means that

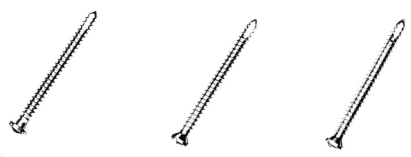

Fig. 23.24   Sherman bone screws. (Full size approx.)
Composition A. Stainless steel, Titanium or Vitallium.
Fine and coarse thread, with self-tapping point and single or cross slotted head.
Supplied in two diameters: 3.6 mm ($\frac{9}{64}$ in) and 4 mm ($\frac{5}{32}$ in).
Lengths available in 10 mm to 51 mm in approx. 3 mm steps, 57 mm, 64 mm, 70 mm, 76 mm, 83 mm, 89 mm, 95 mm and 102 mm.
$\frac{3}{8}$ to 2 in, in $\frac{1}{8}$ in steps, $2\frac{1}{4}$, $2\frac{1}{2}$, $2\frac{3}{4}$, 3, $3\frac{1}{4}$, $3\frac{1}{2}$, $3\frac{3}{4}$ and 4 in.

Technical data —
$\frac{9}{64}$ in (3.6 mm) diameter screws:
   Head diameter: $\frac{15}{64}$ in (.234 in or 5.9 mm).
   Outside thread diameter: $\frac{9}{64}$ in (.140 in or 3.6 mm).
   Root thread diameter: $\frac{7}{64}$ in (.109 in or 2.8 mm).
   Threads per inch (fine thread): 32
   Threads per inch (coarse thread): 20
   Recommended drill size. No. 31 (.120 in or 3 mm).

$\frac{5}{32}$ in (4 mm) diameter screws:
   Head diameter: $\frac{9}{32}$ in (.281 in or 7.1 mm).
   Outside thread diameter: $\frac{5}{32}$ in (.156 in or 4 mm).
   Root thread diameter: just under $\frac{1}{8}$ in (.116 in or 2.9 mm).
   Threads per inch (fine thread): 32.
   Threads per inch (coarse thread): 20.
   Recommended drill size: $\frac{9}{64}$ in (.140 in or 3.6 mm).

A   B   C   D

Fig. 23.25   Varieties of screw heads (enlarged views).

A. Single slot, available in all varieties of screws; composition A Stainless steel, Titanium and Vitallium.
B. Crosss slot, available in Sherman screws composition A. Stainless steel and Titanium.
C. Hexagonal recessed slot.

D. Phillips recessed head, available in Phillips screws Vitallium, which have an identical shaft to $\frac{9}{64}$ in diameter Sherman screws. (These are available as Duo Drive screws on which a single slot, suitable for an ordinary screwdriver, is superimposed over the cross recess.

Supplied in one diameter: 4.4 mm ($\frac{11}{64}$ in).
Lengths available: 45 mm ($1\frac{3}{4}$ in), 51 mm (2 in), 57 mm ($2\frac{1}{4}$ in), and 64 mm ($2\frac{1}{2}$ in), (Vitallium); 45 mm ($1\frac{3}{4}$ in), 51 mm (2 in), 57 mm ($2\frac{1}{4}$ in), 64 mm ($2\frac{1}{2}$ in), 70 mm ($2\frac{3}{4}$ in), and 76 mm (3 in), Composition A.

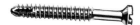

Fig. 23.26   Transfixion screw.

Composition A. Stainless steel, Titanium or Vitallium.
Partially coarse thread with self-tapping point and single slotted head.

Technical data–
Head diameter: $\frac{9}{32}$ in (.116 in or 2.9 mm).
Outside thread diameter: just over $\frac{11}{64}$ in (.177 in or 4.5 mm).
Root thread diameter: just under $\frac{9}{64}$ in (.135 in or 3.4 mm).
Threads per inch: 20 (s/s); 18 (Vitallium).
Recommended drill size: $\frac{9}{64}$ in (.140 in or 3.6 mm).

Figs. 23.24 to 23.26   Bone screws. (Biomet Ltd.)

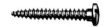

Fig. 23.27 Wood type thread bone screws
Composition A Stainless steel, Titanium or Vitallium.
Fully and partially coarse threaded with tapered point, single slotted head.
  Supplied in two diameters: 2.8 mm ($\frac{7}{64}$ in) Vitallium, and 3.6 mm ($\frac{9}{64}$ in) composition A stainless steel Titanium or Vitallium.
  Lengths available: 2.8 mm ($\frac{7}{64}$ in) diameter, 10 mm ($\frac{3}{8}$ in), 13 mm ($\frac{1}{2}$ in), 16 mm ($\frac{5}{8}$ in) and 19 mm ($\frac{3}{4}$ in);
    3.6 mm ($\frac{9}{64}$ in) diameter, 19 mm ($\frac{3}{4}$ in), 22 mm ($\frac{7}{8}$ in), 25 mm (1 in), 29 mm ($1\frac{1}{8}$ in), 32 mm ($1\frac{1}{4}$ in), 38 mm
    ($1\frac{1}{2}$ in) and 38 mm ($1\frac{1}{2}$ in) and 45 mm ($1\frac{3}{4}$ in).

Technical data —

2.8 mm ($\frac{7}{64}$ in) diameter screws:
Head diameter: $\frac{1}{4}$ in (.25 in or 6.4 mm).
Outside thread diameter: $\frac{5}{64}$ in (.109 in or 2.8 mm).
Root thread diameter: $\frac{5}{64}$ in approx. (.078 in or 2 mm).
Threads per inch: 22.
Recommended drill size: $\frac{3}{32}$ in (.093 in or 2.4 mm).

3.6 mm ($\frac{9}{64}$ in) diameter screws:
Head diameter: $\frac{15}{64}$ in (.234 in or 5.9 mm).
Outside diameter: in (.140 in or 3.6 mm).
Root thread diameter: just under $\frac{7}{64}$ in (.100 in or 2.5 m).
Threads per inch: 20
Recommended drill size: $\frac{7}{64}$ in (.109 in or 2.8 mm).

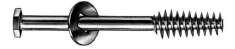

Fig. 23.28 Johannson lag screw
Composition A. Stainless steel or Vitallium.
Very coarse thread for one-third of shaft approximately tapered point, single slotted hexagon head.
Supplied in one shaft diameter: 4 mm ($\frac{5}{32}$ in).
Lengths available: 41 mm ($1\frac{5}{8}$ in), 57 mm ($2\frac{1}{4}$ in) and 76 mm (3 in).

Technical data —
  Head diameter: $\frac{5}{16}$ in A/f hexagon (.312 in or 8 mm).
  Outside thread diameter: $\frac{11}{32}$ in (.343 in or 8.7 mm) tapering to about $\frac{3}{16}$ in (.187 in or 4.8 mm).
  Root thread diameter (shaft): $\frac{5}{32}$ in (.156 in or 3.9 mm).
  Threads per inch: 10.
  Recommended drill size: $\frac{3}{16}$ in (.187 in or 4.8 mm) for about $\frac{1}{8}$ in through the bone cortex followed by $\frac{5}{32}$ in.
    (.156 in or 4 mm) for total depth of screw being inserted.

Figs. 23.27 and 23.28   Bone screws (*cont'd.*)

the weaker the bone, the more space is left for it between the threads, and the thinner the resultant thread profile. In hard bone though, the thread must be pre-cut with a tap which also removes cutting debris.

  The screw slot varies in shape within four varieties: the plain slot, the Phillip's recessed head/Duodrive, the cruciform or cross slot and the hexagonal slot (AO system). A standard shape of screwdriver is used for the first variety but a special 'cross point' screwdriver must be used for the second and third variety, and a screwdriver with a hexagonal head for the AO screws.

  Sherman, Phillips and cruciform screws used for holding bone plates in position are of two main diameters, 3.6 mm ($\frac{9}{16}$ in) and 4 mm ($\frac{5}{32}$ in). AO screws used with bone plates are generally 4.5 mm diameter; other sizes ranging from 3.5 mm to 1.5 mm diameter are for special application. The AO fixation system is described later in this chapter.

As the screw always passes through both cortices in the fixation of bone plates, this type of screw is fully threaded in order that the threads may gain the greatest purchase in both sides of the bone.

Screws used alone for the fixation of bone fragments are partially threaded and termed 'wood or transfixion' screws. In this case the screw is usually inserted through the fragment and into the area of cancellous bone adjacent, e.g., fracture of the medial malleolus. The partially threaded portion of the screw near the head allows the surgeon to 'draw up' the loose fragment against the larger one without causing the bone to split.

The holding power of a screw having conventional Sherman-type threads is almost at its maximum in bone when the size of the hole drilled is approximately equivalent to half the distance between the outside diameter and root diameter of the screw threads. Therefore, the hole drilled in cortical bone should approximate 85 per cent of the outside diameter of the screw. This obviates both the weak holding power of larger holes and the tendency of the screws to split the bone with smaller holes. However, when the bone is of a soft composition, i.e., cancellous bone, the hole drilled should be only slightly larger than the root diameter of the threads.

For a 2.8 mm ($\frac{7}{64}$ in) diameter screw, size No. 9, 2.4 mm ($\frac{3}{32}$ in) diameter drill is used; 3.6 mm ($\frac{9}{64}$ in) diameter screws require a size No. 31 approx. 2.8 mm ($\frac{7}{64}$ in) diameter drill; 4 mm ($\frac{5}{32}$ in) diameter screws require a 3.6 mm ($\frac{9}{64}$ in) or 3.2 mm ($\frac{1}{8}$ in) diameter drill; and 4.5 mm approx. ($\frac{11}{64}$ in) diameter screws require a 4 mm ($\frac{5}{32}$ in) or 3.6 mm ($\frac{9}{64}$ in) diameter drill.

After drilling a hole the surgeon measures its depth with a screw measure. This measure has a hooked end with which he feels the outer edge of the hole in the opposite cortex. The handle of the instrument is then slid down to touch the proximal cortex and the depth read off against a scale engraved on the handle.

If the surgeon does not wish to drill right through the bone, the depth of the hole is determined by probing the bottom with his measure and reading off the scale as before.

A self-retaining or automatic screwdriver is used to insert the screw up to 6.4 mm ($\frac{1}{4}$ in) from the head. The Williams or Burns are probably the ones most popular for standard single-slot screws. Alternatively there are a number of power operated screwdrivers including the Stryker bit which fits into the Stryker power tool and the 3M Air Driver.

The Williams screwdriver is adjustable for various sizes of screw heads by means of the large screw connected to the retaining lever on the handle (illustrated in Figs. 23.38 and 23.57). When loading screws, care must be taken to avoid force as the lever is closed. The adjusting screw must be altered until the lever closes easily with the screw in position. Failure to do this will result in breakage of the sleeve which supports the screw head. Both the Williams and the Burns screwdrivers must be dismantled, cleaned, lubricated regularly and sent for repair when the tip becomes worn and does not fit snugly into the screw head.

The screw is finally tightened home with a plain-end screwdriver, such as Lane's which must fit tightly into the screw slot. Nothing is more irritating than a screwdriver which keeps slipping out of the slot as the screw is driven home, and in addition, there is a grave danger of scratching the screw, with risk of corrosion.

Plates

Bone plates are designed to provide maximum strength with minimal dimensions, although no plate will take full weight bearing until the fracture has almost healed. Plates may be contoured slightly to accommodate the curvature of a bone, but if greater angles are needed, the manufacturer will incorporate these when the implant is cast or machined. Once a plate

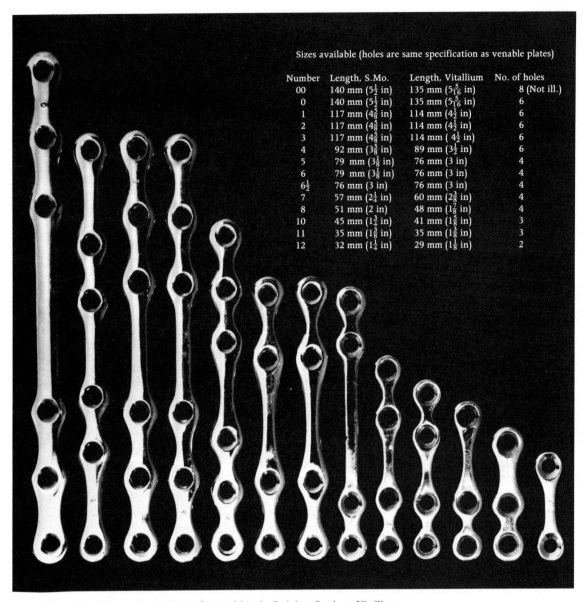

Sizes available (holes are same specification as venable plates)

Number	Length, S.Mo.	Length, Vitallium	No. of holes
00	140 mm ($5\frac{1}{2}$ in)	135 mm ($5\frac{5}{16}$ in)	8 (Not ill.)
0	140 mm ($5\frac{1}{2}$ in)	135 mm ($5\frac{5}{16}$ in)	6
1	117 mm ($4\frac{5}{8}$ in)	114 mm ($4\frac{1}{2}$ in)	6
2	117 mm ($4\frac{5}{8}$ in)	114 mm ($4\frac{1}{2}$ in)	6
3	117 mm ($4\frac{5}{8}$ in)	114 mm ($4\frac{1}{2}$ in)	6
4	92 mm ($3\frac{5}{8}$ in)	89 mm ($3\frac{1}{2}$ in)	6
5	79 mm ($3\frac{1}{8}$ in)	76 mm (3 in)	4
6	79 mm ($3\frac{1}{8}$ in)	76 mm (3 in)	4
$6\frac{1}{2}$	76 mm (3 in)	76 mm (3 in)	4
7	57 mm ($2\frac{1}{4}$ in)	60 mm ($2\frac{3}{8}$ in)	4
8	51 mm (2 in)	48 mm ($1\frac{7}{8}$ in)	4
10	45 mm ($1\frac{3}{4}$ in)	41 mm ($1\frac{5}{8}$ in)	3
11	35 mm ($1\frac{3}{8}$ in)	35 mm ($1\frac{3}{8}$ in)	3
12	32 mm ($1\frac{1}{4}$ in)	29 mm ($1\frac{1}{8}$ in)	2

Fig. 23.29 Sherman bone plates. Composition A. Stainless Steel, or Vitallium.

has been contoured, it must not be re-bent in the reverse direction, otherwise metal fatigue may occur.

Plates such as Sherman's, Venable's, Lane's and AO straight standard plates have round holes for screw fixation, but there are other types such as AO dynamic compression plates (DCP) which have elongated holes to facilitate compression techniques.

In order to minimise bacterial contamination of implants such as screws and plates, etc., these should always be handled with sterile forceps and not the gloved hands.

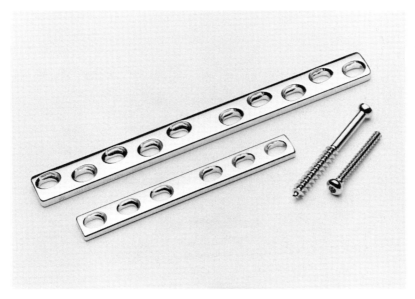

Fig. 23.30   AO Straight bone plates. (Straumann (Great Britain) Ltd.)

ASIF 316L Stainless steel, or Titanium.

Technical data

Semi-tubular plates — used with 4.5 mm Cortex screws and 6.5 mm cancellous bone screws as a tension band on radius and fibula. Compression is exerted by eccentric positioning of the screws.

Profile: half-tube diameter 12 × 1 mm; 16 and 26 mm distance between holes.

Sizes available:

Length:	39 mm	Holes:	2
	55 mm		3
	71 mm		4
	87 mm		5
	103 mm		6
	119 mm		7
	135 mm		8
	151 mm		9
	167 mm		10
	183 mm		11
	199 mm		12

Narrow plates — used with 4.5 mm Cortex screws as a neutralisation and tension band plate on the tibia and ulna. Slots at both ends for use with the tensioning device, or alternatively 6.5 mm Cancellous bone screws can be fitted.

Narrow dynamic compression plates — DCP [TM] — Similar to narrow plates, but all screw holes are designed as self-compressing spherical holes

Profile: 12× 3.8 mm; 16 and 26 mm distance between holes.

Sizes available:

Length:	39 mm	Holes:	2*
	55 mm		3*
	71 mm		4* (*used exceptionally)
	87 mm		5
	103 mm		6
	119 mm		7
	135 mm		8
	151 mm		9
	167 mm		10
	183 mm		11
	199 mm		12
	215 mm		13
	231 mm		14
	247 mm		15
	263 mm		16

Broad plates — used with 4.5 mm Cortex screws as a tension band plate on the femur and for pseudarthrosis of the humerus. Slots at both ends for use with the tensioning device, or alternatively 6.5 mm Cancellous bone screws can be fitted.

Broad dynamic compression plates — DCP [TM] — Similar to broad plates, but all screw holes are designed as self-compressing spherical holes.

Profile: 16 × 4.8 mm; 16 and 26 mm between holes

Sizes available:

Length:	103 mm	Holes:	6*
	119 mm		7* (*used exceptionally)
	135 mm		8
	151 mm		9
	167 mm		10
	199 mm		12
	231 mm		14
	263 mm		16
	295 mm		18

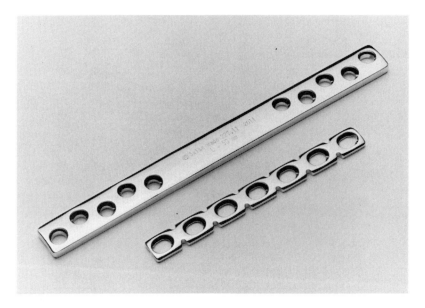

Fig. 23.31 AO Straight lengthening bone plates and reconstruction plates. (Straumann (Great Britain) Ltd.)
ASIF 316L Stainless steel, or Titanium.

Technical data —

Broad and narrow lengthening plates — used with 4.5 mm Cortex screws for internal fixation following lengthening osteotomy. Plates have relieved holes at both ends for use with the tensioning device for distraction. Alternatively 6.5 mm Cancellous bone screws can be fitted into the end holes.

Broad lengthening plates, with 10 or 8 holes — for lengthening osteotomies of the femur.

Profile: width — 16.0 mm; thickness — 4.8 mm; distance between holes — 12.0 mm

Sizes available with 10 holes:

Length:	Amount of lengthening possible:
179 mm	50 mm
189 mm	60 mm
199 mm	70 mm
209 mm	80 mm
219 mm	90 mm
229 mm	100 mm
239 mm	110 mm
249 mm	120 mm

Sizes available with 8 holes:

Length:	Amount of lengthening possible:
135 mm	30 mm
145 mm	40 mm
155 mm	50 mm
165 mm	60 mm

Narrow lengthening plates, with 8 holes — for lengthening osteotomies of the tibia.

Profile width — 12.0 mm; thickness — 3.8 mm; distance between holes — 12.0 mm.

Sizes available:

Length:	Amount of lengthening possible:
135 mm	30 mm
145 mm	40 mm
155 mm	50 mm
165 mm	60 mm
175 mm	70 mm
185 mm	80 mm

AO/ASIF Technique

AO is the abbreviation for 'Arbeitsgemeinschaft fur Osteosynthesfragen' or the Association for the Study of problems in Internal Fixation (ASIF) which was initiated in 1958. The objectives of the group, which consisted of both orthopaedic and general surgeons, were to stem the tide of disability following fracture treatment which existed widely at that time.

The aims of the AO method were clearly defined in 1958 and remain extant since they have proved to be instrumental in obtaining excellent results for over quarter of a century. The overall aim is rapid recovery of the injured limb; (1) anatomical reduction, (2) stable

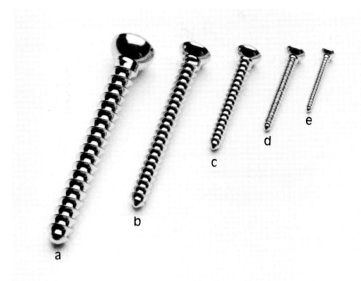

Fig. 23.32 AO Cortex bone screws. (Straumann (Great Britain) Ltd.)

ASIF 316L Stainless steel, or Titanium.

Fully threaded asymmetric thread bone screws, head with recessed hexagonal socket, used in the cortical bone of the *diaphysis*. In hard bone, the thread is pre-cut with a suitable tap which removes cutting debris.

Supplied in five diameters:
    Large – 4.5 mm (A)
    Small – 3.5 and 2.7 mm (B and C)
    Mini – 2.0 and 1.5 mm (D and E)

Technical data —
(Width across flats of recessed hexagonal socket in head: 3.5 mm)

4.5 mm diameter cortex screws:
    Head diameter: 8.0 mm
    Outside thread diameter: 4.5 mm
    Root thread diameter: 3.0 mm
    Threads per 25 mm (1 inch) approx: 14
    Recommended drill size: for threaded hole —
                3.2 mm
                for gliding hole —
                4.5 mm
    Tap diameter: 4.5 mm

3.5 mm diameter small fragment cortex screws:
    Head diameter: 6.0 mm
    Outside thread diameter: 3.5 mm
    Root thread diameter: 1.9 mm
    Threads per 25 mm (1 inch) approx: 20
    Recommended drill size: for threaded hole —
                2.0 mm
                for gliding hole —
                3.5 mm
    Tap diameter: 3.5 mm

2.7 mm diameter small fragment cortex screws:
    Head diameter: 5.0 mm
    Outside thread diameter: 2.7 mm
    Root thread diameter: 1.9 mm
    Threads per 25 mm (1 inch) approx: 25
    Recommended drill size: for threaded hole —
                2.0 mm
                for gliding hole —
                2.7 mm
    Tap diameter: 2.7 mm

2.0 mm diameter mini cortex screws:
    Head diameter: 4.0 mm
    Outside thread diameter: 2.0 mm
    Root thread diameter: 1.3 mm
    Threads per 12 mm (1 inch) approx: 20
    Recommended drill size: for threaded hole —
                2.0 mm
                for gliding hole —
                3.5 mm
    Tap diameter: 3.5 mm

1.5 mm diameter mini cortex screws:
    Head diameter: 3.0 mm
    Outside thread diameter: 1.5 mm
    Root thread diameter: 1.0 mm
    Threads per 12 mm (1 inch) approx: 20
    Recommended drill size: for threaded hole —
                1.1 mm
                for gliding hole —
                1.5 mm
    Tap diameter: 1.5 mm

internal fixation, (3) preservation of the blood supply and (4) early pain-free mobilisation. If these conditions are carefully followed then the fixation will not only provide the best situation for the bone to heal but also offer an environment for the other components of the injury to respond positively.

In collaboration with experts in biomechanics, metallurgy and implant manufacturers, the AO Group in 1961 formed a Technical Committee to develop a standardised instrument and implant system. Factors such as soft tissue problems, choice of implant, where it should be positioned and how it should be applied are critical. An incorrect decision on which aspect of the bone to place the plate could ultimately result in a fatigue fracture of the implant within days of weight bearing. Equally, the wrong choice of implant can have a similar effect since all SYNTHES implants are designed to take into consideration the biomechanical forces existing within the body.

After correct pre-operative decisions have been taken, the instrument procedure also becomes critical. A wrong sequence can destroy the end result if care is not taken. For example, in an oblique mid-shaft fracture of the radius, a plate is contoured and positioned on the tension side of the bone with the central portion of the plate across the fracture site. The length of the plate should ensure that a minimum hold of six good cortices is possible to either side of the fracture line. In an ideal reduction, one side of the plate is secured through the hole nearest the fracture site, then moving to the first convenient hole on the other side of the fracture line the 'load' DCP guide is used. This is the gold banded guide and the arrow must be pointing towards the fracture line. This offsets the drill hole sufficiently to move the bone by 1 mm in a compressive action. When the desired compression is achieved, the neutral DCP guide (green banded) is used in all remaining holes. Any bone loss at the fracture site should be filled using autogenous cancellous bone graft to strengthen the fixation.

There are of course other methods of plate fixation such as 'neutralisation and buttressing', but whatever the name it is paramount that the appropriate technique is followed.

This also holds true for screw fixation for which the most commonly known procedure is the Lag Screw technique, i.e. the screw must glide freely through the fragment adjacent to the screw head and engage only in the opposite fragment.

Table 23.4 Instrument sequence for cortical screw applications

Single lag screw through plate	Lag screw through plate	Non lag screw
4.5 drill near cortex	4.5 drill near cortex	3.2 drill both cortices
3.2 drill far cortex	3.2 drill far cortex	–
countersink	–	–
measure	measure	measure
4.5 short tap	4.5 long tap	4.5 long tap
insert screw	insert screw	insert screw

The lag screw technique can be applied to all screws but it is important to note that as with plates, screws are designed to fulfil a particular function and the right screw for the task in hand should be used, i.e.:

AO cortical screws are designed for the diaphysis and a thread profile should always be cut (tapped) in the bone before inserting the screw.

AO cancellous screws are used only in the epi and metaphysis where the cortex is relatively thin.

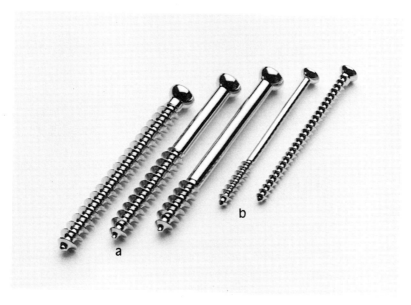

Fig. 23.33 AO Cancellous bone screws. (Straumann (Great Britain) Ltd.)

ASIF 316L Stainless steel, or Titanium.

Partially or fully threaded asymmetric, deep, coarse pitch thread bone screws, head with recessed hexagonal socket, used in the epi- and metaphysis where the cortex is relatively thin. After the hole is drilled, generally only the cortex needs to be tapped, as the screw tip is capable of cutting its own path through the cancellous bone.

Supplied in three diameters:
Large – 6.5 mm (A)
Small – 4.0 and 3.5 mm (B)

Technical data —
(Width across flats of recessed hexagonal socket in head: 3.5 mm)

6.5 mm diameter 16 mm and 32 mm partially-threaded large cancellous bone screws:
Head diameter: 8.0 mm
Outside thread diameter: 6.5 mm
Root thread diameter: 3.0 mm
Diameter of shaft: 4.5 mm
Threads per 25 mm (1 inch) approx: 9
Recommended drill size: for threaded hole —
3.2 mm
for gliding hole in hard bone — 4.5 mm
Tap diameter: 6.5 mm

6.5 mm diameter fully threaded large cancellous bone screws:
Head diameter: 8.0 mm
Outside thread diameter: 6.5 mm
Root thread diameter: 3.0 mm
Diameter of shaft: 4.5 mm
Threads per 25 mm (1 inch) approx: 9
Recommended drill size: for threaded hole —
3.2 mm
Tap diameter: 6.5 mm

4.0 mm diameter 5 to 15 mm partially-threaded small cancellous bone screws:
Head diameter: 6.0 mm
Outside thread diameter: 4.0 mm
Root thread diameter: 1.9 mm
Diameter of shaft: 2.3 mm
Threads per 25 mm (1 inch) approx: 14
Recommended drill size: for threaded hole —
2.0 mm
for gliding hole in hard bone — 4.0 mm
Tap diameter: 3.5 mm

3.5 mm diameter fully-threaded small cancellous bone screws:
Head diameter: 6.0 mm
Outside thread diameter: 3.5 mm
Root thread diameter: 1.9 mm
Threads per 25 mm (1 inch) approx: 14
Recommended drill size: for threaded hole —
2.0 mm
for gliding hole in hard bone — 3.5 mm
Tap diameter: 3.5 mm

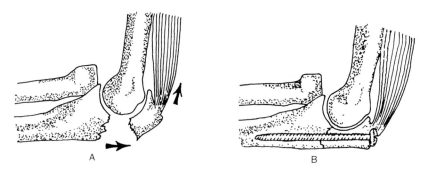

Fig. 23.34 Fracture of the olecranon. (Robinson.)
(A) The displacement due to the pull of the triceps.
(B) Internal fixation by a screw.

Good understanding of preparation and the basic AO techniques is essential. These are best learnt initially through the official AO/ASIF courses and basic literature. Then after the basics have been grasped, greater knowledge can be achieved by the various forms of the more advanced education available.

NB. DCP, SYNTHES and ASIF are trade marks of Synthes AG, Switzerland.

Plating and screwing

Definition

Internal fixation of a fracture by means of plates and screws.

Position

Generally supine, but dependent upon the location of the fracture.

Instruments

General set (Figs. 14.1 to 14.28)
Bone and fracture instruments (p. 624)
2.5 or 3 (2/0 or 0) Synthetic absorbable or plain catgut for ligatures
3, 4 or 5 (0, 1 or 2) Synthetic absorbable, plain or chromic catgut sutures, on appropriate needle for that area of the body
2.5 or 3 (2/0 or 0) Synthetic non-absorbable or silk on a small, medium or large cutting needle for skin sutures
Plaster of Paris or splints may be required
Bone clamp, self-retaining (Hey Grove), 2
Bone clamp, adjustable and self-retaining (Charnley) (Fig. 23.47)
Bone clamp, self-retaining (Lowman)
Bone clamps, self-retaining (Sinclair), large and small
Bone plates, appropriate size
Ordinary screwdriver (Lane)
Automatic screwdriver (Williams)
Plate benders, 2

Figs. 23.35 to 23.37   Self-retaining bone clamps. (Biomet Ltd.)

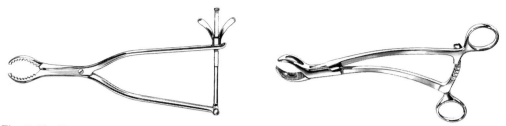

Fig. 23.35   Hey Groves bone holding forceps with self-retaining screw.

Fig. 23.36   Burns bone holding forceps.

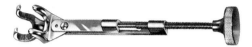

Fig. 23.37   Lowman self-retaining bone holding clamps.

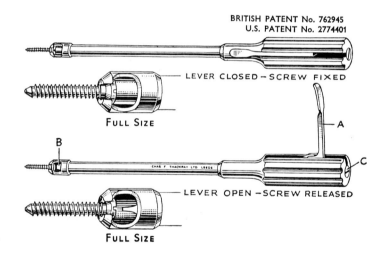

BRITISH PATENT No. 762945
U.S. PATENT No. 2774401

LEVER CLOSED—SCREW FIXED

FULL SIZE

LEVER OPEN—SCREW RELEASED

FULL SIZE

Fig. 23.38   Williams improved automatic screwdriver. (Chas. F. Thackray Ltd.)

The upper illustration shows the screwdriver ready for use; the spring-loaded driving shaft has been pushed forward to engage the slot of the screw head; the lower illustration shows the lever (A) open and the screw head disengaged. The lever (A) is closed or opened to fix or release a screw from the shaped sleeve (B) in the end of the tubular shaft.

Standard screws such as Sherman's or Lane's patterns can be used with this instrument, up to 4 mm ($\frac{5}{32}$ in) external diameter of thread with a head diameter of 7.1 mm ($\frac{9}{32}$ in). The shaped sleeve at the distal end accommodates a wide variation in shapes of screw heads.

It is possible to use the instrument to drive a screw fully home after it has been released, and in this case the lever (A) is closed so that the screwdriver protrudes from the sleeve. However, some surgeons use an ordinary Lane's screwdriver to complete this manoeuvre.

A special feature of the instrument is the adjusting screw (C) in the base of the handle. This screw is adjusted to give the lever (A) a firm fixation on the screw head. Once this screw is set correctly it need not be altered unless a screw with a larger or smaller head is required.

The use of this instrument was described in the *Lancet*, June 15, 1957, p. 1225.

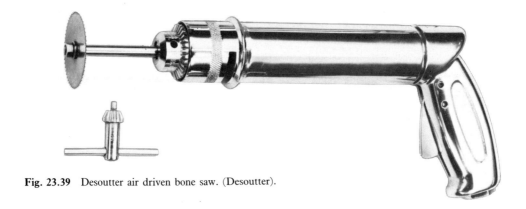

Fig. 23.39 Desoutter air driven bone saw. (Desoutter).

Figs. 23.40 to 23.43 Screwing and plating instruments (Biomet Ltd.)

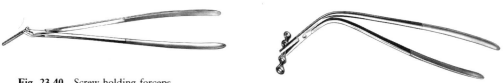

Fig. 23.40 Screw-holding forceps.

Fig. 23.41 Lane plate-holding forceps.

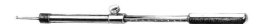

Fig. 23.42 Screw depth gauge.
This is used to determine the length of the screw needed to penetrate the bone. The end of the gauge is inserted in the drilled hole and hooked over the bone surface. By releasing the thumb screw, the sleeve may be advanced snugly against the bone or bone plate. When the screw is tightened, the sleeve will remain in position as the gauge is withdrawn. Calibrations on the stem barrel indicate the length of screw required.

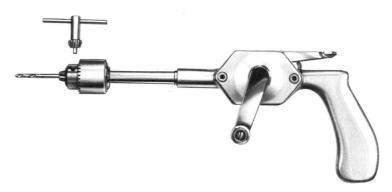

Fig. 23.43 Pistol-grip hand drill with Jacobs Chuck.
This drill has a 2-to-1 gear ratio and is cannulated for the entire length to accommodate Steinmann pins, Kirschner wires, long-shank drills and screwdriver bits. Release of the thumb-operated lever at the top of the drill instantly stops the turning of the gears and locks the chuck.

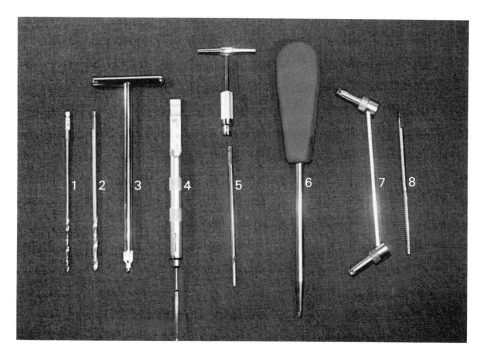

Fig. 23.44 AO/ASIF insertion instruments. (Straumann Great Britain Ltd.)
1. 3.2 mm diameter drill bit
2. 4.5 mm diameter drill bit
3. Countersink
4. Depth gauge
5. Tap handle and 4.5 mm short tap
6. Hexagonal screwdriver
7. Load and neutral DCP™ drill guide
8. 4.5 mm long tap.

Plate-holding forceps
Screw-holding forceps
Screw measuring device (Crawford Adams)
Set of screws and drills
Power drill and chuck key
For AO screws and plates — set (Fig. 23.44)
Rubber air hose or drive-cable for power drill.

Outline of procedure

The fracture is exposed and reduced. If plating is to be performed, the plate is adjusted to the correct contour and applied to the bone subperiosteally, and screwed in position. If screw fixation only is required, one or more screws are introduced obliquely across the fracture line.

The wound is closed in the usual manner and temporary splints applied if required.

Wiring

Definition

Internal fixation of a fracture by means of cerclage wire loops.

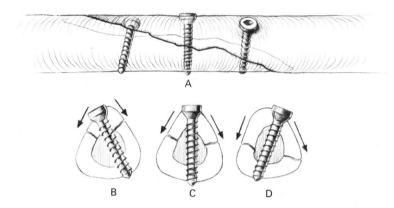

Fig. 23.45   Direction of cortex screws in spiral or long oblique fractures.

At least one screw should be inserted perpendicular to the shaft of the bone. The other screws should be inserted in such a way that some will come to lie anteriorly and others posteriorly to the middle screw in order to exert interfragmental compression at right angles to the fracture plane and overcome all shearing or torsional stresses.

Cross-section demonstrates why screws placed in different directions effect the best compression between fragments. (Hall: *Air Instruments Surgery, Orthopaedics*)

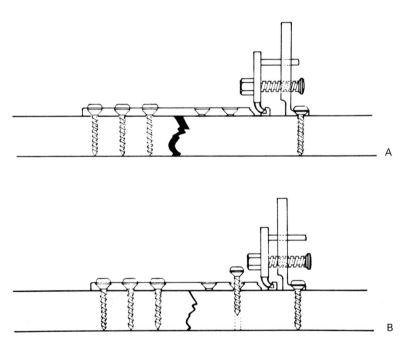

Fig. 23.46   Illustration of compression plating. (A) The compression device hooked into the lowest hole of plate but fracture not yet compressed. (B) Compression applied while lower half of the plate is screwed to the lower fragment.

Figs. 23.47 to 23.50 Charnley adjustable bone holding forceps with range of detachable jaws. (Chas. F. Thackray Ltd.)

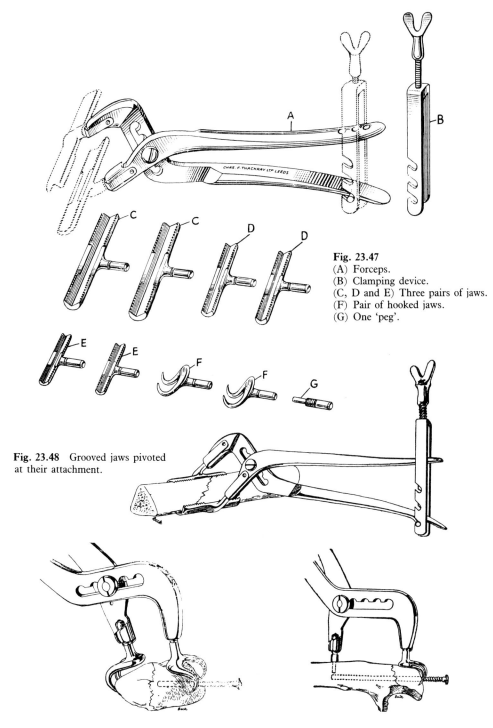

Fig. 23.47
(A) Forceps.
(B) Clamping device.
(C, D and E) Three pairs of jaws.
(F) Pair of hooked jaws.
(G) One 'peg'.

Fig. 23.48 Grooved jaws pivoted at their attachment.

Fig. 23.49 Hooked jaws.　　　　**Fig. 23.50** Hooked jaw and 'peg'.

Position

Generally supine, but dependent upon the location of the fracture.

Instruments

General set (Figs. 14.1 to 14.28)
Bone and fracture instruments (p. 624)
Wiring set (Fig. 23.51)
Bone clamps illustrated on pages 639 and 643 may be required
Bone awl or drill
2.5 or 3 (2/0 or 0) Synthetic absorbable or plain catgut for ligatures
3, 4 or 5 (0, 1 or 2) Synthetic absorbable, plain or chromic catgut sutures on appropriate needles for that area of the body
2.5 or 3 (2/0 or 0) Synthetic non-absorbable or silk on a small, medium or large cutting needle for skin sutures
Plaster of Paris or splints may be required.

Outline of procedure

The fracture is exposed and reduced. Austenitic stainless-steel wire within the range of 29 SWG and 18 SWG (Chapter 8) is generally used, although sizes 20, 24 and 28 SWG are the most useful.

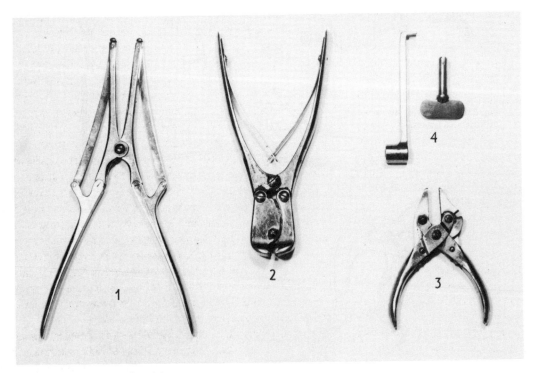

Fig. 23.51 Instruments for wiring.
1. Wire knot-tying forceps (Harris).
2. Wire-cutting forceps, compound action.
3. Pliers and wire-cutting forceps combined.
4. Wire-twisting apparatus (Hey Grove).

The fracture may be immobilised by a circumferential wire loop, e.g. a butterfly fracture of a bone shaft; or a loop is passed through holes drilled in each fragment, e.g., fracture of the patella.

The surgeon will require a bone awl or drill if holes are needed in the bone fragment. If the wire is sufficiently stiff it is passed directly round the bone or through the holes made. If a smaller gauge of wire is used, it is first threaded on to a large suture needle and is twisted back upon itself for about one inch. Alternatively, an aneurysm needle or wire passer (e.g., Sharps) may be used and the wire is threaded through the eye but not twisted back upon itself. Sometimes the surgeon may find it easier to pass the aneurysm needle round the bone first and then thread the wire through the terminal hole.

When the wire is in position, a final check is made on correct alignment of the fragments and the wire is twisted or tied in a knot. If the wire is to be twisted, this is accomplished either with special twisting forceps or two pairs of pliers. If a knot is being tied and unless the wire is very fine, a special forceps for typing wire knots is needed. Fine wire is then cut with heavy scissors reserved for the purpose and heavy wire with wire-cutting forceps.

It is essential the scrub nurse ensures that the wire is free from kinks before she hands it to the surgeon. A kink is a weak point and is very liable to break, either during insertion or after operation.

The wound is closed in the usual manner and splints or plaster of Paris may be applied.

Dynamic axial fixation

Definition

External skeletal fixation for fractures may be employed as an alternative to internal screwing and plating. The principle involves pins or elongated screws being driven through the bone above and below the fracture. These pins/screws are then clamped by an external frame on one or both sides of the limb and form a rigid splint to immobilise the reduced fracture.

Conventional external fixation devices utilising a double or single frame attempt to provide rigidity similar to that of internal fixation and promote primary bone healing without periosteal callus formation. Mechanical limitations of the equipment may preclude such a level of rigidity, and optimum primary healing of the bone may not be achieved (Bastiani et al., 1984). Furthermore, McKibbin (1979) considers that primary bone healing is not an entirely true method of union, but a remodelling process occurring late in the normal healing process. He regards the formation of callus as an important part of the process and this is dependent on some motion occurring at the fracture site during healing (Green, 1981).

The degree of stiffness of rigid frames actually provokes only minimal development of periosteal callus. In addition there may be a problem of pin track infection and loosening. This may be caused by bending of the pins/screws and osteolysis, with subsequent osteitis at the sites of insertion. For these and other reasons a unilateral dynamic axial fixator (DAF) is now commonly used. An example of such apparatus is the Orthofix DAF which achieves stability three ways: partially through alignment of the fixator body with the long axis of the bone, partially through geometry of the screws, and partially the inherent rigidity of the screws and body of the fixator (Chao and Kasman, 1984).

The Orthofix apparatus consists of a single metal body with two articulating ball joint ends in which the bone screws are clamped. These can be locked at the correct angle for axial alignment by a cam system (Fig. 23.52). The body of the fixator incorporates a telescopic device to permit conversion from rigid to dynamic fixation; the dynamic movement is in an axial longitudinal direction — not in rotation. Initially, following reduction of the fracture

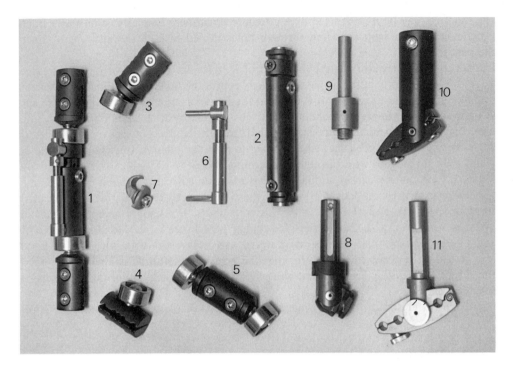

Fig. 23.52 Dynamic axial fixator (DAF) components. (Orthofix, Electro-Biology International (UK) Ltd.)

1. Dynamic axial fixator complete with compression unit and Allen wrench.
2. DAF central body with cams, bushes and locking nut.
3. Straight clamps which allow screws to be fitted parallel to the diaphyseal axis.
4. T clamp allows screws to be fitted at right angles to the diaphyseal axis.
5. Double-coupling clamp which makes it possible to fit two DAF units in series; normally used for central dislocation of the hip.
6. Showing compression unit detached from the body; this enables adjustment of DAF distraction and compression.
7. Supplementary screw holder when fitted to the compression unit, secures supplementary screws which anchor comminuted bone fragments.
8. Articulated body for the distraction of the hip and for progressive correction of angular abnormalities.
9. Accessory for assembling the articulated body.
10. Articulated body for the distraction of the ankle.
11. Accessory for assembling articulated body.

rigid axial fixation is adopted. Partial weight bearing is instituted and increased progressively. Conversion from rigid to dynamic axial loading is usually carried out in about 3–4 weeks in a stable fracture, or when evidence of callus formation is apparent in the radiographs. Following this, as the patient walks, intermittent dynamic compression takes place.

A compressor unit can be attached to the fixator to provide compression or distraction of the fracture site if this is considered necessary. The bone screws which are tapered and self-tapping are inserted so as not to intrude through the distal cortex.

Examples of the fixator in various locations are illustrated in Figure 23.56.

Position

Generally supine but depends on the site and nature of the fracture.

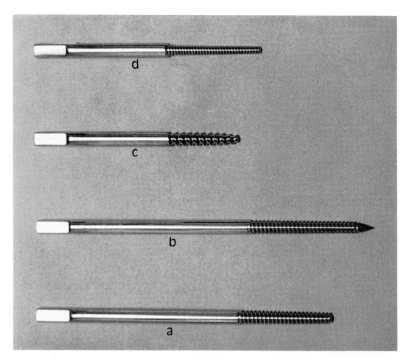

Fig. 23.53 Screws for Orthofix fixator. (Electro Biology International (UK) Ltd.)

Technical data

(a) Cortical screws:

Screw length mm	Thread length mm	Thread diameter mm	Diameter of drill mm
60	20	4.5/3.5	3.2
80	30	4.5/3.5	3.2
80	40	4.5/3.5	3.2
100	40	4.5/3.5	3.2
120	40	4.5/3.5	3.2
110	30	6/5	4.8
110	40	6/5	4.8
110	50	6/5	4.8
130	40	6/5	4.8
150	50	6/5	4.8
150	60	6/5	4.8
180	50	6/5	4.8
200	50	6/5	4.8
200	60	6/5	4.8

(b) Cortical screws:

150	50	6/5	no predrilling
110	30	6/5	no predrilling

(c) Cancellous screws:

90	30	6/5	3.2
100	40	6/5	3.2
110	50	6/5	3.2
120	60	6/5	3.2
130	60	6/5	3.2
140	50	6/5	3.2
150	60	6/5	3.2
160	70	6/5	3.2
160	90	6/5	3.2
170	80	6/5	3.2
180	90	6/5	3.2
180	100	6/5	3.2
200	80	6/5	3.2
200	90	6/5	3.2

Instruments

Open reduction and dynamic axial fixation
    Basic instruments as page 624
    Orthofix set and screws (Figs. 23.54 and 23.53)
    Orthofix DAF (Fig. 23.52)
Closed reduction and dynamic axial fixation
    Sponge-holding forceps (Rampley), 2
    Scalpel handle No. 3 or 9 with No. 15 blade (Bard Parker)
    Scissors, straight, 13 cm (5 in) (Mayo)
    Orthofix set and screws (Figs. 23.54 and 23.53).
    Orthofix DAF (Fig. 23.52).

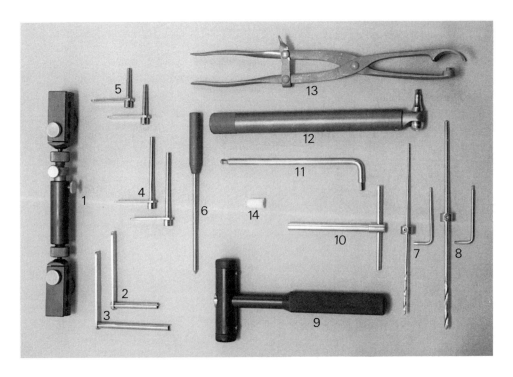

Fig. 23.54 Orthofix instrumentation. (Electro-Biology International (UK) Ltd.)

1. Fixator template
2. Screw guide units 100 mm (6)
3. Screw guide units 60 mm (6)
4. Drill guides 80 mm, size 4.8 mm and 3.2 mm diameter
5. Drill guides 40 mm, size 4.8 mm and 3.2 mm diameter
6. Tapered trocar
7. Drill with adjustable stop, 180 mm and 240 mm, size 4.8 mm diameter
8. Drill with adjustable stop, 200 mm, size 3.2 mm diameter
9. Nylon faced mallet
10. T wrench for securing screws in bone
11. Allen wrench for compressor, clamp and body locking screws
12. Torque wrench for locking cams
13. Fixator manipulation, forceps
14. Screw covers
15. Self-taping cortical and cancellous screws. (Orthofix, EBI Medical Systems Ltd.)

Outline of procedure

Before commencing fitting of the fixator an approximate reduction of the fracture is made. The first screw to be inserted is the one whose position is most critical, e.g. the screw closest to a joint/fracture. When sufficient space is available the distance from the fracture to the closest screw should be at least 4 cm.

A longitudinal incision of 1 cm is made over the screw insertion site on the first bone fragment, and opened with blunt end scissors (Fig. 23.55a). The trocar is inserted into the correct length screw guide which is then positioned along the mid-line of the bone cortex. With the guide perpendicular to the longitudinal axis of the bone and pressed against the cortex, the trocar is withdrawn (Fig. 23.55b and c). Using a mallet, the screw guide is tapped lightly to drive the teeth of the guide into the cortex (Fig. 23.55d).

The correct sized drill guide is inserted into the screw guide. The corresponding drill fitted with a drill stop set at the appropriate depth is used to drill through the proximal cortex up to the distal cortex (Fig. 23.55e and f). The 4.8 mm drill is used for cortical screws, and the 3.2 mm drill for cancellous screws. The 3.2 mm drill is also used for smaller diameter 4.5/3.5 mm screws which are intended for bones of 15 mm diameter or less.

To prevent damage to soft tissue beyond the distal cortex, the drill stop is offset by 5 mm before continuing drilling through the distal cortex (Fig. 23.55g and h). The drill and drill guide are removed from the screw guide which is still kept pressed against the bone. The selected screw is inserted and turned with minimum effort through the cortex with the 'T' wrench. After the screw traverses the proximal cortex and medullary canal, an increase in resistance is encountered as it penetrates the distal cortex. A further 7–8 half turns are then required to ensure that at least two threads of the screw protrude beyond the distal cortex.

The screw guide used for the first screw is left in position and one end of the template applied to it (Fig. 23.55k). Using the grooves on the template clamp as a guide, a second skin incision is made, ideally so that the position of the screws corresponds with the grooves furthest apart. The screw insertion procedure described previously (Fig. 23.55a–j) is repeated. Normally only two screws per clamp are required. In the case of poor quality bone, and/or the fixator is more than 6 cm from the closest cortex, three screws may be needed.

Before the screws are inserted in the second bone fragment, the template body is adjusted to the correct length (Fig. 23.55l) and the screws inserted following the procedure previously described (Fig. 23.55a–j). The template is then removed and the Orthofix DAF attached to the screws (Fig. 23.55m and n). Care is taken to ensure that the body locking screw is on the outside and that the dot and arrow marked on the cam mechanism and the clamp screws are facing upwards. The fixator is fitted at least 1 cm from the skin to allow for post-operative oedema and dressing. The fixator body is adjusted parallel to the diaphyseal axis. The clamp screws are tightened using the Allen wrench (Fig. 23.55o). If the two outside holes of the clamp have not been used, a dummy screw is fitted in each to prevent abnormal stresses when locking the clamp screws.

Final reduction of the fracture is achieved by using manipulation forceps, and the cams and body locking screws are locked to maintain reduction (Fig. 23.55p and q). Final locking of the cams is accomplished using the Torque wrench; a click indicates the correct torque. Compression and distraction can be achieved by fitting a compressor/distractor unit into the cam recesses, and loosening the body locking screw. A 360° turn anticlockwise gives 1 mm distraction; similarly, 360° clockwise gives 1 mm compression. This is not carried out for a fresh fracture; compression is most likely to be used only in hypertrophic delayed or non-unions.

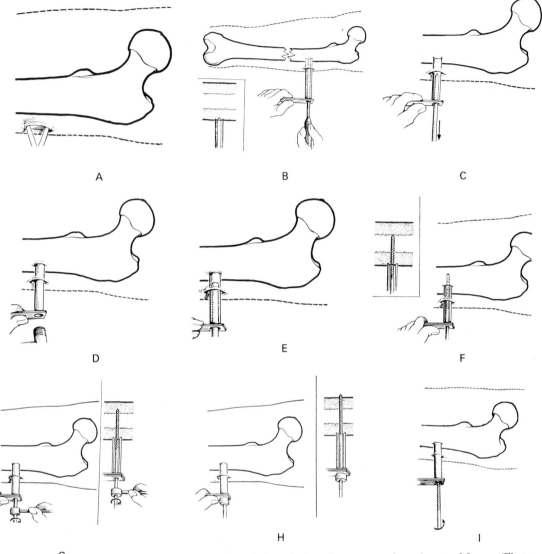

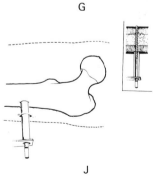

Fig. 23.55 Orthofix technique for inserting screws and attachment of fixator. (Electro-Biology International (UK) Ltd.) (A) Incision made in skin over site of screw in first bone fragment and opened with blunt end scissors. (B) Screw guide positioned aided by trocar. (C) Trocar removed, screw guide pressed against bone cortex. (D) Teeth of screw guide engaged in cortex by lightly tapping guide with mallet. (E) Correct size drill guide inserted into screw guide. (F) Drill fitted with stop used to make hole through proximal cortex only. (G) Drill stop offset by 5 mm before continuing drilling. (H) Drill penetrates through distal cortex. (I) Drill and drill guide removed from screw guide; selected screw inserted and turned into bone with 'T' wrench. (J) Screw full home, at least two threads protruding beyond distal cortex. (K) Template applied, using grooves to determine correct position for second screw in first bone fragment. (L) Template adjusted for length, screws inserted in second bone fragment. (M) Removal of template and screw guides. (N) Attachment of Orthofix Dynamic Axial Fixator in place of template. (O) Fixator positioned, clamp screws tightened with Allen wrench. (P) Final reduction of fracture using manipulation forceps. (Q) Cams and body locking screws being locked. (R) Use of Torque wrench for final locking of the cams. (S) Showing compressor/distractor unit fitted into cam recesses. (Orthofix, EBI Medical Systems Ltd.)

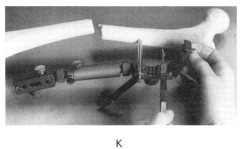

K

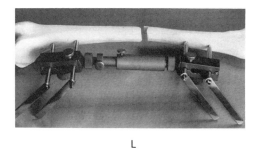

L

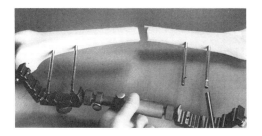

M

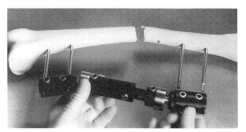

N

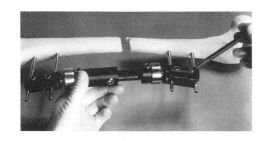

O

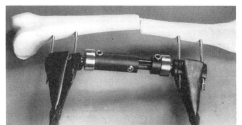

P

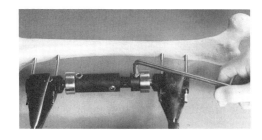

Q

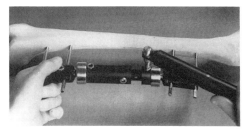

R

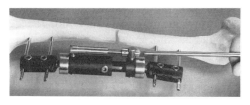

S

Post-operatively, the skin puncture wounds which should be of sufficient size to ensure that the skin is not under tension are sealed with gauze dressings. The screw/pins should be cleaned every 2–3 days with an alcohol-based skin disinfectant (iodine-free) to remove any crust formed, and the gauze dressings replaced.

Femoral neck fractures

Definition

The internal fixation of a subcapital or transcervical fracture of the femoral neck with a trifin pin. This procedure may be used also to immobilise a slipped upper femoral epiphysis in adolescents.

Position

Immobilised on a fracture table (Fig. 5.21).

Instruments

Smith Petersen nail
General set (Figs. 14.1 to 14.28)
Bone and fracture instruments (p. 624)
Set of trifin nails (Smith Petersen) (Fig. 23.57), or four flange nails
Steel rule, 15 cm (6 in)
Plate blenders, 2
3 (0) Synthetic absorbable or plain catgut for ligatures
3 or 4 (0 or 1) Synthetic absorbable or plain catgut on a medium half-circle cutting or
    Mayo needle with a trocar point for muscle sutures
2.5 or 3 (2/0 or 0) Synthetic non-absorbable or silk on a medium curved cutting needle
    for skin sutures.

Outline of procedure

The patient is immobilised on a fracture table and if necessary the fracture is manipulated and reduced. This fracture table may be similar to that illustrated in Fig. 5.21, which is a special orthopaedic attachment on a general operation table, or Bell, Albee, Shropshire horse, or Hawley table. The position of the patient's legs is adjusted to maintain reduction of the fracture during operation, and this usually means in abduction and extension with some degree of internal rotation of the affected limb.

X-ray apparatus is positioned to give anterior and lateral position films during the course of operation.

An incision is made about 25 mm (1 in) below the tip of the trochanter, and is carried 5 cm to 8 cm (2 to 3 in) down the lateral aspect of the thigh parallel with the femoral shaft. Dissection is made down to the fascia lata which is incised and split with scissors in line with the skin incision. The fascia lata is retracted to expose the vastus lateralis which is incised and retracted away from the femur with bone levers. Further blunt dissection with a periosteal elevator exposes the region of the trochanter.

A Smith Petersen nail, like many implants used for the fixation of fractures in the femoral neck region, has a central cannulation to accommodate a guide wire. It is important that

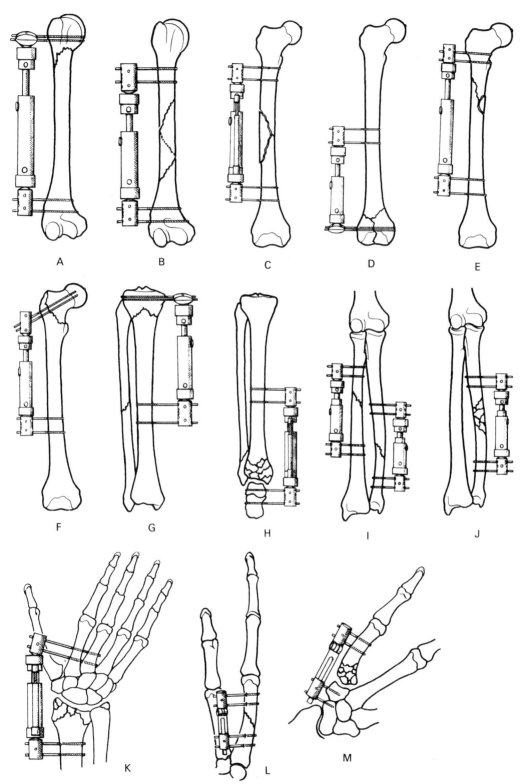

Fig. 23.56   Applications of dynamic axial fixator. (Orthofix, Electro-Biology International (UK) Ltd.)

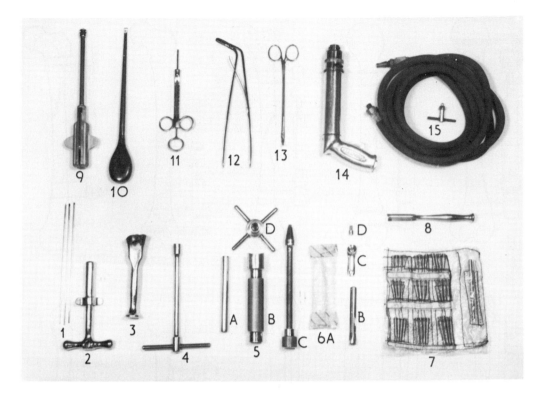

Fig. 23.57 Femoral neck fracture, Smith Petersen nail

1. Three guide wires of exactly the same diameter and length 2.3 cm × 25 cm ($\frac{3}{32}$ in × 10 in).
2. Guide wire hand chuck (Watson-Jones).
3. Fracture impactor (Smith Petersen).
4. Box spanner for bolt (Smith Petersen).
5. Driver/extractor for trifin nail (Smith Petersen).
   A. Tommy bar for additional leverage on capstan during extraction of nail.
   B. Extractor barrel.
   C. Driver/extractor, threaded bar.
   D. Extraction capstain.
6. A. Trifin nail of appropriate size (Smith Petersen), sterile in packet.
   B. Showing Smith Petersen trifin nail.
   C. Small retaining plate (Coventry).
   D. Bolt and spring washer for attaching plate to nail (Coventry).
7. Set of screws and drills in fabric wallet.
8. Trifin nail starter (Smith Petersen).
9. Automatic screwdriver (Williams).
10. Ordinary screwdriver (Lane).
11. Screw measuring device (Crawford Adams).
12. Plate-holding forceps.
13. Screw-holding forceps.
14. Power drill (Desoutter compressed air drill).
15. Rubber air hose for power drill, and chuck key.

a guide wire is checked for correct size by passing it through the cannulation of the nail. If the wire is too tight, or does not run smoothly through it (perhaps due to a bent wire or some manufacturing error), either the wire or the nail must be replaced. There is grave danger of a tight wire being carried through into the pelvis as the nail is driven home.

After drilling a 4.8 mm ($\frac{3}{16}$ in) to 6.4 mm ($\frac{1}{4}$ in) hole in the bone about 25 mm (1 in) below the trochanter along the shaft, the guide wire is inserted into the femoral neck and an X-ray taken to confirm its position. The guide wire may require several adjustments before the correct position is achieved.

The length of the nail required is determined by placing another identical guide wire alongside the portion of the wire which projects from the bone, and the amount projecting is deducted by measurement from the total length of the guide wire. This measurement is the same as that in the femoral neck.

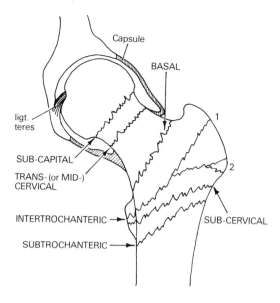

Fig. 23.58   Types of fractures of the upper end of the femur.

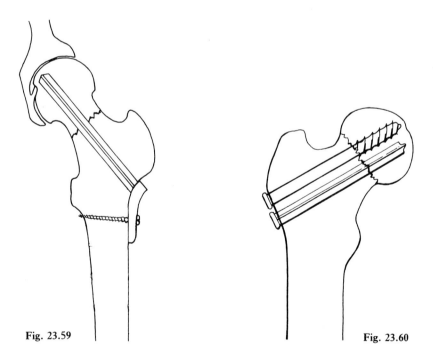

Fig. 23.59

Fig. 23.60

Fig. 23.59   Fixation of transcervical femoral neck fracture with trifin nail and small retaining plate.

Fig. 23.60   Fixation of fractured neck of femur showing trifin nail and cannulated lag screw which gives better fixation than a single device. (Rintoul: *Farquharson's Textbook of Operative Surgery.*)

If a small plate is to be used to retain the nail in position, it is usual to add a 6.4 mm ($\frac{1}{4}$ in) to the required measurement of nail.

A three or four flange nail of appropriate length is hammered home over the guide wire within 13 mm ($\frac{1}{2}$ in) of the cortex. The guide wire is then removed, and the fracture impacted with a blow on a Smith Peterson impactor positioned over the head of the protruding nail. The nail is then driven home either flush with the femoral cortex (no retaining plate) or with approx 6 mm ($\frac{1}{4}$ in) left projecting (small, one hole retaining plate).

If required, the small retaining plate may then be secured to the nail with a threaded bolt and screwed to the femoral shaft. Additionally a cannulated lag screw may be inserted as shown in Fig. 23.60. This gives better fixation than a single device.

The wound is closed in layers and the patient may require a plaster boot which incorporates a short splint across the heel and at right angles to the leg to prevent rotation of the foot after operation.

There are many other types of appliances for immobilising femoral neck fractures, these include compression screws which are described in the next section.

Femoral trochanteric fractures

Definition

The internal fixation of a basal, petrochanteric or subtrochanteric fracture of the upper femur.

Position

As for Smith Petersen nail (Fig. 5.21).

Instruments

McLaughlin appliance
General set (Figs. 14.1 to 14.28)
Bone and fracture set (p. 624)
Femoral neck fracture set (Fig. 23.57)
Set of trifin nails (Smith Petersen type) (Fig. 23.61)
Intertrochanteric plate, five or seven hole, with bolt and locking washer (McLaughlin)
Ligatures and sutures as for Smith Petersen nail

McKee nail and plate
General set (Figs. 14.1 to 14.28)
Bone and fracture set (p. 624)
Femoral neck fracture set (Fig. 23.57 minus items 4, 5 and 6)
Driver/extractor (McKee)
Box spanner (McKee)
Trifin nail of appropriate size (McKee), (Fig. 23.61)
Intertrochanteric plate (McKee), (Fig. 23.61)
Plate benders, 2
Ligatures and sutures as for Smith Petersen nail

Figs. 23.61 to 23.63   Femoral neck nails and plates. (Howmedica, U.K., Ltd.)

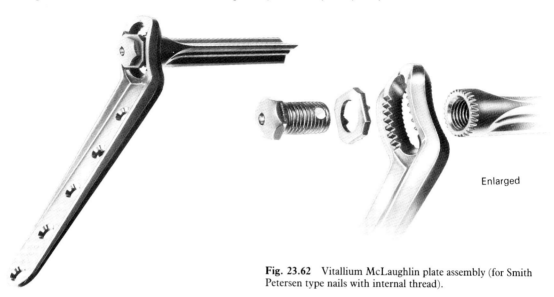

Fig. 23.62   Vitallium McLaughlin plate assembly (for Smith Petersen type nails with internal thread).

Fig. 23.61   Thornton nail, Smith-Petersen type.
Plate Lengths: 38 mm ($1\frac{1}{2}$ in), 57 mm ($2\frac{1}{2}$ in), 82.5 mm ($3\frac{1}{4}$ in), 95 mm ($3\frac{3}{4}$ in), 114 mm ($4\frac{1}{2}$ in), 133 mm ($5\frac{1}{4}$ in), 203 mm (8 in).
Holes: 2, 3, 4, 5, 6, 7, 12.

Nail lengths: 76 mm (3 in), 82.5 mm ($3\frac{1}{4}$ in), 89 mm ($3\frac{1}{2}$ in), 95 mm ($3\frac{3}{4}$ in), 102 mm (4 in), 108 mm ($4\frac{1}{4}$ in), 114 mm ($4\frac{1}{2}$ in), 121 mm ($4\frac{3}{4}$ in), 127 mm (5 in), 133 mm ($5\frac{1}{4}$ in), 140 mm ($5\frac{1}{2}$ in), 146 mm ($5\frac{3}{4}$ in), 152 mm (6 in).
The Vitallium Thornton nail is designed with a serrated head and is cannulated to accept a 2.4 mm ($\frac{3}{32}$ in) guide wire.

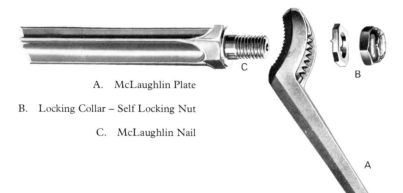

A.   McLaughlin Plate

B.   Locking Collar – Self Locking Nut

C.   McLaughlin Nail

Fig. 23.63   Vitallium McLaughlin plate assembly (for nails with external thread).
Includes:
Plate lengths: 38 mm ($1\frac{1}{2}$ in), 57 mm ($2\frac{1}{4}$ in), 82.5 mm ($3\frac{1}{4}$ in), 95 mm ($3\frac{3}{4}$ in), 114 mm ($4\frac{1}{2}$ in), 133 mm ($5\frac{1}{4}$ in), 203 mm (8 in).
Holes: 2, 3, 4, 5, 6, 7, 12.

Nail lengths: 76 mm (3 in), 82.5 mm ($3\frac{1}{4}$ in), 89 mm ($3\frac{1}{2}$ in), 95 mm ($3\frac{3}{4}$ in), 102 mm (4 in), 108 mm ($4\frac{1}{4}$ in), 114 mm ($4\frac{1}{2}$ in), 121 mm ($4\frac{3}{4}$ in), 127 mm (5 in), 133 mm ($5\frac{1}{4}$ in), 140 mm ($5\frac{1}{2}$ in), 146 mm ($5\frac{3}{4}$ in), 152 mm (6 in).
The Vitallium McLaughlin nail is four-flanged and cannulated to accept a 2.4 mm ($\frac{3}{32}$ in) guide wire.

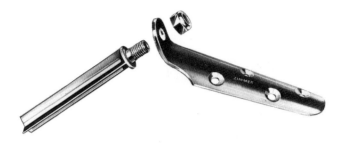

Fig. 23.64 McKee Trifin nail and interochanteric plate. (Biomet Ltd.)
Composition A. Stainless steel, Titanium or Vitallium.
Sizes of nail available:
   75 mm to 150 mm lengths in 5 mm steps. Nail: 3 to 6 in lengths in ¼ in steps; diameter, 13 mm (0.5 in).
   Plates: Available with a single slot, four slots, four holes or six holes. The nail is cannulated to receive a
   2.4 mm (³⁄₃₂ in) guide pin and the male screw thread is 7 mm diameter, 1 mm pitch to take a locking nut.

AO/ASIF Dynamic hip screw
General set (Figs. 14.1 to 14.28)
Bone and fracture set (p. 624)
AO/ASIF Bone screw set (Fig. 23.44)
AO/ASIF DHS set (Fig. 23.66f)
AO/ASIF DHS/DCS hip/screws and plate (Fig. 23.65).
Ligatures and sutures as for Smith Petersen nail.

Outline of procedure

The initial stages of the immobilisation of the patient, fracture reduction and incision are similar to that for Smith Petersen nail. In the case of trochanteric fractures, however, the incision extends several centimeters further down the femoral shaft in order to provide adequate exposure to insert the longer plate.

A McLaughlin plate is bolted to a Smith Petersen nail which is inserted as described previously, with 6 mm (¼ in) of the nail head left protruding from the bone. The plate is secured to the femoral shaft with five or seven screws, depending upon the length of the plate. The design of this plate, which has a curved shoulder, allows adjustment of the angle between the nail and plate without having to actually bend the plate itself.

A McKee plate is bolted to a McKee nail which is inserted in a manner similar to a Smith Petersen nail. The difference between the two nails is that whereas the Smith Petersen nail has a threaded hole in the head portion, the McKee nail has a threaded projection. The plate is fitted over this threaded projection and secured with a hexagonal nut. However, this type of plate may first require adjustment of its angle with the plate benders, in order that the plate lies flush along the shaft when bolted to the nail. The plate is then secured to the shaft by four or six screws, depending upon the length of plate selected.

Dynamic hip screw implant system comprises a DHS lag screw and DHS/DCS plate. The lag screws are supplied in lengths from 50 mm up to 145 mm, with increments of 5 mm between sizes. The standard plates have a 38 mm barrel to accommodate the lag screw; a short 25 mm barrel version is produced but seldom used. DHS plates are available with several barrel angles (135°, 140°, 145° and 150°); the 135° version is generally the most universal and is supplied in various lengths with 2 to 12 screw holes (Fig. 23.65). Although

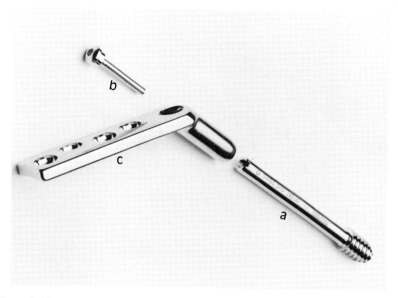

Fig. 23.65 Dynamic hip screws (A) compression screws (B), and plates with dynamic compression holes (C). (Straumann (Great Britain) Ltd.)

ASIF 316L Stainless steel or Titanium.

Technical data —

DHS screws
    Outside thread diameter: 12.5 mm
    Diameter of shaft: 8.0 mm
    Thread length: 22 mm

Sizes available, lengths in mm:
    50, 55, 60, 65, 70, 75, 80, 85, 90, 95, 100, 105,
    110, 115, 120, 125, 130, 135, 140, 145

(Note: sizes 50, 55, and 60 mm lengths are for use only with short barrel DHS compression plate.)

DHS hip screw plates
    Shaft profile: 19 × 5.8 mm
    DCP holes for 4.5 mm AO/ASIF Cortex screw
    Barrel: 12.6 mm diameter

Plates with 38 mm standard barrel:
135° angle

Length	No. of holes
46 mm	2
78 mm	4
94 mm	5
110 mm	6
142 mm	8
174 mm	10

206 mm	12
238 mm	14
270	16

150° angle:

46 mm	2
78 mm	4
94 mm	5
110 mm	6
142 mm	8
176 mm	10
206 mm	12

140° and 145° angle

78 mm	4
94 mm	5
110 mm	6

Plates with 25 mm short barrel:

135° angle:

78 mm	4
94 mm	5
110 mm	6

DHS Compressing screw:
    36 mm long, with 3.5 mm hexagonal head for
    AO/ASIF screw driver

designed mainly for the intertrochanteric to subtrochanteric fractures, the DHS can be used also for femoral neck fractures in conjunction with a short plate (Fig. 23.66 A and B).

With the aid of the DHS angle guide and radiographic visualisation, a guide pin is inserted in the middle of the femoral neck (Fig. 23.66A and B). The direct measuring device is slid over the guide wire to determine the length of lag screw required (Fig. 23.66C). The triple reamer, set to a depth of 10 mm short from the distal point of the guidewire (joint surface),

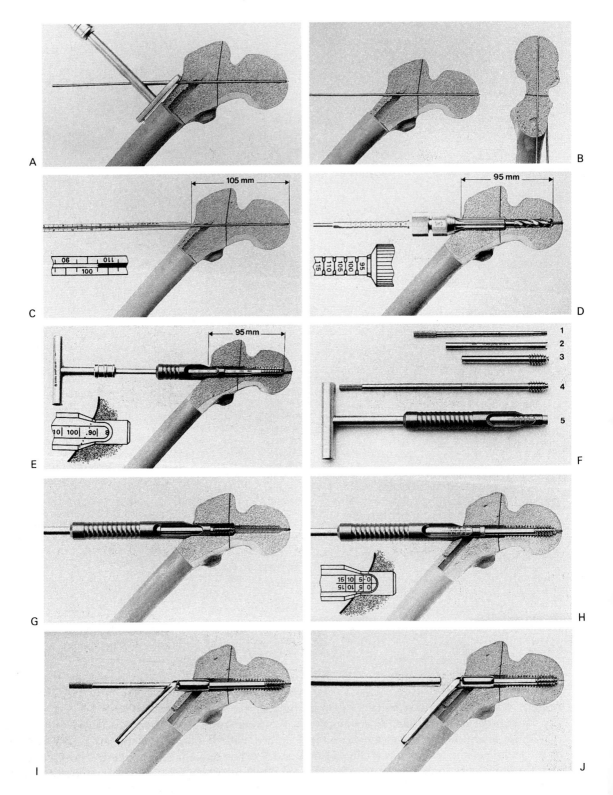

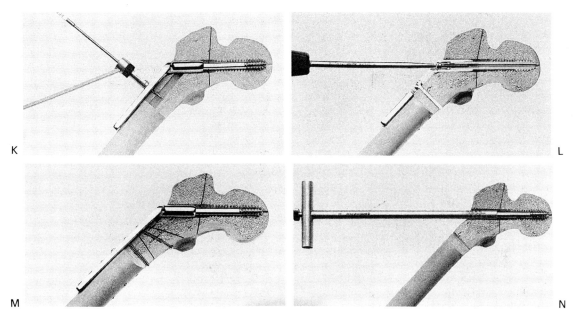

K

L

M

N

Fig. 23.66 Dynamic hip screw technique for insertion. (Straumann (Great Britain) Ltd.) (A) Initially, Kirschner wires may be inserted into the upper part of the femoral neck for temporary fixation following reduction of the fracture. Another Kirschner wire may be slid over the front of the femoral neck to determine degree of anteversion, and then hammered gently into the femoral neck. The DHS angle guide is used to insert a guide pin centred in the femoral neck to the level of subchondral bone. (B) Showing guide lying in centre of femoral neck. (C) The depth of guide pin in the femoral neck is determined with the measuring device. (D) Drilling holes to accommodate hip screw, screw barrel and barrel plate junction, using a triple reamer which completes procedure in one operation. (E) The hip screw thread may be pre-cut with a tap if the cancellous bone appears hard. (F) Preparing the DHS/DCS screw for insertion (see text for steps 1–5). (G and H) Whole screw assembly is slid over the guide wire and screwed into the bone until the O mark on the wrench reaches the lateral cortex. This means that the lag screw is 10 mm from the joint. In osteoporotic bone, the screw can be inserted some 5 mm deeper. (I) The wrench is removed with its centering sleeve and the appropriate DHS plate slid onto the assembly. The coupling screw is loosened and the guide shaft removed. The guide pin is removed using a power drill set to reversed rotation. (J) The plate is gently seated with the impactor. (K) AO/ASIF 4.5 mm cortex screws are used to fix the DHS plate to the femur. (L) Final impaction of the fracture if necessary is achieved with a DHS/DCS compressing screw. (For the compressing screw to achieve full effect the hip screw must not touch the bone cortex. (M) Additional subtrochanteric fragments can be fixed with lag screws through the DHS plate. (N) Implant removal. After removal of the DHS plate, the wrench is placed over the DHS/DCS screw. The long coupling screw allows traction to be exerted whilst unscrewing the screw.

is threaded over the guide wire and the hole drilled. This reamer makes appropriate holes in one operation for the lag screw, screw barrel and the plate/barrel junction (Fig. 23.66D). If the guide pin is inadvertently withdrawn with the reamer, it is reinserted immediately before proceeding further.

Before inserting the lag screw, for extremely hard cancellous bone, the bone screw thread is precut with a tap (Fig. 23.66E). The DHS/DCS screw is prepared for insertion in five steps (Fig. 23.66F): the coupling screw (1) is inserted through hollow guide shaft (2), and the male screw thread is screwed into the female thread of the DHS/DCS screw (3). The ridge and the slot between the guide shaft and the DHS/DCS screw must interdigitate (4). The longer of the two centering sleeves is slid over the wrench (5), the whole assembly screwed into the wrench (Fig. 23.66G), and the screw is driven into the bone until the O mark on the wrench reaches the proximal cortex (Fig. 23.66H). The wrench with its

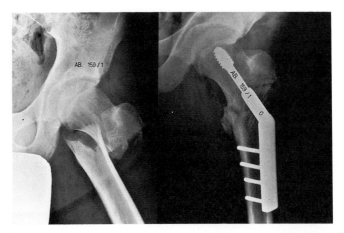

Fig. 23.67 X-ray of pertrochanteric fracture before reduction and following fixation with DHS screw.

centering sleeve is removed, and the appropriate DHS plate slid onto the assembly (Fig. 23.66I). The coupling screw is loosened and the guide shaft removed, followed by the guide pin. The DHS plate is gently tapped in position (Fig. 23.66J), and fixed to the femur with 4.5 mm AO/ASIF cortex screws (Fig. 23.66K). The fracture is finally impacted with a DHS/DCS compressing screw (Fig. 23.66L), which may be left in position. Additional subtrochanteric fragments can be fixed with lag screws through the plate.

Slipped upper femoral epiphysis

It has been mentioned that the Smith Petersen trifin nail can be used to immobilise a slipped upper femoral epiphysis. Alternatively, Austin Moore pins, Knowle's pins or fine Steinmann pins may be used for this procedure.

These pins resemble guide wires but are made from composition A austenitic stainless steel or Vitallium. The procedure is similar to Smith Petersen nail up to the insertion of the guide wire, but in this case an Austin Moore pin, Knowle pin or Steinmann pin is drilled into the femoral neck and across the epiphyseal line.

The position and length of the pin are checked radiologically and when satisfactory, several other pins, up to four, may be inserted alongside the first pin within the neck but generally at slightly different angles. Any excess pin projecting from the bone is cut off and the wound is closed in the usual manner.

One of the advantages of this technique is said to be that these pins occupy less space within the femoral neck than the conventional trifin nail, and there is consequently less interference with bone formation. It is also less traumatic.

Intramedullary fixation of the femoral shaft fracture, Kuntscher nail

Definition

Intramedullary fixation of fractures of the middle and upper shaft of the femur.

Position

Either supine, with a sandbag under the affected buttock, or full lateral.

Instruments

General set (Figs. 14.1 to 14.28)
Bone and fracture set (p. 624)
Kuntscher nail set (Fig. 23.68)
Diathermy leads, electrodes and lead anchoring forceps
Power drill
Intramedullary reamers, appropriate size
3 and 4 (0 and 1) Synthetic absorbable or plain catgut for ligatures
4 or 5 (1 or 2) Synthetic non-absorbable, chromic catgut or silk, etc., on a large half-circle
    cutting or Mayo's needle with a trocar point for muscle sutures
3 (0) Synthetic non-absorbable or silk on a large curved or straight cutting needle for skin
    sutures.

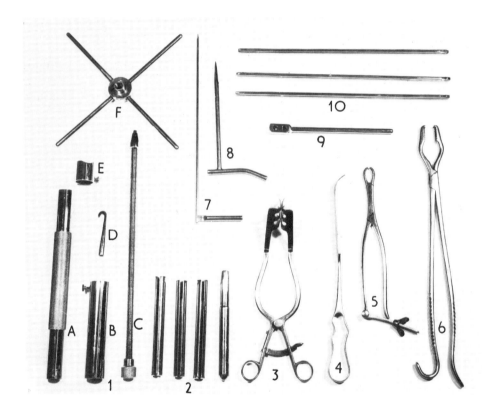

Fig. 23.68   Femoral shaft fracture, Kuntscher nail
1. Extractor for Kuntscher nails (Brigden).
   A. Extractor barrel.
   B. Extension tube for extractor barrel (long
      nails).
   C. Threaded extractor bar.
   D. Extractor hook.
   E. Sleeve designed for contact with trochanter or
      end of fractured bone.
   F. Extractor capstan.
2. Drivers and set for Kuntscher nails, one driver for
   each diameter of nail in use.

3. Retractor, self-retaining (Adson).
4. Large bone-levers (Lane), 2.
5. Bone clamp, self-retaining (Hey Grove), 2.
6. Large bone-holding forceps (Lane), 2.
7. Guide for Kuntscher nails.
8. Reamer for Kuntscher nails.
9. Nail bender.
10. Femoral shaft nail (Kuntscher). Those illustrated
    show 8.5 mm, 9 mm and 9.5 mm diameter.

Outline of procedure

There are several surgical approaches to the femur but the one most used for Kuntscher nailing is the lateral approach.

The leg is angulated at the fracture site, and a short incision made over the fracture on a line which extends between the greater trochanter and the external condyle of the femur. The superficial and deep fascia are incised and the vastus lateralis and vastus intermedius are divided in the direction of their fibres.

The upper and lower fragments of the fracture are exposed by retraction with bone levers, and the fracture is reduced. The fracture is then disimpacted and the upper fragment elevated out of the wound. Some surgeons ream out the medullary canal with a hand or power-reamer before inserting the nail to obviate a tendency for the nail to jam (Fig. 23.70A). A clover leaf nail, slotted and pointed at both ends and of appropriate length, is inserted into the upper fragment. This nail is driven through the trochanter into the buttock and through a small skin incision made overlying, until the distal end is flush with the fracture surface. The fracture is then reduced and the nail driven from the upper end into the lower fragment (Fig. 23.70B). The nail is inserted so that the slot at the upper end just projects above the trochanter for removal of the nail at a later date.

The wound is closed in layers and the patient may be immobilised temporarily on a Thomas splint.

Intramedullary fixation of tibial shaft fractures, Kuntscher nail

Definition

Intramedullary fixation of tibial shaft fractures with a nail.

Position

Supine, with leg flexed over a triangular support (optional).

Instruments

General set (Figs. 14.1 to 14.28)
Bone and fracture set (p. 624)
Kuntscher nail set (Fig. 23.68)
Power drill
9.6 mm ($\frac{3}{8}$ in) diameter twist drill
Intramedullary reamers, appropriate size
3 (0) Synthetic absorbable or plain catgut for ligatures
4 (1) Synthetic absorbable or plain catgut on a medium half-circle cutting or Mayo needle with a trocar point for muscle and fat sutures
2.5 (2/0) Synthetic non-absorbable or silk on a medium curved or straight cutting needle for skin sutures.

Outline of procedure

Some surgeons perform this operation as a 'blind' procedure by inserting the nail into the upper end of the tibia and controlling the position of the fracture and insertion of the nail

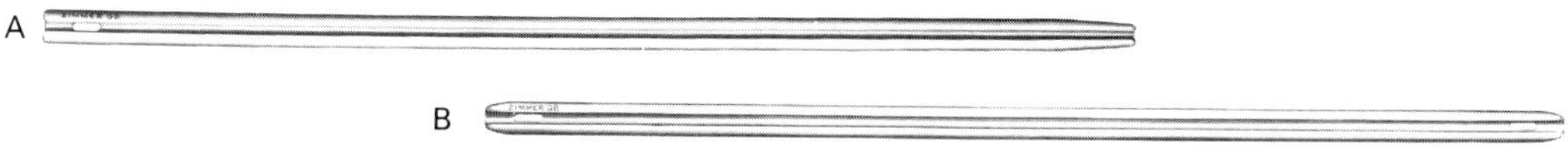

A

B

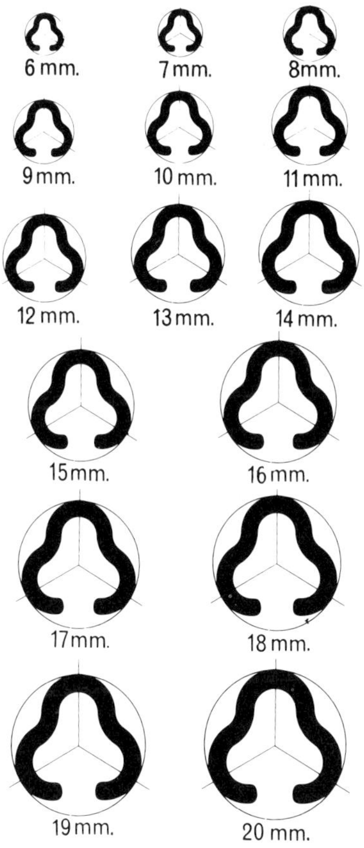

6 mm. 7 mm. 8mm.

9 mm. 10 mm. 11 mm.

12 mm. 13mm. 14 mm.

15mm. 16 mm.

17mm. 18 mm.

19mm. 20 mm.

Cross section.

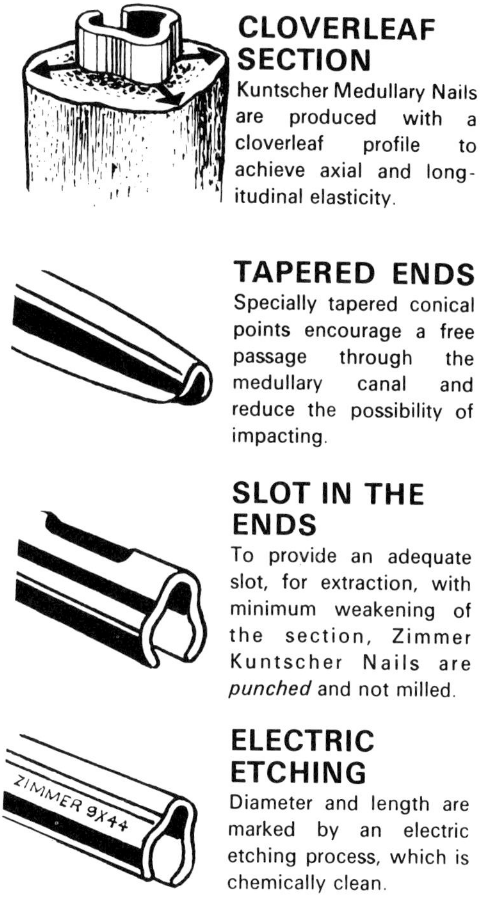

CLOVERLEAF SECTION

Kuntscher Medullary Nails are produced with a cloverleaf profile to achieve axial and longitudinal elasticity.

TAPERED ENDS

Specially tapered conical points encourage a free passage through the medullary canal and reduce the possibility of impacting.

SLOT IN THE ENDS

To provide an adequate slot, for extraction, with minimum weakening of the section, Zimmer Kuntscher Nails are *punched* and not milled.

ELECTRIC ETCHING

Diameter and length are marked by an electric etching process, which is chemically clean.

ZIMMER 9X44

Characteristics.

Fig. 23.69 Kuntscher intramedullary femoral nails (Biomet Ltd.)
Composition A. Stainless steel
A. Single slot
B. Slotted and pointed each end.
These are clover-leaf in section and are supplied either slotted and pointed at one or both ends, the latter being essential if the nails are to be inserted by the retrograde method.
Standard sizes available:
  12 mm width; lengths of 36 to 52 cm in 2 cm steps.
  9, 10 and 11 mm width; lengths of 32 to 52 cm in 2 cm steps.
  8 mm width; lengths of 14 to 42 cm in 2 cm steps.
  6 mm width; lengths of 14 to 34 cm in 2 cm steps.

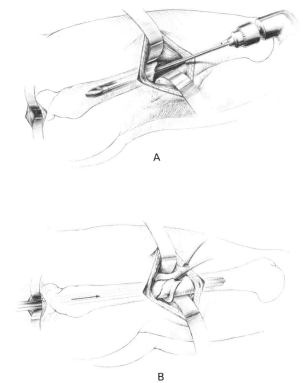

A

B

Fig. 23.70 Insertion of Kuntscher nail.
A. Reaming of the upper fragment before inserting nail.
B. Nail being driven from upper end of femur into lower fragment, (Hall: *Air Instrument Surgery, Orthopaedics*)

radiologically. However, the method generally used is to expose and reduce the fracture before 'nailing'.

A curved incision is made over the fracture site on either side of the anterior border of the tibia. The skin is reflected and the periosteum incised and retracted with bone levers. The fracture is reduced under direct vision and the reduction maintained with bone clamps.

A small incision is made medially at the upper part of the tibia and a 10 mm ($\frac{3}{8}$ in) hole is drilled with the drill pointing in the direction of the tibial tubercle. The nail is inserted and driven along the inside of the tibial shaft past the fracture and into the lower fragment. The nail may be bent slightly before insertion. The wounds are closed in the usual manner.

A useful bending tool can be fabricated from two lengths of tubular stainless-steel.

A splint is generally unnecessary unti the patient commences weight bearing, and then a light plaster cast may be applied.

Osteotomy — of the femur

Definition

Division of the upper shaft of the femur and displacement in order to alter the line of weight bearing of the extremity, e.g., in cases of osteoarthritis, certain femoral neck fractures and persistent valgus and subluxation of the hip in children.

Position

Supine, with leg abducted and supported by an assistant, or as Figure 5.21, Smith Petersen nail.

Instruments

General set (Figs. 14.1 to 14.28)
Bone and fracture set (p. 624)
Power drill or hand drill

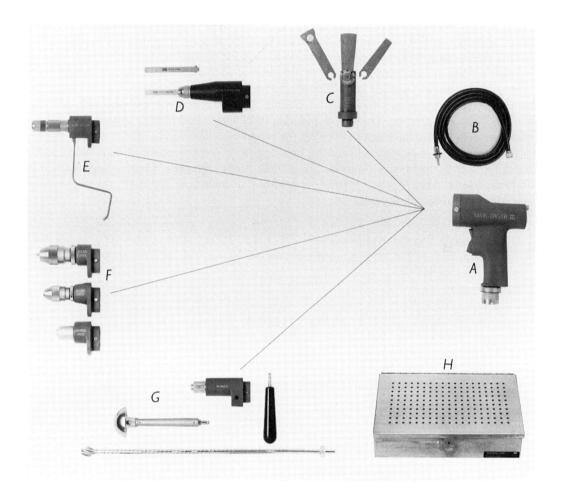

Fig. 23.71 The 3M Maxi-Driver III with attachments. (Orthopaedic Products — 3M Health Care Ltd.)
(A) The handpiece is an air vane motor with a maximum speed of 18,000 r.p.m. There is a speed selector ring at the base of the handle which can be used to vary the speed. The speed can be further controlled by the throttle lever. The handpiece is also cannulated to accept wires and pins. (B) Return air hose with a swivel to prevent the hose from twisting. (C) Oscillating saw attachment with blades that can be set in five positions. (D) Reciprocating saw attachment with blades. The saw has four blade positions. (E) Automatic pin driver — quick release mechanism that allows for easy pin insertion and advancement. The internal cannulation accommodates wires and pins from 1.58 mm–3.96 mm. (F) Universal chuck — designed to power intramedullary reamers with Hudson/Zimmer arbors. The 2.55 mm cannulation keyless chuck accepts straight shank wires and pins from 0.3 mm–2.4 mm, and straight shank twist drills from 0.8 mm to 6 mm.
(G) 250 r.p.m. reamer drive attachment for intramedullary acetabular reamers. (H) Stainless steel steam sterilizer case.

Twist drills, 3.2 mm ($\frac{1}{8}$ in) to 4.8 mm ($\frac{3}{16}$ in) diameter

Osteotomes 16 mm ($\frac{5}{8}$ in), 19 mm ($\frac{3}{4}$ in) and 38 mm ($1\frac{1}{2}$ in)

Bone punches (Smillie straight and angled), 2

(A high-speed air turbine and burr or oscillating saw may be used for performing the osteotomy (Fig. 23.71))

3 (0) Synthetic absorbable or plain catgut for ligatures

4 or 5 (1 or 2) Synthetic absorbable or plain or chromic catgut on a medium half-circle cutting or Mayo needle with trocar point for muscle sutures

2.5 or 3 (2/0 or 0) Synthetic non-absorbable or silk on a large curved or straight cutting needle for skin sutures.

Osteotomes, chisels and gouges generally are made from carbon or martensitic stainless-steel. Although carbon steel is the better material for a sharp edge, stainless-steel is less brittle, and there is less risk of a fragment breaking off during use (p. 626).

These cutting instruments are made in a variety of shapes and sizes as can be seen from Figure 23.72, but are classed according to the basic shape of the blade. An osteotome has two bevelled sides curving towards the cutting edge; a chisel has one flat side and one bevelled side; and a gouge has a curved cutting edge and is hollowed or grooved in section, being concave on one side and convex on the other.

Theoretically an osteotome is used for splitting as in the procedure of osteotomy, and a chisel for slicing; but many surgeons use a thick blade osteotome for splitting and a thin blade type for slicing. A gouge is used for grooving or hollowing and is of special use when saucering an osteomyelitis cavity or cyst.

If plate fixation is contemplated

Twist drill, No. 31 for 3.6 mm ($\frac{9}{64}$ in) screws, or 3.6 mm ($\frac{9}{64}$ in) for 4 mm ($\frac{5}{32}$ in) screws

Set of bone screws

Screw measure

Plate and screw-holding forceps, 2

Various bone clamps (Figs. 23.35 to 23.37 and 23.47)

Automatic screwdriver (Williams or Burns)

Plain screwdriver (Lane)

Osteotomy plates e.g. Müller

Appropriate osteotomy driver/extractor.

Outline of procedure

The trochanteric region of the femur is exposed as previously described for Smith Petersen nail.

A hole is drilled across the shaft below the level of the trochanter but just above the level of the lesser trochanter. Sometimes this drill is left in position whilst a radiographic check is made. Several holes are then drilled in the line of the osteotomy and the femur is cleanly divided with an osteotome. Alternatively, the femoral shaft is divided with a high-speed turbine and burr.

The leg is abducted and pressure applied to the proximal portion of the lower fragment until the shaft is displaced inwards. If no plate is being inserted, the wound is closed and the patient immobilised in a double plaster of Paris spica.

Some surgeons utilise metallic blade plates to fix the osteotomy, and these are driven into the upper fragment and screwed to the femoral shaft. The plate may incorporate a com-

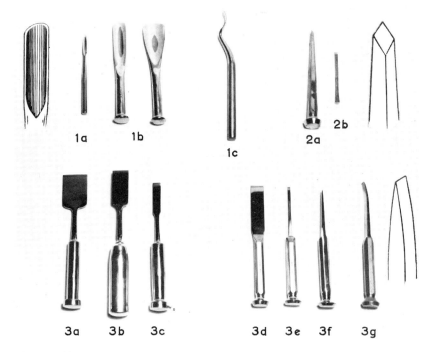

Fig. 23.72 Gouges, chisels and osteotomes
1a. Hahn gouge.
1b. Jones gouges, medium and large.
1c. Smith Petersen hip gouge.
2a. MacEwan chisel, side view.
2b. Hahn chisel.
3a. Whitchurch Howell osteotome, large.

3b. Bristow osteotome, medium.
3c. Whitchurch Howell osteotome, small.
3d. MacEwan osteotome, medium.
3e. MacEwan osteotome, small.
3f. MacEwan osteotome, side view.
3g. Platt osteotome, curved on flat.

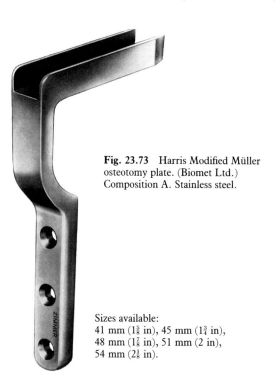

Fig. 23.73 Harris Modified Müller osteotomy plate. (Biomet Ltd.) Composition A. Stainless steel.

Sizes available:
41 mm ($1\frac{5}{8}$ in), 45 mm ($1\frac{3}{4}$ in),
48 mm ($1\frac{7}{8}$ in), 51 mm (2 in),
54 mm ($2\frac{1}{8}$ in).

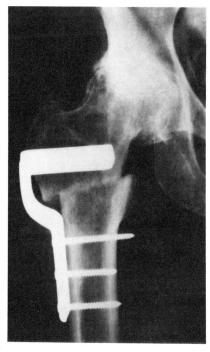

Fig. 23.74 Post-operative radiograph.

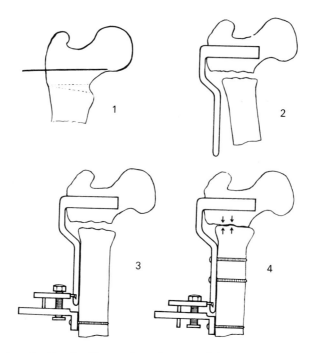

Fig. 23.75 1 Insertion of guide wire. Note wedge to be removed for varus osteotomy.
2 Appliance inserted parallel to proximal cut surface of the osteotomy and at least 2.5 cm (1 in) above it.
3 Müller clamp in position. Note the gap at the osteotomy.
4 Osteotomy compressed.

pression device to draw together the fragments on either side of the osteotomy, e.g., Müller, Figure 23.75, Coventry Infant lag screw and plate for varus osteotomy in children Figure 23.88. If this fixation is secure, the plaster spica is omitted.

Osteotomy of the tibia, with metallic fixation

Definition

Division of the shaft of tibia and excision of a wedge in order to alter the line of the shaft (especially performed for tibial deformities) and fixation with a plate or screws.

Position

Supine.

Instruments

General set (Figs. 14.1 to 14.28)
Bone and fracture set (p. 624)
Plating and screwing set (p. 638)
Circular saws
Osteotomes 16 mm ($\frac{5}{8}$ in), 19 mm ($\frac{3}{4}$ in) and 38 mm ($1\frac{1}{2}$ in)

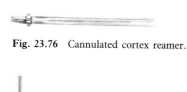

Fig. 23.76 Cannulated cortex reamer.

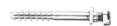

Fig. 23.77 Cannulated lag screw with nut.

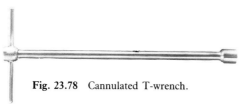

Fig. 23.78 Cannulated T-wrench.

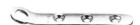

Fig. 23.79 Standard plate.

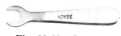

Fig. 23.80 C-spanner.

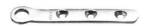

Fig. 23.81 Standard plate — straight.

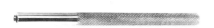

Fig. 23.82 Cannulated threaded handle.

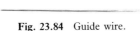

Fig. 23.84 Guide wire.

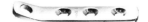

Fig. 23.83 Heavy duty plate.

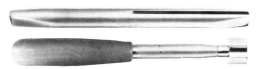

Fig. 23.85 Plate benders.

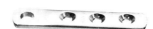

Fig. 23.86 Heavy duty plate — straight.

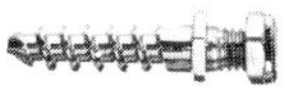

Fig. 23.87 Cannulated lag screw with nut.

Figs. 23.76 to 23.87 Coventry infant lag screw composition A Stainless steel (Reduced size). (D. Howse & Co.)

Developed by R. J. Brigden for Mr J. H. Penrose, FRCS, formerly consultant orthopaedic surgeon at Coventry and Warwickshire Hospital, England.

The use of a rigid blade plate for varus and valgus osteotomies in children has two disadvantages. Firstly the blade component has to be hammered home into the neck which is unnecessarily traumatic in a child, and secondly when performing a varus osteotomy the osteotomy has to be completed first. This subsequently involves driving the blade into the now mobile upper fragment which can prove difficult. Both these difficulties can be overcome by the use of a coarse threaded screw and plate as illustrated. The screw is cannulated and can be introduced over a guide wire if desired. When the screw has been satisfactory placed in the neck the osteotomy is performed.

During the application of the plate complete control of the angle of the upper fragment can be maintained by temporarily screwing a threaded handle on to the screw in place of the nut. When the plate has been screwed onto the shaft of the femur the handle is removed and the nut applied, giving rigid fixation. No hammering is necessary and the ease of application and subsequent removal is striking.

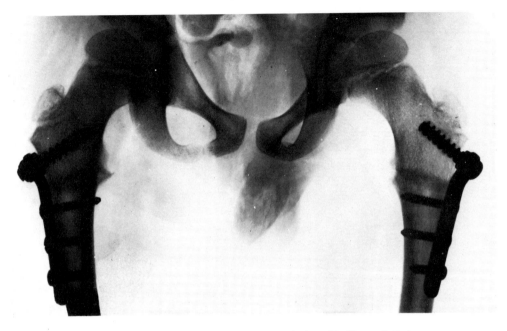

Fig. 23.88 Insertion technique for Coventry infant lag screw and plate. (D. Howse & Co.)

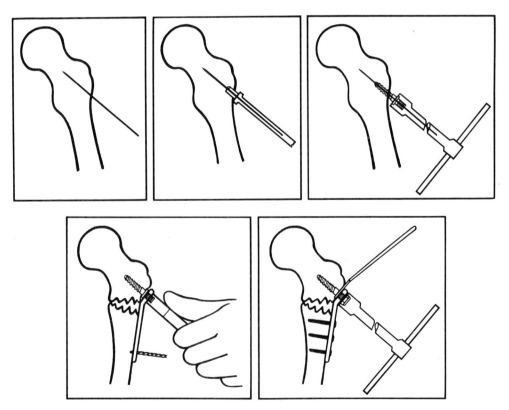

Fig. 23.89 Radiograph taken after insertion of Coventry infant lag screw and plate.

3 (0) Synthetic absorbable or plain catgut for ligatures

4 (1) Synthetic absorbable or plain catgut on a medium half-circle cutting or Mayo needle with a trocar point for muscle sutures

2.5 (2/0) Synthetic non-absorbable or silk or a medium curved or straight cutting needle for skin sutures.

Outline of procedure

The area for osteotomy is exposed with minimal periosteal stripping. A wedge of bone is excised, either with a circular saw or an osteotome, and the tibial shaft is re-aligned. The osteotomy is fixed by screws alone, or a plate contoured to the shape of the tibial shaft and secured with several screws.

The wound is closed in the usual manner; plaster of Paris may or may not be applied. This technique can be used for almost any bone shaft where it is necessary to excise a wedge of bone in order to alter the contour of the shaft.

Femoral and tibial epiphyseal arrest

Definition

Arrest of epiphyseal growth by inserting staples across the epiphyseal line of the lower femur and upper tibia. This retards growth of a normal leg in a child so that the short leg is allowed to grow and the two are equal in length when maturity is reached.

Position

Supine.

Instruments

General set (Figs. 14.1 to 14.28)

Bone and fracture set (p. 624)

Staples, stainless-steel or Vitallium (Müller)

Staples driver/inserter

2.5 mm (2/0) Synthetic absorbable or plain catgut for ligatures

3 (0) Synthetic absorbable or plain catgut on a medium half-circle cutting needle for deep sutures

2.5 (2/0) Synthetic non-absorbable on a medium curved cutting needle for skin sutures.

Outline of procedure

The epiphyseal lines of the lower end of the femur, upper end of the tibia and fibula are exposed through medial and lateral incisions which extend above and below the joint line on each side.

A 4 to 5 cm (1½ to 2 in) longitudinal incision is made along the central axis of the bone over the epiphyseal line, and the periosteum is reflected slightly. Two or more staples are inserted so that they bridge the epiphyses. This procedure is repeated on the other side of the femur and at both sides of the upper tibial epiphyses. The number of staples inserted, and whether femoral and tibial epiphyses are dealt with at the same operation, depends upon

Figs. 23.90 to 23.93 Epiphyseal staple sizes and insertion instruments. (Biomet Ltd.).

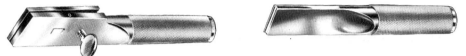

Fig. 23.90 Staple Driver/Inserter.

Fig. 23.91 Staple Punch or Set.

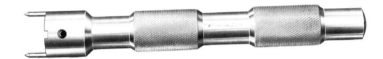

Fig. 23.92 Müller Staple Driver Inserter. (Staple fitted in position for insertion.)

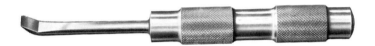

Fig. 23.93 Staple Extractor.

2.4 mm ($\frac{3}{32}$ in) diameter
16 mm ($\frac{5}{8}$ in) width × 19 mm ($\frac{3}{4}$ in) length
22 mm ($\frac{7}{8}$ in) width × 19 mm ($\frac{3}{4}$ in) length
Vitallium
16 mm ($\frac{5}{8}$ in) width × 16 mm ($\frac{5}{8}$ in) or 22 mm ($\frac{7}{8}$ in) length
22 mm ($\frac{7}{8}$ in) width × 16 mm ($\frac{5}{8}$ in) or 22 mm ($\frac{7}{8}$ in) length
10 mm ($\frac{3}{8}$ in) width × 16 mm ($\frac{5}{8}$ in), 22 mm ($\frac{7}{8}$ in) or 29 mm ($1\frac{1}{8}$ in) length

1.2 mm ($\frac{1}{16}$ in) diameter
16 mm ($\frac{5}{8}$ in) width × 19 mm ($\frac{3}{4}$ in) length
22 mm ($\frac{7}{8}$ in) width × 19 mm ($\frac{3}{4}$ in) length

the degree of shortening required. The epiphyseal line of the proximal fibula may be curetted to obliterate the growth centre. This operation is generally performed under radiological control.

The wound is closed in the usual manner. Growth of the bone continues after the staples are removed at a later date.

Bone grafts

Autogenous bone grafts (from the patient himself) are usually removed from either the tibia, fibular or ilium. These three provide cortical grafts, whole bone transplants or cancellous chips and strips respectively, although, of course, there is some of each type of bone in all.

Homogenous bone grafts (from another human donor) are obtained usually from non-infected amputated limbs and are stored in deep freeze, or are freeze dried in pieces of a size suitable for grafting.

In deep freeze, grafts are stored at $-15\,°C$ and then thawed in warm saline just before use. A small fragment of bone must be cultured a few days before use to confirm sterility of the specimen.

In the case of freeze dried specimens these are reconstituted by submerging in sterile saline before use.

In all cases, before the bone is stored, all soft tissue and cartilage is removed from the specimen and a Wassermann reaction performed on the donor, together with a check on the medical history to exclude other transmissible diseases.

Autogenous onlay graft, tibia to other long bone

Definition

The removal of a cortical bone graft from the anterior surface of the tibia for transplantation as an onlay graft, which is screwed into position to bridge a non-united fracture of another long bone. This type of graft may be used also for other procedures such as spinal fusion.

Position

Generally supine.

Instruments

General set (Figs. 14.1 to 14.28)
Bone and fracture set (p. 624)

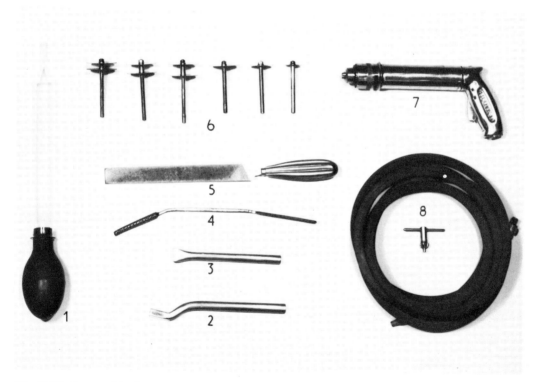

Fig. 23.94 Bone-grafting instruments
1. Irrigation syringe.
2. Bone punch, angled (Smillie).
3. Bone punch, straight (Smillie).
4. Bone rasp (Tubby).
5. Bone file (Tubby).
6. Circular saws, twin and single.
7. Power drill (Desoutter compressed air).
8. Rubber air hose for power drill and chuck key.

Bone grafting set (Fig. 23.94)
Bone clamps shown in Figures 23.35 to 23.37
Twist drill of appropriate size
Set of bone screws
Screw measure
Screw-holding forceps
Automatic screwdriver (Williams or Burns)
Plain screwdriver (Lane)
2.5 or 3 (2/0 or 0) Synthetic absorbable or plain catgut for ligatures
Appropriate size of synthetic absorbable or catgut and needles for muscle sutures in that area of the body
2.5 or 3 (2/0 or 0) Synthetic non-absorbable on a medium curved or straight cutting needle for skin sutures
Plaster of Paris.

Outline of procedure

The tibia is exposed through a curved incision and the periosteum is stripped off carefully from the graft area.

An oblong graft is removed from the anterior surface of the tibia with a circular or oscillatory bone saw. Ordinarily the borders are not violated as this would considerably weaken the tibia. The circular saw is driven by a power drill, and may be a medium 38 mm ($1\frac{1}{2}$ in) to 40 mm ($1\frac{5}{8}$ in) single or twin blade for the sides, and a small 19 mm ($\frac{3}{4}$ in) to 20 mm ($\frac{3}{4}$ in +) single blade for the ends. Saline irrigation provides lubrication for the saw, and the assistants must ensure that swabs and their hands are kept as far away from the blade as possible. In the first case, the gauze may foul the saw and become entwined with it; and in the second case, the saw may jerk during use with risk of injury to the assistant's hand. The use of an oscillatory bone saw reduces the danger of the blade 'jumping'. The oscillating movement of the blade from side to side permits cuts in either direction in bone but does not tear soft tissue, which if touched moves with the blade. Furthermore, it is considered that the amount of burning of the bone due to friction is reduced considerably.

The wound is closed in layers and the limb may be placed in a plaster cast. Sometimes if two teams are operating, one may cut the graft and the other insert it to reduce the operating time. In this case the instruments are split into two sets.

The non-united fracture area is exposed and the periosteum stripped off for the extent of the graft. The fracture ends are freshened, the bone re-aligned, and the cortical graft screwed in position on either side with two or more screws. The wound is closed in layers and a plaster cast applied.

Autogenous inlay or sliding graft

Definition

Sliding an oblong-shaped graft cut from the affected bone itself across a non-united fracture.

Position

Generally supine.

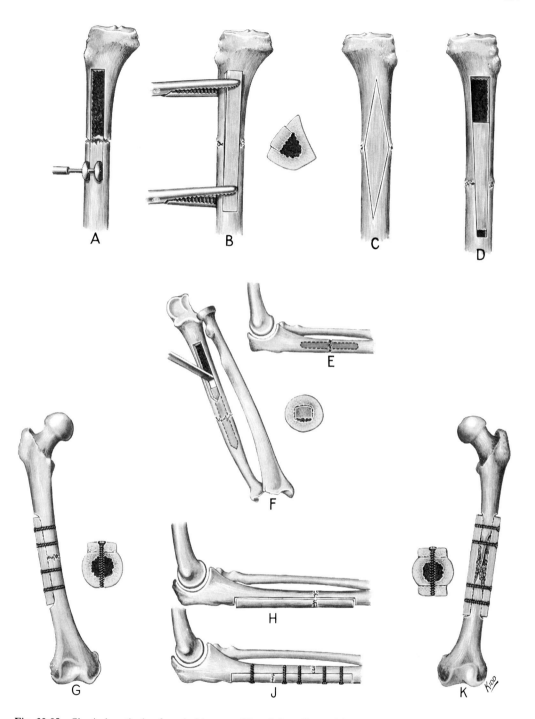

Fig. 23.95 Classical methods of cortical bone grafting. Inlay, diamond inlay, intramedullary peg. Onlay, sliding onlay, and double onlay grafts. A, B — inlay grafting by the Albee technique; C — diamond inlay grafting; D — sliding inlay grafting; E — intramedullary peg grafting; F — sliding intramedullary peg grafting; G — onlay grafting; H, J — sliding onlay grafting; K — double onlay grafting. (Wilson: *Watson–Jones Fractures and Joint Injuries*)

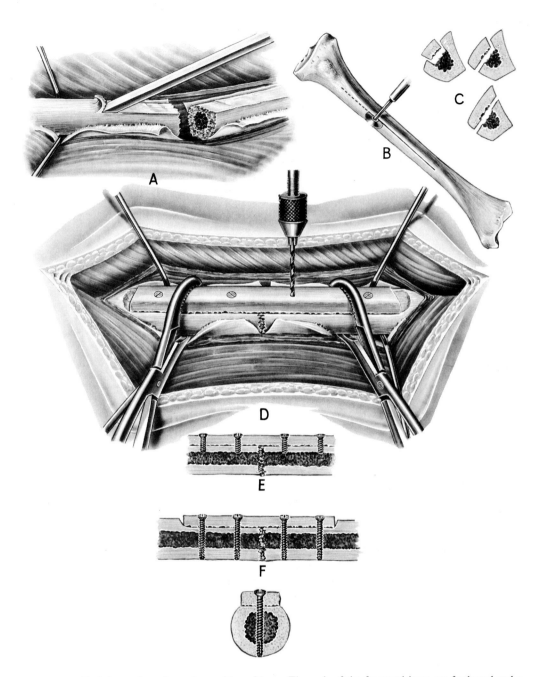

Fig. 23.96 Technique of massive onlay grafting of bone. The ends of the fractured bone are freshened and a bed is prepared on the surface of each fragment with a chisel (A). The graft cut from the tibia may include one or both cortical margins (B, C). The graft is fixed to the host bone by screws and inserted after a track has been drilled. (D). The screws must engage the opposite cortex (F) and the length should be measured accurately. Incorrect fixation with screws only engaging one cortex is also shown (E). (Wilson: *Watson–Jones Fractures and Joint Injuries*)

Instruments

As for onlay graft.

Outline and procedure

The fracture area is exposed and the periosteum stripped off for the extent of the graft. The fractured ends are freshened and fibrous tissue excised.

Using a twin saw, the surgeon cuts an oblong slot about 13 mm ($\frac{1}{2}$ in) wide, with one-third of its length at one side of the fracture line and two-thirds at the other. The grafts are levered from their bed and are re-inserted into the slot, but reversed so that the longer of the two bridges the fracture line. The two grafts are secured with screws and the wound is closed in the usual manner.

Either a plaster of Paris cast or a splint is applied.

Autogenous cancellous iliac grafts

Definition

The removal of cancellous strips or wedges from the ilium as a bone graft for non-united fractures or in fusion procedures, e.g., spine.

Position

Supine.

Instruments

General set (Figs. 14.1 to 14.28)
Bone and fracture set (p. 624)
Osteotomes, 16 mm ($\frac{5}{8}$ in), 19 mm ($\frac{3}{4}$ in) and 25 mm (1 in)
Diathermy leads, electrodes and lead anchoring forceps
Suction tubing, nozzles and tube anchoring forceps
Power saw may be required
Corrugated drainage tubing
4 (1) Synthetic absorbable or plain catgut for ligatures
4 or 5 (1 or 2) Synthetic absorbable, plain or chromic catgut on a large half-circle cutting or Mayo needle with a trocar point for muscle sutures
2.5 or 3 (2/0 or 0) Synthetic non-absorbable or silk on a large curved cutting needle for skin sutures.

Outline of procedure

An incision is made along the subcutaneous border of the iliac crest and carried down to bone. The muscles are reflected off the bone subperiosteally to expose the graft area.

For sliver or chip grafts, these are removed with an osteotome parallel to the iliac crest. For wedge grafts, the graft is outlined with an osteotome and then peeled up with slight prying movements of a broad osteotome.

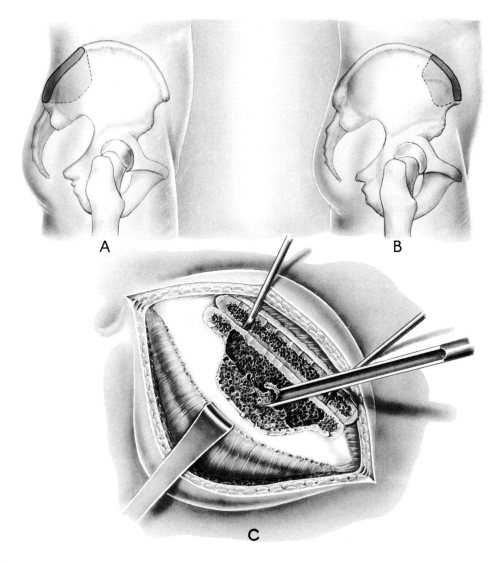

Fig. 23.97 Cancellous chip grafting of bone. Cancellous chip grafts should usually be cut from the ilium in the region of the posterior superior spine and the crest (A) or from near the anterior superior spine (B). The crest is reflected with its attached muscles and the grafts are then cut with a gouge (C). (Wilson: *Watson–Jones Fractures and Joint Injuries*).

The wound is closed in the usual manner, occasionally with drainage. The graft is then transferred to the host area either as strips, chips, or a wedge which may be screwed into position.

Aspiration of a joint

Definition

The removal of fluid from a joint by suction, using a syringe and hollow needle.

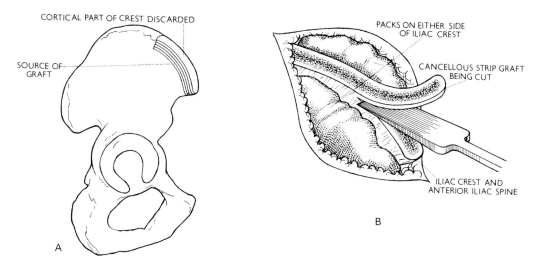

Fig. 23.98 Bone for Phemister grafting should be cut as cancellous strips from the anterior part of the iliac crest (A), the cortical top of the crest being discarded. Both sides of the crest must be displayed (B). To close the donor site the gluteal muscles are sutured to the abdominal muscles. Suction drainage should be used for 24 to 48 hours after taking the graft. (Wilson: *Watson–Jones Fractures and Joint Injuries.*)

Position

Depends upon the joint being aspirated.

Instruments

As Figure 23.99.

Outline of procedure

Basically the same set of instruments is required for the aspiration of any joint. Wide-bore aspirating needles are used with a syringe of at least 20 ml capacity.

The area is prepared and draped, and the needle attached to the syringe is inserted into the cavity. If the needle is large, a scalpel will be used to make a stab incision. The fluid is aspirated and a specimen sent to the laboratory for microbiological examination. The puncture wound is sealed with cotton-wool and Nobecutane, and a pressure dressing may be applied in conjunction with a splint or guarding plaster.

Arthroscopy

Definition

Endoscopic examination of a joint; generally the knee joint.

Position

Supine with leg straight or flexed over the bottom section of the operation table, which is lowered or removed.

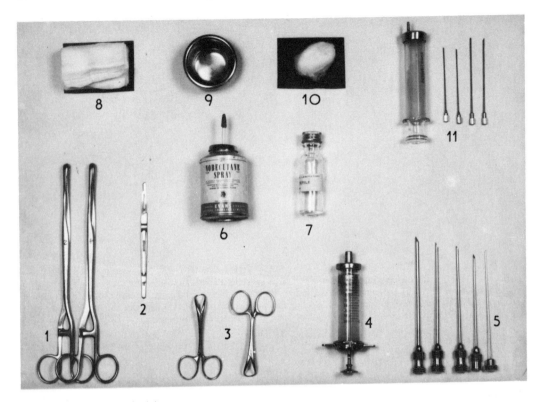

Fig. 23.99   Aspiration of a joint
1. Sponge-holding forceps (Rampley), 2.
2. Scalpel handle No. 9 with No. 15 blade (Bard Parker).
3. Towel clips, 2.
4. Aspiration syringe (Martin).
5. Wide-bore needles for Martin aspiration syringe, 3 assembled needles and 1 dismantled to show needle and obturator.
6. Nobecutane for sealing puncture wound.
7. Specimen bottle.
8. Swabs.
9. Gallipot containing skin antiseptic.
10. Cotton-wool for sealing over puncture wound.
11. 20 ml syringe and aspiration needles.

Instruments

Sponge-holding forceps (Rampley), 3
Scalpel handïe No. 3 with No. 10 blade (Bard Parker)
Artery forceps, curved on flat (Dunhill), 2
Dissecting forceps, toothed fine (Gillies)
Scissors, straight, 15 cm (6 in) (Mayo)
Needle holder (Kilner)
Arthroscope, fibre light cable, irrigation tube, trocar and cannulae for arthroscope
Biopsy forceps
Irrigation fluid in plastic bags (Ringer's lactate or saline) and irrigation set
Aspiration needles/cannula 14 g, 7.5 cm (3 in)
Towel clips (Backhaus), 6
Syringes, 100 ml, 2
2.5 (2/0) Synthetic non-absorbable or silk on a small curved cutting needle for skin sutures.

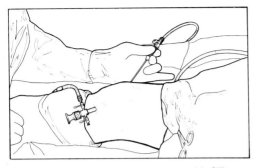

Fig. 23.100 Arthroscope in knee joint with filling tube plus drainage tube.

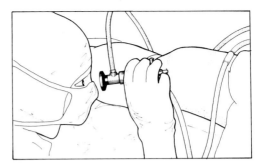

Fig. 23.101 Viewing medial meniscus. (Down's Surgical Ltd.)

Outline of procedure

The operation is carried out under tourniquet and with continuous irrigation. Irrigation is generally provided from two pre-warmed three or five litre bags of saline or Ringer's lactate solution which are coupled via a Y connector and tubing to an inlet on the arthroscope sheath. The outflow of fluid is channeled through a separate tube attached to an irrigating cannula. Fluid flow though the knee may be by continuous irrigation and suction, or with intermittent independent drainage. With suction, this is applied to the outflow tubing; with dependent drainage, the outflow tubing is directed into a bucket.

The solution bags are prepared and the inflow irrigation tubing is temporarily occluded with clamps at the instrument end. The arthroscope, lighting, and various instruments are checked. The operation site is prepared in the usual manner and the lateral aspect of the knee covered with a plastic skin barrier drape (Steridrape, OpSite etc).

The most commonly used portal is anterolateral; the central and anteromedial approaches are also used. Saline or Ringer's lactate solution (80 mm) may first be injected to distend the knee joint. A stab incision is made and an irrigation cannula inserted; this is coupled to the outflow tubing (which may be connected to suction or directed to a bucket). Another stab incision is made and the trocar and cannula are inserted to pierce the joint capsule. The sharp trocar is removed and if the knee has not been distended with fluid beforehand, replaced with a blunt obturator to avoid damage to the articular cartilage as the cannula is

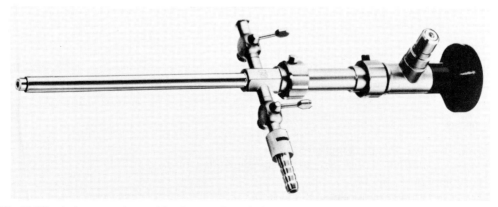

Fig. 23.102 Arthroscope, sleeve with telescope. (Down's Surgical Ltd.)

advanced. The inflow irrigation tubing is connected to the cannula, and the obturator replaced with the arthoscope which is locked into the protective sheath. The light cables are connected to the arthroscope and the clamps removed from the inflow tubing to commence irrigation.

The patella-femoral articulation and the supra condylar pouch are examined. The medial compartment, lateral femoral tibial articulation and medial meniscus are readily visualised by flexing the knee with a valgus strain. A blunt right-angled probe may be inserted into the joint through a separate stab incision. This is used to manipulate and explore structures within the joint. A variety of instruments are available for diagnostic and operative arthroscopy procedures (Aiello, 1986); these include:

Grasping forceps for the removal of loose bodies and tissue fragments

Punches to resect portions of meniscus, plicae or articular cartilage which may then be irrigated from the joint

Scissors to cut away portions of menisci or tissue

Synovial biopsy forceps

Knives to cut torn meniscus, lateral retinacular release of the patella

Curettes

Guillotine forceps for cutting meniscus or resecting tissue

Magnetic suction retrieval for removing metallic objects from the knee

Motorised intra-articular shaver for trimming torn menisci, articular cartilage and other soft tissue

Instruments for anterior ligament repairs.

These instruments may be passed through the same incision or through a second cannula, visualisation taking place through the arthroscope. A camera or television fibre cable can be attached to the telescope at any stage of the procedure.

At the end of the procedure the knee joint is drained of fluid, the outflow draining cannula and arthroscope cannula removed, and the small incisions closed with a suture if not proceeding to an arthrotomy. A plaster wool and crepe pressure bandage is applied and the tourniquet removed.

Arthrotomy, meniscectomy or removal of loose bodies (knee)

Definition

Removal of a torn semilunar cartilage, or removal of loose bodies which are usually osteo-cartilaginous in nature.

Position

Supine, with leg straight or flexed over the bottom section of the operation table, which is lowered or removed.

Instruments

Sponge holding forceps (Rampley), 5
Scalpel handles No. 4 with No. 20 blades (Bard Parker), 2
Dissecting forces, toothed (Lane), 2
Dissecting forces, non-toothed, 15 cm (6 in), 2
Scissors, straight, 15 cm (6 in) (Mayo)

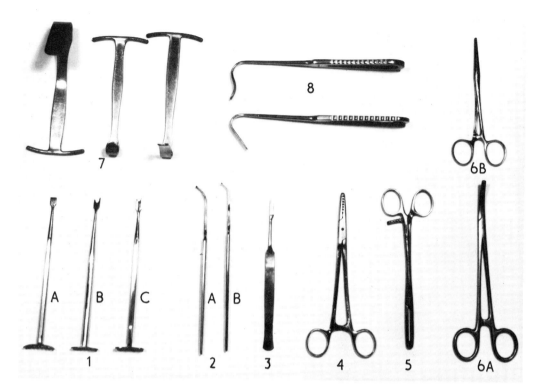

Fig. 23.103 Meniscectomy
1. Cartilage knives (Smillie).
   A. Chisel-shaped blade.
   B. and C. With probe-shaped lateral projections.
2. Meniscectomy knives (Fairbank).
   A. Blade for cutting to the left.
   B. Blade for cutting to the right.
3. Cartilage knife (Munro).

4. Cartilage-holding forceps.
5. Cartilage-holding forceps (Martin).
6. A. Cartilage-holding forceps, curved on flat (Mayo-Oschner), 3.
   B. Cartilage-holding forceps, straight (Kocher), 2.
7. Cartilage retractors (Smillie), set of 3.
8. Cartilage retractors (Jackson Burrow).

Scissors, curved on flat, 15 cm (6 in) (Mayo)

Retractors, double hook, 2

Small retractors, single hook, 2

Artery forceps, curved on flat (Kilner), 5

Tissue forceps (Allis), 5

Needle holder (Kilner)

Meniscectomy set (Fig. 23.103)

2.5 (2/0) Synthetic absorbable or plain catgut for ligatures

3 or 4 (0 or 1) Synthetic absorbable or plain catgut on a medium half-circle cutting needle for deep sutures

2.5 (2/0) Synthetic non-absorbable on a medium curved cutting needle for skin sutures.

Outline of procedure

The long slender knives used for removing a torn cartilage need to be resharpened frequently. However, care must be taken to ensure that the knife is discarded when its

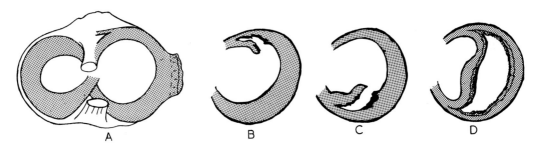

Fig. 23.104   The upper end of tibia and menisci. (A) The medial meniscus is attached to the medial ligament. (B) Anterior horn tear. (C) Posterior horn tear. (D) Bucket-handle tear. (Macfarlane *Textbook of Surgery*)

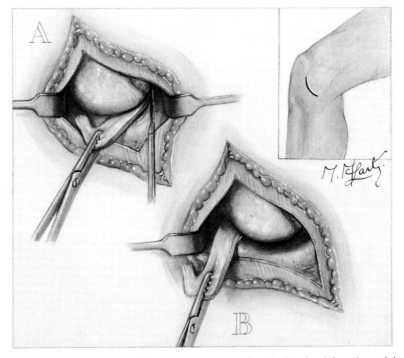

Fig. 23.105   Removal of semilunar cartilage of the knee. The cartilage is first freed from its peripheral attachment (A), and at its anterior end. It is then dislocated, if possible, into the intercondyloid space (B), before being detached posteriorly. (Top inset) Incision. (Farquharson and Rintoul *Textbook of Operative Surgery, 6th Ed*)

dimensions and strength have been reduced considerably by grinding. A very thin, weak knife is dangerous in the knee joint, for if it breaks in the back of the knee, the surgeon may have to make an additional incision in order to remove the broken piece.

A curved or straight incision is made just medial or lateral to the patella, depending upon the location of the torn meniscus or loose bodies. Occasionally it may be necessary to make a posterior approach from the back of the knee. The incision is deepened through the fascia and the capsule and synovium is incised.

In the case of meniscectomy, the semilunar cartilage is detached from the tibial plateau,

utilising the special clamps and cartilage knives. In the case of loose bodies, these are removed with forceps or a curetting spoon.

The wound is closed in layers and the knee is immobilised with a padded metal back splint, wool and bandages.

Synovectomy (knee joint)

Definition

Excision of a diseased synovial membrane.

Position

Supine.

Instruments

General set (Figs. 14.1 to 14.28)
Tissue forceps, curved (Fagge), 5
Long scalpel, solid variety
Scissors, curved on flat 15 cm (6 in) (Mayo)
3 (0) Synthetic absorbable or plain catgut for ligatures
4 (1) Synthetic absorbable or plain catgut on a large half-circle cutting or Mayo needle with trocar point for capsule sutures
4 or 5 (1 or 2) Synthetic absorbable or non-absorbable, or silk on a large half-circle cutting or Mayo needle with trocar point for muscle sutures
3 (0) Synthetic non-absorbable or silk on a large curved cutting needle for skin sutures.

Outline of procedure

The joint is exposed through an anteromedial incision, which generally commences about 10 cm (4 in) above the knee joint on the medial border of the quadriceps tendon, curves round the inner border of the patella, and continues in the midline down to or below the tibial tubercle. The fascia is incised and retracted and the capsule exposed by dissection between the medial border of the quadriceps tendon and the vastus medialis muscle. The capsule and synovial membrane are incised and the patella retracted laterally.

The entire synovial membrane is excised by block dissection from the inner, outer and anterior aspects of the joint. The prepatellar pad of fat is excised and any other pathological tissue on the femoral condyles is removed with a scalpel or gauze swab. Care is taken to avoid damage to the posterior capsule of the knee and the popliteal vessels in the midline.

After all the pathological tissue has been excised the wound is closed. If the ligaments have been divided they are apposed and sutured. The capsule is sutured, followed by the fascia and skin. The leg is immobilised either with a padded metal back splint, wool and bandages, or a plaster of Paris cast.

Patellectomy

Definition

Excision of the patella for hypertrophic arthritis and fractures.

Position

Supine.

Instruments

As for synovectomy
Bone-holding forceps (St Thomas')
Bone awl
Ligatures and sutures as for synovectomy.

Outline of procedure

A longitudinal or transverse incision is made over the patella and deepened down to the bone. The whole patella (or fragments in the case of a fracture) is dissected free from the tendon.

The knee is closed in the usual manner, repairing the defect in the quadriceps mechanism by overlapping the tendon with synthetic absorbable chromic catgut, or silk sutures. The leg is immobilised in a plaster of Paris cast.

Arthrodesis of toes

Definition

Fusion of the proximal phalangeal joints of the toes.

Position

Supine.

Instruments

Sponge-holding forceps (Rampley), 5
Towel clips, 5
Scalpel handles No. 3 with Nos 10 and 15 blades (Bard Parker), 2
Scalpel, solid variety
Fine dissecting forceps, toothed (Gillies), 2
Fine dissecting forceps, non-toothed (McIndoe)
Fine retractors, double hook, 2
Scissors, curved on flat, 13 cm (5 in) (Mayo)
Small bone cutting forceps (Liston)
Small bone nibbling forceps, curved
Bone levers (Trethowan ring spikes), 2
Small rugine (Faraboeuf)
Small gouges, 6 mm, 10 mm and 12 mm (Jenkins or Hahn), 3
Small mallet (Rowland)
Bone awl (optional)
Austenitic traction wires (Kirschner), 1.6 mm (0.062 in) diameter, 9 cm (3½ in) long, and sterile corks

Hand chuck or Kirschner wire drill, if wires are to be used
Wire-cutting forceps
Small needle holder
2 (3/0) Synthetic non-absorbable on a small curved cutting needle for skin sutures
Ribbon gauze and plastic dressing (Nobecutane) to form individual toe splints.

Outline of procedure

A transverse or longitudinal incision is made over the joint to be fused. The joint is exposed and the cartilage removed from the bone surfaces with bone cutters, gouges or the solid scalpel. Fusion is achieved either with a 'spike' arthrodesis or intramedullary wires.

With a 'spike' arthrodesis, the distal end of the proximal or middle phalanx is fashioned into the shape of a spike and a hole made with an awl in the proximal end of the middle or distal phalanx. This spike is wedged into the hole and the skin incision sutured before immobilising the toe with a Nobecutane splint.

For Kirschner wire fixation, the wire is drilled retrograde fashion from the joint through the distal phalanx and out through the toe pulp just below the nail, so that one end is flush with the joint surface being fused. The two bone ends are brought into apposition and the wire is drilled back across the joint surface and into the proximal phalanx. If an excess amount of wire is left protruding from the toe, this is cut short or turned over before attaching a cork to cover the point. The skin incision is sutured and the toe immobilised further with a Nobecutane splint.

Arthrodesis of ankle (sliding fibula graft)

Definition

Fusion of the ankle utilising fibula graft.

Position

Supine, with a sandbag placed under the buttock on the affected side.

Instruments

General set (Figs. 14.1 to 14.28)
Bone and fracture set (p. 624)
Plating and screwing set (p. 638)
Osteotomes, 13 mm ($\frac{1}{2}$ in), 16 mm ($\frac{5}{8}$ in) and 19 mm ($\frac{3}{4}$ in)
Gouges, 13 mm ($\frac{1}{2}$ in), 16 mm ($\frac{5}{8}$ in) and 19 mm ($\frac{3}{4}$ in)
Circular saws, medium and small, single blades
Wire saw and handles (Gigli or Olivecrona), optional
2.5 (2/0) Synthetic absorbable or plain catgut for ligatures
3 or 4 (0 or 1) Synthetic absorbable or plain catgut on a medium half-circle cutting or
   Mayo needle with a trocar point for muscle sutures
2.5 (2/0) Synthetic non-absorbable or silk on a medium curved cutting needle for skin
   sutures
Plaster of Paris.

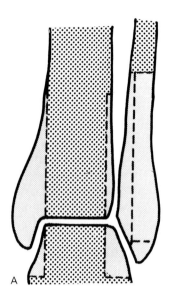 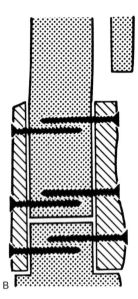

Fig. 23.106 Arthrodesis of ankle. (A) White area outlines the bone to be removed. The part of the fibula depicted by the broken line is preserved for use as an onlay graft. (B) The operation completed. The lower part of the tibia and the talus are sandwiched between the two bone grafts. (Crawford Adams: *Standard Orthopaedic Operations*)

Outline of procedure

An incision is made along the line of the fibula starting about 15 cm (6 in) above the ankle joint, curving slightly as it reaches the heel.

The superficial and deep tissues are incised to expose the fibula and ankle joint. The fibula is divided across about 13 cm (5 in) above the external malleolus and excised, and is placed in a sterile saline. The cartilage is excised from the joint surfaces of the tibia and talus. The lateral surface of the tibia adjoining the excised portion of the fibula is roughened and a groove cut in the lateral surface of the talus bone.

All periosteum and cartilage is removed from the fibula graft and the medial aspect is smoothed to ensure a close fit when the fibula is re-inserted below its original position. This graft is then screwed to the tibia and talus and any gaps which may be left are packed with cancellous bone chips which can be obtained either from the bone bank or the patent's iliac crest.

The wound is closed in the usual manner and the leg is immobilised in a plaster of Paris cast.

Tripe arthrodesis. Stabilisation of the foot

Definition

Stabilisation of the foot by removing the cartilaginous surfaces of the subtaloid, calcaneocuboid and talonavicular joints.

Position

Supine, with a sandbag under the buttock on the affected side.

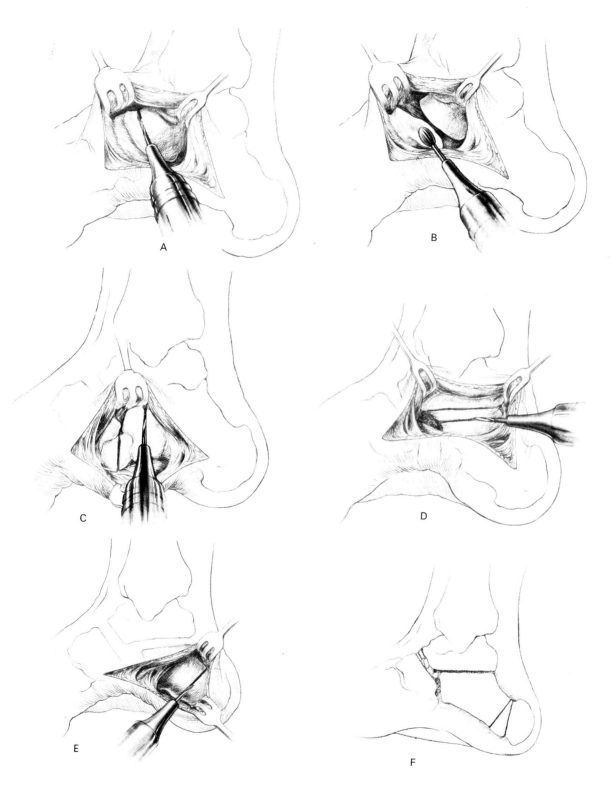

Fig. 23.107 Triple arthrodesis of the ankle carried out with air tool and burr. (A) Excision of head of talus. (B) Removing navicular cartilage. (C) Excision of bone from both surfaces of calcaneo cuboid joint. (D) Removal of both surfaces of subtalar joint. (E) Osteotomy of calcaneus. (F) Completed operation. (Hall: *Air Instrument Surgery, Orthopaedic.*)

Instruments

General set (Figs. 14.1 to 14.28)
Bone and fracture set (p. 624)
Osteotomes, 16 mm ($\frac{5}{8}$ in), 19 mm ($\frac{3}{4}$ in) and 25 mm (1 in)
Gouges, 16 mm ($\frac{5}{8}$ in), 19 mm ($\frac{3}{4}$ in) and 25 mm (1 in)
2.5 (2/0) Synthetic absorbable or plain catgut for ligatures
3 or 4 (0 or 1) Synthetic absorbable or plain catgut on a medium half-circle cutting or
Mayo needle for deep sutures.
2.5 (2/0) Synthetic non-absorbable or silk on a medium curved cutting needle for skin
sutures.

Outline of procedure

The subtaloid, talo-navicular and calcaneo-cuboid joints are generally exposed through a curved dorsolateral incision which is deepened through the fascia and ligaments. The foot is dislocated medially at mid-tarsal level.

The cartilage is removed from the joint surfaces in such a manner that the three bones can be brought in good contact with each other in the position chosen for fusion. The wound is closed and a plaster of Paris cast applied to the leg.

Some surgeons utilise metallic staples across the calcaneocuboid joint.

Arthrodesis of knee (Charnley's operation)

Definition

Fusion of the knee joint by compression arthrodesis.

Position

Supine.

Instruments

General set (Figs. 14.1 to 14.28)
Bone and fracture set (p. 624)
Amputation saw with detachable guard (Sergeant) or power driven saw
Large tissue forceps (Fagge or Lane), 4
Traction pins (Steinmann), 2 of size 4.8 mm ($\frac{3}{16}$ in) diameter by 20 cm to 25 cm (8 to
10 in) long, with diamond points and square or triangular chuck ends
Hand or power drill
Compression clamps (Charnley), 2
Pin caps or small corks, 2
3 (0) Synthetic absorbable or plain catgut for ligatures
4 and 5 (1 and 2) Synthetic absorbable or plain catgut on a medium half-circle cutting
or Mayo needle with a trocar point for capsule, etc.
2.5 or 3 (2/0 or 0) Synthetic non-absorbable or silk on a medium curved or straight cutting
needle for skin sutures.

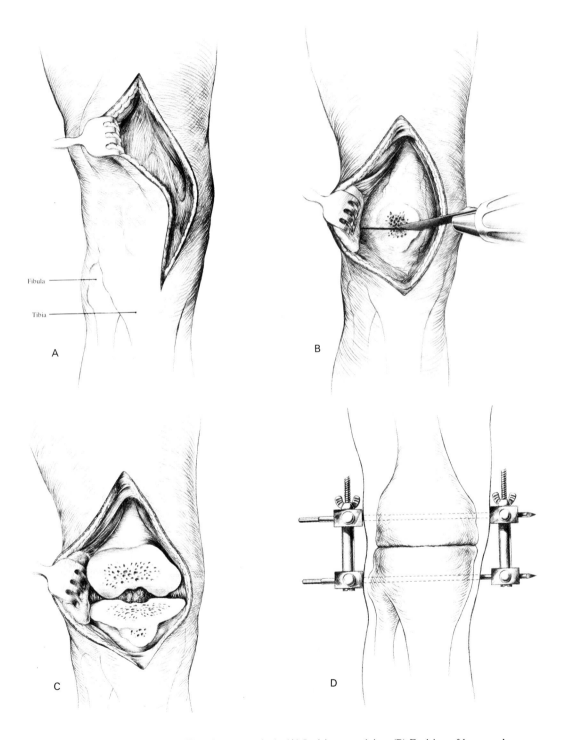

Fig. 23.108 Arthrodesis of knee (Charnleys operation). (A) Incision over joint. (B) Excision of bone wedge from superior aspect of upper tibia. (C) Similar amount of bone excised from lower end of femur so that both surfaces fit together with the knee in 10 degrees of flexion to full extension. (D) Steinmans pins inserted and compression clamps applied. (Hall: *Air Instrument Surgery, Orthopaedic*.)

Outline of procedure

The joint is exposed through a longitudinal anterolateral incision or a transverse incision similar to patellectomy but with wider exposure.

The patella is either excised or the cartilage from the undersurface is removed with the amputation saw. The joint is flexed and a small amount of the upper end of the tibia and condyles at the lower end of the femur, together with the joint cartilage, are removed with the saw. The saw cuts are placed almost parallel to each other so that when the raw surfaces of the two bones are brought together, the knee is in the correct position for fusion (that is usually with about 10 degrees of flexion).

Two stout Steinmann's pins are inserted parallel to each other through the lower end of the femur and the upper end of the tibia. These are clamped together with Charnley's compression clamps on the medial and lateral aspect of the leg, with sufficient compression to maintain good contact between the two surfaces of raw bone.

The wound is closed and the leg is immobilised on a Thomas splint or in a plaster of Paris cast.

Arthrodesis of hip (Brittain extra-articular fusion)

Definition

Extra-articular fusion of the hip by means of cortical bone graft which is driven through an osteotomy of the upper femur and into the ischium.

Position

As for Smith Petersen nail (Fig. 23.57).

Instruments

General set (Figs. 14.1 to 14.28)
Bone and fracture set (p. 624)
Bone grafting set (Fig. 23.94)
Osteotomes, 13 mm ($\frac{1}{2}$ in), 25 mm (1 in) and 38 mm ($1\frac{1}{2}$ in)
Twin chisels (Brittain) for positioning of graft (optional)
Twist drills, 4.8 mm ($\frac{3}{16}$ in) and 6.4 mm ($\frac{1}{4}$ in) diameter, 13 cm (5 in) long
Bone punches (Smillie), angled and straight, 2
3 (0) Synthetic absorbable or plain catgut for ligatures
4 (1) Synthetic absorbable, plain or chromic catgut on a large half-circle cutting or Mayo needle with trocar point for muscle sutures
3 (0) Synthetic non-absorbable or silk on a large curved or straight cutting needle for skin sutures.

Outline of procedure

The upper third of the femur is exposed through a lateral longitudinal incision as for Smith Petersen nail. A drill is introduced at a predetermined point through the femur and into the ischium. Its position is verified radiologically and, if correct, a number of holes are drilled along a transverse line each side of it.

Either a suitable piece of cortical bone about 13 mm ($\frac{1}{2}$ in) wide by 15 cm (6 in) long is cut from the tibia (see bone grafting) or removed from the bone bank. The graft is bevelled to a point at one end and denuded of any adherent soft tissue. An osteotomy of the femur is made in line with the drill holes and the osteotome is driven on until it has penetrated the ischium. A slot is created in the ischium by levering the osteotome backwards and forwards and the graft is inserted along the blade until it enters this slot. The osteotome is then removed and the graft is driven home. Some surgeons use the Brittain twin chisel to assist this manoeuvre but in either case the graft is inserted so that its endosteal portion lies distally.

The distal portion of the femur just below the osteotomy, is then displaced inwards with the bone punch and the wound is closed in layers. The patient is immobilised in a double hip spica.

Arthrodesis of the hip (Charnley's central dislocation fusion)

Definition

Intra-articular fusion of the hip by planing the head and neck of the femur into a tubular shape which fits into a corresponding size of hole in the acetabulum.

Position

Supine.

Instruments

General set (Figs. 14.1 to 14.28)
Bone and fracture set (p. 624)
Artery forceps, curved on flat (Kelly Fraser), 20
Large tissue forceps (Fagge or Lane), 5
Large retractors (Hibb), 2
Scissors, heavy, curved on flat, 20 cm (8 in) (Mayo)
Long scalpel, solid variety
Osteotomes, 16 mm ($\frac{5}{8}$ in), 22 mm ($\frac{7}{8}$ in) and 28 mm ($1\frac{1}{8}$ in)
Osteotomes, 13 mm ($\frac{1}{2}$ in) and 16 mm ($\frac{5}{8}$ in) (curved)
Gouges, 13 mm ($\frac{5}{8}$ in), 22 mm ($\frac{7}{8}$ in) and 38 mm ($1\frac{1}{2}$ in)
Hip levers (Judet), 2
Reamers for shaping the femoral head (32 mm [$1\frac{1}{4}$ in] and 38 mm [$1\frac{1}{2}$ in]. Crawford Adam head shapers are suitable)
Perforator drills for acetabular hole (32 mm [$1\frac{1}{4}$ in] and 38 mm [$1\frac{1}{2}$ in])
Hip brace
Irrigation syringe and warm sterile saline
Suction tubing, wide nozzles and tube anchoring forceps
Diathermy leads, electrodes and lead anchoring forceps
3 and 4 (0 and 1) Synthetic absorbable or plain catgut for ligatures
4 or 5 (1 or 2) Synthetic absorbable, chromic catgut or silk on a large half-circle cutting needle for muscle sutures
3 (0) Synthetic non-absorbable or silk on a large curved cutting needle for skin sutures.

Outline of procedure

There are several approaches to the hip joint, including anterior, lateral or posterior. Only one approach will be described and that is the anterolateral approach.

An incision is made commencing about 8 cm (3 in) below the trochanter, continuing to a point over the trochanter where it curves anteriorly to complete the flap. The fascia lata is incised in line with the longitudinal portion of the wound and the gluteus medius and minimus are divided transversely. The capsule of the hip joint is incised and the hip dislocated forwards.

The size of the femoral head is reduced to that of the femoral neck by gouging and planing away the cartilage and cortex of the bone. A hole of corresponding size is drilled in the acetabulum and all joint cartilage is removed. The cavity is irrigated to remove debris and the hip is returned to its normal position, but with the reconstructed head and neck jammed in the hole made in the acetabulum. Any gaps remaining in the joint cavity are filled with bone shavings obtained when drilling the acetabular hole.

The wound is closed with the leg supported in the optimum position for fusion, and a double hip plaster spica is applied for immobilisation

Arthrodesis of the wrist (Brittain fusion)

Definition

Fusion of the wrist by inserting a bone graft between the lower end of the radius and the base of the third metacarpal bone.

Position

Supine, with affected arm extended on an arm table.

Instruments

General set (Figs. 14.1 to 14.28)
Bone and fracture set (p. 624)
Bone grafting set (p. 675)
Power driven burr may be used
2.5 (2/0) Synthetic absorbable or plain catgut for ligatures
3 (0) Synthetic absorbable or plain catgut on a small half-circle cutting needle for deep sutures
2.5 (2/0) Synthetic non-absorbable or silk on a medium curved cutting needle for skin sutures.

Outline of procedure

A longitudinal incision is made on the dorsal aspect of the wrist extending just distal to the base of the third metacarpal to about 8 cm (3 in) above the lower end of the radius. This incision is deepened and the tendons retracted to each side.

A circular saw or burr is used to cut a longitudinal slot for the graft, extending from a point 5 cm (2 in) above the end of the radius to the proximal third of the third metacarpal bone. This graft bed, which is prepared about 13 mm ($\frac{1}{2}$ in) in width, includes the carpal bones between the radius and third metacarpal without respect to their identity. A small

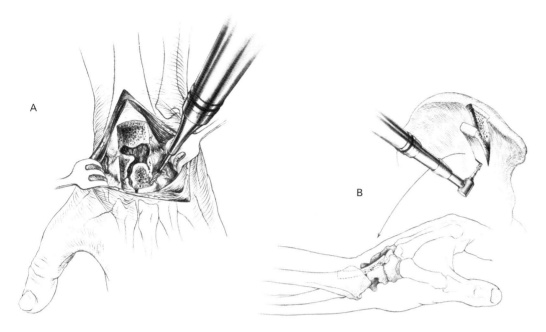

Fig. 23.109 (A) Arthrodesis of wrist. Preparation of graft bed in distal radius and carpals. (B) Removal of graft from illium and insertion of graft in wrist to maintain arthrodesis. (Hall: *Air Instrument Surgery Orthopaedics.*)

osteotome is introduced into each end of the bed of the raft to open the medullary cavity for about 10 mm ($\frac{3}{8}$ in).

A graft is taken from the bone bank or cut from the tibia and is the same width as the graft bed, but 13 mm ($\frac{1}{2}$ in) longer. This graft is pointed at both ends before introducing it into the radius for about 6 mm ($\frac{1}{4}$ in). Traction is exerted on the fingers and the other end of the graft is levered into the prepared hole in the third metacarpal bone. Release of traction will ensure a snug fit and good immobilisation of the graft.

The wound is closed in layers and a plaster of Paris cast is applied.

Arthroplasty of the hip (Austin Moore, McKee Farrar, Arden, Charnley and Wrightington F-C operations)

Definition

The reconstruction of new joint surfaces in the hip by replacing the femoral head with a metallic or metallic/plastic prosthesis.

Position

Lateral or supine, with a sandbag under the buttock on the affected side.

Instruments

General set (Figs. 14.1 to 14.28)
Bone and fracture set (p. 624)

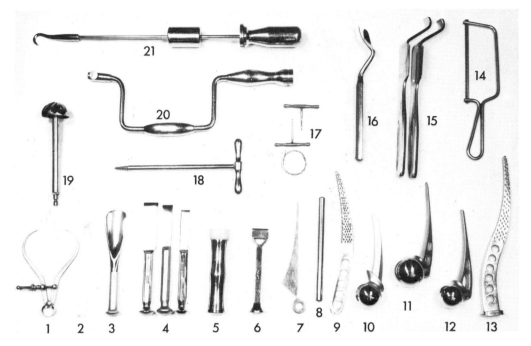

Fig. 23.110 Basic arthroplasty instruments
 1. Measuring calipers.
 2. Steel rule 15 cm (6 in).
 3. Large gouge or skid (for reduction of hip).
 4. Straight osteotomes 16 mm ($\frac{5}{8}$ in), 19 mm ($\frac{3}{4}$ in), 25 cm (1 in).
 5. Impactor (with nylon insert) for prosthesis.
 6. Box chisel.
 7. Template guide.
 8. Tommy-bar for shaft of rasps.
 9. Thompson rasp for femoral shaft.
10. Thompson prosthesis.
11. Austin Moore prothesis, standard stem.
12. Austin Moore prosthesis modified, narrow stem.
13. Austin Moore rasp.
14. Hacksaw.
15. Hip Levers (Judet).
16. Femoral head skid (Smith Petersen).
17. Wire saw (Gigli) with handles.
18. Auger for extracting femoral head (Judet).
19. Acetabular reamer (Duthie).
20. Brace for acetabular reamer.
21. Extractor for Austin Moore heads.

Arthroplasty set (Fig. 23.110)
Bone cement powder
Bone cement liquid
Bone cement mixer (Fig. 23.116)
Bone cement gun (Fig. 23.117)
Additional instruments for prosthesis
  McKee Farrar-Arden
  Hand drill and chuck key
  Twist drills, No. 32 (for screws), 6.4 mm ($\frac{1}{4}$ in), 9 mm ($\frac{5}{16}$ in), 10 mm ($\frac{3}{8}$ in)
  Bone screws (stainless steel)
  Automatic screwdriver (Williams)
  Ordinary screw driver (Lanes)
  Instrument for holding acetabular cup in position during setting of bone cement
  Charnley operation (Fig. 23.112)
  Wrightington operation (Fig. 23.113)
Artery forceps, curved on flat (Kelly Fraser), 20

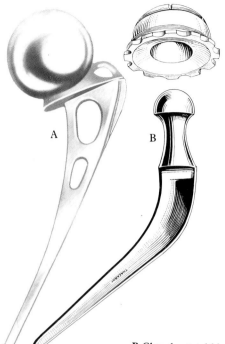

A Austin Moore self locking hip prosthesis (*Example: fenestrated regular curved stem*) (Sterile packet) (Howmedica U.K. Ltd.)

Vitallium composition B stainless steel, Titanium

Head diameter		Stem length	
mm	in	mm	in
38	$1\frac{1}{2}$	130	5
40		130	
41		130	
42	$1\frac{5}{8}$	130	5
43	$1\frac{11}{16}$	130	5
44	$1\frac{3}{4}$	130	5
45		140	
46	$1\frac{13}{16}$	140	$5\frac{1}{2}$
47	$1\frac{7}{8}$	140	$5\frac{1}{2}$
48		140	
49	$1\frac{15}{16}$	140	$5\frac{1}{2}$
50		150	
51	2	150	6
52	$2\frac{1}{16}$	150	6
53		150	
54	$2\frac{1}{8}$	150	6
55		150	
56		150	6
57	$2\frac{1}{4}$	150	6
60	$2\frac{3}{8}$	150	6
63	$2\frac{1}{2}$		

B Charnley total hip prosthesis (Chas. F. Thackray Ltd)

	Head diameter		Stem length		Cup O.D.	
	mm	in	mm	in	mm	in
w/small Cup	22	$\frac{7}{8}$	117	$4\frac{5}{8}$	43	$1\frac{11}{16}$
straight narrow stem	22	$\frac{7}{8}$	117	$4\frac{5}{8}$	40	$1\frac{9}{16}$
straight narrow stem small cup	22	$\frac{7}{8}$	121	$4\frac{3}{4}$	43	$1\frac{11}{16}$
	22	$\frac{7}{8}$	121	$4\frac{3}{4}$	40	$1\frac{9}{16}$

The Charnley Type Total Hip Prosthesis is a low friction replacement prosthesis for arthroplasty of the hip joint. A two-piece appliance, it combines the tissue compatibility of a Vitallium femoral prosthesis with the low friction characteristics of an ultra-high molecular weight polyethylene cup. The femoral head portion is ground to a virtually perfect spherical shape and polished to an optical mirror finish. Shaped and polished to an optical mirror finish. The cup is double wrapped and sterilized by gamma radiation. A radiopaque Vitallium wire over the cup permits determination of the position of the cup post-operatively.

C. McKee-Farrar-Arden hip prosthesis (Biomet Ltd)
Sizes available:
McKee-Farrar femoral stem
Alivium® (Cobalt Chrome alloy)/Sterile packed.

Sizes available:	Head diameter	Stem length
Standard neck	39.5 mm	115 mm
Standard neck	35.0 mm	115 mm
Elongated neck	35.0 mm	115 mm

Arden acetabular component
U.H.M.W. polyethylene/sterile packed.

Sizes available:	Inside cup diameter	Outside cup diameter
Arden cup	39.5 mm	51.0 mm
Arden cup	35.0 mm	44.5 mm
Arden cup	35.0 mm	57.0 mm
Arden cup	35.0 mm	51 mm

Fig. 23.111 Hip prostheses for arthroplasty operations (*continued overleaf*).

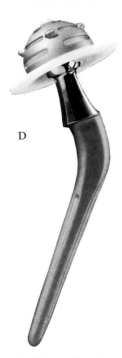

D

D. Wrightington F-C total hip system (Howmedica (UK) Ltd)
Sizes available:

Wrightington femoral stem
Vitallium® (cobalt chrome alloy)

All heads = 22 mm outside diameter

Sizes available:	Neck length	Offset	Stem no.
Short neck (i) standard stem	25.0 mm	26.6 mm	1
Short neck (ii) standard stem	25.5 mm	35.0 mm	2
Standard neck (i) standard stem	32.0 mm	33.4 mm	3
Standard neck (ii) standard stem	32.0 mm	38.0 mm	4
Standard neck (i) large stem	32.0 mm	33.0 mm	5
Standard neck (ii) large stem	32.5 mm	40.0 mm	6
Standard neck, extra large stem	34.5 mm	40.0 mm	7
Long neck, large stem	42.0 mm	40.0 mm	8
Extra long neck, large stem	49.5 mm	40.0 mm	9
Long neck, extra large stem	42.0 mm	45 mm	10
Mini stem	25.4 mm	26 mm	11
CDH stem	23.5 mm	20 mm	12

Wrightington acetabular component
U.H.M.W. Polyethylene.
All cups = 22 mm inside diameter

Sizes available:	Outside cup diameter
U.H.M.W.P.E. Cups	40.0, 42.0, 44.0, 46.0 mm
U.H.M.W.P.E. metal backed Cups	sizes as above

Fig. 23.111 Hip prostheses for arthroplasty operations.

Fig. 23.112 Additional instruments for Charnley low friction arthroplasty of the hip. (Chas. F. Thackray Ltd.)
1. Brace, wide throw.
2. Starting drill, 12.5 mm (½ in) diameter with centering ring.
3. Deepening reamer, spigot is 12.5 mm (½ in) diameter and engages with the pilot hole made by the starting drill in the floor of the acetabulum. The reamer produces a concave surface of 25 mm (1 in) radius.
4. Expanding reamer, this completes the cutting of a 5 cm (2 in) hemisphere after the deepening reamer has thinned the floor of the acetabulum. The profile of the hemisphere is a circle of 2.5 cm (1 in) radius with a 6.25 mm (¼ in) parallel section near the mouth.
5. Socket size gauge, small and large size gauges are used.
6. Cement restrictor.
7. Socket holder and guide; the plastic socket both small and large is held in position by an interference fit with three pins on the holder. The holder permits an orientation of 45 ° of the face of the socket to be made with precision. The plastic socket is clipped to the holder with the plane of the radiological marker in the same plane as the introducer handle. This enables the orientation of the radiological marker to be correct in an anteroposterior radiograph.
8. Socket pusher, is used to exert pressure in the centre of the socket holder where it engages in a depression. It enables the acrylic cement to be impacted in the cancellous bone by two blows of a mallet delivered through the socket pusher. This is done when the cement is nearly hard, and coins the cement to the cancellous bone and gets rid of any blood clot which may be interposed.
9. Pin retractor, used in the superior lip of the acetabulum to 'stake' back the abductor muscles improving the exposure of the acetabulum.
Instruments used for reattachment of the trochanter (Nos. 10–14).
10. Wire holding forceps.
11. Wire passer.
12. Drill and wire guide forceps for trochanter.
13. Lightweight brace with female trochanter reamer.
14. Male trochanter reamer, used on the inner surface of the detached trochanter in preparation for reattachment in the correct position.
Instruments required in the preparation of the acetabulum site and cementing of the plastic socket (Nos. 15–20).
15. Femoral prosthesis punch, designed to avoid damage to surface of head.
16. Femoral prosthesis pusher.
17. Femoral prosthesis with standard prosthesis mounted.
18. Tommy bar for broach.
19. Femoral broach.
20. Taper reamer for medullary canal.

Arthroplasty of hip, instruments cont'd:

Large tissue forceps, curved (Fagge), 5
Deep retractors (Hibb), 2
Osteotomes, 16 mm ($\frac{5}{8}$ in), 19 mm ($\frac{3}{4}$ in) and 38 mm ($1\frac{1}{2}$ in) (straight)
Osteotomes, 16 mm ($\frac{5}{8}$ in) and 19 mm ($\frac{3}{4}$ in) (curved)
Gouges, 16 mm ($\frac{5}{8}$ in), 19 mm ($\frac{3}{4}$ in) and 38 mm ($1\frac{1}{2}$ in)
Wire saw and handles (Gigli or Olivecrona), optional
Femoral neck saw
Scissors, curved on flat 20 cm (8 in) (Mayo)
Long scalpel, solid variety
Syringe 20 ml, and 18 gauge filling needle
Simplex bone cement
Diathermy leads, electrodes and lead anchoring forceps
3 and 4 (0 and 1) Synthetic absorbable or plain catgut for ligatures

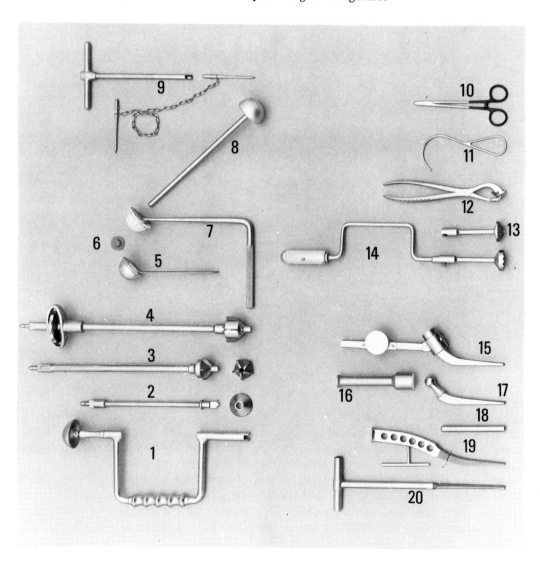

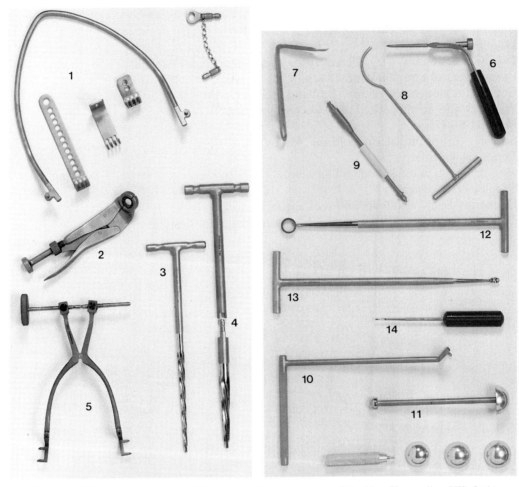

Fig. 23.113 Additional instruments for Wrightington F-C arthroplasty of the hip. (Howmedica (UK) Ltd.)

1. Initial incision retractor
2. Stem introducer
3. Femoral reamer, standard
4. Femoral reamer, extra large
5. Horizontal retractor
6. Superior capsule retractor
7. Anterior capsule rectractor

8. Dislocation hook
9. Acetabular drill
10. Cup holder
11. Cup positioning instrument
12. Ring curette
13. Long handle curette.
14. Wire passer

Outline of procedure

There are a number of alternative approaches to the hip joint. The approach may be postero-lateral for a McKee Farrar-Arden procedure (Fig. 23.114A to C), lateral for a Wrightington F-C prosthesis or for a Charnley prosthesis. The surgeon may dislocate the hip and remove the femoral head with a saw or large osteotome, or may prefer to divide the femoral neck before dislocation, and extract the head with a large corkscrew instrument. This latter method is applicable when a prosthesis is being inserted for the treatment of a subcapital fracture of the femoral neck which is not suitable for nailing, and when the head is separated and loose in the acetabulum.

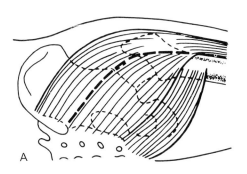

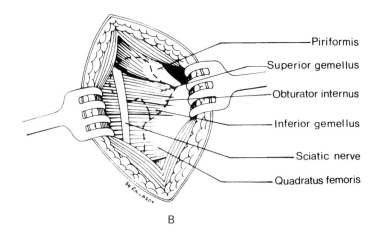

- Piriformis
- Superior gemellus
- Obturator internus
- Inferior gemellus
- Sciatic nerve
- Quadratus femoris

B

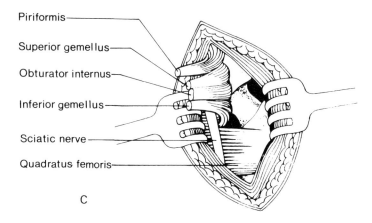

Piriformis—
Superior gemellus—
Obturator internus—
Inferior gemellus—
Sciatic nerve—
Quadratus femoris—

C

Fig. 23.114 Postero-lateral approach to the hip.
(A) The gluteus maximus is split in the direction of its fibres. The dotted outline shows the underlying bony landmarks.
(B) The short transverse lateral rotator muscles deep to the gluteus maximus. Note that the sciatic nerve lies upon the superficial aspect of the obturator internus, gemelli and quadratus femoris, but deep to the piriformis.
(C) The piriformis, obturator internus and gemelli have been divided close to the greater trochanter and reflected backwards, thus protecting the sciatic nerve. (In most cases sufficient access can be gained without reflecting the piriformis.) (Crawford Adams.)

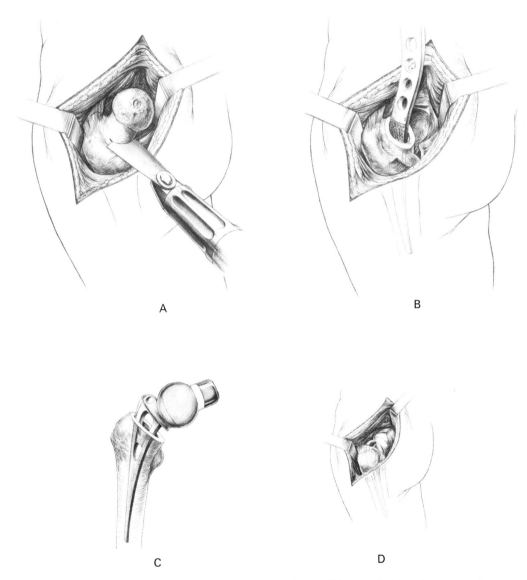

A   B

C   D

Fig. 23.115   Insertion of Austin Moore prosthesis. (A) Femoral head dislocated, division of femoral neck. (B) Reaming femoral shaft. (C) Insertion of prosthesis. (D) Hip reduced. (Hall: *Air Instrument Surgery*, *Orthopaedics*.)

The extent to which the acetabulum is prepared depends on whether a 'total hip replacement' is to be carried out; if not an Austin Moore prosthesis is generally inserted. With this type of prosthesis, which is made from stainless steel or Vitallium, the stem projects along the femoral neck and curves into the femoral shaft. The femoral channel is made with a long curved rasp and small gouges.

The McKee Farrar Arden F-C total hip prosthesis. This consists of a two-part ball and socket appliance; the metallic* femoral part being basically similar to a Thompson prosthesis, and

* Titanium, Vitallum or composition B stainless steel.

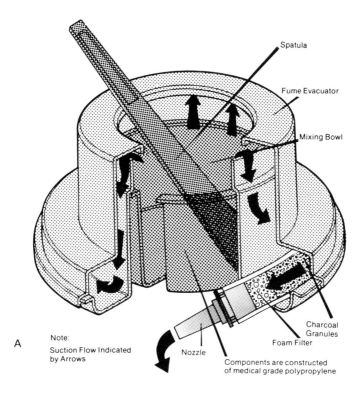

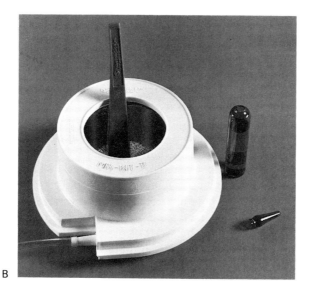

Fig. 23.116 Bone cement mixing system. (Mix-KitI, Howmedica (UK) Ltd.) This is a sterile, disposable unit which provides monomer vapour scavenging ability. Made from medical grade polypropylene and sterilized by gamma irradiation, the MikKitI system comprises an evacuator element which is good for two full dose cement mixings, and one mixing bowl and spatula. Monomer vapour liberated during the mixing of the cement is extracted through a pipeline suction tubing connected to the unit. (A) Exploded view of the unit showing principles of use; (B) unit assembled for use.

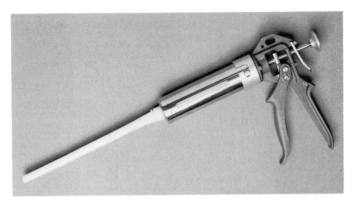

Fig. 23.117   Exeter bone cement gun. (Biomet Ltd.)

the acetabular part a polyethylene hemispherical cup which is manufactured to extremely fine limits and is interchangeable with any femoral stem of corresponding head diameter. The outer surface of the cup is covered with linear lugs. The purpose of these linear lugs is to provide a positive hold when the cup is embedded in acrylic cement in the acetabulum.

The acrylic cement mix consists of two parts, a powder (the polymer) and a liquid (the monomer). These are available as a sterile pack containing the correct amount of each. They are mixed together ideally in a mixing device which scavenges the chemical fumes to minimise liberation into the theatre atmosphere (Fig. 23.116) until within 2 or 3 minutes the plastic assumes a soft, workable consistency and no longer sticks to gloved fingers. The dough mix is pushed into the prepared acetabulum either by hand or with a cement gun (Fig. 23.117) and the cup inserted in the correct position. The cup is held firmly by a special dome-shaped instrument until the cement has set, usually about 5 minutes.

The Charnley total hip prosthesis. This also is a metal to plastic bearing prosthesis which was the original design of this type.

The essential difference between this and the McKee Farrar-Arden is that the Charnley femoral head component is smaller and does not have the Thompson type extended seating area at the base of the neck.

The Wrightington F-C total hip system is a development from the Charnley approach. It comprises a metallic femoral fluted frusto-conical stem which it is claimed provides an all round resistance to the anatomical loading taking place on a hip prosthesis stem (Fig. 23.111D). Uniformity of the thickness of cement mantle associated with more rectangular stems can lead to the risk of incorporating stress raisers in cement. The Wrightington F-C prosthesis has a rounded contour which more evenly fills the medullary cavity, leaving a cement mantle of greater uniformity (Fig. 23.119).

During preparative stages the Charnley technique consists of detaching the great trochanter which subsequently is reattached after the prosthesis has been inserted. This together with the lateral approach to the hip is said to prevent dislocation after operation. The Wrightington procedure may or may not include trochanteric osteotomy.

The acetabulum is prepared by removing all remnants of articular cartilage and roughening the walls with a gouge. Three or four 6 mm ($\frac{1}{4}$ in) to 10 mm ($\frac{3}{8}$ in) wide holes are made with a drill. These holes provide anchoring points for the acrylic cement. The outer cortex of the ilium immediately above the acetabulum is cleaned of soft-tissue attachments.

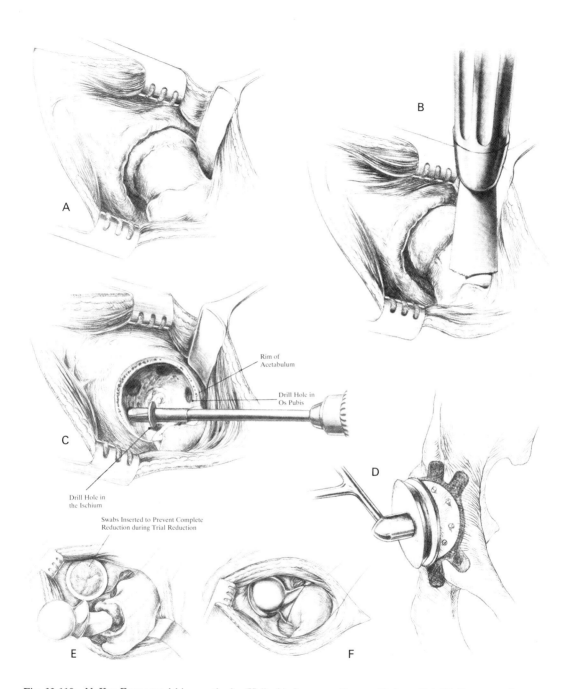

Fig. 23.118 McKee-Farrar total hip prosthesis. (Hall: *Air Instrument Surgery, Orthopaedics*) (A) Exposure of acetabulum and femoral neck. (B) Excision of femoral head with osteotomy saw. (C) Preparation of acetabulum, soft tissue excised, 9.3 mm (⅜ in) holes drilled in acetabulum. (D) Cement applied to acetabulum, insertion of cup. (E) Cement inserted in femoral medullary cavity, prosthesis being driven home so that shaft of prosthesis sits firmly upon the femoral neck. (F) When cement is firmly set artificial joint is reduced.

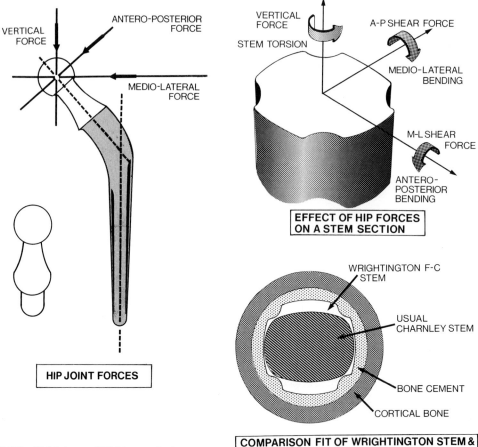

Fig. 23.119   Wrightington F-C hip prosthesis.

The femoral neck is prepared in the usual way with gouges and a rasp, although care is taken that the stem of the prosthesis lies accurately within the femoral shaft with adequate room for introduction of the acrylic cement.

The appropriate size femoral stem of the prosthesis is inserted and a trial reduction of the hip performed. After removing the prosthesis, a second mix of acrylic cement is made and inserted into the femoral shaft. The prosthesis is re-inserted and the cement allowed to set. The hip is then finally reduced.

Following insertion of the prosthesis the wound is closed in layers. Some surgeons may tie the legs together until the patient recovers consciousness. Russell traction of 3.2 to 4.5 kg (7 to 10 lb) may then be applied to the affected limb.

There are many types of arthroplasty of hip but the reader will find that these examples are currently in use at present. It must be understood that only an outline of the procedures has been described. Each of the operations requires a special technique and the reader is recommended to consult the appropriate literature for further information.

Arthroplasty of the knee

Definition

The reconstruction of the new joint surfaces in the knee by replacing the femoral condyles and tibial plateau with a metallic/plastic prosthesis.

Position

Supine.

Instruments

General set (Figs. 14.1 to 14.28)
Bone and fracture set (p. 624)
Osteotomes, 39 mm ($1\frac{1}{2}$ in) and 26 mm (1 in)
Power driven saw (optional)
Large tissue forceps (Fagge or Lane), 4
Irrigation syringe and saline
Suction tubing, nozzles and tube anchoring forceps
Venting tubes
Mixing bowl and spoon for cement
Simplex bone cement
Syringe 20 ml, and 18 gauge filling needle
3 (0) Synthetic absorbable or plain catgut for ligatures
4 and 5 (1 and 2) Synthetic absorbable or plain catgut on a medium half-circle cutting or Mayo needle with a trocar point for capsule etc.
2.5 or 3 (2/0 or 0) Silk or nylon on a medium curved or straight cutting needle for skin sutures.

Outline of procedure

Most knee arthroplasty operations consist of either a hinged or a gliding prosthesis.

The hinged prosthesis consists of two components which can be disassembled for insertion into the femoral and tibial shafts and then reconnected to form a hinged joint. The gliding prosthesis also consists of two components, one of which is either inserted into the femoral shaft or fitted over the femoral condyles, and the other fitted in place of the tibial plateau.

It would not be practicable to describe the multitude of operations available. The description of the procedure will therefore be confined to the Stanmore hinged total knee replacement. The operation is performed under tourniquet.

The knee joint is exposed through a lateral para-patella skin incision and a medial para-patella incision in the joint capsule. The stem of the femoral component is aligned with the femoral shaft and the femoral condyles resected (Fig. 23.121A).

The articular surface of the tibia is resected immediately above the tibial tubercle (Fig. 23.121B) and a gauge block is used to check that the correct amount of the bone has been resected. Sufficient cancellous bone is curetted from both bone surfaces to take the stems of the prosthesis and the cement. A trial reduction is made, after inserting the femoral and tibial components and connecting them with a temporary axle. A check is made that the joint will flex through its full range of flexion/extension movements; if necessary additional bone is trimmed from the tibia (Fig. 23.121C).

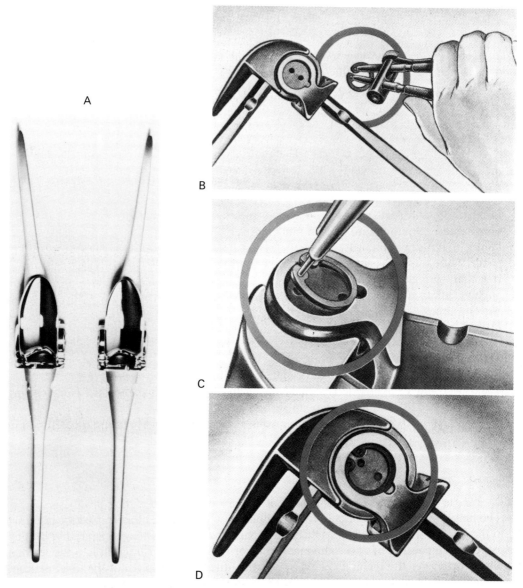

Fig. 23.120 Stanmore Titanium hinged total knee prosthesis.
(A) Left and right prosthesis. (B) Components joined with axle, circlip fixing device ready for insertion.
(C) Circlip being positioned. (D) Circlip in position and instrument removed. (Biomet Ltd.)

Debris is washed away from the medullary and joint cavities. Both medullary cavities are then packed with cement (see page 706 for preparation) using venting tubes connected to suction. The tibial and femoral components are inserted whilst the cement is still soft, and the temporary axle used to check articulation. The trial axle is replaced with the permanent axle, which is secured with a special circlip (Fig. 23.120).

The incision is closed in the normal way and a Redivac, Activac or Portovac suction drain inserted. Before the tourniquet is removed, a pressure bandage is applied over cotton wool and a plaster of Paris or polyethylene back splint applied.

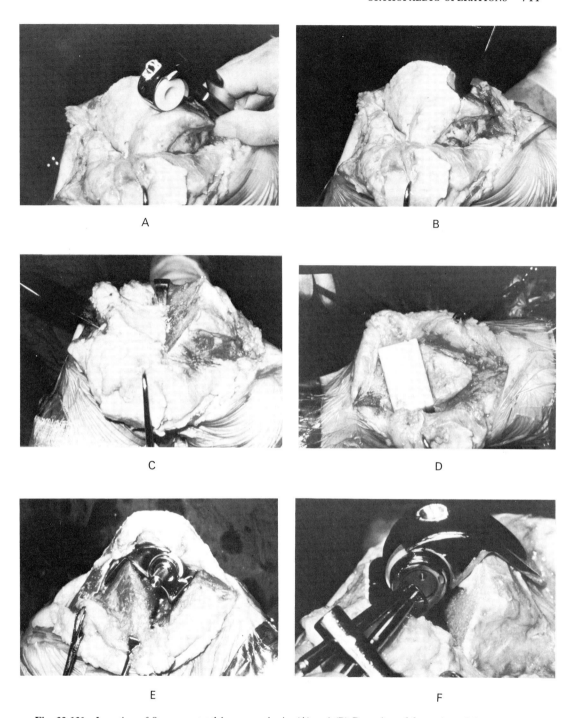

Fig. 23.121 Insertion of Stanmore total knee prosthesis. (A) and (B) Resection of femoral condyles. (C) Resection of tibial plateau. (D) Application of gauge block to check extent of resection. (E) Trial reduction. (F) Prosthesis inserted, locking axle. (Biomet Ltd.)

Congenital dislocation of hip (shelf operation)

Definition

To deepen the acetabulum by constructing a shelf of bone over the top of the femoral head.

Position

Lateral or supine, with a sandbag under the buttock on the affected side.

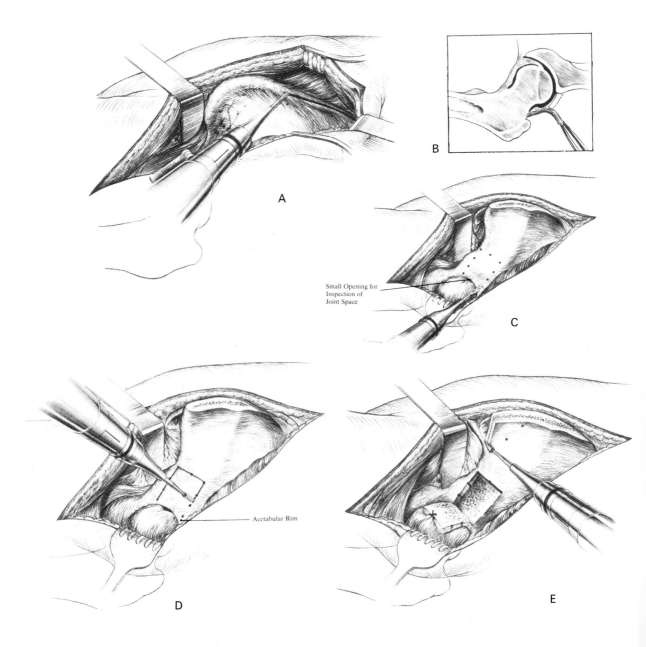

Instruments

As for Charnley's central dislocation arthrodesis of the hip
 As for skeletal traction, insertion of Steinmann pin or Kirschner wire (Fig. 23.5).

Outline of procedure

The hip joint is exposed through an anterolateral or lateral incision; the head of the femur is stripped of soft tissue structures which interfere with mobility.
 (After shelf operations, it is essential that continuous traction be applied to the leg until the bone shelf has healed, as the femoral head tends to displace the grafts. This may be accomplished by skin or skeletal traction which is sometimes applied before operation.)

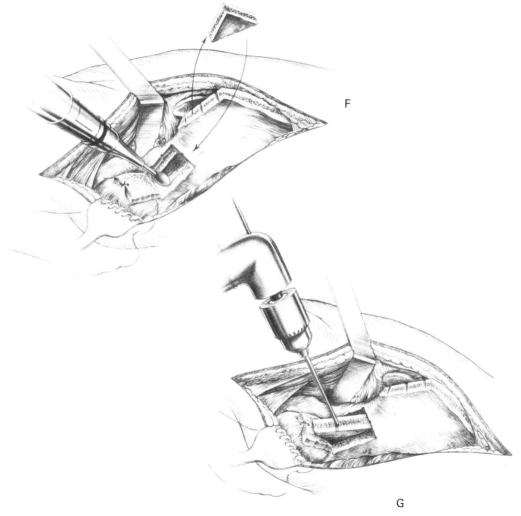

Fig. 23.122 Modified Gill operation for congenital dislocation of the hip. (A) Iliac crest exposed, reflection of the iliac apophysis. (B and C) Subtotal capsulectomy, outline of shelf made with drill holes. (D) Cutting of bone shelf from ilium. (E) A 12 mm ($\frac{1}{2}$ in) osteotome is used to turn down bone flap which is sutured to margin of capsule with catgut or Dexon. (F) Wedge graft removed from iliac crest. (G) Wedge graft in position, held with fine Steinmann pin through inner table of ilium, pin cut off subcutaneously. (Hall: *Air Instrument Surgery, Orthopaedics*)

The shelf of bone on the acetabular rim may be constructed in several ways. The Albee technique involves the division of the acetabular rim with a thin blade osteotome in a semi-circular line following the natural curve of the acetabulum. This segment of bone is prised outward and downward and secured with triangular shaped cortical grafts from the tibia or bone bank.

The Gill operation is similar, but the shelf is made by turning down a bone flap from the outer table of the ilium, sufficiently wide to cover the portion of the femur which projects beyond the acetabulum. This flap is secured with bone wedges from the crest of the ilium or bone bank (Fig. 23.122).

The wound is closed in layers and the patient is immobilised in a double plaster of Paris hip spica with traction on the affected limb.

Recurrent dislocation of the shoulder (Bankart's and Putti-Platt capsulorraphy)

Definition

A plastic procedure on the capsule and ligaments of the shoulder joint to prevent recurrent dislocation.

Position

Supine, with a sandbag under the scapula on the affected side.

Instruments

General set (Figs. 14.1 to 14.28)
Bone hooks, 2

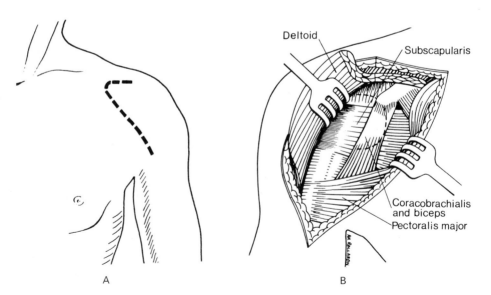

A   B

Fig. 23.123 Anterior exposure of shoulder. (A) The skin incision. (B) After separation of the deltoid and pectoralis major the conjoined coracobrachialis and biceps muscles are seen attached to the coracoid process. Deep to them lies the subscapularis, the fibres of which become tendinous as they approach their insertion into the humerus. The broken line shows the position of the head of the humerus. (Crawford Adams: *Standard Orthopaedic Operations*)

Small bone levers (Lane), 2

Small mallet (Rowland)

Small rugine, curved (Farabeouf)

Osteotome, 13 mm ($\frac{1}{2}$ in)

Bone awl

Contra-angle power drill (Bankart's operation only)

Bone graft set. (Instruments as in Fig. 23.94) may be required for graft to deficient glenoid rim.)

Staples and insertion punch, optional

Diathermy leads, electrodes and lead anchoring forceps

Suction tubing, nozzles and tube anchoring forceps

2.5 and 3 (2/0 and 0) Synthetic non-absorbable or silk for ligatures.

3 or 4 (0 or 1) Synthetic absorbable, plain or chromic catgut on a small fish hook, half-circle cutting 6, or Mayo needle with trocar point for capsulorrhaphy, etc.

3 or 4 (0 or 1) Synthetic absorbable or chromic catgut on a medium half circle cutting needle for deltoid muscle sutures

2.5 (2/0) Synthetic non-absorbable or silk on a medium curved cutting needle for skin sutures.

Outline of procedure

Bankart operation. An incision is made commencing at the outer border of the clavicle, curving medially to the coracoid process and continuing along the inner border of the deltoid muscle in line with the cephalic vein.

The interval between the deltoid and the pectoralis muscle is developed and the cephalic vein is retracted medially after dividing branches which may interfere with the exposure of the joint. The deltoid origin is reflected from the clavicle and the muscle retracted laterally. A hole about 3 mm ($\frac{1}{8}$ in) by 25 mm (1 in) deep may be drilled in the coracoid process with an awl or twist drill, to facilitate subsequent suture. The coracoid process is divided with an osteotome, and its tip, together with muscle attachments, is retracted medially and downwards.

The shoulder is then placed into external rotation and the subscapularis tendon is identified. A plexus of veins on the lower border of the tendon is usually ligated or diathermised and divided. Two synthetic non-absorbable or silk sutures are placed in the medial part of the tendon and are left long for retraction. The tendon is incised, and medial portion of the tendon allowed to retract, and the capsule then opened by a vertical incision 6 mm ($\frac{1}{4}$ in) lateral to the glenoid rim.

The glenoid rim is freshened with a curette and three holes are drilled in it with an angled drill. The shoulder is placed in internal rotation and abduction, and the cartilaginous labrum which is invariably detached from the glenoid rim is sutured (or stapled) back to its original position, utilising the three holes in the bone. In order to reinforce this, the medial part of the capsule *may* be plicated over the area of repair as in the Putti-Platt procedure. The subcapularis tendon is approximated with sutures, the coracoid process is re-attached, and the rest of the wound closed in layers. The arm is immobilised to the chest with cotton-wool and crêpe bandages.

Putti-Platt operation. The exposure is essentially the same as the Bankart's operation as far as the subscapularis tendon. This tendon is incised about 25 mm (1 in) medial to its insertion, and the joint is opened. The lateral portion of the subscapularis tendon is sutured either to the anterior rim of the glenoid cavity or the deep surface of the stripped capsule

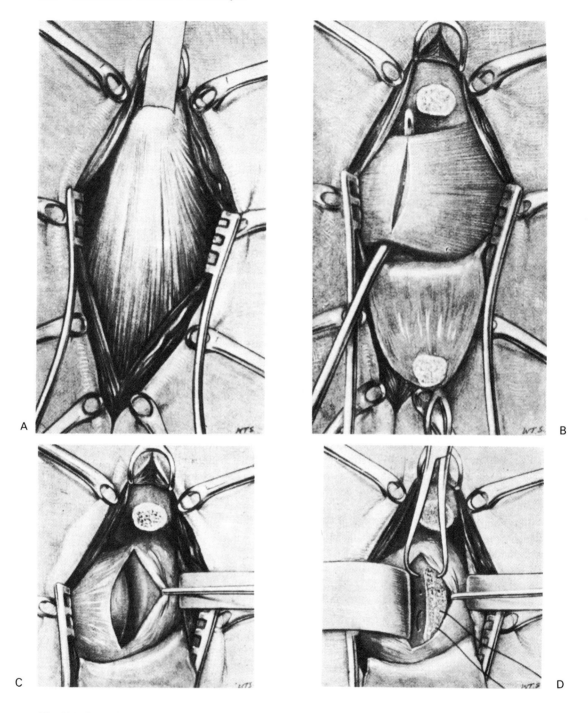

Fig. 23.124 Bankhart's operation for recurrent dislocation of the shoulder. (Wilson: *Watson–Jones Fractures and Joint Injuries*) (A) Division of coracoid process of deltoid with an osteotome. (B) Division of subscapularis tendon. (C) Incision of joint capsule. (D) Three holes are made in glenoid rim, either using an angled drill or towel forcep. (E) Reattachment of cartilaginous labrum with sutures which utilise holes in glenoid rim. (F) Reattachment of coracoid process with sutures.

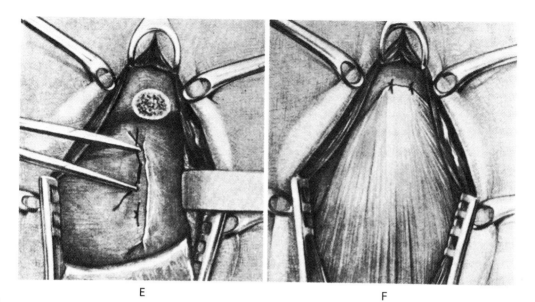

E   F

and subscapularis. The medial portion of the capsule is plicated over this lateral part of the subscapularis tendon, and finally the medial portion of the subscapularis tendon is plicated over all the previous suture lines, being attached to the bicipital groove or tendinous cuff over the greater tuberosity. This is in effect an overlapping of the medial and lateral parts of the capsule and subscapularis tendon so that a barrier to redislocation is formed.

The wound is closed as before, with immobilisation of the arm to the side.

Spinal fusion

Definition

Fusion of the spine in the treatment of tuberculosis, spondylolisthesis, idiopathic scoliosis (particularly adolescent) and some fracture dislocations.

Position

Knee/elbow, as Figure 5.23, or prone position of extension.

Instruments

As in laminectomy (Chapter 21, Neurosurgery, page 580)
Bone grafting set (Fig. 23–96)
Spinal rasps (Wheeler and Tubby), 2
Osteotomes, 13 mm ($\frac{1}{2}$ in), 16 mm ($\frac{5}{8}$ in), 19 mm ($\frac{3}{4}$ in) and 38 mm ($1\frac{1}{2}$ in) (straight)
Osteotomes, 13 mm ($\frac{1}{2}$ in), 16 mm ($\frac{5}{8}$ in) and 19 mm ($\frac{3}{4}$ in) (curved)
Gouges, 16 mm ($\frac{5}{8}$ in), 19 mm ($\frac{3}{4}$ in) and 25 mm (1 in).

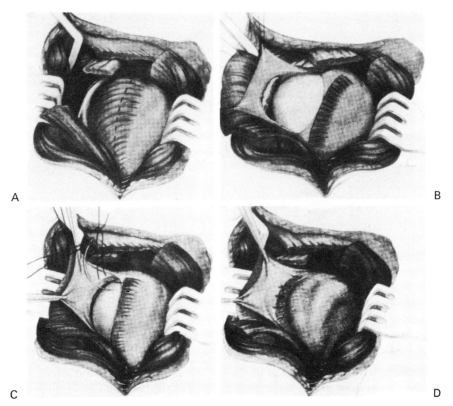

Fig. 23.125 Putti-Platt operation for recurrent dislocation of shoulder. (A) The coraco-brachialis has been divided by osteomising the coracoid process (as in Fig. 23.124). (B) The medial part of scapularis and the capsule being retracted inwards, the detachment of the glenoid labrum (Bankhart's lesion) is exposed. (C) The tissues in front of the neck of the scapula, including labrum periosteum and deep capsule, are sutured to the lateral stump of subscapularis. (D) The four or five sutures have been tied while the limb was in internal rotation. The medial part of the capsule and subscapularis are then overlapped and sutured to the region of the tuberosity. After repair of the coraco-brachialis and the closure of the wound the limb is held in internal rotation for four weeks. (Sir Henry Osmond-Clarke.)

For Harrington rod fixation
Wiring set (Fig. 23.51)
Harrington distraction rods
Sharp and blunt hooks for ratchet and collar end of distraction rod
Sharp hooks, for compression rod
Compression rod assemblies
Distraction/fusion rods and hooks (used in pairs)
Rod bender
Outrigger distraction unit
Angled and straight drivers for hooks
Pin cutters
Hook/rod spreader
Rod and hook clamps
Wrench to turn hexagonal nuts on compression rods
Harrington rod extractor

Figs. 23.126 to 23.138 Selection of Harrington Rod instruments (Downs Surgical Ltd.)

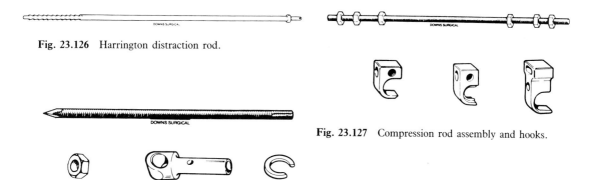

Fig. 23.126 Harrington distraction rod.

Fig. 23.127 Compression rod assembly and hooks.

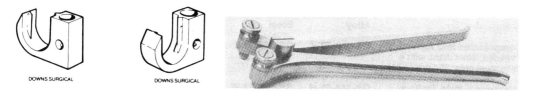

Fig. 23.128 Sacral rod, nut, eyelet and 'C' washer for ratchet end of distraction rod.

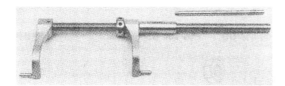

Fig. 23.129 Distraction fusion hooks.   **Fig. 23.130** Rod bender.

Fig. 23.131 Outrigger distraction unit for straightening the spine.

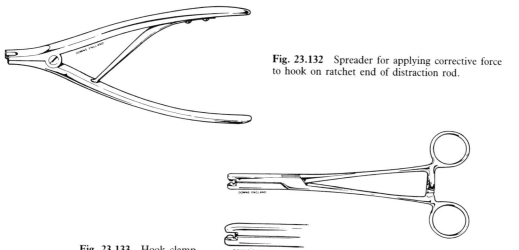

Fig. 23.132 Spreader for applying corrective force to hook on ratchet end of distraction rod.

Fig. 23.133 Hook clamp.

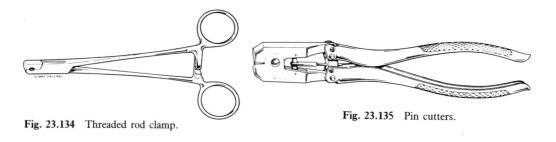

Fig. 23.134 Threaded rod clamp.

Fig. 23.135 Pin cutters.

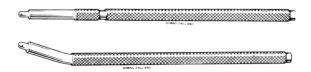

Fig. 23.136 Straight and angled drivers for round collar end hooks.

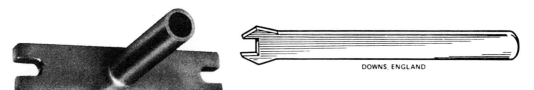

Fig. 23.137 Berkin-Harrington rod extractor.

Fig. 23.138 Flat wrench to turn hegagonal nuts when on compressor rods.

Plating and screwing set (p. 638), optional
Ligatures and sutures as for laminectomy.

Outline of procedure

The initial stages of the operation follow that for laminectomy, but with a wider exposure at both sides of the vertebrae. In the case of Harrington rod insertion, the entire subperiosteal area to be fused is exposed and cleaned of soft tissue. The tips of the spinous processes are removed. Usually two vertebrae above and two below the spinal lesion are fused.

Bone graft. Fusion is accomplished by a bone graft which can be taken from the patient himself or the bone bank. Cortical grafts, i.e., from the tibia, may be screwed or bolted in position either singly or as a twin graft on each side of the spine. The spinous processes and laminae are carefully prepared before the graft is inserted by removing periosteum and generally freshening the bone surfaces. Sometimes the spinous processes are removed completely and the area bridged with an 'H' bone graft. In addition to preparing the graft bed, the surgeon may perform a laminectomy and explore the intervertebral disc spaces.

Following the insertion of a cortical graft, the area is packed with cancellous bone chips or strips. Wire loops may be used also, in conjunction with cortical or cancellous bone grafts.

Another method of spinal fusion consists of removing soft tissue from the lamellae surfaces, excising the tips of the spinous processes and packing a large quantity of cancellous bone chips and shavings in the graft bed.

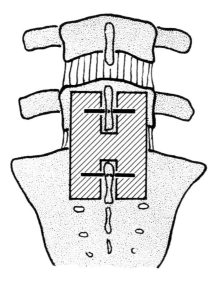

Fig. 23.139   H-shaped graft for posterior lumbar fusion. The graft is retained in position by cross pins transfixing the spinous processes. (Crawford Adams: *Standard Orthopaedic Operations.*)

Harrington distraction rods (stainless steel or Titanium) The technique involves insertion of a series of hooks or wire loops along the spinal column, through which a rod is threaded and fixed under tension to straighten the spine and provide correction for scoliosis (Fig. 23.140 and 23.141).

There are a number of variations to the basic operation but most first involve the insertion of an upper anchor hook under T4 lamina, and a lower hook under T12 lamina (Figs. 23.142 and 23.143). Where six further hooks are employed these are first threaded onto the Harrington distraction rod (Fig. 23.144A). Three hooks are inserted around the transverse process of T5, T6 and T7, and three inserted under the lamina of T10, T11 and T12 (Fig. 23.144B). Tension is applied to the rod which is secured to the hooks.

Alternatively, a series of stainless steel wire loops around the lamina may be used. These are tightened to draw the spine towards a stainless steel rod, secured at the upper and lower ends of the spine with hooks as described above. The fusion procedure is completed by packing cancellous bone grafts around the spine.

The wound is closed in the usual manner, the patient may be immobilised on a plaster of Paris bed which has been prepared to measurement before operation.

Hallux valgus (Keller's operation)

Defintion

Removal of an exostosis of the first metatarsal head and a portion of the proximal phalanx in the treatment of hallus valgus or bunions.

Position

Supine.

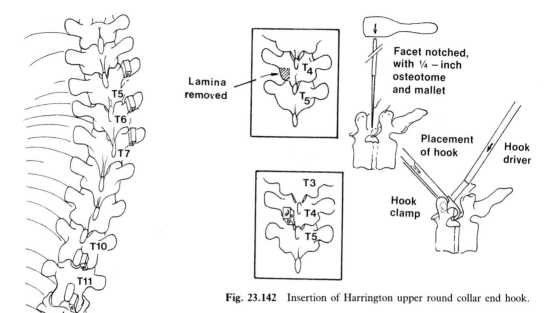

Fig. 23.140   Showing levels for inserting hooks or wire loops in scoliotic spine.

Fig. 23.142   Insertion of Harrington upper round collar end hook.

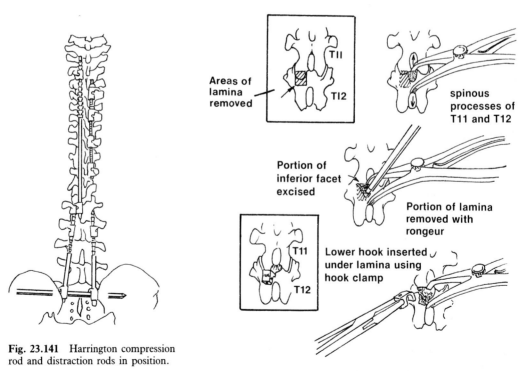

Fig. 23.141   Harrington compression rod and distraction rods in position.

Fig. 23.143   Insertion of Harrington lower round collar end hook.

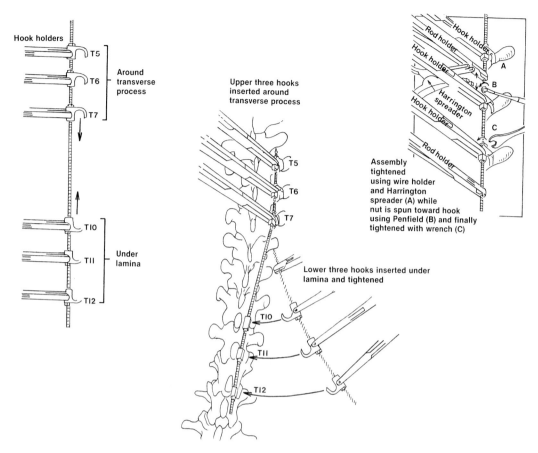

Fig. 23.144 Harrington rod insertion. (A) Assembly of hooks on compression rod, (B) Insertion of six hooks between T5–T7, and T10–T12.

Instruments

Sponge-holding forceps (Rampley), 5
Towel clips, 5
Scalpel handles No. 3 and No. 10 blades (Bard Parker), 2
Scalpel, solid variety
Dissecting forceps, toothed (Lane), 2
Scissors, curved on flat, 13 cm (5 in) (Mayo)
Scissors, straight, 13 cm (5 in) (Mayo)
Small retractors, double hook, 2
Artery forceps, curved on flat (Kilner), 5
Tissue forceps (Allis), 5
Bone levers (Trethowan), 2
Small rugine (Faraboeuf)
Bone-cutting forceps, compound action (Horsley)
Small bone-cutting forceps, single action (Liston)
Bone hook (Lane)

Mallet (Heath)
Osteotomes, 13 mm ($\frac{1}{2}$ in) and 16 mm ($\frac{5}{8}$ in)
Small needle holder (Kilner)
2.5 (2/0) Synthetic absorbable or plain catgut for ligatures
3 (0) Synthetic absorbable or plain catgut on a small half-circle cutting needle for subcutaneous structures
2 (3/0) Synthetic non-absorbable or silk on a small curved cutting needle for skin sutures.

Outline of procedure

A curved incision is made over the medial aspect of the first metatarsophalangeal joint, and the skin reflected with bone levers placed on either side of the base of the proximal phalanx.

The base of the phalanx is divided with bone-cutting forceps and removed. The bursa which usually lies over the bunion is excised and the exostosis on the medial aspect of the first metatarsal is removed with an osteotome.

The subcutaneous structures are approximated with a synthetic absorbable or catgut and the skin closed in the usual manner.

Arthroplasty of the metacarpophalangeal and proximal interphalangeal joints (Swanson operation)

Definition

Excision of the metacarpophalangeal joint or interphalangeal joint and replacement with an intramedullary prosthesis having an integral hinge joint.

Instruments

Sponge-holding forceps (Rampley), 5
Towel clips, 5
Scalpel handles No. 3 with No. 10 blades (Bard Parker), 2
Scalpel handle No. 9 with No. 15 blade (Bard Parker)
Scalpel, solid variety
Dissecting forceps, toothed 13 cm (5 in) (Lane), 2
Dissecting forceps, fine toothed (Gillies), 2
Scissors, curved on flat 13 cm (5 in) (Mayo)
Scissors, curved on flat, 14.5 cm (5¾ in) (Lahey)
Small retractors, double hook (Lane rake), 2
Skin hooks, single hook (Gillies), 2
Artery forceps, curved on flat (Kilner), 5
Tissue forceps (Allis), 5
Bone levers (Trethowan), 2
Small rugine (Faraboeuf)
Small bone-cutting forceps (Stamms)
Swanson Silastic HP 100 Finger joint implant (appropriate size)
Swanson finger joint grommet (Fig. 23.148)
Set of blue trial prostheses
Power bone saw or Hall drill
Small needle holder (Kilner)

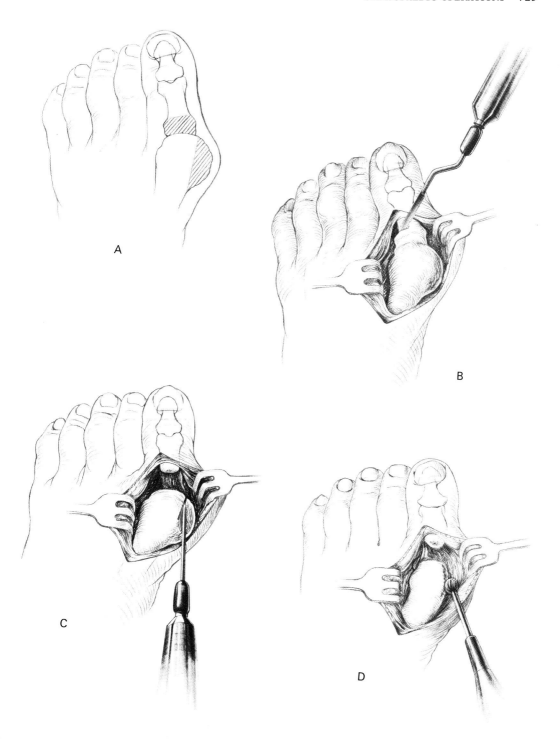

Fig. 23.145 Kellers operation using power saw. (A) Area of bone to be removed. (B) Excision of base of proximal phalanx. (C) Removal of exostosis. (D) Smoothing plantar surface of metatarsal. (Hall: *Air Instrument Surgery, Orthopaedics*)

2.5 (2/0) or 2 (3/0) Synthetic absorbable or plain catgut for ligatures

2 (3/0) or 1.5 (4/0) white synthetic non-absorbable on small curved cutting needle for extensor expansion and capsular tissues

1.5 (4/0) or 1 (5/0) Synthetic non-absorbable or silk on small curved cutting needle for skin sutures

2 ml syringe and needle for antibiotic solution

Malleable aluminium or plaster of Paris splints.

Outline of procedure

Metacarpophalangeal joint implant arthroplasty

The joints are approached through a transverse dorsal skin incision made over the necks of the metacarpals and carried down through subcutaneous tissue to expose the extensor tendons. The dorsal veins are freed and retracted laterally. After exposing the extensor hood to the base of the proximal phalanx, the extensor tendon is dislocated towards the ulna (Fig. 23.146). Exposure of the joint in the index finger is by an incision between the extensor digitorium communis and the indicis proprius tendons. A longitudinal incision in the extensor hood parallel to the extensor tendon on its ulnar aspect is used for the middle and ring fingers. Approach in the little finger is made between the extensor communis and proprius tendons.

The metacarpal head transected subperiostally leaving part of the metaphyseal flare, is removed together with hypertrophied synovial material. A comprehensive soft tissue release is undertaken so as to permit the base of the proximal phalanx to be displaced dorsally above the metacarpal.

The base of the proximal phalanx is resected, and the intramedullary canal of the metacarpal reamed in a rectangular fashion with rasp, curette, broach and air drill burr. A trial implant fit is then carried out using special blue sizers; this enables the appropriate size of proximal stem to be selected, usually 4 through 9. A rectangular hole is made in the base of the proximal phalanx and the medullary canal reamed as before to accept the distal stem of the implant. A further trial fit to verify the size of implant is carried out (Fig. 23.147).

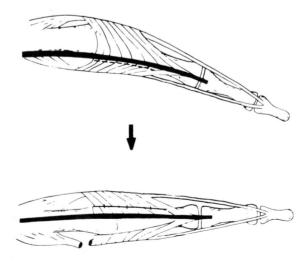

Fig. 23.146 Swanson Silastic finger joint implant; release of the dislocated extensor tendon by incision on its ulnar border. (Dow Corning.)

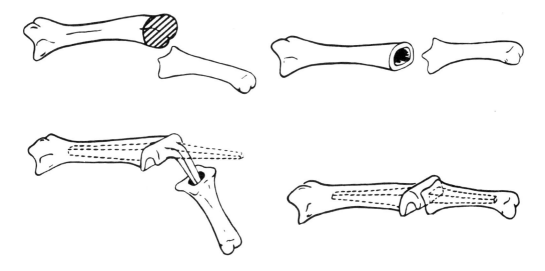

Fig. 23.147 Swanson Silastic finger joint implant; resection of metacarpal head, trial fit of implant. (Dow Corning.)

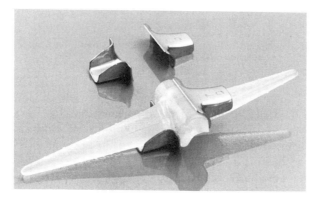

Fig. 23.148 Swanson Silastic finger joint implant with Titanium grommets. (Dow Dorning.)

With joint in extension, care is taken to avoid any impingement of its mid-section; if necessary, further reaming may be carried out to correct this. The implant is then inserted with blunt instruments, using a non-touch technique.

Titanium Swanson grommets may be used to prevent damage to the implant from the biomechanical shearing forceps of sharp bone edges during joint motion (Fig. 23.148). In this case the resected surfaces of the metacarpal and proximal phalanx are shaped to obtain a precise fit of the grommet sleeve, and of its slightly curvilinear flanges which prevent contact with overlying soft tissue. The grommet must be accurately centred else it may impinge on one side of the bone and cause bone absorption. The distal grommet is generally used on the dorsal surface, and the proximal grommet on the palmar surface. The grommet sizing corresponds to the implant sizing; the principle of the flexible hinge as a joint spacer must be followed (Figs. 23.149 and 23.150).

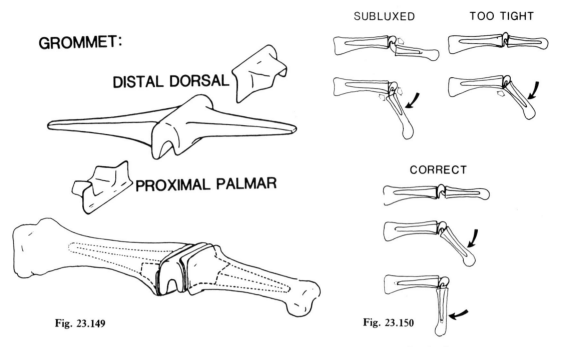

GROMMET:

DISTAL DORSAL

PROXIMAL PALMAR

SUBLUXED   TOO TIGHT

CORRECT

Fig. 23.149

Fig. 23.150

Fig. 23.149   Swanson Silastic finger joint implant and grommets inserted. (Dow Corning.)

Fig. 23.150   Swanson Silastic finger joint implant, showing joint relationship and spacer concept. (Dow Corning.)

Reconstruction of the radial collateral ligament is carried out by the technique of reefing. This is done by passing a 2 (3/0) synthetic non-absorbable suture through one or two 0.5 mm drill holes made in the dorsal radial side of the cut end of the metacarpal, to re-attach the ligament to bone (Fig. 23.151). The extensor hood mechanism is repaired with three to five synthetic non-absorbable buried knot sutures, followed by meticulous approximation of the juncturae tendinae using sutures with inverted knots. Small drains may be inserted in the wound and the skin incision closed with interrupted 1 (5/0) synthetic non-absorbable sutures.

Immediately postoperatively a padded dressing and conforming bandage is applied, together with a palmar plaster of Paris splint secured with a conforming bandage. After about two days, if swelling is minimal a dynamic brace is fitted to enable the patient to start finger movements in a protected arc (Fig. 23.153).

Exostosectomy

Definition

The excision of an abnormal bony prominence.

Position

ndent upon the location of the exostosis.

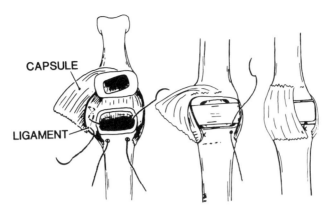

Fig. 23.151 Reconstruction of radial collateral ligament following metacarpophalangeal arthroplasty. (Dow Corning.)

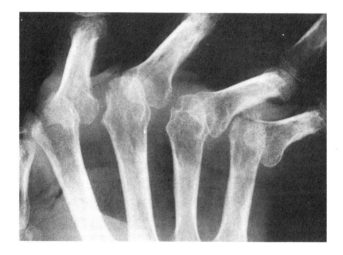

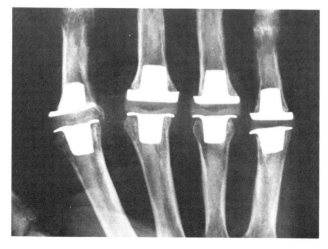

Fig. 23.152 Pre- and post-operative radiographs, metacarpophalangeal arthroplasty. (Dow Corning.)

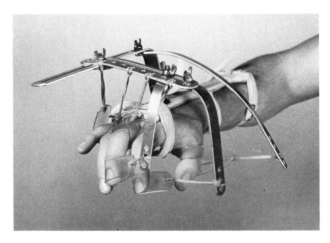

Fig. 23.153 Dynamic brace applied following metacarpophalangeal arthroplasty. (Dow Corning.)

Instruments

General set (Figs. 14.1 to 14.28)
Bone and fracture set (p. 624)
Osteotomes, 13 mm ($\frac{1}{2}$ in), 19 mm ($\frac{3}{4}$ in) and 25 mm (1 in)
Appropriate ligatures and sutures for that area of the body.

Outline of procedure

The exostosis is exposed and the periosteum elevated. An osteotome is used to excise the bony prominence and the wound is closed in the usual manner.

Bone tumours

The technique involved depends upon the location and extent of the lesion. If amputation of a limb is contraindicated, the surgeon may excise the tumour and replace the defect with a bone graft. This graft may be purely a question of filling in a cavity with cancellous chips, or may mean transplant of a large wedge of bone.

Instruments required vary but as a guide the surgeon will probably require a general set (Figs. 14.1 to 14.28); a bone and fracture set (p. 624); with the possible addition of instruments for bone grafting (Fig. 23.94) and instruments for plating and screwing (p. 638).

Amputation, forearm

Definition

Amputation through the forearm, preferably at a level which is a few centimetres above the wrist.

Position

, with the affected arm extended on an arm table.

Instruments

General set (Figs. 14.1 to 14.28)

Rugine (Mitchell)

Bone-cutting forceps, compound action (Horsley)

Amputation saw (Sergeant) or power driven saw/cutting burr, connecting tubing or drive cable

Bone levers, small (Lane), 4

Fine rubber or plastic drainage tubing

Suction drain (Redivac, Activac or Portovac), optional

2.5 and 3 (2/0 and 0) Synthetic absorbable or plain and chromic catgut for ligatures

3 (0) Synthetic non-absorbable or silk etc., for ligatures

2.5 (2/0) Synthetic non-absorbable or silk on a medium curved cutting needle for skin sutures.

Outline of procedure

Equal anterior and posterior skin flaps are cut, together with the underlying fat and muscle fascia. These are reflected up and the radial and ulnar nerves are sectioned above the level for dissection of the bone.

The muscles are divided across just below the level of bone resection and are retracted proximally. The radius and ulna are divided across with a saw and the hand removed. The major vessels are identified and ligated with a synthetic absorbable, catgut or silk and the two fascial flaps are approximated with a synthetic absorbable or catgut sutures. If the operation is being performed without a tourniquet, the major vessels are identified and clamped before transection of the muscles and bone.

A drain may or may not be inserted and the wound is closed.

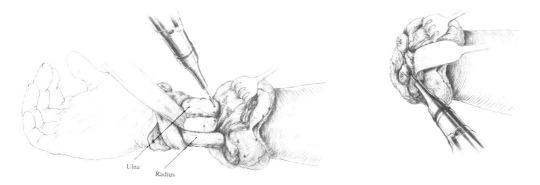

Fig. 23.154 Amputation through the forearm using a power driven cutting burr. (Hall: *Air Instrument Surgery, Orthopaedics*)

Amputation through the humerus

Definition

Amputation of the arm through the humerus.

Position

Supine, with affected limb extended on an arm table initially.

Instruments

As for amputation of forearm.

Outline of procedure

Equal anterior and posterior skin flaps are cut, but may be modified in order to effect a plastic closure. These flaps are reflected with the fat and muscle fascia, and the anterior muscles are divided across just below the level for bone section. The major vessels are ident-ified and clamped, and the posterior muscles are divided. The bone is divided with a saw and the arm removed.

The nerves are divided at the level of bone section and the major vessels are ligated with double ligatures. The muscles are bevelled to form a thin myofascial flap and are approxi-mated with a synthetic absorbable or catgut sutures. A drainage tube is inserted and the skin closed in the usual manner.

Amputation below the knee

Definition

Amputation of the leg through the upper or middle tibia.

Position

Supine.

Instruments

General set (Figs. 14.1 to 14.28)
Large tissue forceps (Fagge or Lane), 5
Rugine (Mitchell)
Bone-cutting forceps, compound action (Horsley)
Amputation saw (Sergeant)
Bone file (optional)
Wire saw and handles (Gigli or Olivecrona), or rib shears optional
Amputation knife
Bone-holding forceps (Fergusson lion)
Medium rubber or plastic drainage tubing
Suction drain (Redivac, Activac or Portovac), optional
2.5 and 3 (2/0 and 0) Synthetic absorbable or plain catgut for superficial ligatures
3 and 4 (0 and 1) Synthetic absorbable, chromic catgut or silk for deep ligatures
4 (1) Synthetic absorbable or plain catgut on a medium half-circle cutting needle for muscle sutures
2.5 (2/0) Synthetic non-absorbable or silk on a medium curved cutting needle for skin sutures.

Outline of procedure

Unequal skin flaps are cut, with the anterior flap slightly longer than the posterior one at the selected level for amputation.

These incisions are carried down to muscle fascia and the flaps are reflected up on each aspect. The periosteum overlying the point for division of the bone is reflected and the anterior muscles are sectioned. During this stage the anterior tibial vessels are ligated and divided and the superficial perioneal and tibial nerves are divided at the level of bone section.

The tibia and fibula are sawn across about a quarter of an inch proximal to the divided anterior muscles. The posterior muscles are divided with an amputation knife and the posterior vessels identified, clamped and divided. The leg is removed and the vessels ligated. The fibula is exposed by subperiosteal dissection and is divided with bone-cutting forceps, a Gigli saw or rib shears at a point which is about 25 mm (1 in) to 40 mm (1½ in) above the level of the sectional tibia. The crest of the tibia is bevelled with a saw or file to prevent a sharp edge pressing on the skin. A flap of fascia is sutured over the stump, a drain is inserted and the skin closed in the usual manner.

Amputation, mid-thigh

Definition

Amputation of the leg through the middle part of the femur.

Position

Supine, or with the knee flexed over the lower part of the table which is lowered or removed.

Instruments

> General set (Figs. 14.1 to 14.28)
> Mid-thigh amputation set (Fig. 23.155)
> Rugine (Mitchell)
> Bone hook (Lane)
> 2.5 and 3 (2/0 and 0) Synthetic absorbable or plain catgut for superficial ligatures
> 3 and 4 (0 and 1) Synthetic absorbable or chromic catgut or silk for deep ligatures
> 4 (1) Synthetic absorbable or chromic catgut on a large half-circle cutting needle for muscle sutures
> 3 (0) Synthetic non-absorbable or silk on a large curved or straight cutting needle for skin sutures.

Outline of procedure

Equal skin flaps are cut at the level for amputation and are reflected up with the fascia. If a tourniquet is in position, the muscles are severed by the circular sweep of an amputation knife which commences its cut on the anteriomedial aspect of the thigh, cuts posteriorly, then laterally and finally anterolaterally. The muscles are then retracted with the amputation shield to a point about 25 mm (1 in) above the level for bone section. The femur is sawn across and the leg removed. The major vessels are picked up with forceps and ligated before release of the tourniquet. The tourniquet is released, hot packs applied and the smaller vessels picked up and ligated. The sciatic nerve is divided at the level of bone section.

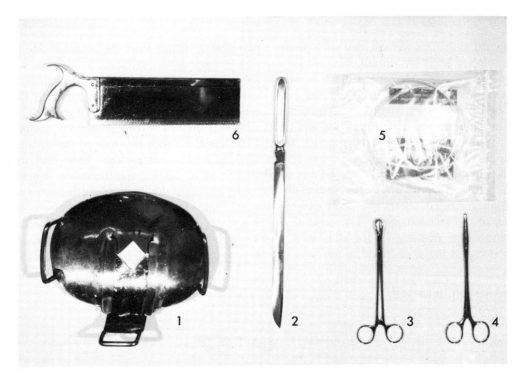

Fig. 23.155 Mid-thigh amputation
1. Amputation shield.
2. Amputation knife (Liston).
3. Tissue forceps (Lane or Fagge).
4. Artery forceps, straight, 20 cm (8 in) (Spencer Wells).
5. Long drainage tube, plastic, pre-packed sterile for use with Redivac, Activac, Portovac or similar suction device.
6. Amputation saw.

If a tourniquet cannot be used, perhaps due to a high level of amputation, the femoral vessels are identified, ligated and divided before the muscles are cut across. The procedure then follows that described previously.

The muscles and fascia are sutured together over the end of the femur, a drain is inserted and the skin closed in the usual manner.

(*Alternatively the limb may be amputated by disarticulation through the knee joint. In this procedure the skin flaps are fashioned at a lower level, but the basic technique is similar to that described.*)

Tendon suture (end to end anastomosis and free grafts)

Defintion

The repair of a divided tendon either as an end to end anastomosis with or without tendon lengthening or tansplant; free tendon grafts.

Position

Supine, with affected hand extended on an arm table.

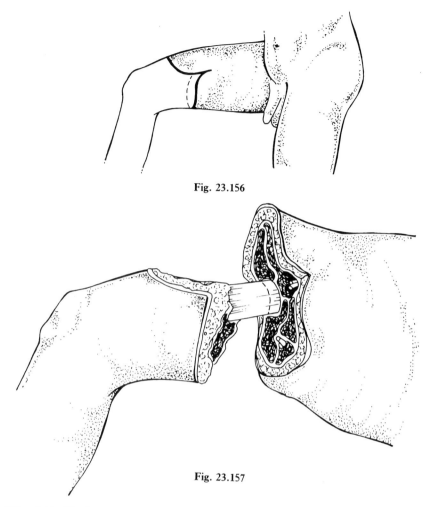

Fig. 23.156

Fig. 23.157

Figs. 23.156 and 23.157   Amputation through the middle third of the thigh. (Rintoul: *Farquharson's Textbook of Operative Surgery*)

Instruments

    Sponge-holding forceps (Rampley), 5
    Scalpel handles No. 3 with No. 10 blades (Bard Parker), 2
    Scalpel handles No. 9 with No. 15 blades (Bard Parker), 2
    Fine artery forceps, straight, mosquito, 5
    Fine artery forceps, curved on flat, mosquito, 10
    Fine dissecting forceps, toothed (Gillies), 2
    Fine dissecting forceps, non-toothed (McIndoe), 2
    Fine scissors, curved on flat, 10 cm (4 in) (Kilner)
    Fine scissors, straight, 10 cm (4 in) (Strabismus)
    Scissors, stitch, 13 cm (5 in)
    Fine tissue forceps (McIndoe), 6
    Fine retractors, double end, 'rake' (Lane), 2

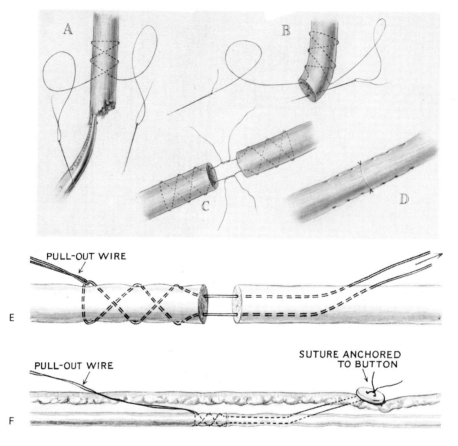

PULL-OUT WIRE

SUTURE ANCHORED
TO BUTTON

PULL-OUT WIRE

Fig. 23.158 (A to D) The classical method of tendon suture. Note the manner in which the suture material, with a needle at each end, is 'spliced' into the tendon, and that the knots are buried between the cut ends. (E and F) Tendon repair by the use of withdrawable sutures of stainless steel wire (*After Bunnell*). (Farquharson and Rintoul: *Textbook of Operative Surgery*)

Skin hooks (Gillies or McIndoe), 4
Probe, malleable silver
Crocodile or tendon passing forceps
Fine bowl awl
Fine needle holder (West)
Lead hand splint or similar, for immobilisation of hand during operation
6 cm ($2\frac{1}{2}$ in) straight round-bodied needles for transfixion of tendon during operation (optional)
2 (3/0) Synthetic absorbable or plain catgut for ligatures
2 or 2.5 (3/0 or 2/0) Synthetic absorbable or plain catgut on a small half-circle cutting needle for subcutaneous sutures
33 SWG or 40 SWG stainless-steel wire or 1.5 (4/0) silk, polyester or polyethylene on a small curved non-traumatic needle for tendon sutures
Pearl button may be required for a 'pull through' suture
1.5 and 2 (4/0 and 3/0) Synthetic non-absorbable or silk on small curved cutting needles for skin sutures
Malleable aluminium or plaster of Paris splint will be required.

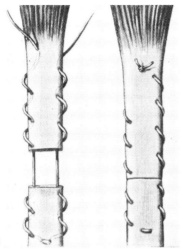
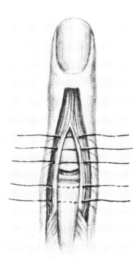

Fig. 23.159
Fig. 23.160

Fig. 23.159   Method of uniting a large flat tendon. (Farquharson and Rintoul: *Textbook of Operative Surgery*)

Fig. 23.160   Method of repairing an extensor tendon severed over the proximal phalangeal joint. (Bailey.)

Outline of procedure

For an end to end anastomosis, the cut tendon is exposed and fibrous tissue excised to effect mobility. The ends are approximated and straight round-bodied needles may be used to transfix the tendons and prevent the ends from retracting. The ends may or may not be trimmed with a knife, before suturing with stainless-steel wire or silk sutures, which are generally placed as modified mattress sutures.

Some surgeons use a 'pull through' wire technique in which a short strand of wire is included in the loop on one side of the anastomosis and is used to pull the wire suture out after the tendon has healed. This strand of wire is threaded on to a needle and passed through the skin at a point proximal to the anastomosis, and tied over a small pad of gauze. After the wire suture used for the anastomosis has been inserted in the distal part of the tendon, it is passed through the skin distal to this point (about 13 mm ($\frac{1}{2}$ in) to 25 mm (1 in) away) and is tied over a pearl button. This 'pull through' technique of Bunnell may be used also to take the tension off a suture line. In this case the tendon is approximated in the usual manner with fine stainless-steel wire synthetic non-absorbable or silk sutures, and a 'pull through' wire inserted proximal to the point of anastomosis is tied over a button, with slight tension. This relieves the strain on the anastomosis until healing is complete. The technique is applied mainly to the repair of extensor tendons although it may be used equally well for flexor tendons, especially transposition procedures.

In the case of injuries to flexor tendons in the fingers, it is generally preferable to make the anastomosis in the palm. Although an end to end anastomosis may be possible, a length of tendon is usually transplanted from the forearm or foot to bridge the gap between the palm and the distal phalanx of the finger.

A mid-lateral incision is made in the affected finger, the flexor tendons identified and removed completely, or leaving a small tag where the profundus is inserted into the terminal phalanx. The tendon pulleys are preserved if possible. The palm is incised and the proximal portion of the tendon identified and drawn into the palm with tissue forceps.

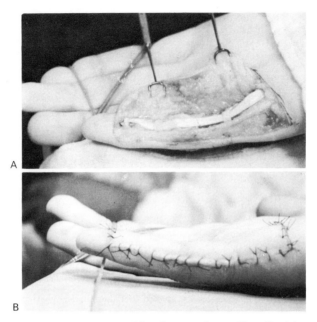

Fig. 23.161   Successive stages in the operation of free flexor tendon grafting. (Rank.)
(A) The free graft placed in position and sutured to the terminal profundus tendon stump after resection of the damaged tendons and most of the tendon sheath. Note the two pulleys retained to prevent prolapse of the graft.
(B) The flap sutured back before proceeding to the proximal graft junction.

A tendon graft of suitable length is removed from the flexor aspect of the forearm and wrist (palmaris longus), or a plantaris tendon or extensor tendon to the toe and is threaded through the tendon tunnel from the palm and under the finger pulleys to the terminal phalanx. At this point it is either sutured to the remaining tag of tendon or a hole is drilled through the terminal phalanx and the tendon approximated to its insertion with a suture which passes through the bone. This suture is tied over a pearl button for subsequent removal. The skin wounds of the finger and forearm or foot are closed in the usual manner.

The finger is placed in the correct degree of flexion and an anastomosis made with the proximal tendon and graft in the palm. This is achieved either by simple side to side suture, or by interweaving the tendons before suturing. The palm wound is closed and the finger, as for all tendon sutures, is immobilised with a malleable splint or plaster of Paris back slab, wool and bandages.

REFERENCES AND FURTHER READING

AIELLO, D. H. (1986) Arthroscopy of the knee, *AORN Journal* **43**, No. 4, 824–847
BASTIANI, R., ALDEGHERI, R. AND RENZI BRIVIO, L. (1986) Dynamic axial fixation. *International Orthopaedics* (SICOT), **10**, 95–99.
CHAO, E. Y. S. AND KASMAN R. A. (1984) The mechanical performance of the orthofix axial external fixator. *Recent Advances in Traumatology — Symposium*, Venice, Paris, 1984.
CRAWFORD ADAMS J. (1976) *Standard Orthopaedic Operations*. Edinburgh: Churchill Livingstone.
FARQUHARSON, E. L. AND RINTOUL R. F. (1972) *Textbook of Operative Surgery*. Edinburgh: Churchill Livingstone.
GREEN, S. A. (1981) *Complications of External Skeletal Fixation*, p. 89. Springfield, Illinois: Charles C. Thomas.

HALL, R. M. (1972) *Air Instrument Surgery Orthopaedics*. New York: Springer Verlag. (Courtesy Surgical Products 3M United Kingdom Limited.)

MACFARLANE, D. A. & THOMAS, L. P. (1972) *Textbook of Surgery*. Edinburgh: Churchill Livingstone.

MCKIBBON, B. (1978) The biology of fracture healing in long bones. *Journal of Bone and Joint Surgery*, **60**, 150–162.

RANK, Sir B. *et al.* (1973) *Surgery of Repair as applied to Hand Injuries*. Edinburgh: Churchill Livingstone.

RINTOUL, R. F. (1986) *Farquharson's Textbook of Operative Surgery*. Edinburgh: Churchill Livingstone.

ROBINSON, J. O. (1965) *Surgery*. London: Longman.

SPACEY, M. (1985) Tourniquets. *Orthopaedic Surgery Supplement, British Journal of Theatre Nursing, NATNews*, February.

WILSON, J. N. (1976) *Watson Jones: Fractures and Joint Injuries*. Edinburgh: Churchill Livingstone.

24

Plastic operations

Repair of cleft lip and cleft palate

Definition

Closure of a cleft to establish continuity of muscle which is important for modelling the underlying bone and to produce a cosmetically acceptable lip; closure of a cleft palate and pushing back the soft palate so that it can approximate with the posterior pharyngeal wall.

Position

Harelip — supine. Cleft palate — supine, with sandbag between the shoulder blades and the neck in extension.

Instruments

Sponge-holding forceps (Rampley), 2
Scalpel No. 9 with Nos. 11 and 15 blades (Bard Parker), 2
Scalpel handles No. 5 with Nos. 11 and 15 blades (Bard Parker), 2
Long fine dissecting forceps, toothed (Waugh), 2
Long fine dissecting forceps, non-toothed (Waugh), 2
Fine dissecting forceps, toothed (Gillies), 2
Fine dissecting forceps, non-toothed (McIndoe), 2
Artery forceps, curved on flat (Micron)
Fine scissors, curved on flat, sharp points
Fine scissors, straight, sharp points
Fine tissue forceps (McIndoe), 2
Skin hooks (Gillies)
Angled tongue depressor
Mouth gag with appropriate size of blade (Dott)
Cleft palate raspatory, left and right patterns will be required, 2
Cleft palate sharp hook; blunt hook may also be needed
Raspatory (Howarth or Heath)
Cleft palate sharp hook and raspatory
Dissector (Macdonald)
Harelip traction bow (Denis Browne)
Cleft palate needle (Reverdin)

Figs. 24.1 to 24.8   Examples of instruments for cleft lip and cleft palate. (Chas. F. Thackray Ltd.)

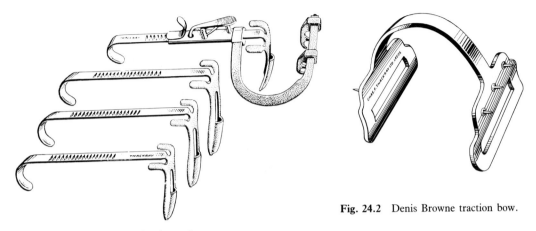

Fig. 24.2   Denis Browne traction bow.

Fig. 24.1   Kilner Dott insulated mouth gag
with East Grinstead blades.

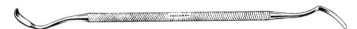

Fig. 24.3   Double end cleft palate elevator (angled to side and on flat).

Fig. 24.4   Cleft palate sharp hook and raspatory.

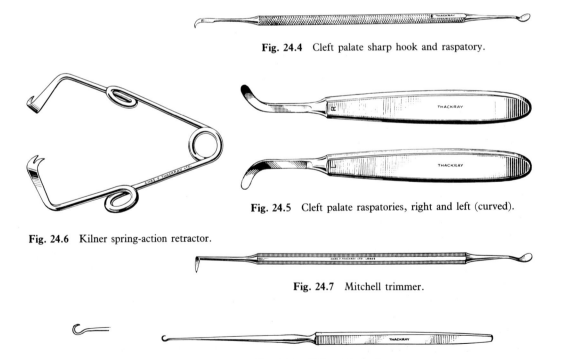

Fig. 24.5   Cleft palate raspatories, right and left (curved).

Fig. 24.6   Kilner spring-action retractor.

Fig. 24.7   Mitchell trimmer.

Fig. 24.8   Gillies skin hook.

Figs. 24.9 to 24.11   Instruments for cleft lip and cleft palate (*cont'd*). (Chas. F. Thackray Ltd.)

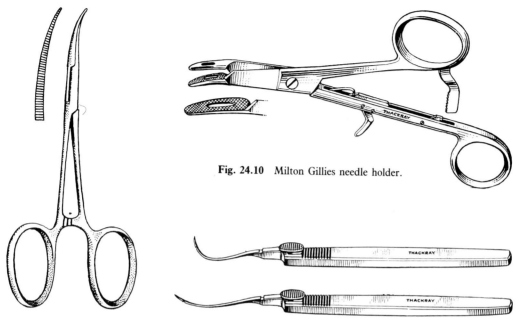

Fig. 24.10   Milton Gillies needle holder.

Fig. 24.9   Micron artery forceps.

Fig. 24.11   Reverdin needles.

Retractor, spring action (Kilner)
Fine needle holder, fulcrum lever type with ratchet
Fine needle holder (Gillies)
Skin pen and sterile ink (e.g. Bonney's blue)
Diathermy leads, electrodes and lead anchoring forceps
Suction tubing, fine nozzles and tube anchoring forceps.
2 (3/0) Plain or chromic catgut or synthetic absorbable on cleft palate needles for cleft palate and harelip (mucosa)
1.5 or 1 (4/0 or 5/0) Synthetic non-absorbable on small curved non-traumatic cutting needles for harelip repair (skin).

Outline procedure

Cleftlip. There are a number of alternative operations that can be undertaken for unilateral cleft. Rotational-advancement (Milland) and triangular flap procedures which are essentially a modified Z-plasty can be used (Fig. 24.12). A Z-plasty type of incision is made, extending from the apex of the cleft to the mucosal edge of the lip. The tissues are undermined at each side of the cleft and if this extends up to the nose, the tissues of the cheek will be undermined towards the orbit in order to lessen tension when the wound is closed. The edges of the cleft are excised, drawn together and a fine silk suture inserted at the mucocutaneous junction in the centre. The muscles are approximated with catgut or synthetic absorbable sutures before completing the suture line with interrupted sutures of a synthethic non-absorbable for the skin and fine plain or chromic catgut or synthetic absorbable for the mucosa. (Some surgeons apply a traction bow to relieve the tension on the suture line.)

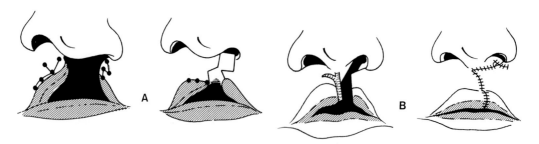

Fig. 24.12 Cleft lip, methods of repair. (A) The triangular-flap method of repair. (Tennyson.) (B) The rotation-advancement method of repair. (Millard.)

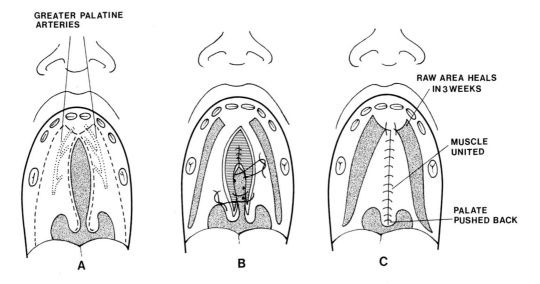

Fig. 24.13 Cleft palate repair. (Wardill-Kilner.) (A) The defect showing lines of incisions. (B) Two mucoperiosteal flaps are raised, conserving the greater palatine arteries. These are transposed medially and are joined in the midline with three layers of sutures. (C) Completed repair with gap left on either side of hard palate, which may be left open or filled with a Whitehead's varnish pack. The pack is generally removed in seven days under sedation or general anaesthesia. The raw area usually heals in two to three weeks.

Bilateral cleft can be corrected by using an Abbé flap which consists of the transfer of a full thickness 'V' of the rather excessive lower lip to the deficiency of the upper lip.

Cleft palate. A suitable mouth gag is inserted, an incision made on each side of the cleft soft palate and the edges of the cleft are freshened. Two flaps of mucosa and muscle with their bases posteriorly are raised on each side from the underlying hard palate.

These two flaps are transposed and sutured together in the midline, thereby leaving a raw area which heals in three weeks.

N.B. *Cleftlip* cleft palate operations may be done as a combined procedure; or the lip is repaired at about 12 weeks of age and the palate before the development of speech.

SKIN GRAFTS

Split-thickness Thiersch-type graft

Definition

This is a graft which does not include all layers of the skin but only the epidermis and the tips of the papilla of the dermis. It is a useful type of graft which takes well and is therefore very widely used by surgeons. However, as healing takes place it contracts because it does not contain elastic fibres, does not have any sweat glands or hair, and may not, therefore, be cosmetically acceptable.

Position

This depends upon the location of the donor and recipient areas. In most cases where the graft is taken from the thigh for transference to an anterior area of the body, supine is suitable.

Instruments

Sponge holding forceps (Rampley), 4
Scalpel handles No. 3 with Nos. 10 and 15 blades (Bard Parker), 2
Fine dissecting forceps, toothed (Gillies), 2
Fine dissecting forceps non-toothed (McIndoe), 2
Fine dissecting scissors, curved on flat, 10 cm (4 in) (Kilner)

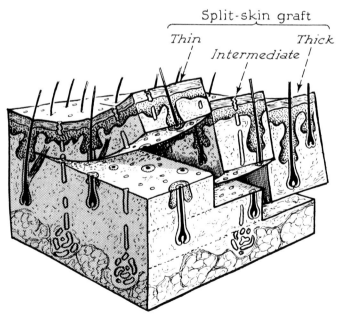

Fig. 24.14 The varying thickness of the split-skin graft, showing the constituents of each. (McGregor: *Fundamental Techniques of Plastic Surgery.*)

Figs. 24.15 to 24.17   Skin grafting instruments. (Down's Surgical Ltd.)

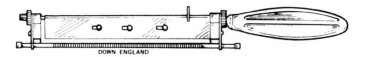

Fig. 24.15   Braithwaite modified Humby skin graft knife, disposable blade.

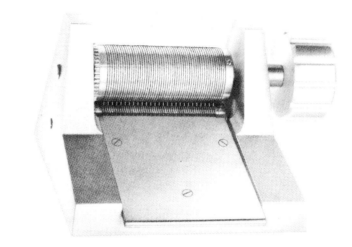

Fig. 24.16   Net graft cutter.

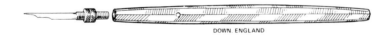

Fig. 24.17   Eckhoff mapping pen.

Scissors, curved on flat 13 cm (5 in) (Mayo)
Long fine scissors, curved on flat 17 cm (7 in)
Fine artery forceps, straight or curved on flat (Mosquito), 10
Skin hooks (Gillies), 2
Skin graft boards (teak), 2
Skin grafting razor (Blair) or
Skin grafting knife (Braithwaite modified Humby)
Net skin graft-cutter
Graft manipulators
Skin pen and sterile ink (e.g. Bonney's blue)
Towel clips (Backhaus or cross action), 6
Needle holders (Gillies), 2
Steel rule 15 cm (6 in)
Irrigation syringe and normal saline
Diathermy leads, electrodes and anchoring forceps
Thrombin, 5 ml syringe and hypodemic needles

1.5 (4/0) or finer, synthetic absorbable or non-absorbable on fine curved cutting needles sizes 12 to 16

Sterile gamgee tissue impregnated with proflavine emulsion, or polyurethane foam

Paraffin gauze dressing or similar

Cotton wool and crêpe bandages

Plaster of Paris may be required.

Outline of procedure

Unless it forms part of a fresh surgical defect, e.g., excision of tumour, debrided traumatic area, the recipient area is prepared by trimming excess granulation tissue to provide a smooth vascular bed for the graft. Haemostasis is secured by picking up blood-vessels and twisting them off or utilising diathermy.

The donor area is prepared by smearing lightly with sterile liquid paraffin or petroleum jelly and the graft is taken with a hand knife or dermatome.

A hand knife consists of a slender blade about 24 cm (9 in) long fitted to a handle which also includes a guide, which is adjustable for various graft thicknesses. Examples of these are the Watson and Braithwaite knives. When using a hand knife the skin is flattened by pressing a graft board at each end of the donor area.

There are two basic types of dermatome, the Paget's drum type and the mechanical oscillating blade type (Figs. 24.20 and 21). The Paget's dermatome is prepared by adjusting the 'depth of graft' mechanism and coating the half cylinder with skin graft adhesive. Adhesive is applied also to the donor area, and the edge of the cylinder is placed at the point on the skin selected for the commencement of the graft. As the cylinder is rotated slightly, the skin adheres and is lifted so that the graft may be taken by oscillating the cutting blade. This manoeuvre is continued until the whole surface of the cylinder is covered with skin. The graft is then detached from the donor area and removed from the drum.

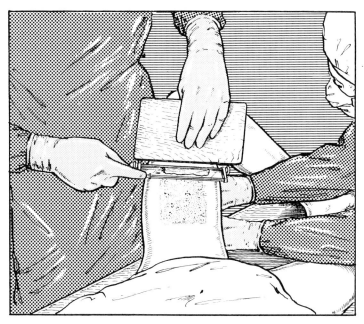

Fig. 24.18 Cutting a graft with the Braithwaite knife. (McGregor: *Fundamental Techniques of Plastic Surgery.*)

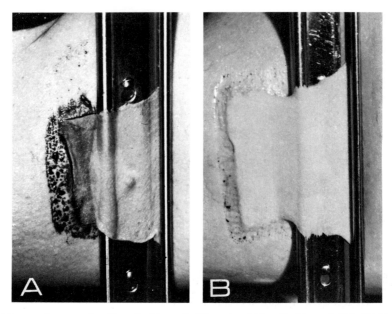

Fig. 24.19 The translucency of a thin split-skin graft (A), and a thick split-skin graft (B). (McGregor: *Fundamental Techniques of Plastic Surgery*.)

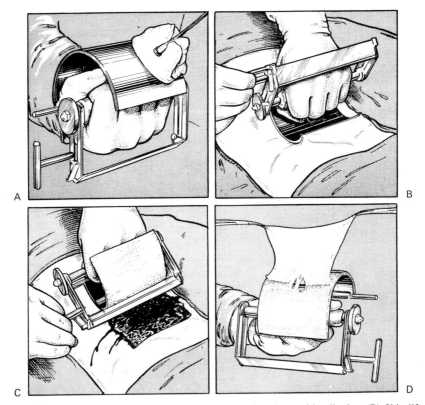

Fig. 24.20 Cutting a graft with the drum dermatome. (A) Painting drum with adhesive. (B) Skin lifted by drum. (C) Cutting the graft. (D) Stripping graft from drum. (McGregor: *Fundamental Techniques of Plastic Surgery*.)

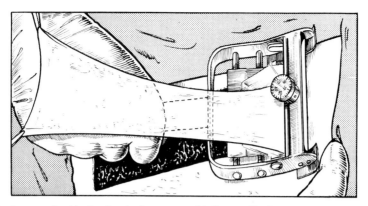

Fig. 24.21   Cutting a graft with the electric dermatome. (McGregor: *Fundamental Techniques of Plastic Surgery.*)

The mechanical type dermatome is adjusted for depth of graft and is operated with a 'planning action' over the selected donor area (Fig. 24.21). A small amount of lubricant may be applied to the skin and under-surface of the dermatome before taking the graft. If a very thin graft is required, sterile adhesive tape or polyvinyl can be applied to the skin, which is cut with the tape still attached. This provides support to aid manipulation of the graft afterwards.

The graft is applied as a sheet, sutured at its periphery to the skin around the recipient area.

When insufficient skin is available or where fixation is difficult, as in the perineum or axilla, 'mesh grafting' may be employed. The graft is passed through an instrument which shreds it into a regular meshwork of skin (Fig. 24.22). Applying traction to the four corners of the mesh increases the areas, and although the final cosmetic result varies greatly, it allows skin to be applied to surfaces where other methods may fail. The meshing also increases the success of the 'take rate' by allowing blood to seep out of the perforations (Fig. 24.23).

Firm pressure is applied over the graft for a few minutes, and layer of petroleum jelly gauze is then placed over the whole area. A pad of polyurethane sponge or cotton-wool impregnated with proflavine emulsion is very useful for exerting localised pressure on the graft and the dressing is completed with gauze and wool and crêpe bandages applied firmly.

Some surgeons inject a solution of thrombin under the skin graft before applying pressure. This serves to encourage adherence of the graft to the underlying tissues and helps to avoid accumulation of fluid which can prevent the graft taking. Alternatively grafts may be fixed in position with a biological glue (fibrinogen or histacryl). Finally, the operation is completed by dressing the donor area with petroleum jelly gauze, gauze, wool and bandages.

Unused portions of skin can be stored in a refrigerator at 1°C (34°F), spread on petroleum jelly gauze, and be placed in a sterile container with a few drops of normal saline. The grafts are then available for application as required in theatre or ward without administering an anaesthetic. Normal storage is up to three weeks.

Sometimes there is only limited skin available for auto-grafting, as for example in major burns involving 35–40 per cent of the body surface area. In such cases temporary skin cover may be provided with homografts from a skin bank.

Rejection of a skin homograft usually takes place in 8–10 days in a healthy individual, although this rejection may be delayed for 21 days in a burned patient. The development of tissue typing has enabled rejection to be postponed for up to 90 days for correctly matched skin (Roberts, 1976).

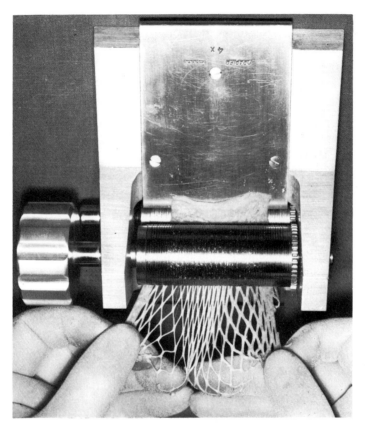

Fig. 24.22 Meshing a skin graft. The split-skin graft, fed between the rollers, emerges meshed so that, stretched, it can be expanded to cover a much larger area. (McGregor: *Fundamental Techniques of Plastic Surgery.*)

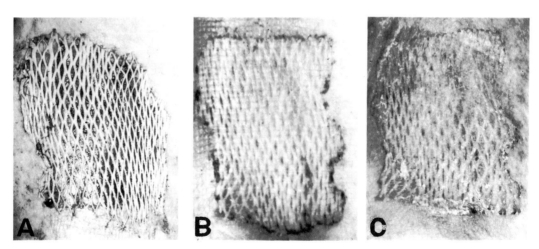

Fig. 24.23 The use of a mesh graft. (A) Shows the mesh graft applied to a granulating area. (B) Shows the intermediate stage of healing by epidermal spread from the graft, seen by the increased blurring of the outline of the mesh. (C) The healed result, showing how the background of the original mesh is still visible. (McGregor: *Fundamental Techniques of Plastic Surgery.*

Application of homografts extends the period available to cover a burned area with autografts; a donor site on a patient can be used every 10–14 days. Ideally, eventually perfect matched skin from a skin bank will provide permanent cover, but present technology has not yet achieved this.

Skin bank. Skin for the bank is removed from cadavers under sterile conditions within 6–16 hours of death. Blood and spleen samples are also taken for tissue typing of the skin.

The homograft is spread and suspended in a film of 15 per cent glycerol with antibiotics, in a sealed nylon envelope. The envelope is mounted in a metal frame and the whole cooled with liquid nitrogen in a programmed freezing apparatus to −100°C, and then stored in liquid nitrogen at −196°C.

To use the graft, the frame is immersed in sterile water at 37°C. Once thawed the viable graft cannot be re-frozen.

Full-thickness Wolfe-type graft

Definition

This is a free graft which includes all layers of the skin. Although it does not 'take' as easily as the Thiersch graft, it does not contract, contains sweat glands and hair and is therefore more cosmetically acceptable.

Position

This varies with the area to be grafted.

Instruments

As for Thiersch graft (but minus skin graft knives)
Sterile jaconet or polyvinyl sheet for patterns.

Outline of procedure

The recipient area is prepared as described previously by trimming excess or damaged tissue. A pattern of the recipient area is made with a piece of sterile jaconet and this is used to outline the graft on the donor area with pen and ink.

An incision is made round this ink outline and deepened to the subcutaneous tissues. Starting at one end, the graft is undermined, held up with skin hooks and dissected free from the underlying fat. It is important that very little or no fat be included with the graft.

The graft is sutured at its periphery to the skin surrounding the recipient area. Fine synthetic absorbable or non-absorbable is used to obtain close approximation.

Pressure dressings are applied as for Thiersch graft.

Skin flaps and pedicles

These are grafts composed of skin and subcutaneous tissue which has an intact and functioning arterial and venous blood circulation.

The successful transfer of skin flaps is dependent on retaining an attachment to the body, so that an active blood circulation can be maintained in the graft at the recipient site. This means these grafts, having their own blood supply, can be used to cover avascular areas such

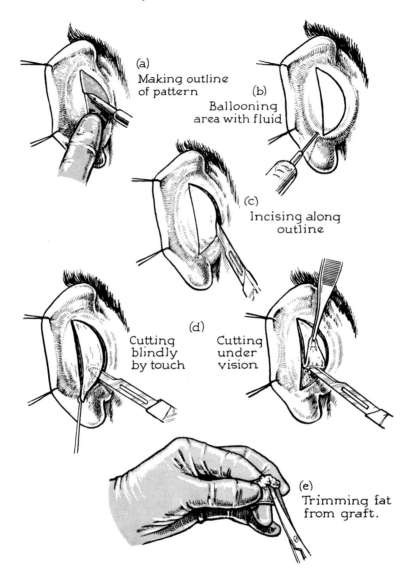

(a)
Making outline
of pattern

(b)
Ballooning
area with fluid

(c)
Incising along
outline

(d)
Cutting
blindly
by touch

Cutting
under
vision

(e)
Trimming fat
from graft.

Fig. 24.24 The method of cutting a full thickness graft. (McGregor: *Fundamental Techniques of Plastic Surgery.*)

as exposed cortical bone, tendon or an open joint. The texture of a flap generally remains unaltered, and as the skin does not contract it is suitable for use over areas where shrinking could create problems, such as the front surface of joints. Flaps can be classified in four main types:

Random pattern flaps obtain their blood supply from the subdermal plexus of vessels. For this reason, in order that an adequate flow of blood to the flap is maintained, the width of the pedicle base is made approximately equivalent to the length of the flap, i.e. a 1:1 ratio (Fig. 24.26A).

Axial pattern flaps can be made much longer than the width of the pedicle base, as they contain a sizable artery and vein running axially within it to provide vascularisation (Fig. 24.26B).

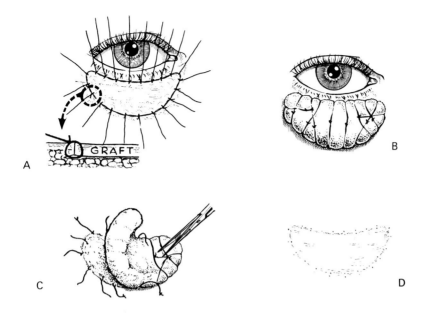

Fig. 24.25   The suturing and dressing of a skin graft. (McGregor: *Fundamental Techniques of Plastic Surgery.*)

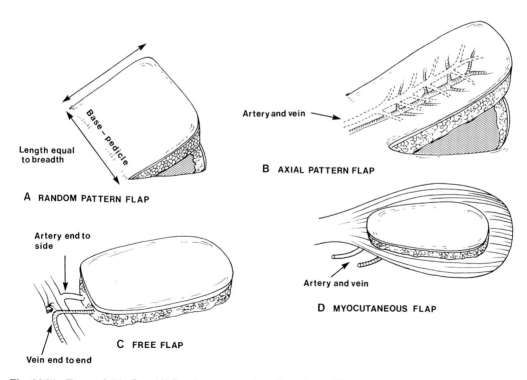

Fig. 24.26   Types of skin flap. (A) Random pattern flap; dimensions of base are made equal to breadth. (B) Axial pattern flap; contains vascular pedicle, can be much longer in proportion to the width of the base. (C) Free flap; artery and vein in flap anastomosed to artery and vein at recipient site. (D) Myocutaneous flap; comprises skin flap together with underlying muscle and attached blood supply.

Free flaps. These function in a similar fashion to axial flaps except that the main blood vessels are divided before the flap is transferred. The vessels are anastomosed, using microsurgical techniques, to an appropriate artery and vein at the recipient site (Fig. 24.26C).

Myocutaneous flaps consist of transferring a skin flap still attached to underlying muscle. Vascularisation is through the multitude of small vessels which pass from the surface of the muscle to he overlying skin. The muscle can be detached at one or both ends retaining its vascular pedicle, and swung into position on the recipient site. Alternatively, the flap may be divided and treated as a free flap with anastomosis of the muscle vessels to a suitable artery and vein at the recipient site (Fig. 24.26D).

Random pattern flaps

Rotation flap. A half circle of skin is rotated on to a triangular defect. This requires a sizeable length of flap; to advance the skin 25 mm (1 in) requires about 20 cm (8 in) along the edge of the flap (Fig. 24.27A).

Transposition flap consists of a square of skin slid over a triangular defect (Fig. 24.27B). The secondary defect resulting in the area from which the flap has been transposed is generally covered with a split skin graft.

Direct or distant flap consists of a flap transferred from a donor site not normally adjacent to the recipient site. Examples of these include hand to abdomen (Fig. 24.27C) and cross-leg flap (Fig. 24.32).

Tubed pedicle flaps, although not commonly used nowadays, enable the transfer of flaps when the donor area cannot be brought close enough to the recipient site. In this instance

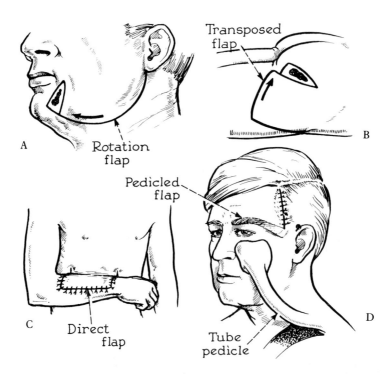

Fig. 24.27 The basic types of flap transfer. (McGregor: *The Fundamental Techniques of Plastic Surgery.*)

the skin flap is raised along two sides as a tube. After approximately three weeks one end of the tube is detached and sutured to the defect; the wound remaining in the donor site is closed with sutures. A further three weeks later the skin tube is severed from the flap which is trimmed and then sutured into its final position (Fig. 24.27D).

Z-plasty may be used for lengthening a contracted scar, or in combination with other procedures, e.g. rotational flaps, for the closure of defects (Fig. 24.28).

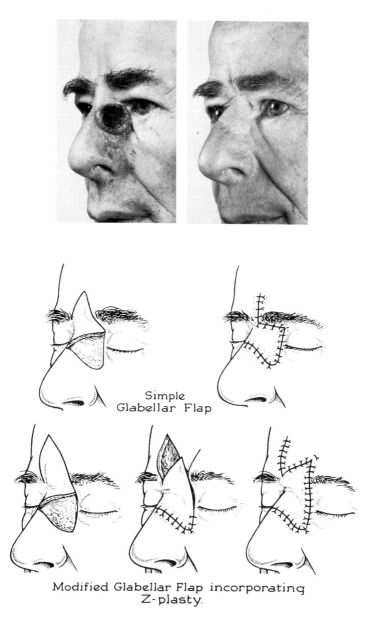

Fig. 24.28 Very extensive molluscum sebaceum (confirmed by biopsy) excised and repaired by simple rotational flap. A modification is also shown which is useful when there is difficulty in closing the secondary defect of forehead. (McGregor: *Fundamental Techniques of Plastic Surgery.*)

Axial flaps

This type of flap can be used for direct or distant flap techniques, or as a free flap.

Free flaps

The successful use of free flaps has become possible only since the development of the operating microscope and microsurgical techniques (Chapter 12, page 367).

An example of this is the groin flap (Fig. 24.29), which can be used to cover defects on the hand or arm. A long length of skin which includes the superficial circumflex artery, is raised over the ilium. The vessels are divided at the point where they join the femoral artery and vein and are anastomosed to suitable vessels at the recipient site.

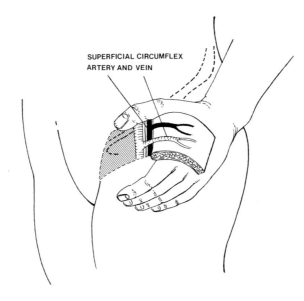

SUPERFICIAL CIRCUMFLEX
ARTERY AND VEIN

Fig. 24.29   Groin flap; example of an axial pattern flap to provide skin cover or defect on the hand.

Myocutaneous flaps

Many of these types of flaps are being developed; two examples are as follows:

Latissimus dorsi myocutaneous flap is particularly useful for defects of the breast or chest wall. The muscle, and overlying skin, is detached from its wide origin at the back and swung across the front of the chest. Blood supply is maintained via the vessels which supply it from the axilla (Fig. 24.30).

Gastrocnemius flap is used to cover defects in front of the knee or over the shin by moving one or both heads of the gastrocnemius from the calf (Fig. 24.31).

Position

This varies with the location of donor and recipient site.

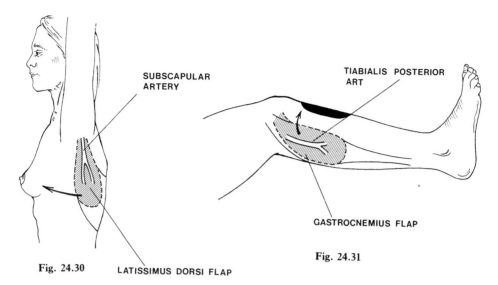

SUBSCAPULAR
ARTERY

TIABIALIS POSTERIOR
ART

GASTROCNEMIUS FLAP

Fig. 24.30   LATISSIMUS DORSI FLAP

Fig. 24.31

Fig. 24.30   Latissimus dorsi myocutaneous flap to cover defects of the chest wall or breast.

Fig. 24.31   Gastrocnemius myocutaneous flap to cover defects on the shin or over the front of the knee.

Instruments

Basic skin graft (page 745)
   Sterile jaconet or polyvinyl sheet for patterns.

Outline of procedure (example)

The number of stages necessary for this procedure depends upon the distance of the donor site from the recipient area and also whether the two areas can be brought together into direct contact with each other, e.g., hand to abdomen.

Two-stage operation, e.g., hand to abdomen and cross leg flap

Abdominal flap. A large defect in the skin of the hand may be replaced by raising an abdominal skin flap and attaching it to the hand which is immobilised on the abdominal wall until healing is complete.

A pattern of the defect is made on a piece of sterile jaconet and the outline transferred to the selected abdominal area, e.g., inguinal region, with pen and ink. The outlined flap and underlying fat are raised on three sides and a Thiersch graft applied to the raw area beneath.

The hand defect is prepared in the usual manner, is approximated to the donor site, and the flap sutured at its periphery to the skin surrounding the recipient area. Pressure dressings of petroleum jelly gauze, gauze, polyurethane sponge, proflavine wool, white wool and crêpe or adhesive bandages are applied.

Two or three weeks later, the fourth side of the flap is detached and sutured to the adjacent recipient skin edge. The donor site is trimmed at its periphery and if a defect remains where the flap has been detached, a further Thiersch graft is applied. Dressings are applied as before.

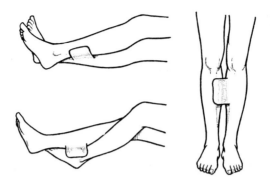

Fig. 24.32 The classical cross-leg flap positions. (McGregor.)

Cross leg flap. The recipient area, e.g., over the tibia, is prepared by excising excess granulation tissue and surrounding skin. A pattern of the defect, usually oblong in shape, is prepared on sterile jaconet. The outline of the pattern is transferred with pen and ink on to the calf of the other leg and an incision made round three sides of the outline. The base of the flap is always more anterior so that when the leg is crossed over the recipient site, the flap covers the defect without kinking.

The flap is sutured at its periphery to the skin surrounding the recipient area. The area underneath the raised flap on the donor leg is covered with a Thiersch graft from the thigh. Pressure dressings are applied in the usual way and the legs are immobilised with plaster of Paris bandages.

Three weeks later the flap is detached from its base and the fourth side sutured to the adjacent skin edge, followed by the application of dressings as before.

Rhinoplasty

Definition

This term describes a wide variety of corrective procedures on the nose, any combination or all of the following may be carried out; excision of nasal hump, correction of sunken bridge, adjustment of length of the nose, narrowing of the nose, remodelling of the nasal tip, rotation or pedicle flap (with or without Z-plasty) to cover nasal defect. The operation is generally undertaken to restore to normal contour anatomy, deviations from the normal e.g., those arising from trauma, familial or racial characteristics.

Position

Supine.

Instruments

Scalpel handles No. 3 with Nos. 10 and 15 blades (Bard Parker), 2
Fine dissecting forceps, toothed (Gillies), 2
Fine dissecting forceps, non-toothed (McIndoe), 2
Fine artery forceps, straight, mosquito, 10
Fine artery forceps, curved or flat, mosquito, 10

Fine tissue forceps (McIndoe), 5
Skin hooks (Gillies), 4
Fine scissors, curved on flat, 10 cm (4 in) (Kilner)
Scissors, curved on flat, 13 cm (5 in) (Mayo)
Dissector (MacDonald or Durham)
Small retractors, double hook, 2
Small retractors, double end, 'rake' (Lane), 2
Fine needle holder (Gillies or Kilner)
Stent composition material or plaster of Paris moulded into a splint
2 and 1.5 (3/0 and 4/0) Plain catgut or synthetic absorbable for ligatures
2 (3/0) Plain catgut or synthetic absorbable on a half-circle cutting needle for subcutaneous sutures
1.5 or 1 (4/0 or 5/0) Synthetic non-absorbable, on a small curved cutting needle (preferably non-traumatic) for skin sutures.

If a bone graft is contemplated
Cancellous bone from the bone bank (with bone-cutting forceps, etc.) *or* instruments for taking a bone graft (Fig. 23.94).

If nasal correction is contemplated
Nasal saw (Joseph)
Nasal rasp
Scissors, angled (Heyman)
Nasal septum forceps (Jansen Middleton)
Nasal raspatory (Hill or Howarth)
Nasal punch forceps, small and medium (Luc), 2
Nasal speculum, long (St Clair Thompson)
Dressing forceps, angled
Small gouges, 4 mm, 6 mm, 8 mm, 10 mm (Jenkins)
Small chisels, 4 mm, 6 mm, 8 mm, 10 mm
Ribbon gauze impregnated with 1 in 10,000 adrenaline.

If prosthesis is contemplated
Autogenous septal or costal cartilage or rhinoplasty implant e.g. Silastic™ silicone elastomer implant designed for augmenting the sunken bridge of the nose (available in three sizes).

Outline of procedure

With the exception of external tissue defects (i.e. skin loss — excisions of tumours), the surgical approach is always from within the nasal cavity. The incisions are made on both sides between the upper and lower lateral cartilages, extending towards the top of the nasal septum. They are pushed through the membranous septum to separate the columella and septum. The skin of the nose is elevated with scissors up to the level of the nasal bones. The periosteum is then elevated from the nasal bones with a long raspatory.

A nasal saw or osteotone and cartilage scissors is used to remove a nasal bump, and the surfaces are smoothed with rasps. A sunken bridge can be corrected with a bone graft autogenous cartilage or Delatic™ rhinoplasty implant.

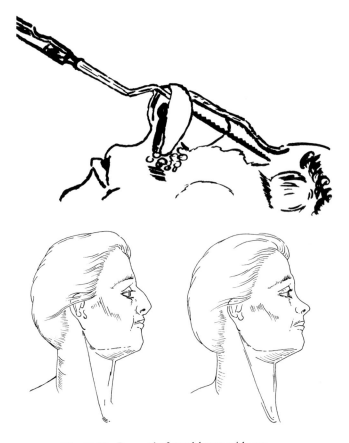

Fig. 24.33 Removal of nasal hump with saw.

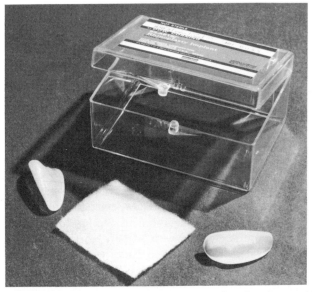

Fig. 24.34 Silastic™ nasal implants and Safian technique for correction of sunken nasal bridge. (Dow Corning International.)

The nose may be narrowed by detaching the nasal bones from the septum in the midline and the maxilla laterally. These bones are then infractured and repositioned medially, thereby narrowing the nose. Shortening of the nose necessitates a triangular resection of the nasal septum.

Plastic remodelling of the nasal tip involves excision of the alar cartilage through a second incision at the junction of the skin and mucous membrane.

After evacuation of any blood clots from beneath the skin, subcutaneous sutures may be inserted followed by suture of the skin edges with synthetic non-absorbable or silk. A nasal pack is usually inserted in both nasal cavities; external splints of Stent or plaster of Paris may be applied.

Operation for protruding ears

Definition

The removal of segments of aural cartilage and reconstruction of antihelix.

Position

Supine, with the head turned to one side.

Instruments

Scalpel handles No. 9 with Nos. 10 and 15 blades (Bard Parker), 2
Fine dissecting forceps, toothed (Gillies)
Fine dissecting forceps, non-toothed (McIndoe)
Fine artery forceps, curved on flat, mosquito, 5
Skin hooks (Gillies), 2
Fine tissue forceps (McIndoe), 2
Fine scissors, curved on flat, 10 cm (4 in) (Kilner)
Small retractors, double end, 'rake' (Lane), 2
Dissector (MacDonald)
Fine needle holder (Gillies or Kilner)
1.5 (4/0) Plain catgut or synthetic absorbable for ligatures
1.5 or 1 (4/0 or 5/0) Synthetic non-absorbable, on a small curved cutting needle
  (preferably non-traumatic) for skin sutures.

Outline of procedure

There are a number of procedures which can be adopted. Essentially, an oval shaped piece of skin behind the ear is excised. The skin is separated from the anterior surface of the cartilage to allow it to bend back in a smooth curve. The cartilage stays in its new position when the skin is closed behind it with continuous sutures (Morgan and Wright, 1986).

Cosmetic breast surgery — mammoplasty

Definition

Reduction of enlarged breasts may be undertaken as a result of conditions such as virginal hypertrophy, macromastia and benign breast disease, e.g. fibrocystic disease

Reconstruction is used where a deformity exists following mastectomy.

Augmentation may be combined with reconstructive procedures or carried out for mammary hypoplasia.

Position

Generally supine or sitting.

Instruments

General set (Figs. 14.1 to 14.28)

Local infiltration set (Fig. 11.60) plus 22 g spinal needle, with 0.5 per cent lignocaine (Xylocaine) and 1: 200,000 adrenaline (optional)

Scissors, curved on flat, long Metzenbaum

Retractors, Deaver, 25 mm (1 in), 2

Retractors, rake, medium, 2

Diathermy leads, electrodes and lead anchoring forceps

Irrigation syringe and saline or topical antibiotic solution

Suction drainage tubes (Redivac, Activac, Portovac)

Mammary prosthesis if appropriate

2.5 (2/0) or 3 (0) synthetic absorbable sutures on half circle round bodied or cutting needles for muscle and subcutaneous tissue

2 (3/0) or 1.5 (4/0) synthetic non-absorbable sutures on curved cutting needles (preferably non-traumatic) for skin.

Outline of procedure

As there are many different procedures adopted in all three categories of cosmetic breast surgery, it is possible only to give examples.

Breast reduction. Most procedures consist of excising skin, fat and breast tissue from the lower half of the breast. If possible, the nipple is preserved on a vascular pedicle based superiorly, laterally, or inferiorly (Fig. 24.35). Alternatively, in massive reduction the nipples and areola are not preserved, but replaced at a second stage operation by free grafts taken generally from either the vulva or medial groin skin. Scars are kept to the inferior half of the breast (Fig. 24.36).

Breast reconstruction. This is generally carried out following mastectomy procedures which, although now more commonly less radical in extent (Chapter 16), often result in a significant skin deficiency. This may require either that the skin be stretched by an inflatable implant or well vascularised flaps used to create an adequate skin envelope. Reconstruction is usually delayed for six months following the mastectomy to allow the tissues to settle, the patient to adjust to the new situation and to determine the best method of reconstruction.

Breast augmentation follows procedures similar to that adopted for breast reconstruction, although in most instances implants are inserted.

Outline of procedure

The method of choice for breast reconstruction is influenced by such factors as the extent of skin shortage, whether the pectoralis muscle remains, the degree of damage to the tissues from radiation therapy, and surgical preferences. These methods include the use of implants

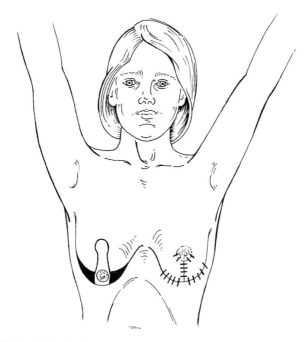

Fig. 24.35 Method of breast reduction; nipple preserved on a pedicle.

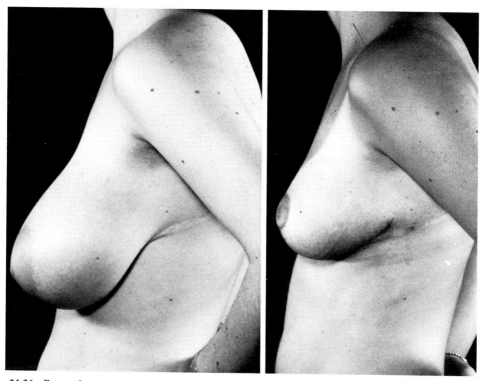

Fig. 24.36 Pre- and post-operative breast reduction using a medially based, unilateral pedicle. (Breach, In *Recent Advances in Surgery*, ed Russell.)

alone, if necessary with tissue stretching beforehand; myocutaneous flaps such as the latissimus dorsi flap (Fig. 24.30); or possibly adjustment of the remaining breast to achieve acceptable symmetry.

Most surgeons prefer to use autogenous tissue rather than implants to reconstruct the breast, in addition to the latissimus dorsi flap just mentioned, new methods of utilising vascularised flaps are constantly being developed. One such technique is the transverse abdominal island flap (TAIF) which produces a reconstructed breast of near normal appearance (Dinner and Coleman, 1985).

The TAIF consists of the transfer of redundant lower abdominal skin and fat to the chest wall to form the new breast. This is carried out in a first stage procedure, followed by nipple-areola reconstruction about three months later. A circumferential-type incision is made in the lower abdomen (Fig.24.37), and the rectus abdominus muscle raised from the posterior rectus sheath after incising the anterior sheath. The myocutaneous flap consisting of an island of skin attached to the rectus muscle is then tunnelled deep to the anterior abdominal wall and then delivered through a submammary incision on the chest wall (Fig. 24.38). To avoid hernia formation, the abdominal defect is repaired with a synthetic non-absorbable mesh. The myocutaneous flap is sutured in position as illustrated in Figure 24.39 and the suction drains inserted into the wound.

Where it is not possible to utilise autogenous tissue, the surgeon may decide to insert an implant (mammary prosthesis). The types of implant available include a sealed silcone bag containing silcone gel; a double lumen bag, the inner containing slicone gel and the outer filled with saline through a valve at time of operation; or one which can be filled entirely with saline. Although the procedure has become a routine operation it is not without problems and complications. The insertion of a mammary implant stimulates the formation of a surrounding capsule which can lead to hardening of the breast, deformity of contour, and subsequent pain. It is not normally undertaken for any patient who has an infection in the breasts, nipple/areola region or other parts of the body; exhibits psychological instability; has a history of repeated failures following subcutaneous mastectomy or cosmetic augmentation; exhibits a lack of skin and tissue viability; or has a history of repeated breast malignancy which has metastasised.

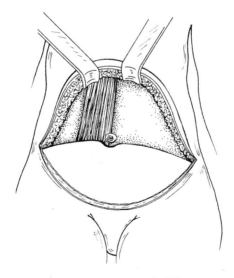

Fig. 24.37   Tranverse abdominal island flap; incision of abdominal flap, rectus muscle exposed.

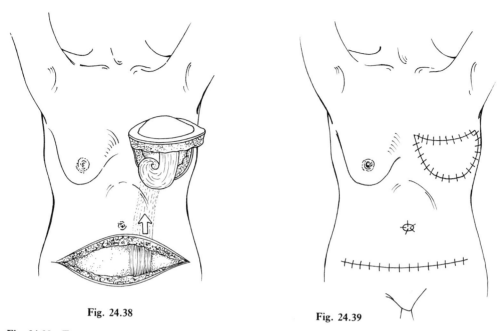

Fig. 24.38

Fig. 24.39

Fig. 24.38 Transverse abdominal island flap; transfer of flap on to chest wall.

Fig. 24.39 Transverse abdominal island flap; procedure completed, the flap has been moulded into a breast form, and the abdominal defect repaired.

At one time manufacturers offered mammary implants with thin walls in the belief that this reproduced the feel of the normal breast. However, there is evidence that during capsule formation the implant may be associated with a tissue reaction to particles of silcone gel which leak though the wall of the implants, and that this is more likely to occur with the thin walled variety. To reduce the leakage of silicone particles there is now a tendency to select thick walled implants or the double lumen variety mentioned previously (Breach, 1986). This permits removal if necessary of quantities of saline to 'soften' the implant if a significant capsule develops.

Another development is the Silastic™ II mammary implant which is a sterile, silicone gell-filled implant made with a laminated silicone envelope (Figs. 24.40 and 24.41). The Silastic™ II is claimed to be a high performance material which provides greater tear resistance than ordinary silicone elastomer; imparts a barrier to gel bleed; closely approximates the weight and consistency of normal breasts; and is essentially non-reactive to body tissue if sterile and uncontaminated.

Special care is necessary when handling mammary implants to avoid damage or contamination. Information given by the manufacturers of the Silastic™ II, Dow Corning make recommendations which include:

1. The implant should be inspected bcfore implantation to check the envelope integrity; if *any* damage is apparent the implant should not be used.

2. Care should be taken to avoid contact of any sharp edges or pointed objects with the implant; it should be inserted by hand and *not* utilising any instrument or blunt object.

3. The incision should be adequate for the size of implant to minimise stress on the implant during surgical insertion.

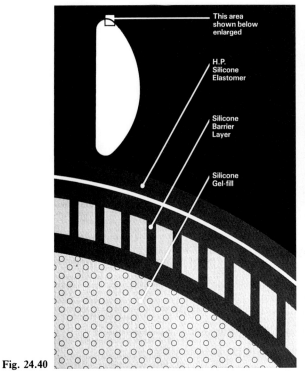

This area
shown below
enlarged

H.P.
Silicone
Elastomer

Silicone
Barrier
Layer

Silicone
Gel-fill

Fig. 24.40

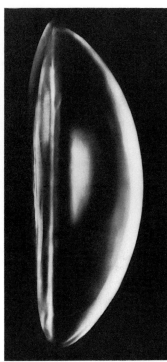

Fig. 24.41

Fig. 24.40 Silastic™ II mammary implant, diagrammatic. This is a sterile, silicone gel-filled breast implant with a laminated silicone envelope. The laminate consists of medical-grade high performance (HP) silicone elastomer, and a special silicone barrier layer. The envelope is soft and seamless; the gel is responsive and transparent. (Technical leaflet 51-160-01, Dow Corning.)

Fig. 24.41 Silastic™ II mammary implant. (Dow Corning.)

4. Should the implant become accidentally punctured during insertion, e.g. nicked with a sharp instrument or caught with a suture needle, it should be replaced.

5. Great care should be taken if it is necessary to evacuate haematomas or aspirate serious fluid accumulation following operation, as this may result in implant puncture.

The surgical technique for inserting an implant depends on many factors, but the following gives an example of an augmentation procedure.

With the patient in a sitting position, the infra-mammary fold is marked symmetrically beneath each breast. The small size can be inserted through a 6 cm (2½ in) incision, while shorter or longer incisions can be made for other sizes as appropriate. The line should be scratched in lightly with a needle prior to the skin prep. The template may be used as a guide to mark area of dissection.

Extending the patient's arms at right angles to her sides extends the pectoral muscles and facilitates dissection of the breast from the muscles. Bringing the arms to the sides of the body relaxes the skin and muscle and may ease the insertion of the implants. However, the complete operation can be done with the arms in either position.

Anaesthesia is usually general but the procedure may also be performed under local anaesthesia. One half per cent lignocaine with 1:200,000 adrenalin is infiltrated, fan-shaped between the breast and the pectoralis major muscle using a 22 gauge spinal needle.

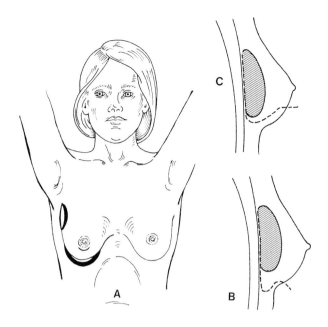

Fig. 24.42 Breast augmentation procedures. (A) Incisions
Insertion of implants:
(B) Infra-mammary approach. (C) Sub-aerolar approach.

An appropriate incision is made through the skin and subcutaneous tissue down to the
loose superficial fascia over the rib cage (Fig. 24.42). The upper edge of the wound is lifted
with a rake retractor and with sharp dissection, the anterior surface of the fascia over the
pectoralis major muscle is exposed. From this point, blunt dissection with a tonsil sponge
in a ring forceps or the gloved fingers may be efficacious. However, the use of long handled
scissors will often be needed. Dever or Harrington retractors are helpful and sometimes the
Trendelenburg position may help the illumination of the cavity. Some surgeons have used
a headlight.

Of greatest importance is that the cavity be made of *generous* size, directing particular
attention to dissection of the anterior axillary fold superiorly and medially. Forcing the
implant into a small cavity will result in undue firmness of the breast due to the pressure
of the surrounding tissues. Hemostasis should be meticulous and is best accomplished by
electrocoagulation. The space should be irrigated with saline, or, if preferred, with an antibiotic mixture such as neomycin — 0.5 gm, or Bacitracin — 10,000 units.

The breast is retracted with a Dever retractor. The implant is gradually forced through
the small sub-mammary or sub-pectoral incision with the fingers, the thin flattened part
inserted first. The retractors are then removed and the exact positioning of the implant is
completed by the manipulation.

The wounds are closed in layers, the final skin closure generally being with a continuous
2 (3/0) synthetic non-absorbable intradermal suture which can be left in for 2 weeks without
leaving suture marks.

As with any large wound, serum accumulation may sometimes be troublesome, so a
suction drainage tube is usually inserted (Redivac, Activac, Portavac).

Note: Dow Corning Silastic™ II prostheses are among the most non-reactive implant materials available. However, dust, lint, talc, skin oils and other surface contaminants deposited on the prosthesis in handling can evoke foreign body reactions with subsequent fluid and fibrous tissue buildup. Extreme care with strict adherence to aseptic techniques must be employed to prevent contamination of the prosthesis and the possible resultant complications.

The implant is supplied sterilized, but if for some reason it becomes contaminated or is not used when the pack is opened at operation, resterilization can be undertaken a maximum of three times. The prosthesis should be scrubbed gently, but thoroughly with a clean, soft-bristled brush in a hot water-soap solution to remove possible surface contaminants. *Use a non-oily cleaner or mild soap. Do not use synthetic detergents or oil-based soap, as these soaps may be absorbed and may subsequently leach out to cause a tissue reaction.* Rinse copiously in hot water and follow with a thorough rinse in distilled water.

To sterilise: Autoclave by one of the following methods:
1. High speed instrument (flash) sterilizer — Place on surgical towel in clean open tray. Sterilize 3 minutes at 130°C (270°F) at 28 p.s.i.
2. Standard gravity sterilizer — Wrap in surgical towel and place in clean open tray. Sterilize 30 minutes at 120°C (250°F) at 15 p.s.i.

Do *not* use a prevacuum high temperature sterilizer as this type of unit will cause the silicone gel to bubble and the prosthesis to swell.

Fasciectomy for Dupuytren's contracture

Definition

Excision of hypertrophied palmar fascia which has contracted, thereby causing contracture of the fingers.

Position

Supine, with the hand extended on an arm table and the fingers separated by securing with a lead hand or similar splint.

Instruments

Scalpel handle No. 3 with No. 10 blade (Bard Parker)
Scalpel handle No. 9 with No. 15 blade (Bard Parker)
Fine dissecting forceps, toothed (Gillies), 2
Fine dissecting forceps, non-toothed (McIndoe), 2
Fine scissors, curved (Kilner). Skin hooks (Gillies), 4
Small retractors, double end, 'rake' (Lane), 2
Fine artery forceps, curved on flat, mosquito, 10
Fine artery forceps, straight, mosquito, 10
Fine tissue forceps (McIndoe), 5
Dissector (MacDonald). Probe, malleable silver
Diathermy electrode, forceps, lead and lead anchoring forceps
2 and 1.5 (3/0 and 4/0) Synthetic non-absorbable on small curved cutting needles for skin sutures.
(Instruments for skin graft (p. 745) may be required.)

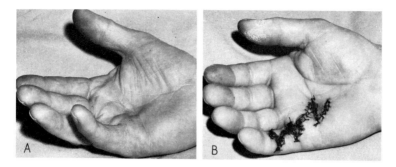

Fig. 24.43   A continuous multiple Z-plasty used in Dupuytren's contracture confined to the little finger ray. The stages of the procedure are shown diagrammatically in Figure 24.44. (McGregor: *Fundamental Techniques of Plastic Surgery*.)

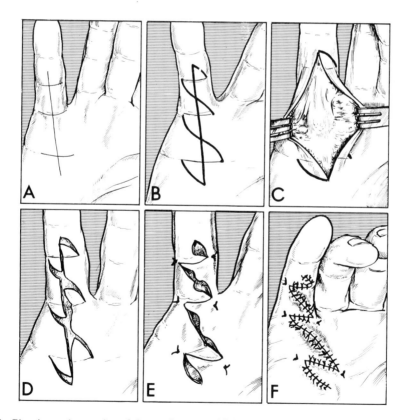

Fig. 24.44   Planning and execution of the continuous multiple Z-plasty of the type used in the Dupuytren's contracture shown in Figure 24.43. The line of the long incision indicating the extent of the contracted fascia and the intended lines of the transverse limbs of the Z-plasty is shown (A). B shows the Z-plasty drawn to place the transverse limbs in the creases as planned. The good exposure obtained by the longitudinal incision is seen C. D shows the Z-plasty flaps incised, transposed for suture, E, and sutured (F). (McGregor: *Fundamental Techniques of Plastic Surgery*.)

Outline of procedure

A tourniquet is always used for this operation (Chapter 23, page 615).

An incision is made in line with the mid-palmar crease from one side of the hand to the other. The skin on each side of the incision is undermined and freed from the palmar fascia, care being taken to avoid 'button holding'.

Beginning proximally, the hypertrophied fascia is dissected from the underlying blood-vessels, nerves and tendons which supply the fingers. If the scar tissue extends to the fingers themselves, a mid-lateral or multiple Z-plasty incision is made and all the hypertrophied fascia excised.

Sometimes the fascia is so adherent to the skin that a segment must be excised, and in this case the defect may require skin grafting.

After fasciectomy is complete the tourniquet will be released and the divided blood-vessels diathermized.

The wounds are closed with fine synthetic non-absorbable sutures and petroleum jelly gauze applied followed by a pressure pad to the palm of sponge rubber, or wool impregnated with proflavine emulsion. The dressing is completed with wool and crêpe bandages applied firmly, so that the fingers are immobilised in the position of function.

Hypospadias operation (Denis Browne's procedure)

Definition

The correction of a congenital abnormality where the urethral meatus lies at a point on the penis proximal to its normal position.

Position

Supine, with the legs separated.

Instruments

Sponge-holding forceps (Rampley), 5
Hypospadias set (Fig. 24.45) and diathermy lead anchoring forceps.

There is usually a contracted undersurface of the penis in addition to a displaced meatus. The first stage of the operation consists of freeing this contraction before making a new urethra.

A transverse incision is made in the skin just below the glans and extended into the prepuce on each side. The rudimentary corpus spongiosum is then peeled away from the main erectile tissue and reflected towards the penile base. The short fibrous bands which exist on each side of the chordee are divided and the transverse skin incision is closed longitudinally with fine plain catgut or synthetic absorbable to effect a lengthening of the penis.

The second stage of the operation follows at a much later date. A fine Malecot's catheter is inserted into the bladder with a fine introducer. A more rigid sound is then passed along this catheter and used to press its mid-shaft towards the perineum. A diathermy knife is then used to cut down on to the catheter which, when seen, is thrust out with the sound. This diverts urine from the operative area until healing has taken place, i.e., perineal urethrostomy.

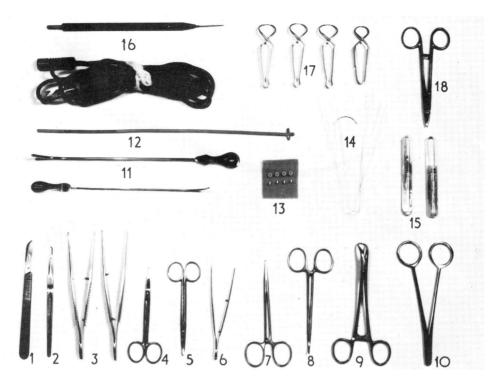

Fig. 24.45 Hypospadias operation.

1. Scalpel handle No. 3 with No. 10 blade (Bard Parker).
2. Scalpel handle No. 9 with No. 15 blade (Bard Parker).
3. Fine dissecting forceps, toothed and non-toothed (Gillies and McIndoe)
4. Iris scissors, straight, sharp points.
5. Fine scissors, curved on flat, 10 cm (4 in) (Kilner).
6. Fine dissecting forceps, toothed, fixation.
7. Fine artery forceps, straight, mosquito, 6.
8. Fine artery forceps, curved on flat, mosquito, 6.
9. Towel forceps for penile holding.
10. Clamping forceps for aluminium collars (Denis Browne).
11. Catheter introducers, flexible and rigid (Denis Browne).
12. Catheter, self-retaining (Malecot), size 12 Charrière gauge.
13. Glass beads and aluminium collars (Denis Browne).
14. Size 5(2) synthetic monofilament non-absorbable and curved cutting needle.
15. 2 and 1.5 (3/0 and 4/0) chromic catgut or synthetic non-absorbable on 16 mm non-traumatic cutting needles.
16. Diathermy electrode and lead.
17. Towel clips, 4.
18. Fine needle holder (Kilner multiple joint).

A U-shaped insertion is made, commencing at one side of the glans, continuing along the undersurface of the penis, around and proximal to the displaced meatus and finishing at the other side of the glans. The skin edges are reflected widely on each side, leaving a central strip of skin extending from the the glans to the displaced meatus. The skin edges are brought together to cover the strip of skin in a manner similar to closing a single-breasted coat.

Approximation is achieved by using synthetic non-absorbable monofilament tension sutures held with a lead stop and glass bead at each side of the wound. The procedure is as follows; a glass bead is threaded on to stout monofilament synthetic non-absorbable monofilament suture material at the end of which has been placed a short piece of crushed lead or aluminium tubing. The suture material is threaded on to a needle and introduced

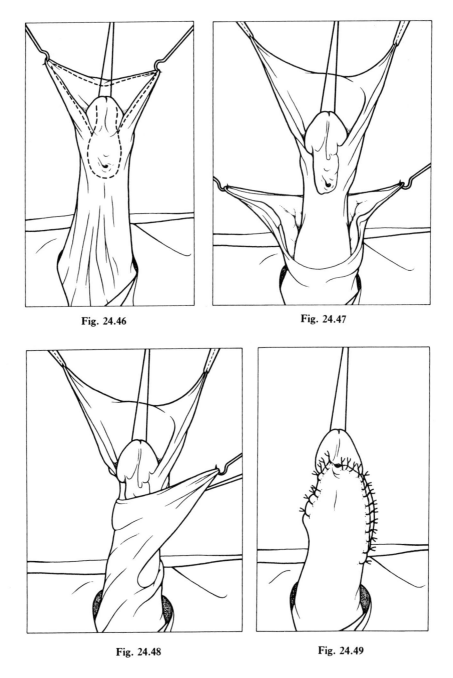

Fig. 24.46

Fig. 24.47

Fig. 24.48

Fig. 24.49

Figs. 24.46–24.49 Van de Meulin's operation for correction of hypospadias (Rintoul: *Farquharson's Textbook of Operative Surgery*, 7th Edn.)

through both skin flaps to emerge on the opposite side. Another bead is threaded on to the suture material followed by an aluminium stop, and both are pushed down the suture material until the correct tension is achieved. The aluminium stop is crushed and excess suture material cut off. The skin edges are then sutured together with very fine catgut or synthetic absorbable on a non-traumatic needle, and a longitudinal relaxing incision is made down the whole of the dorsum of the penis to prevent tension to the suture line and swelling.

If the operation area involves the scrotum, it is usual to make a small incision or incisions on each side of it, leading down to the central wound, so as to allow drainage and prevent accumulation of fluid in the scrotal tissues.

Van de Meulen's procedure

Another procedure for correction of hypospadias is the Van de Meulen's operation which makes use of excessive skin from the dorsum of the prepuce (Fig. 24.46). The skin along the length of penis shaft is undermined and rotated so that dorsal skin from the prepuce can cover the ventral surface of the glans (Figs. 24.47 and 24.48). An oblique incision on the dorsum of the penis facilitates this procedure. Two triangular areas of skin from the ventral surface on either side are excised thereby extending the skin strip from the ectopic meatus. The skin flap is then sewn to the outer margin of the triangles (Fig. 24.49). The deficiency left on the dorsum of the penis is filled by folding back the inner layer of the prepuce, and the skin margins remaining around the circumference are sutured.

REFERENCES AND FURTHER READING

ROBERTS, M. (1976) The skin bank. *Nursing Mirror*, Sept. 2.
McGREGOR, I. A. (1977) *Fundamental Techniques of Plastic Surgery*. Edinburgh: Churchill Livingstone.
MORGAN, B and WRIGHT, M. (1986) *Essentials of Plastic and Reconstructive Surgery*. London: Faber and Faber
BREACH, N. M. (1986) Breast reconstruction, In *Recent Advances in Surgery*. Edited by R.C.G. Russell.
   Edinburgh, Churchill Livingstone
DINNER, M. I. and COLEMAN, C. (1985) Breast reconstruction, *AORN J*, **42** No 4, 410–496.

25

Urological operations

Circumcision

Definition

Partial excision of the penile foreskin.

Position

Supine.

Instruments

Scalpel handle No. 3 with No. 10 blade (Bard Parker)
Fine dissecting forceps, toothed (Gillies)
Fine dissecting forceps, non-toothed (McIndoe)
Probe, malleable silver
Artery forceps, straight, 18 cm (7 in) (Spencer Wells) *or*
Bone cutters or sinus forceps
Scissors, straight, blunt points (Mayo 13 or 15 cm (5 or 6 in))
Fine scissors, curved on flat, dissection points (Kilner)
Fine artery forceps, straight, mosquito, 5
2 (3/0) Chromic catgut or synthetic absorbable for ligatures
2 (3/0) Chromic catgut or synthetic absorbable on a small curved cutting needle, pref-
    erably non-traumatic, for prepuce sutures
Dressing of gauze impregnated with petroleum jelly, Tinct. Benz. Co., or Whiteheads
    varnish.

Outline of procedure

Two artery forceps are clipped to each side of the prepuce opening, and a probe inserted
to separate the glans from the prepuce. More traction is applied to the foreskin and a pair
of artery forceps or bone cutters is placed obliquely across the prepuce, but distal to the
underlying glans. The excess foreskin is excised with a knife and the cut edge allowed to
retract. The inner layer of the prepuce has to be slit up the dorsum of the penis to the glans
and the redundant piece of skin excised. Any bleeding vessels are picked up and ligated
before the cut edge of the skin is sutured to the inner layer of the prepuce.

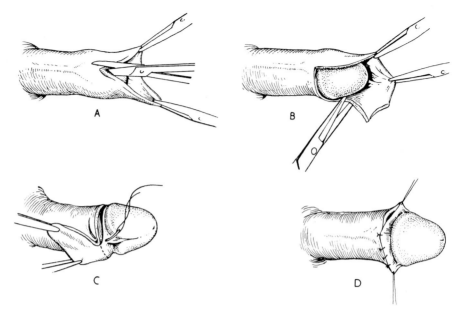

Fig. 25.1 Circumcision. (Swinney and Hammersley: *A Handbook of Operative Urological Surgery.*)

Excision of hydrocele or encysted hydrocele of the cord

Definition

Removal of a hydrocele sac (formed by the tunica vaginalis surrounding the testicle) or removal of an encysted hydrocele of the cord (formed by the prolongation of the tunica vaginalis from the testicle along the spermatic cord).

Position

Supine.

Instruments

General set (Fig. 14.1 to 14.28)
Hydrocele trocar and cannula
Diathermy leads, electrodes and lead anchoring forceps
Corrugated drain
2 and 2.5 (3/0 and 2/0) Chromic catgut or synthetic absorbable for ligatures
2.5 and 3 (2/0 and 0) Chromic catgut or synthetic absorbable on a small half-circle round-bodied needle for deep sutures
2 (3/0) Synthetic non-absorbable or silk on a small or medium curved cutting needle for skin sutures.

Outline of procedure

Hydrocele. The testicle is exposed through an incision made over the external inguinal ring, extending downwards and inwards towards the pubis. Unless the testicle is very large

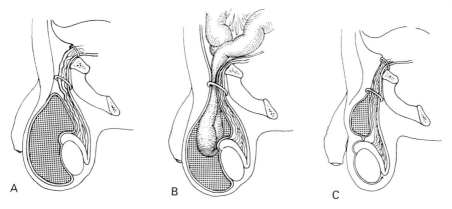

Fig. 25.2   Three types of hydrocele. (A) Simple. (B) With Hernia. (C) Hydrocele of the Spermatic Cord.
(Swinney and Hammersely: *A Handbook of Operative Urological Surgery.*)

the incision stops just short of the scrotal skin. The spermatic cord is dissected free and
traction applied until the hydrocele sac appears in the lower part of the wound. A trocar
and cannula may then be inserted to drain the fluid, and the collapsed tunica vaginalis is
cut away with scissors or a diathermy needle, and the innumerable vessels which have been
divided during dissection are ligated or diathermized. When haemostasis is complete, a
corrugated drain is inserted through a stab wound in the bottom of the scrotum, and the
testicle is returned to its normal position.

The wound is closed in layers. Some surgeons remove a hydrocele through an upper
scrotal incision, and instead of excising the sac it may be slit up the front, turned back and
sutured behind the testicle.

An encysted hydrocele of the cord. The incision, which generally is made over the swelling,
usually lies over the inguinal canal, which is incised. The distended sac is freed from other
structures of the cord, and ligated above and below before excision. The surgeon will search
towards the internal ring in case there is an extension to the sac, which may form a hernia
at a later date. Any sac so found is treated as a hernial sac (Chapter 15). The wound is closed
in layers.

Orchidectomy

Definition

Removal of the testicle.

Position

Supine.

Instruments

General set (Figs. 14.1 to 14.28)
Corrugated drain
2.5 and 3 (2/0 and 0) Chromic catgut, synthetic absorbable or non-absorbable for
ligatures

3 or 4 (0 or 1) Chromic catgut or synthetic absorbable on a small half-circle round-bodied needle for muscle (inguinal incision)

2.5 (2/0) Synthetic non-absorbable or silk on a small or medium curved cutting needle for skin sutures.

Outline of procedure

The testicle is exposed through an inguinal (or scrotal) incision. The spermatic cord is dissected up and the vessels and vas deferens ligated individually, and the testicle is removed. A corrugated drain is inserted into the scrotum through a stab incision and the wound is closed. A pressure dressing is applied.

Vasectomy

Definition

Excision of part of the vas deferens.

Position

Supine.

Instruments

Sponge-holding forceps (Rampley), 2
Towel clips, 4
Scalpel handle with No. 10 blade *or*
Diathermy scalpel with ball attachment
Fine dissecting forceps, toothed (Gillies), 2
Fine dissecting forceps, non-toothed (McIndoe), 2
Fine scissors, curved on flat (McIndoe or Lahey), 1
Scissors, curved on flat, 13 cm (5 in) (Mayo), 1
Fine artery forceps, curved on flat (Mosquito), 5
Artery forceps, curved on flat (Criles), 2
Tissue forceps, 15 cm (6 in) (Allis), 2
Special vasectomy mobilisation clamp (Tinkler), 1 (Optional)
Diathermy leads and electrodes
Local anaesthesia requisites (Fig. 11.60)
2.5 and 3 (2/0 and 0) Chromic catgut or synthetic absorbable for ligatures
2 or 2.5 (3/0 or 2/0) synthetic non-absorbable or silk on straight or curved non-traumatic cutting needle for skin sutures.

Outline of procedure

The skin and underlying tissues are infiltrated with local anaesthetic. The vas is palpated and either mobilised between the fingers or with a special vasectomy clamp. The skin overlying the vas is incised longitudinally for a few centimetres and the vas is picked up out of the incision with tissue forceps. It is usual to infiltrate the covering sheath of the vas with a few millilitres of local anaesthetic before proceeding further.

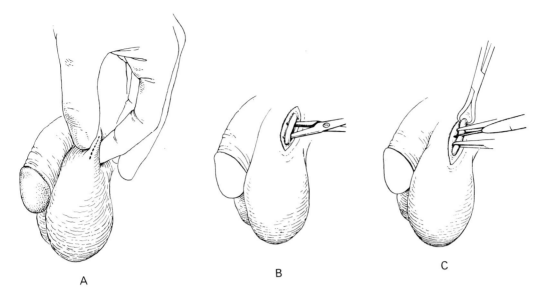

Fig. 25.3 Vasectomy. (Swinney and Hammersley: *A Handbook of Operative Urological Surgery.*)

The spermatic cord coverings are incised to display the vas deferens proper, a white avascular structure similar in appearance to a strand of spaghetti. The vas is gently lifted and the sheath teased away to free about 5 or 6 cm of vas. The vas is clamped at each end with an artery forceps and the segment between excised and sent for histological examination. The severed ends are ligated with catgut, synthetic absorbable or silk and a careful inspection made for haemostasis.

The skin is closed with mattress sutures of synthetic non-absorbable or silk (some surgeons use catgut or synthetic absorbable to avoid having to remove the sutures) and the wound dressed with plastic spray solution such as Nobecutane.

Excision of varicocele

Definition

The ligation and excision of varicose veins in the spermatic cord.

Position

Supine.

Instruments

General set (Figs. 14.1 to 14.28)
2.5 and 3 (2/0 and 0) Chromic catgut or synthetic absorbable for ligatures
3 or 4 (0 or 1) Chromic catgut or synthetic absorbable on a small half-circle cutting needle for muscle tendon suture
2.5 (2/0) Synthetic non-absorbable or silk on a small or medium curved on straight cutting needle for skin sutures.

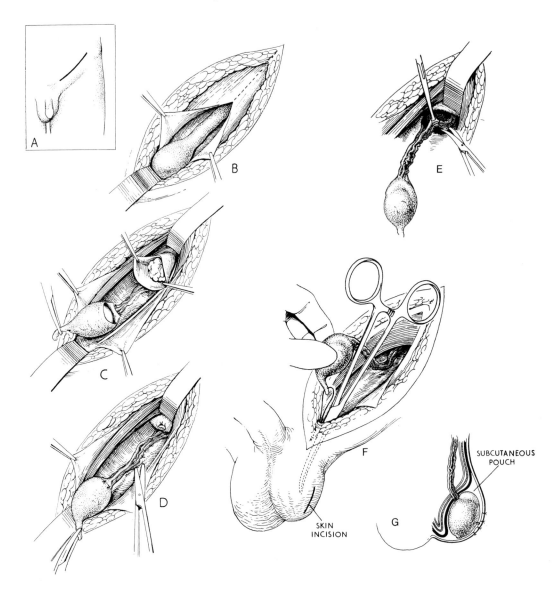

Fig. 25.4 Orchidopexy. (A) Groin incision. (B) Mobilisation of testicle. (C) Excision of hernial sac. (D and E) Dissection of cord structures. (F) Testicle being brought down into scrotum. (G) Operation completed. (Swinney and Hammersley: *A Handbook of Operative Urological Surgery.*)

Outline of procedure

An incision is made over the external inguinal ring and the spermatic cord dissected out. Some of the varicose veins are isolated from the rest of the spermatic vessels and are separated from the cord for about 8 cm (3 in) of their length. These vessels are ligated above and below the varicocele which is then excised. Some surgeons leave these ligatures long and tie them together, so pulling the testicle a little away from the scrotum. The wound is closed.

Orchidopexy

Definition

Placing an undescended testicle into the scrotum (in a child).

Position

Supine.

Instruments

General set (Figs. 14.1 to 14.28)
Fire artery forceps, curved on flat, mosquito, 10
Fine tissue forceps (McIndoe), 5
Fine-toothed dissecting forceps (Gillies), 2
Fine scissors, curved on flat, 10 cm (4 in) (Kilner or strabismus)
2 and 2.5 (3/0 and 2/0) Chromic catgut or synthetic absorbable for ligatures
2.5 (2/0) Chromic catgut or synthetic absorbable on a small half-circle or curved
   non-traumatic round-bodied needle for testicle fixation and hernial sac transfixion
2.5 or 3 (2/0 or 0) Chromic catgut or synthetic absorbable on a small half-circle
   round-bodied needle for muscle sutures
2 (3/0) Synthetic non-absorbable on a small or medium curved cutting needle for skin
   sutures.

Outline of procedure

Through a groin incision, the testicle is mobilised and the hernial sac is excised and the neck transfixed. By dissecting the structures of the cord from the extraperitoneal tissues, the testicle is eventually brought down into the scrotum. It is retained there either by transposing the organ into the opposite side of the scrotum, or by sewing the testicle to the fascia lata in a tunnel constructed between the scrotum and thigh. A second operation is needed three months later, to separate the scrotum and thigh.

Bougies, catheters and sounds (Figs. 25.5 to 25.20)

These are available in a number of materials — rubber, plastic, metal (silver or stainless steel). Some catheters have one lumen, whereas others have several for the purpose of irrigation. They are obtainable with inflatable cuffs or balloons at their distal tip which prevent accidental withdrawal. Catheters at present are measured in the Charrière gauge, size being three times the nominal external diameter expressed in millimetres, usually stated to be a certain French size, e.g. 18FG, which equals 6 mm external diameter. Details of care and sterilization of catheters are given in Chapter 7.

Cystourethroscopy

Definition

Examination of the interior of the urethra or urinary bladder with an endoscope.

Figs. 25.5 to 25.20   Examples of bougies, sound, and catheters. (Eschmann)

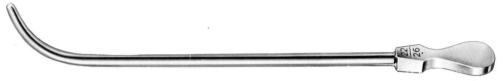

Fig. 25.5   Clutton bougie. Sizes available: 00/1, 0/2, ½/3, 1/4, 2/5, 3/6, 4/7, 5/8, 6/9, 7/10, 8/11, 9/12, 10/13, 11/14, 12/15, 13/16, 14/17, 15/18 Charrière gauge. Stainless steel.

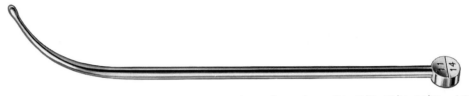

Fig. 25.6   Lister bougie. Sizes available: 6/10, 8/12, 10/14, 12/16, 14/18, 16/20, 18/22, 20/24, 26/30 and 2½ Charrière gauge. Stainless steel.

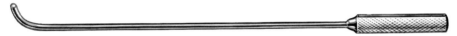

Fig. 25.7   Clutton bladder sound. Sizes available: 9, 12, 15 and 18 Charrière gauge. Stainless steel.

Fig. 25.8   Nélaton catheter. Sizes available: 8 to 30 Charrière gauge. Rubber or plastic.

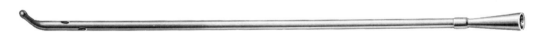

Fig. 25.9   Tiemann catheter. Sizes available: 10 to 26 Charrière gauge. Rubber or plastic.

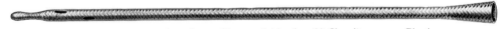

Fig. 25.10   Olivary tip catheter. Sizes available: 5 to 30 Charrière gauge. Plastic.

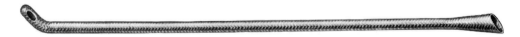

Fig. 25.11   Coudé catheter. Sizes available: 5 to 30 Charrière gauge. Plastic.

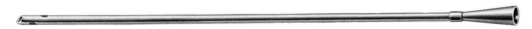

Fig. 25.12   'Whistle tip' catheter. Sizes available: 9 to 45 Charrière gauge. Rubber or plastic.

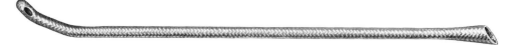

Fig. 25.13 Bicoudé catheter. Sizes available: 5 to 30 Charrière gauge. Plastic.

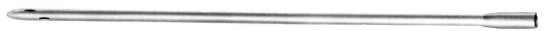

Fig. 25.14 Harris catheter. Sizes available: 9 to 45 Charrière gauge. Rubber or plastic.

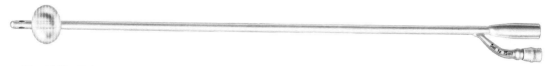

Fig. 25.15 Foley self-retaining catheter. Sizes available: 5 to 15 ml balloon, 14 to 26 Charrière gauge. Latex or plastic.

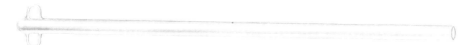

Fig. 25.16 Malecot self-retaining catheter. Sizes available: 9 to 48 Charrière gauge. Rubber.

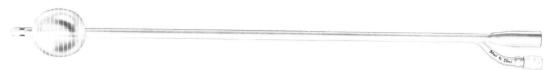

Fig. 25.17 Foley self-retaining catheter, haemostatic. Sizes available: 30 to 50 ml balloon, 14 to 26 Charrière gauge. Latex or plastic.

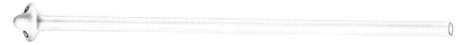

Fig. 25.18 De Pezzer self-retaining catheter. Sizes available: 12 to 39 Charrière gauge. Rubber.

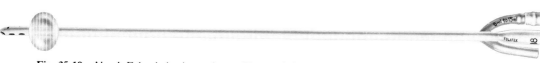

Fig. 25.19 Alcock-Foley irrigating catheter. Sizes available: 14 to 26 Charrière gauge. Latex or plastic.

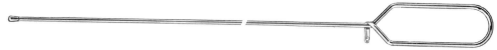

Fig. 25.20 Catheter introducer. (Chas. F. Thackray Ltd.)

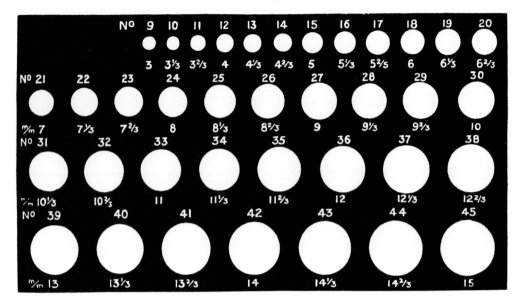

Fig. 25.21 Charrière catheter gauge.

Position

Lithotomy or supine.

Instruments

    Cysto-urethroscope sheath with obturator (of appropriate diameter) (e.g., Stortz, Canny Ryall, Brown Beurger, Braäsch direct vision Geiringer, etc)
    Sponge holding forceps (Rampley), 3
    Telescopes (Forward oblique, lateral, straight forward retrospective)
    Catheter deflecting mechanisms (may be integral with sheath)
    Irrigating stopcocks and tubing
    Biopsy or grasping forceps
    Fibre light or electric cable, and light or low voltage source
    Kidney dish
    Penile clamp (if local analgesia being used).
    Towel clips (Bachaus), 4.

A supply of sterile water, normal saline or 1.5 per cent w/v glycine solution (see Chapter 7, chemical disinfection) at a temperature of 34.5° to 35.5°C should be available to fill the bladder and provide irrigation. This fluid should be dispensed from closed inverted containers 1 or 2 litre, via a suitable connector, tubing and the cystoscope irrigation connection. If large quantities of fluid are required several containers can be interlinked with one another (Fig. 25.23). The flasks should be renewed for each operation.

Outline of procedure

    Cystoscope optics. Since the first practical cystoscope was devised by Nitze and Leiter in

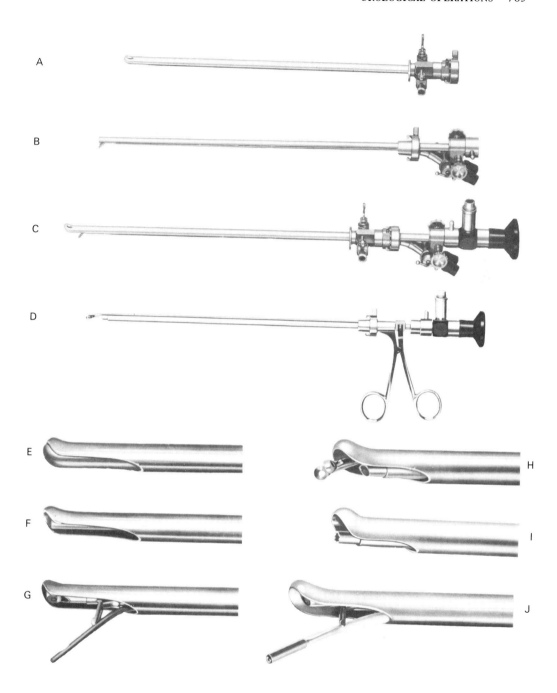

Fig. 25.22 Cystourethroscope and accessories. (Stortz-Rimmer Bros.)

(A) Sheath with obturator.
(B) Catheter deflecting mechanism.
(C) Sheath with catheter deflecting mechanism and telescope in position.
(D) Biopsy or grasping forceps.

(E) Distal end of sheath with obturator.
(F) Telescope in 'position'.
(G) Catheter deflecting mechanism.
(H) Biopsy or grasping forceps.
(I) Ultra sonic suction tube.
(J) Diathermy electrode.

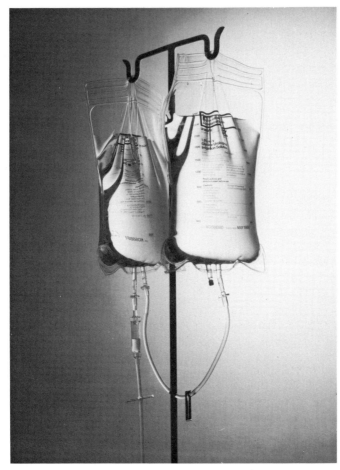

Fig. 25.23 Uromatic 'linked' 3 litre plastic irrigation containers. (1.5% w/v glycine solution) set up for cystoscopy. (Travenol Laboratories Ltd.)

1879, and until recently, the basic design of cystoscopes has consisted of a small distal lamp and a telescope comprised of a series of small lenses. (Fig. 25.24a) (Wallace, 1975).

Two inventions in the last decade by Professor H. H. Hopkins of Reading University have resulted in considerable improvements in the optics of cystoscopes and other endoscopic instruments. These are the application of fibre-optics the development of the rod lens system.

The first invention of Professor Hopkins was a redesign of the telescope to incorporate a rod lens system. A good deal of optic transmission is lost by the conventional lens system, because the light is dispersed on the sheath walls between the groups of lens. The Hopkins lens system, utilises a series of glass rods which reduces the light loss by the same principal of reflecting light from the surface of the rods. The ends of the rods are ground to reproduce the lens effect (Fig. 25.24C).

A number of significant advantages are claimed for the rod lens system, and these include wide viewing angle, bright and better light transmissions, natural colour reproduction, lens system occupies less space therefore smaller diameter instruments are possible, and more versatility in inter-changeability of telescopes between sheaths.

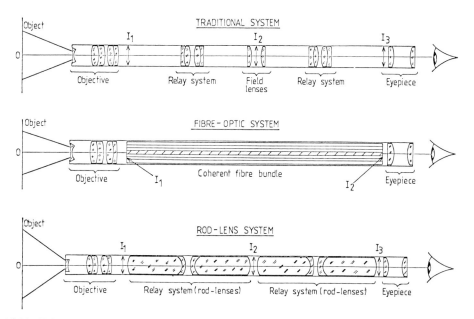

Fig. 25.24 Telescope optical systems. The symbols I_1, I_2, I_3 refer to the successive images that are formed. (Courtesy: Professor H. H. Hopkins, University of Reading.)

The second and most important invention by Professor Hopkins was that of fibre-optics, the principles of which have already been described in Chapter 13. The reader will recall that two types of flexible glass fibres are utilised to convey light or images. When the glass fibres are arranged in any order in a bundle or in an annular fashion around a rigid cysto-scope tube, they are said to be incoherent, and are used to transmit light to the distal end of the instrument (Fig. 25.25). When the glass fibres are arranged carefully so that the fibres

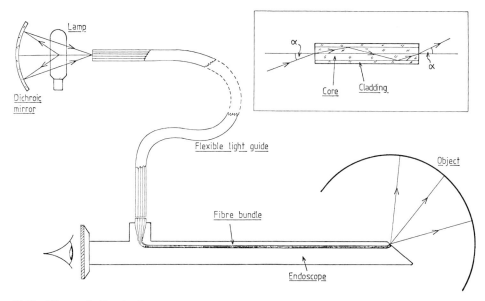

Fig. 25.25 Fibre optic illumination system. (Courtesy: Professor H. H. Hopkins, University of Reading.)

at one end correspond with the fibres at the other, they are termed coherent and can transmit a visual image (Fig. 25.24B and 13.2).

The rigid cystoscopes mentioned previously often incorporate incoherent optical glass fibres to transmit 'cool' illumination from a high intensity halogen light source. More recently, small calibre flexible fibrescopes (4.5–5 mm, 14–16 Ch) have been developed for urethrocystoscopy. These instruments are particularly useful when carrying out procedures under local anaesthesia (Fowler, 1984; Blandy and Fowler, 1986). An example of this instrument is illustrated in Figure 25.26.

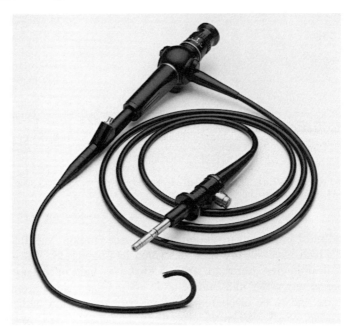

Fig. 25.26   Flexible cystoscope. (Olympus CYF, Key Med.)

For anterior urethroscopy an instrument similar to the cystoscope shown in Figure 25.22A and having a concave tip is used. Alternatively an instrument incorporating a straight closed-end sheath, or a straight open-end sheath may be used e.g., the Canny Ryall or Geiringer respectively. For posterior urethroscopy, the end of the sheath is convex in shape, although the straight open-end instrument can be used for this also.

The lubricated instrument is inserted and if urethral constrictions are present, these are dilated first in the usual manner with sounds. The telescope is inserted, the light cable attached and the irrigation commenced.

Three types of telescopes are available, the fore-oblique, the right wide-angled field, and the direct vision. The fore-oblique telescope is similar to the one used for simple cystoscopy, when the surgeon generally wishes to examine a field of view which lies in front of, and a little to one side of the distal tip of the instrument. This type of instrument can be used for urethroscopy, but it is preferable to use a wide-angle lens telescope, which gives a field of view at right angles to the aperture in the tip of the instrument. The direct vision telescope can be used if the instrument has an open-end sheath.

The Braasch cystoscope does not incorporate a telescope and the surgeon views the interior of the urethra through a glass window in the proximal part of the instrument.

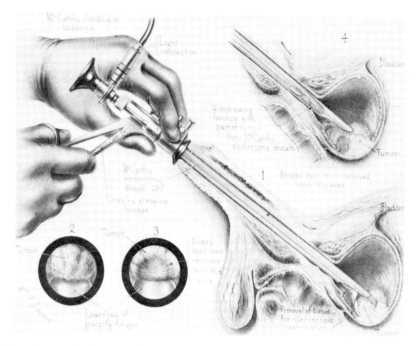

Fig. 25.27   Lowsley grasping forceps being used with a fibre optic for oblique telescope. (A.C.M.I.)

After the urethra has been examined, the instrument may be passed into the bladder, which is filled with solution and a general examination is carried out, unless this was performed at the beginning of the procedure.

A biopsy may be taken with biopsy forceps (Figs. 25.22D and 25.27). If bleeding is persistant after biopsy, the surgeon may complete the procedure by leaving an indwelling catheter.

During cystoscopy the dye excretion test may be carried out. In this instance intravenous 0.4 per cent indigo carmine is used.

Illumination of urological endoscopes is now generally accomplished by fibre optic systems and high intensity light sources. The reader is referred to Chapter 13 which describes the concept applied to gastroenterology and which is also applicable to urological instruments.

Ureteric catheterisation and retrograde pyelography

Definition

The insertion of a ureteric catheter into the ureter and the kidney pelvis to obtain a specimen of urine from the kidney, or for the retrograde injection of a radio-opaque fluid for X-ray examination of the kidney.

Position

Lithotomy.

Instruments

As for cystourethroscopy (p. 784) plus ureteric catheters and specimen tubes.

Outline of procedure

A lubricated catheterising cystoscope is inserted, the obturator removed and the telescope inserted to visualise the ureteric orifices. A ureteric catheter of appropriate size is passed into each orifice in turn by using the movable platform at the distal end of the instrument. The stilette is left in the catheters until it has been advanced a few centimetres into the ureter, and it is then removed before the catheter is advanced any further. The bladder is emptied, the light cable detached and the cystoscope carefully removed, leaving the catheters in position.

The instrument nurse must ensure that the ureteric catheter marked with a red band at its proximal end is used for the right kidney. Similarly, the left ureter is catheterised with a catheter marked blue or green at its proximal end. Two test tubes are marked Right and Left and strapped to the right and left thighs respectively to collect urine specimens from the kidneys. The catheters are each passed, either through the holes of a rubber teat which fits over the test tube, or through a cotton-wool plug in the neck of each tube. In the X-ray department, a radio-opaque medium such as iopamidol or omnipaque will be injected into each catheter before making a radiographic examination of the kidneys.

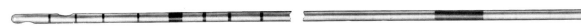

Fig. 25.28 Ureteric catheter cylindrical. Marked with blue or red bands to distinguish right and left. Sizes available: 3 to 12 Charrière gauge. Plastic.

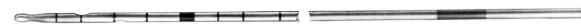

Fig. 25.29 Ureteric catheter olivery. Marked with blue or red bands to distinguish right and left. Sizes available: 3 to 12 Charrière gauge. Plastic.

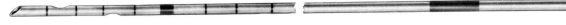

Fig. 25.30 Ureteric catheter flute end. Marked with blue or red bands to distinguish right and left. Sizes available: 3 to 12 Charrière gauge. Plastic.

Transurethral prostatectomy

Definition

Transurethral removal of the prostate gland.

Position

Lithotomy.

Instruments

Bladder sounds or bougies (Lister, Clutton, etc.), set
Supply of sterile water, etc., for irrigation (see cystoscopy)
Connecting tubing and nozzles for resectoscope

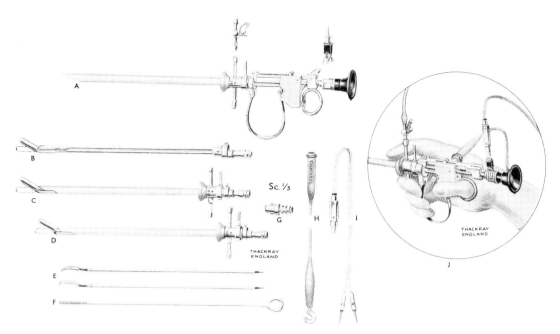

Fig. 25.31 Rapier resectoscope. (Chas. F. Thackray Ltd.)

(A) Resectoscope assembled in insulated sheath, 30 Charrière gauge. *Note.* Double-prong connector for light lead: small irrigating nozzle with tap.
(B) Obturator for above.
(C and D) Insulated sheaths, 28 and 26 Charrière gauge, with obturators.
(E) Cutting loops (active diathermy electrode slides inside sheath).

(F) Probe for cleaning.
(G) Large irrigation nozzle.
(H) Diathermy lead.
(I) Light lead.
(J) Resectoscope ready for use. *Note.* Irrigation tube attached to side nozzle; light lead coupled to double-prong connector.

Electro-resectoscope (Fig. 25.31A) or 'cold punch' instrument
Fibre light or electric cable and light or low voltage source. Electric cable and batteries
Diathermy leads, lead anchoring forceps and diathermy apparatus
Urethral catheter, self-retaining (Foley size 18, 20 or 22 Charrière gauge)
20 ml syringe and sterile water for inflating cuff of catheter.

Outline of procedure

The indifferent diathermy electrode is applied to the patient's thigh with the usual precautions. (Alternatively the resectoscope sheath incorporates bipolar diathermy electrodes.) Progressively larger sizes of sounds are passed into the urethra followed by the resectoscope. The obturator is removed and the telescope/resecting loops inserted. Irrigation and diathermy connections are made and the interior of the bladder examined together with the prostatic area.

The prostate is resected by advancing and withdrawing the diathermy loop with the current switched on. It may be necessary to change the diathermy loops several times during operation as they become charred.

A special electrode is used to coagulate bleeding vessels. A self-retaining catheter is inserted and the bladder irrigated until the water returns clear.

Alternatively, the 'cold punch' instrument is used for prostatic resection via the urethra. In this case the instrument is introduced in a similar manner to the electro-resectoscope, but the hypertrophied prostate gland is excised with a punch mechanism at the distal end of the instrument.

Fulguration of bladder tumours

Definition

Removal of bladder tumours or lesions by diathermy.

Position

Lithotomy.

Intruments

As for cysto-urethroscopy (p. 784)

Operating cystoscope, preferably an irrigating instrument, having channels through which flexible diathermy electrodes can be introduced and manipulated: *or* an operating cystoscope which incorporates its own electrode at the distal end.

Diathermy electrodes, set of flexible variety leads and anchoring forceps

(Self-retaining urethral catheter occasionally required (e.g., Foley 18, 20 or 22 Charrière gauge).)

Outline of procedure

The indifferent diathermy electrode is applied to the patient's thigh with the usual precautions. The lubricated cystoscope is inserted, the obturator removed, the irrigation tubing and diathermy connections are made and the telescope inserted to visualise the lesion.

The electrode is applied to the tumour and diathermy used until fulguration is complete. The bladder is emptied, the cystoscope removed and if necessary the catheter is inserted.

Lithotrity or litholapaxy

Definition

Crushing and removal of bladder stones via the urethra.

Position

Lithotomy, with the head of the table slightly lowered.

Instruments

As for cystoscopy
    Lithotrite and sheath
    Obturator
    Evacuator (Ellik or Bigelow)
    Fibre light or electric cable and light or low voltage source

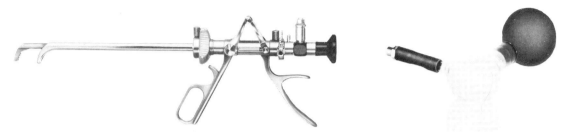

Fig. 25.32 Lithotrite and Ellik evacuator. (Stortz-Rimmer Bros.)

Outline or procedure

A cystoscopy is performed. When the stones have been visualised, the cystoscope is removed and progressively larger sizes of sounds are inserted followed by the lithotrite. The stone or stones are crushed, the lithotrite removed and an evacuation catheter inserted. The Ellik evacuator is used to irrigate the bladder and extract the fragments of stone by suction. It may be necessary to repeat this procedure several times before all the stone or stones have been completely crushed and removed.

Suprapubic cystostomy

Definition

Temporary or permanent suprapublic drainage of the bladder.

Position

Supine, with some Trendelenburg.

Instruments

General set (Figs. 14.1 to 14.28)
Suprapubic trocar
Catheter introducer
Catheter, self-retaining (De Pezzer, 30 to 34 Charrière gauge)
Spigot
Urethral catheter (Jaques or Nélation size 18 Charrière gauge). To distend bladder if
    required.
Catheter lubricant
Bladder syringe and warm irrigation solution
Corrugated drain and safety-pin
Suction tubing, nozzles and tube anchoring forceps
2.5 and 3 (2/0 and 0) Chromic catgut or synthetic absorbable for ligatures
3 or 4 (0 or 1) Chromic catgut or synthetic absorbable on a medium half-circle cutting
    needle for bladder and muscle sutures
2.5 (2/0) Synthetic non-absorbable on a medium or large curved or straight cutting needle
    for skin sutures.

Outline of procedure

If the bladder is not distended, it is first filled with irrigation solution. A 7–10 cm (3–4 in) midline incision is made just above the pubis. The incision is deepened and the rectus sheath opened in the midline, followed by a transverse opening in the transversalis fascia. The fascia and peritoneum are pushed upwards, and two stay sutures are inserted into the bladder wall and left long. Any veins in the vicinity of the proposed opening into the bladder are under-run and tied off. A stab incision is made, the bladder fluid suctioned away and a De Pezzer catheter inserted. The stay sutures are used to secure the catheter in position and these are reinforced if necessary with further interrupted sutures of chromic catgut or synthetic absorbable.

Some surgeons make a smaller incision in the abdomen and use a large trocar and cannula to insert the catheter. The wound is closed in layers with a corrugated drain in the lower part. The catheter is secured to the skin with a suture which is tied round the catheter near to the point where it emerges from the wound.

Transvesical prostatectomy

Definition

Removal of the prostate gland via a suprapubic incision into the bladder.

Position

Trendelenburg.

Instruments

General set (Figs. 14.1 to 14.28)
Artery forceps, 20 cm (8 in) (Spencer Wells), 10
Long scissors, curved on flat (Nelson's)
Long dissecting forceps, toothed, 25 cm (10 in)
Long dissecting forceps, non-toothed
Deep retractors, narrow blade (Deaver or Paton), 2
Illuminated bladder retractor, self-retaining (Morson)
Vulsellum forceps (Teale), 2
Boomerang needles (Harris or Millin) for reconstruction of prostactic bed, 3 sizes
Ligature-carrying forceps (Harris or Millin), 2
Bladder syringe and irrigation solution at 43.3° to 46°C
Urethral catheter (Harris or Jaques size 18 Charrière gauge)
Large drainage tube or self-retaining catheter (De Pezzer size 36 Charrière gauge)
Catheter lubricant
Corrugated drain
Suction tubing, nozzles and tube anchoring forceps
Diathermy leads, electrodes and lead anchoring forceps
2.5 and 3 (2/0 and 0) Chromic catgut or synthetic absorbable for ligatures, and on ligature-carrying forceps for prostatic bed sutures
3 (0) Chromic catgut or synthetic absorbable on a small half-circle round-bodied needle for bladder sutures
3 or 4 (0 or 1) Chromic catgut synthetic absorbable a medium half-circle cutting needle for muscle

2.5 (2/0) Synthetic non-absorbable or silk on a large curved or straight cutting needle for
skin sutures
2.5 (2/0) Synthetic monofilament non-absorbable on a large Colts needle for catheter
suture.

Outline of procedure

There are several prostatectomy operations via this route and the following is a description
of the Harris procedure:

If the bladder is not distended, it is first filled with sterile irrigation solution. A 13 cm
(5 in) or longer midline incision is made just above the pubis. The incision is deepened and
the rectus sheath opened in the midline, followed by a transverse opening in the transversalis
fascia. The fascia and peritoneum are pushed upwards and two stay sutures are inserted into
the bladder wall and left long. Any veins in the vicinity of the proposed opening into the
bladder are under-run and tied off. A stab incision is made, the bladder fluid suctioned
away, the incision extended and a self-retaining bladder retractor inserted.

The mucous membrane over the prostate is incised under direct vision with a pair of scissors. The retractor is removed and the gland shelled out with two fingers. The retractor is
reinserted and any bleeding points picked up with forceps and diathermised. Using the
boomerang needle, the torn mucous membrane is sutured well down into the prostatic cavity
so that its posterior wall is covered.* A urethral catheter is inserted into the bladder and

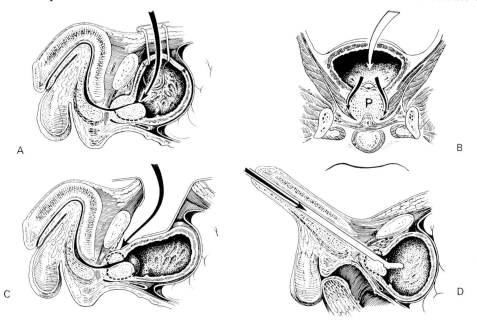

Fig. 25.33 Surgical approaches to the prostate. (A and B) Suprapubic transvesical approach. (C) Retropubic
approach. (D) Transurethral approach. (Swinney and Hammersley: *A Handbook of Operative Urological Surgery.*)

---

* The Harris or Millin boomerang needle (Fig. 25.33) consists of a spring-loaded holder to which the needle is
attached. The needle has an open eye at its distal point and can be rotated through about 60 degrees by depressing
the handle. In operation the surgeon approximates the needle to the tissues being sutured, and advances it through
them by depressing the handle. The assistant positions a loop of suture material (usually catgut) in the open eye
of the needle by means of ligature-carrying forceps and the surgeon releases the tension on the spring-loaded handle.
The needle rotates back through track created by it, withdraws the catgut and thereby completes the suture. The
boomerang needle may be used for single or continuous sutures.

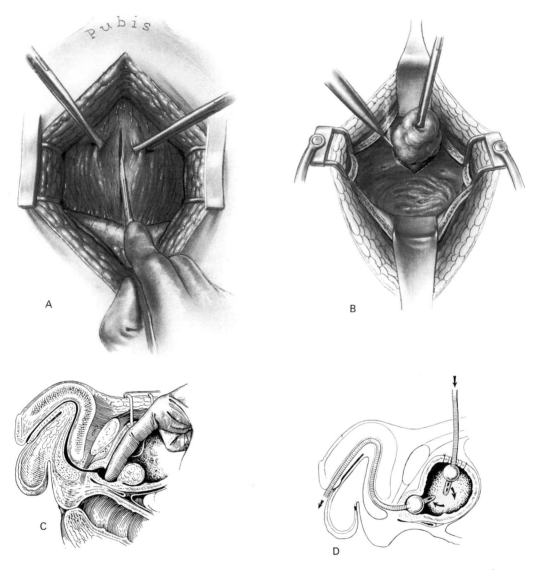

Fig. 25.34 Transvesical prostatectomy. (A) Incision in bladder. (B and C) The prostatic adenoma being freed from the false capsule with diathermy and blunt dissection. (D) Irrigation of the bladder. (Swinney and Hammersley: *A Handbook of Operative Urological Surgery*.

a figure-of-eight suture introduced in front of the catheter so that when it is tied, the side walls of the prostatic cavity are brought together. This manoeuvre largely obliterates the cavity and acts as a haemostatic suture also.

A long nylon suture is inserted through the abdominal wall at one side of the incision and passes into the bladder, through the tip of the catheter, and out again through the abdominal wall at the opposite side of the incision. When the incision has been closed, these ends are tied together over a gauze pad or are threaded through a short length of rubber tubing in the manner described for tension sutures (Chapter 15). This suture serves to suspend the catheter in the bladder until it is withdrawn about the tenth day post-operatively.

When all bleeding has stopped, the bladder drainage tube is inserted and the wound closed in layers around this tube. A corrugated drain extending down to the bladder is left at the lower end of the wound. The suprapubic drain and corrugated drain are usually removed on the fourth or fifth day post-operatively.

Millin's retropubic prostatectomy

Definition

Removal of the prostate gland through a suprapubic incision but without opening the bladder.

Position

Trendelenburg.

Instruments

General set (Figs. 14.1 to 14.28)
Millin's prostatectomy set (Fig. 25.35)

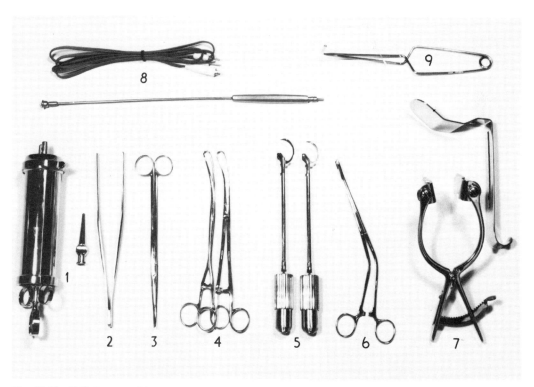

Fig. 25.35 Millin's retropubic prostatectomy.
1. Bladder syringe.
2. Long dissecting forceps, toothed (Millin).
3. Long scissors, curved, 23 cm (9 in) (Nelson).
4. Vulsellum forceps, 2.
5. Boomerang needles (Millin or Harris), 2.
6. Ligature-carrying forceps (Young).
7. Retractor self-retaining (Millin).
8. Malleable light with electric lead.
9. Bladder-neck spreader (Millin).

Artery forceps, 20 cm (8 in) (Spencer Wells), 10
Long artery forceps, curved on flat (Gordon Craig), 5
Deep retractors, narrow blade (Paton or Deaver 25 mm (1 in))
Irrigation solution at 43.3° to 46°C
Urethral catheter (whistle tip or similar, Foley, size 20 Charrière gauge)
Catheter lubricant and Spigot
Suction tubing, nozzles and tube anchoring forceps
Diathermy leads, electrodes and lead anchoring forceps.

Outline of procedure

A transverse suprapubic incision is made and the prostate exposed behind the pubis. Blood-vessels running across the anterior aspect of the gland are ligated before opening the capsule in the front. The gland is enucleated, haemostasis secured with diathermy and sutures and a urethral catheter inserted into the bladder. The prostatic capsule is sutured and the wound closed in the usual manner with a corrugated drain down to the prostate capsule in the lower end of the wound.

With any form of prostatectomy the vas deferens may be ligated on both sides to prevent any possibility of infection reaching the testicles by this route.

Total cystectomy and ureterosigmoidostomy

Definition

Removal of the urinary bladder, ureteric transplantation into the sigmoid colon.

Position

Trendelenburg.

Instruments

General set (Figs. 14.1 to 14.28)
Laparotomy set (Figs. 15.1 to 15.7)
Fine tissue forceps (McIndoe), 5
Fine dissecting forceps, non-toothed (McIndoe), 2
Fine dissecting forceps, toothed (Gillies), 2
Scalpel handle No. 9 with No. 15 blade (Bard Parker)
Fine artery forceps, straight, mosquito, 10
Fine artery forceps, curved on flat, mosquito, 10
Intestinal occlusion clamps, curved (Doyen), 2
Suction tubing, nozzles and tube anchoring forceps
Diathermy leads, electrodes and lead anchoring forceps
Laparotomy ligatures and sutures
2 (3/0) Chromic catgut or synthetic absorbable on a small curved non-traumatic intestinal
    needle size 20 mm for ureteric anastomosis.

Outline of procedure

Sometimes the ureters are transplanted as a first procedure and the cystectomy follows at a later date.

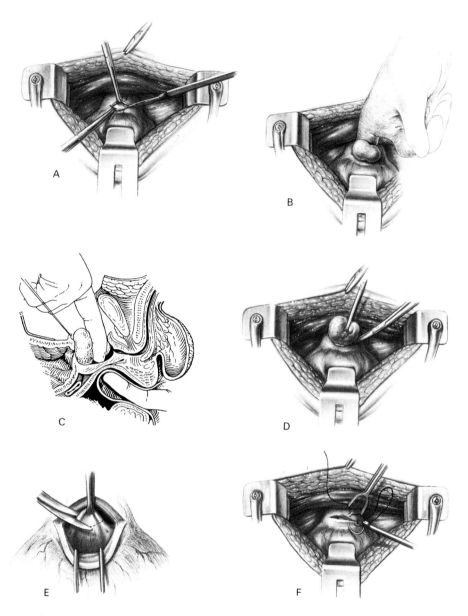

Fig. 25.36 Millin's retropubic prostatectomy. (A) Incision of prostatic capsule. (B and C) Prostatic adenoma being freed within false capsule. (D) Adenomatous mass is delivered through the capsular incision and dissected from overlying trigone. (E) Trigone seized with Vulsellum forceps; bladder neck and trigone excised. (F) Capsular incision sutured with boomerang needle. (Swinney and Hammersley: *A Handbook of Operative Urological Surgery*.)

Ureterosigmoidostomy. Through a lower midline incision, the sigmoid colon is mobilised. The posterior peritoneum is incised and the ureters are mobilised for a considerable length. A ligature is placed at the junction of each ureter with the bladder and they are divided proximal to this ligature.

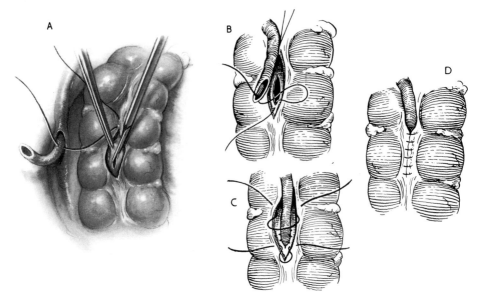

Fig. 25.37   Ureterosigmoidostomy — Leadbetter's technique. (Swinney and Hammersley: *A Handbook of Operative Urological Surgery.*)

Curved occlusion clamps are applied longitudinally to the colon at the point selected for the anastomosis. A small longitudinal incision is made in the bowel wall through the serosa, muscle and mucosa. The ureters are united to the colon mucosa by direct mucosa to mucosa sutures, using fine non-traumatic chromic catgut or synthetic absorbable sutures (Leadbetter's operation). The ureters may be immobilised further by suturing the serosa over them for a short distance from the anastomosis, and the sigmoid colon is immobilised to the wing of the pelvis. The wound is closed and a rectal tube inserted.

Cystectomy. If this is done as a second stage, the approach is as before. The peritoneum is stripped off the bladder, which is then dissected free from the surrounding tissue. The urethra is ligated and severed and the blood-vessels divided between forceps to complete mobilisation so that the bladder can be removed. The blood-vessels are diathermised or ligated, and when haemostasis is complete, the peritoneum is sutured to reconstruct the pelvic floor. The wound is closed in layers.

It may be mentioned here that the ureters can be transplanted into a loop of ileum (uretero-ileostomy) instead of the sigmoid colon. In this case 15 cm (6 in) or so of ileum is transected with the mesentery left intact, and the remaining proximal and distal bowel are anastomosed to re-establish intestinal continuity. The short section of ileum is closed at one end and the ureters transplanted in the manner previously described for ureterosigmoidostomy. The open end of the ileum is brought through the abdominal wall as for ileostomy (Chapter 15) and the urine drains into this, so forming an artificial bladder. It is usual to leave a small Paul's tube in the ileostomy, or apply an ileostomy bag immediately after operation.

Partial cystectomy

Definition

Removal of part of the urinary bladder, and if necessary transplantation of one or both ureters to another part of the bladder.

Position

Trendelenburg.

Instruments

As for cystectomy

Urethral catheter (Jaques or Nélation or Foley, size 18 Charrière gauge)

Bladder syringe and irrigation solution

3 or 4 (0 or 1) Chromic catgut or synthetic absorbable on a small half-circle round-bodied needle for bladder sutures.

Outline of procedure

The bladder is distended with irrigation solution and an approach made through a lower midline incision.

Two stay sutures are inserted into the bladder wall and left long. Any vessels which are overlying the area for incision are under-run with chromic catgut or a synthetic absorbable and tied. The bladder is opened and the fluid evacuated with the suction tube. The segment of bladder for removal is excised either by diathermy or by the clamp and cut method,

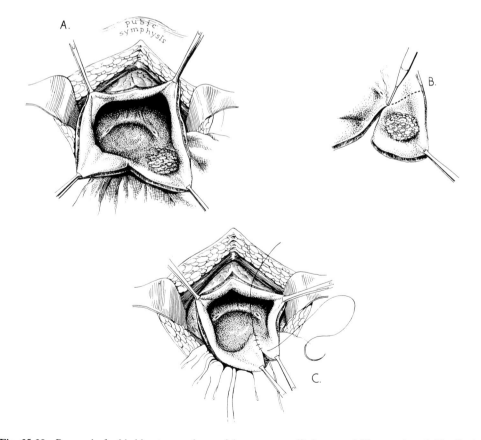

Fig. 25.38 Removal of a bladder tumour by partial cystectomy. (Swinney and Hammersley: *A Handbook of Operative Urological Surgery*.)

whereby artery forceps are applied across the tissue before excision. If the ureter or ureters are involved in this area, they are divided and immobilised for sufficient of their length to enable transplantation into another part of the bladder by the direct mucosa to mucosa anastomosis. The bladder is closed with two layers of chromic catgut or a synthetic absorbable sutures and a urethral catheter inserted. The wound is closed as before with drainage.

Adrenalectomy

Definition

Removal of whole or part of one or both adrenal glands.

Position

Supine (the operation may also be performed through a posterolateral incision, and in this case the position is that for kidney operations).

Instruments

Abdominal approach
  General set (Figs. 14.1 to 14.28)
  Laparotomy set (Figs. 15.1 to 15.7)
  Long scissors, curved on flat, 23 cm (9 in) (Nelson)
  Long dissecting forceps, non-toothed, 25 cm (10 in)
  Long dissecting forceps, toothed, 25 cm (10 in)
  Silver ligature clips and insertion forceps (McKenzie)
  Suction tubing, nozzles and tube anchoring forceps
  Diathermy leads, electrodes and lead anchoring forceps
  Laparotomy ligatures and sutures.

Posterolateral approach
  As nephrectomy, minus stone forceps, ureteric bougies and catheters.

Outline or procedure

Abdominal. A midline or paramedian approach is made and the upper pole of the kidney visualised by incising the posterior peritoneum and mobilising and retracting the overlying organs. The gland is palpated and grasped with tissue or sponge-holding forceps. It is carefully dissected free from the vena cava if it is on the right side. The adrenal vessels are clamped with long artery forceps or metal ligature clips and divided with the long scissors. The gland is removed and haemostasis secured either by ligatures, metal clips, chromic catgut or synthetic absorbable sutures or diathermy. The posterior peritoneum is reconstructed with chromic catgut or synthetic absorbable sutures and the wound closed in the usual manner.

Posterolateral. A posterolateral incision is made and the kidney exposed through the bed of the twelfth rib. Removal of the gland follows that described above except that the peritoneum is not opened. The wound is closed as for nephrectomy.

KIDNEY AND URETERIC OPERATIONS

Nephrectomy

Definition

Removal of the kidney.

Position

Lateral, with kidney bridge elevated (Fig. 5.14).

Instruments

General set (Figs. 14.1 to 14.28)
Nephrectomy set (Fig. 25.39)
Artery forceps, 20 cm (8 in) (Spencer Wells), 10
Long artery forceps, curved on flat (Moynihan gall-bladder), 5

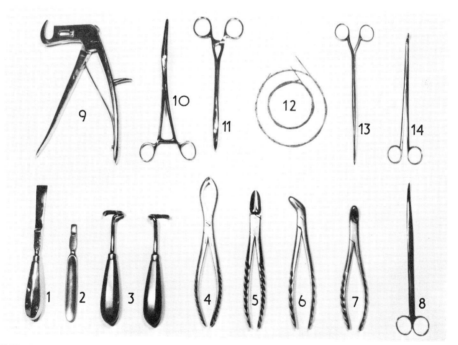

Fig. 25.39 Nephrectomy and other kidney operations.
1. Rugine (Mitchell).
2. Rugine (Faraboeuf).
3. Rib raspatories (Doyen), left and right side.
4. Bone-holding forceps (Fergusson).
5. Bone-cutting forceps (Liston).
6. Bone-nibbling forceps, angled on side.
7. Bone-nibbling forceps, angled on flat.
8. Long-scissors, curved on flat, 23 cm (9 in) (Nelson).
9. Rib shears (Exner).
10. Kidney pedicle clamp.
11. Long artery forceps, curved on flat (Moynihan gall-bladder), 8.
12. Ureteric catheters.
13. Renal calculi forceps (Desjardin).
14. Renal calculi forceps (Thompson Walker).

Long artery forceps, curved on flat (Gordon Craig), 5

Long dissecting forceps, non-toothed, 25 cm (10 in)

Long dissecting forceps, toothed, 25 cm (10 in)

Deep retractors, narrow blade (Deaver), set of 4

Deep retractors, broad blade (Winsbury-White and Worrall), 2

Long, medium-diameter drainage tube and safety-pin

2.5, 3, 4 and 5 (2/0, 1 and 2 Chromic catgut or a synthetic absorbable or non-absorbable for ligatures

4 or 5 (1 or 2) Chromic catgut or synthetic absorbable on a large half-circle cutting needle for muscle sutures

2.5 (2/0) Synthetic non-absorbable or silk on a large curved needle for skin sutures.

Outline of procedure

An oblique incision is made commencing just below the mid-point of the last rib and continuing downwards and forwards towards the anterior superior iliac spine. The external oblique, transversus and internal oblique muscles are divided in line with the incision and the twelfth rib may or may not be excised.

The kidney is separated from its surrounding fat by blunt dissection and is delivered into the wound. The ureter and renal vessels are either clamped separately and divided distal to each forcep; or double ligatures are passed round each vessel and the ureter, which are divided between these ligatures. The kidney is removed and if artery forceps have been applied, the vessels and ureter are ligated. A drainage tube is inserted, the kidney bridge lowered and the wound closed in layers.

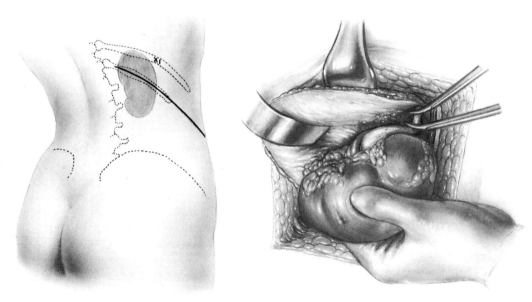

Fig. 25.40   **Fig. 25.41**

Fig. 25.40 Incision along the Line of the Twelfth Rib. (Swinney and Hammersley: *A Handbook of Operative Urological Surgery.*)

Fig. 25.41 Nephrectomy — clamping the ureter. (Swinney and Hammersley: *A Handbook of Operative Urological Surgery.*)

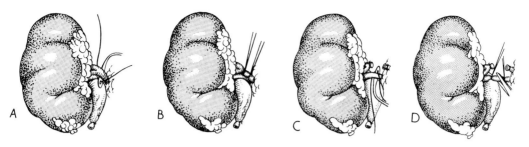

Fig. 25.42 Nephrectomy — dividing the renal pedicle. (Swinney and Hammersley: *A Handbook of Operative Urological Surgery.*)

Nephrolithotomy, pyelolithotomy or partial nephrectomy

Definition

Removal of a stone from the kidney, or pelvis of the ureter; excision of part of the kidney.

Position

Lateral, with kidney bridge elevated (Fig. 5.14).

Instruments

As for nephrectomy
Arterial clamps, bulldog, 2
Self-retaining retractor (e.g., Ring)
Kidney cooling coils and temperature probe
Netalast sling
20 ml syringe, fine catheter and 1 litre plastic container with sterile irrigation solution
  (cooled in refrigerator).

Outline of procedure

Hypothermia. This technique is being used with increasing frequency for operations on the kidney; it enables the surgeon to occlude the blood supply to the kidney for an extended period whilst complicated intra pelvic procedures are undertaken. (Ward and Wickham, 1976). Normally, at body temperature of 37°C, ischaemia time of more than 30 minutes can cause kidney injury, whereas if the kidney *in situ* is cooled to 15°–20°C the ischaemia time can be extended for up to two hours. This allows sufficient time in a 'non-bloody' operative field, for the removal of tumours or multiple calculi — particularly those of the staghorn type, which requires great care in searching through the kidney for all fragments. There will also be a need to take X-rays of the kidney, during the operation, to locate the stones and check that all have been found.

Renal hypothermia is achieved by using cooling coils applied directly to the surface of the kidney. Utilising good exposure (Fig. 25.43A) the kidney is mobilized so that it is attached only by its pedicle of renal artery, vein and ureter. It is suspended by a Netalast sling (Fig. 25.43B) and the renal artery clamped with bulldog forceps. The sterile saucer-shaped coils are applied as illustrated in (Fig. 25.44B).

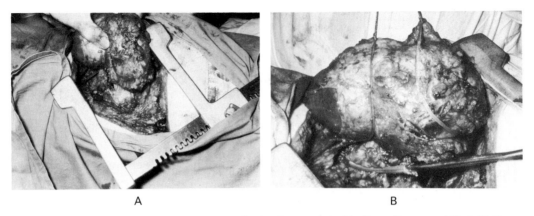

Fig. 25.43 (A) Kidney exposed. (B) Kidney mobilised and suspended with slings. (Courtesy of Mr J. H. B. Yule, M. Ch., F.R.C.S., Consultant Surgeon and Mr J. R. Jenkins, Senior Medical Photographer, Victoria Hospital, Blackpool.)

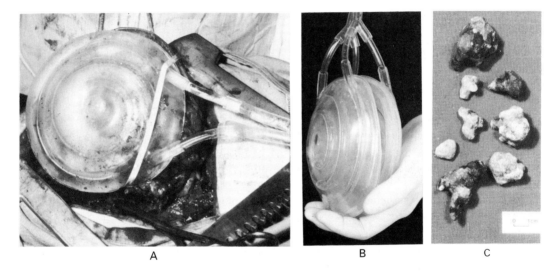

Fig. 25.44 (A) Cooling coils positioned around kidney. (B) Kidney cooling coils. (C) Calculi removed from kidney. (Courtesy of Mr J. H. B. Yule, M.Ch., F.R.C.S., Consultant Surgeon and Mr J. R. Jenkins, Senior Medical Photographer, Victoria Hospital, Blackpool.)

Cooling is achieved by pumping cold water through the coils and this is done by connecting the coils to the renal hypothermia unit (Fig. 25.45). The temperature of the kidney is monitored by using a needle probe which is connected to a telethermometer fitted in the hypothermia unit.

Operative procedure. The kidney is exposed in the usual manner and freed from surrounding fat. For *nephrolithotomy*, the calculus is palpated by holding the kidney between the finger and thumb. The calculus is steadied carefully through the kidney substance and an incision made over it starting on the convex border of the organ. When the knife reaches the calculus it is removed and an examination made for others. Small fragments may be removed by irrigation. The incision is closed with two or three stout chromic catgut or

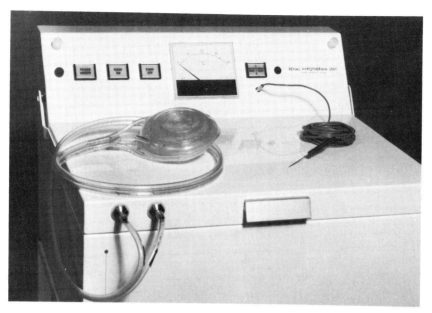

Fig. 25.45 Hypothermia apparatus for kidney cooling coils. (Courtesy of Mr J. H. B. Yule, M.Ch., F.R.C.S., Consultant Surgeon and Mr J. R. Jenkins, Senior Medical Photographer, Victoria Hospital, Blackpool.)

synthetic non-absorbable sutures placed through the kidney substance, followed by several fine sutures to approximate the capsule. A drainage tube is inserted down to the kidney, the bridge is lowered and the wound closed in layers.

For *pyelolithotomy* exposure and mobilisation are the same as above, but care is taken to free the pelvis of the ureter by rotating the kidney forwards, as all the vessels pass in front of the ureter in their normal course. The calculus is palpated, steadied between the forefinger and thumb, and an incision made into the pelvis. The stone is extracted and the kidney probed for other stones, finally irrigating with sterile irrigation solution (e.g., saline). The incision is closed with fine non-traumatic sutures of chromic catgut or synthetic non-absorbable which may be reinforced with a piece of fat. A drainage tube is inserted down to the kidney, the operation table levelled and the wound closed in layers.

The operation of nephrolithotomy may be replaced by by partial nephrectomy in suitable cases. In this procedure, the approach, dissection and closure follow that for nephrolithotomy. Hypothermia of the kidney may be carried out. The stone is located and the overlying capsule incised and carefully peeled off the area of excision. As bleeding is usually profuse, a vascular occlusion clamp is applied across the renal pedicle for a limited time. A segment of kidney is removed together with the stone contained and the kidney pelvis may be irrigated. The stump of the calyx is closed with fine catgut and the substance of the kidney with several mattress sutures of strong chromic catgut which are so placed that when they are tied, the cut edges of the kidney tend to invaginate slightly. When haemostasis is complete, the capsule is sutured over the kidney with fine chromic catgut on a non-traumatic needle (Figs. 25.46F to 25.47A).

(Note: *The conventional procedures for removal of renal stone have been described. Approximately 10 per cent of patients requiring removal of stones are treated in this way. The remaining 90 per cent are generally treated by lithotrity or percutaneous endoscopy.*)

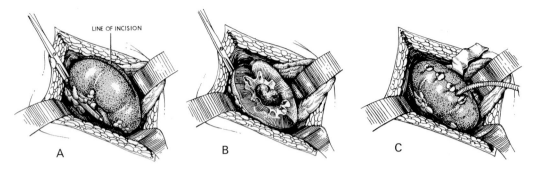

Fig. 25.46 (A to C) *Nephrolithotomy* (A) Vertical incision. (B) Exposure of calculus. After removal of main calculus fragments are washed out by irrigation. (C) Suture and drainage.

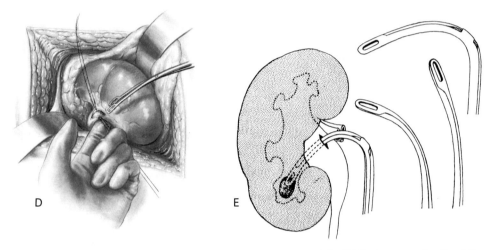

Fig. 25.46 (D and E) *Pyelolithotomy* (D) Incision in posterior wall of pelvis. (E) Pyelotomy, using Randal's forceps.

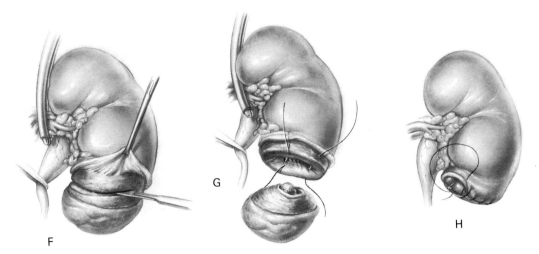

Fig. 25.46 (F to H) *Partial nephrectomy* (F) Incising renal cortex. (G) Suturing renal parenchyma. (H) Closing the renal capsule. (Fig. 25.46A to H, Swinney and Hammersley: *A Handbook of Operative Urological Surgery.*)

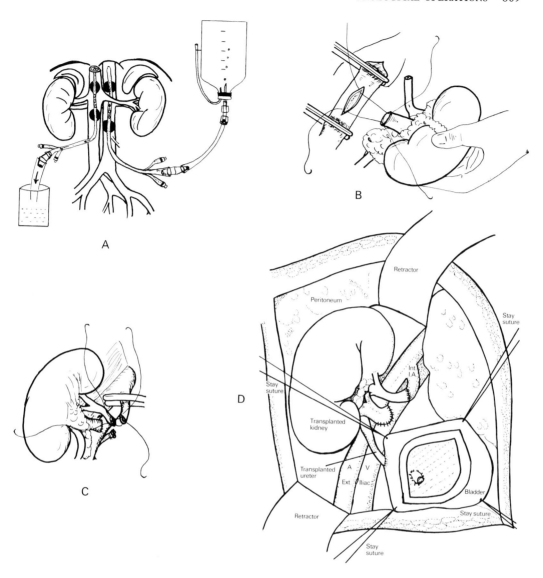

Fig. 25.47 (A) *In situ* perfusion. (B) Anastomosis of renal vein to external iliac vein. (C) Anastomosis of renal artery to internal iliac artery. (D) Uretero-vesical anastomosis following revascularisation of kidney. (Courtesy of Mr O. N. Fernando and Miss. A. Adams, and *Nursing Times*.)

Ureterolithotomy

Definition

Removal of a stone from the ureter.

Position

Supine, or lateral as for nephrectomy.

Instruments

As for nephrectomy
20 ml syringe, fine catheter and irrigation solution
Fine rubber or plastic tubing, or nylon tape
2 (3/0) Chromic catgut or synthetic absorbable (or plain catgut at the surgeon's discretion)
on a small curved rounded-bodied non-traumatic needle.

Outline of procedure

The ureter is approached either through an extension of the kidney incision, or through a paramedian incision. In the former case, the kidney incision is continued forwards to the centre of Poupart's ligament, deepened through the muscles to the peritoneum which is not opened but reflected inwards from the posterior abdominal wall.

The ureter lies on the psoas muscle and may be adherent to the peritoneum from which it is dissected free.

In the latter case, a lower midline incision is made and the peritoneum not opened but peeled inwards from the anterior and lateral abdominal wall. The ureter is then mobilised as before and the stone palpated.

A piece of tubing or nylon tape is passed around the ureter just above and below the stone, which is manoeuvred a little beyond the point of impaction. An incision is made into the ureter, the stone removed and the incision closed with fine non-traumatic catgut or synthetic absorbable sutures which pass through the muscular coats only. A drain is inserted down to the ureteric incision and the wound closed in layers. Some surgeons irrigate the ureter and probe with fine ureteric bougies to search for other stones.

Renal transplantation

Definition

Transplantation of a kidney from a living related donor, or a suitable cadaver.

Position

Supine.

Instruments

General set (Figs. 14.1 to 14.28)
Laparotomy set (Figs. 15.1 to 15.7)
Long scissors, curved on flat, 23 cm (9 in) (Nelson)
Long dissecting forceps, fine, non-toothed, 25 cm (10 in), 2
Long dissecting forceps, fine, toothed, 25 cm (10 in), 2
Long dissecting forceps, fine toothed, 20 cm (8 in) (Waugh), 2
Long dissecting forceps, fine, non-toothed, 20 cm (8 in) (Waugh), 2
Vascular clamps (Potts, De Bakey or Satinsky), 2
Large bulldog clamps (Potts), 4
Small bulldog clamps (Potts), 4
Long needle holders (Potts, Smith etc), 2
Heparinised saline, and syringes with cannulae

Suction tubing, nozzles and tube anchoring forceps
Diathermy leads, electrodes and lead anchoring forceps
Tantalum marker clips and insertion forceps
Laparotomy ligatures and sutures
1 and 0.75 (5/0 and 6/0) Synthetic non-absorbable or silk on small fine curved arterial
needles for anastomosis.

Outline of procedure

Live donor transplant. A classical nephrectomy will usually be carried out through a lumbar
or trans-abdominal incision. Instruments and procedure are similar to that described on page
803. Great care is taken when mobilising the renal pedicle, to avoid damage to the blood
vessels and ureter. After removal of the kidney, excess perureteric tissue is dissected away
and the kidney perfused with cold irrigating solution (Collins *et al.*, 1969; Sacks *et al.*, 1973;
Fernando and Adams, 1976). The kidney is double-wrapped, and transferred to the recipient
operating room for grafting.

Cadaveric donor nephrectomy. Kidneys from cadavers are used more frequently for transplants. They must be removed and perfused within one hour of cessation of renal blood
flow.

Both kidneys are removed from a cadaver through a transverse or vertical transperitoneal
incision. The aorta and inferior vena cava and ureters are carefully isolated, and mobilized
from the diaphragm to the pelvic brim. The aorta and vena cava are clamped above and
below the kidneys, which are then removed *en bloc* following careful perureteric dissection.
The kidneys are then perfused with cold Collin's solution or Sack's solution through the
aorta, or separately through the left and right renal artery. After separate dissection, and
ligation of small blood vessel branches, each kidney is double-wrapped in sterile plastic bags
and placed in ice for transplantation to the appropriate recipient hospital.

The kidneys can be perfused *in situ* with a special balloon catheter (Fernando and Adams,
1976). This permits an unhurried dissection of the kidneys following death (Fig. 25.47A).
Gentle handling, meticulous aseptic techniques and observation of any anatomical abnormality are important at every stage of the procedure.

A collaborative scheme in Europe ensures that each available kidney is matched in terms
of ABO and HLA compatibility, and the most suitable recipient is thereby chosen for
transplantation.

Transplantation. The iliac fossa is used for transplantation, preferably the right side
because of the sigmoid colon on the left.

An oblique, muscle-cutting incision is made from above the iliac spine to the suprapubic
region. The peritoneum is pushed medially and the iliac vessels are exposed carefully. The
internal iliac artery is mobilised and its terminal branches ligated. If this artery is found to
be unsuitable due to calcification or atheroma the external iliac artery is prepared.

The external iliac vein is mobilised and dissected in a similar fashion, and isolated between
two vascular clamps. An incision is made anterolaterally between the clamps, the kidney
removed from its storage bag and the renal vein is anastomosed to the window that has been
created in the vein. An end to side anastomosis is carried out with fine synthetic absorbable
sutures or silk (Fig. 25.47B).

A distal ligature is applied to the internal iliac artery, which is then clamped at its origin
from the common iliac artery. The vessel is divided obliquely, close to the ligature, and an
end to end anastomosis made to the renal artery (Fig. 25.47C). Should the external iliac have
been selected, an end to side anastomosis is carried out.

Before the anastomoses are completed, the vessels are flushed with heparinised saline to prevent embolisation of the kidney. The vascular clamps are released, and the kidney perfused to regain its normal colour and tension.

The procedure is completed by joining the ureter to the bladder, using an anastomosis similar to the anti-reflux technique of Leadbetter (Fig. 25.37A to D), except that a cystotomy is made in the bladder rather than colon.

Marker clips are placed at each pole of the kidney, to indicate the size and position, especially with a view to facilitating radiological control of X-ray therapy that may be given following transplantation. The kidney is placed in the iliac fossa and the wound closed with drainage. It is essential to make sure that there is no kinking of the anastomosis before wound closure.

FURTHER READING AND REFERENCES

BLANDY, J. P. and FOWLER, C. G. (1986) Lower tract endoscopy, *British Medical Bulletin*, **42** (3), 280–283
COLLINS, G. M., BRAVO-SHUGARMAN, M. AND TERASAKI, P. I. (1969) *Lancet*, **ii**, 1219.
FERNANDO, O. N. AND ADAMS, A. (1976) *Nursing Times*, 1598.
FOWLER, C. G. (1984) Fibrescope urethrocystoscopy, *British Journal of Urology*, **56**, 304–307
LEADBETTER, G. W., JR., MONACO, A. P. AND RUSSEL, P. S. A. (1966) *Surg. Gynae. Obstet.* **123**, 839.
SACK, S. A., PETRITSCH, P. H. AND KAUFMAN, J. J. (1973) *Lancet*, **i**, 1024.
SWINNEY, J. AND HAMMERSLEY, D. P. (1963) *A Handbook of Operative Urological Surgery*. Edinburgh: Churchill Livingstone.
WALLACE, D. M. (1975) *Nursing Mirror*, July 17, 60.
WARD, J. P. AND WICKHAM, J. E. (1976) *Nursing Times*, 91.

26

Operations on the thyroid and neck

Radical cervical node dissection

Definition

Removal of the submental, submaxillary and deep cervical glands, together with the sterno-mastoid muscle.

Position

Supine, with a support under the shoulder blades, and the neck in extension (Fig. 5.18).

Instruments

General set (Figs. 14.1 to 14.28)
Long scissors, curved on flat (McIndoe)
Large aneurysm needle
Artery forceps, curved on flat (Kelly Fraser), 10
Artery forceps, curved on flat (Dunhill), 25
Retractors, self-retaining (Travers and West), 2
Corrugated drainage tube and safety-pin or long plastic drainage tubing and
    suction system (Redivac, Activac, Portovac)
Suction tubing, nozzles and tube anchoring forceps
Diathermy leads, electrodes and lead anchoring forceps
2, 2.5 and 3 (3/0, 2/0 and 0) Chromic catgut, synthetic absorbable or silk for ligatures
3 (0) Chromic catgut or synthetic absorbable on a medium half-circle round-bodied needle
    for muscle sutures
2.5 (2/0) Synthetic non-absorbable on a small or medium curved cutting needle for skin
    sutures
(Staples, Michel or Kifa clips may be used.)

Outline of procedure

An oblique incision is made from the mastoid process to the sternum. This incision is extended Y-fashion to the chin just beyond the midline. The skin flaps are reflected and the platysma incised at the lower end of the sternomastoid muscle which is then divided across. This muscle is dissected up and the lower part of the internal jugular vein clamped and ligated. Dissection is continued, turning up the sternomastoid muscle and jugular vein and removing all tissue which lies behind as far as the trapezius muscle. When the dissection

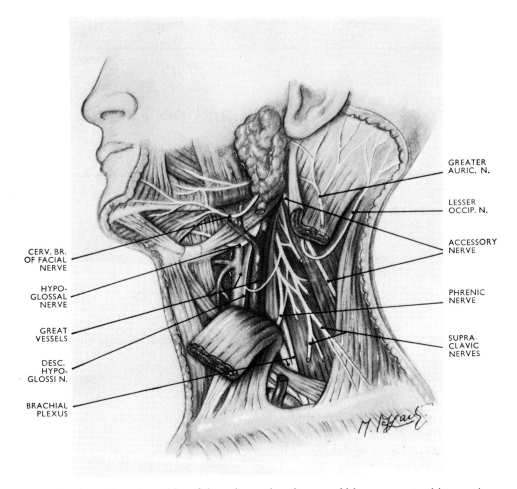

GREATER
AURIC. N.

LESSER
OCCIP. N.

ACCESSORY
NERVE

PHRENIC
NERVE

SUPRA-
CLAVIC
NERVES

CERV. BR.
OF FACIAL
NERVE

HYPO-
GLOSSAL
NERVE

GREAT
VESSELS

DESC.
HYPO-
GLOSSI N.

BRACHIAL
PLEXUS

Fig. 26.1 Drawing to show the position of the main vessels and nerves which are encountered in operations on the cervical lymph glands. (Farquharson and Rintoul: *Textbook of Operative Surgery.*)

reaches the bifurcation of the common carotid artery, the tissues below the chin, including the submaxillary gland, are then dealt with and reflected towards the carotid bifurcation also. The insertion of the sternomastoid muscle into the skull is severed and the mass of tissue removed, together with the lower pole of the parotid gland. During this dissection the facial artery and vein and the upper part of the jugular vein will be ligated, but the carotid vessels and the vagus and other essential nerves are carefully preserved. The wound is closed with drainage after haemostasis is complete.

Excision of parotid tumour

Definition

Removal of a tumour in the parotid gland.

Position

As radical cervical dissection.

Instruments

As radical cervical dissection, except
2 (3/0) Synthetic non-absorbable or silk on a small curved cutting needle for skin sutures.

Outline of procedure

An incision is made commencing near the lobe of the ear and extending along the crease of the neck. The parotid gland is exposed and the tumour freed by dissection. Haemostasis is secured, a drain inserted and the wound is closed.

Excision of thyroglossal duct or cyst

Definition

Removal of a congenital duct between the thyroid gland and the pharynx, which may be cystic, and have an external opening in the neck.

Position

As radical cervical dissection.

Instruments

As radical cervical dissection
Small bone cutting forceps.

Outline of procedure

Sistrunk's operation consists of a transverse curved incision which is made over the site of the cyst, or an elliptical incision around the sinus opening. The cyst and sinus tract are grasped with tissue forceps and dissected down to the hyoid bone, the centre of which is removed, thereby dividing the bone. Dissection is continued down to the base of the tongue and the extent of this dissection confirmed by palpating through the mouth. The sinus and cyst are removed and the tissues of the tongue are closed with chromic catgut or synthetic absorbable sutures. The hyoid bone is approximated with chromic catgut or synthetic absorbable, a drain inserted and the wound closed.

Partial thyroidectomy or excision of adenoma of thyroid

Definition

Removal of part of the thyroid gland or removal of thyroid adenoma.

Position

As radical cervical dissection.

Instruments

General set (Figs. 14.16 to 14.28)
Thyroidectomy set (Fig. 26.2)
Long scissors, curved on flat (McIndoe)
Corrugated drainage tube and safety-pin
Suction tubing, nozzles and tube anchoring forceps
Diathermy leads, electrodes and lead anchoring forceps
Local infiltration requisites and adrenaline 1 in 400,000 in saline (Optional)
2.5 and 3 (2/0 and 0) Chromic catgut or synthetic absorbable and silk for ligatures
2 and 3 (3/0 and 0) Chromic catgut or synthetic absorbable on small half-circle
   round-bodied needles for muscle and subcutaneous sutures
2 (3/0) Synthetic non-absorbable or silk on a medium curve cutting needle for skin
   sutures *or* staples, or Michel or Kifa clips.

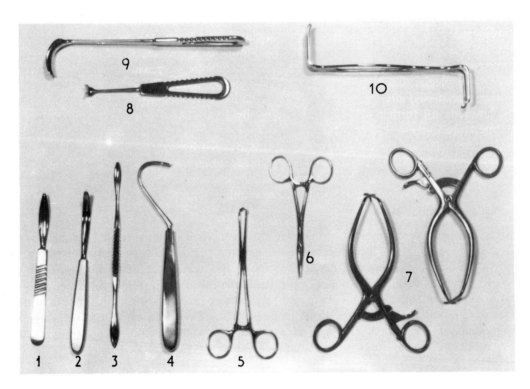

Fig. 26.2 Partial thyroidectomy, etc.
1. Thyroid dissector with eye at point (Kocher).
2. Thyroid dissector (Kocher).
3. Dissector (Durham).
4. Large aneurysm needle.
5. Thyroid-holding forceps (Laney), 2.
6. Artery forceps, curved on flat (Dunhill), 36.
7. Retractors, self-retaining, thyroid, 2 (Jackson Burrow, or alternatively one Joll type).
8. Small, short blade retractors, thyroid (Kocher), 2.
9. Small, long blade retractors, thyroid (Kocher), 2.
10. Medium retractors (Czerny), 2.

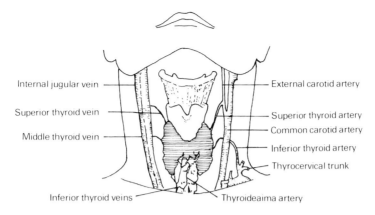

Fig. 26.3   Arterial supply and venous drainage of thyroid gland. (After Robinson.)

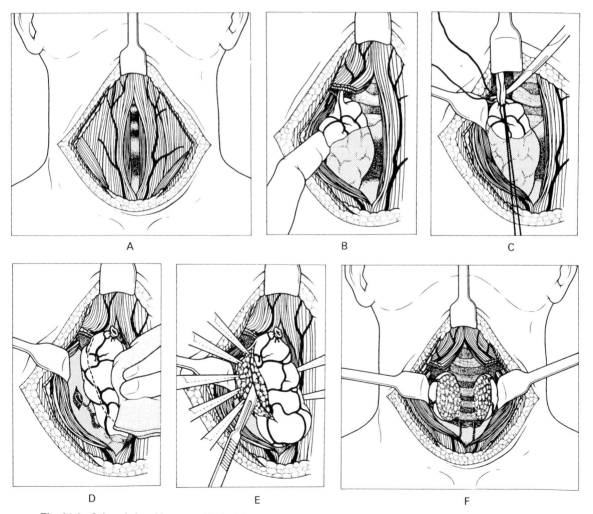

Fig. 26.4   Subtotal thyroidectomy. (A) Incision of deep fascia in the mid line. (B) Mobilisation of the right lobe. (C) Ligating of superior thyroid vessels. (D) Exposure of the inferior thyroid artery. (E) Division of the gland. (F) Appearances after the subtotal removal. (Rintoul: *Farquharson's Textbook of Operative Surgery.*)

Outline of procedure

Some surgeons infiltrate the skin of the incision area and the platysma with a solution of 1 in 400,000 adrenaline in saline which acts as a vasoconstricting agent, lessens bleeding and provides a plane of cleavage between the platysma and the deeper structures.

A low transverse incision is made in the neck, in line with the skin creases. The skin flaps and platysma are reflected widely and a self-retaining retractor or retractors inserted. The deep cervical fascia is incised in the midline and the infra-hyoid muscles retracted laterally or divided. The gland is carefully freed one lobe at a time by first clamping and dividing the middle thyroid vein, and then elevating the upper pole with a gland enucleator and ligating the superior thyroid artery. The lower lobe of the gland is then dislocated forwards and the inferior thyroid artery is ligatured in continuity.

This process may then be repeated on the other lobe before any glandular tissue is excised. A small portion of the posterior part of one or both lobes which contains the parathyroid glands is left and the remainder excised, first clamping with forceps as the excision proceeds. These divided vessels and tissue are ligated to secure haemostasis, a drain is inserted through a stab incision in the deep fascia on each side, and the muscles and fascia are sutured. The skin is closed with sutures or skin clips.

For excision of adenoma, the gland is exposed in the usual manner, and artery forceps are placed along the line where the tumour has caused the gland tissue to thin out. An incision is made just in front of these into the adenoma capsule. The tumour is then shelled out and the resultant cavity sutured over. The wound is closed as above.

REFERENCE AND FURTHER READING

FARQUHARSON, E. L. AND RINTOUL, R. F. (1972) *Textbook of Operative Surgery*. Edinburgh: Churchill Livingstone.

27

Thoracic operations

Bronchoscopy

Definition

Examination of the trachea and main bronchi by means of an endoscope which is passed into their lumens.

Position

This will depend on whether a rigid or flexible instrument is used. It may be supine with flexion, or extension of the head as required, or sitting.

Instruments

Bronchoscope (Flexible — Fig. 27.6 or rigid — Fig. 27.3)
Biopsy or grasping forceps (Flexible or rigid)
Cytology brush
Suction nozzles (long) (for rigid instruments only)
Suction tubing, tube anchoring forceps
Fibre light or electric cable
Light or electrical source
Pharyngeal spray and topical anaesthetic (lignocaine [xylocaine]) 2, and 4 per cent liquid, or 2 per cent gel.
Silicone liquid
Camera
Specimen tubes.

Outline of procedure

The introduction of the flexible fibreoptic bronchoscope has resulted in a safer procedure. The basic principles of this instrument have been described in Chapter 13, and the reader referred to page 389 for further information. In comparison with the rigid instrument the fibreoptic bronchoscope is about one third slimmer than the former (Fig. 27.6). This enables the instrument to be introduced through the nose under local analgesia. The bronchial tree can be examined to subsegmental level in all lobes; the upper lobes are not visible when using a rigid instrument.

The fibreoptic bronchoscope can be used in several ways. In addition to passing the instrument through the nose or mouth under premedication and local analgesia, it can be

Figs. 27.1 to 27.5 Rigid bronchoscope, laryngoscope and grasping forceps (Down's Surgical Ltd.)

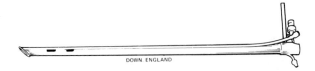

Fig. 27.1 Negus aspirating bronchoscope — fibre lighting.

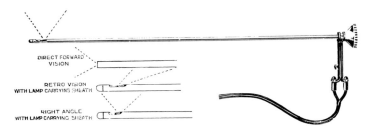

Fig. 27.2 Poppers telescope.

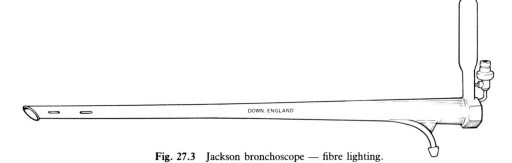

Fig. 27.3 Jackson bronchoscope — fibre lighting.

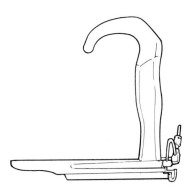

Fig. 27.4 Negus laryngoscope fitted with fibre light carrier.

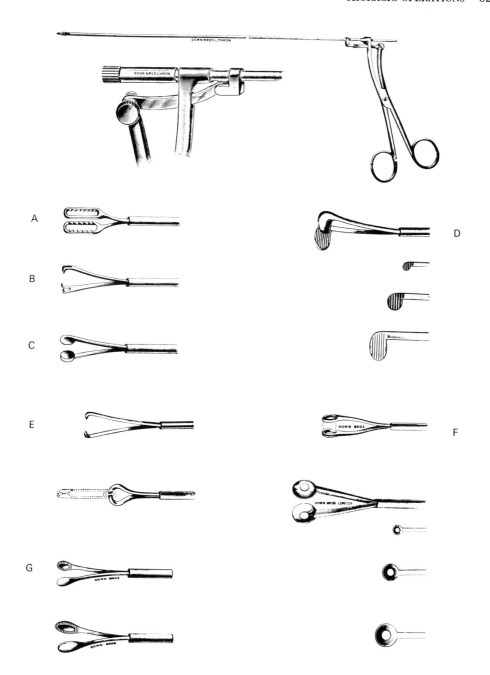

Fig. 27.5 Chevalier Jackson grasping forceps with Negus handle. (Downs Surgical Ltd.)

A. Forward grasping forceps.
B. 2/2 teeth claw forceps (Brünings).
C. Scoop cutting biopsy forceps (Brünings).
D. Side grasping forceps.

E. Rotation forceps.
F. Bronchial fenestrated biopsy forceps (Brünings).
G. Round foreign body forceps.

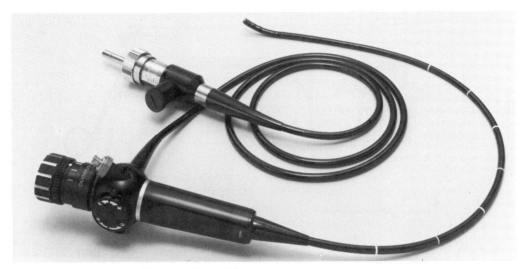

Fig. 27.6   Olympus bronchofibrescope. (Keymed.)

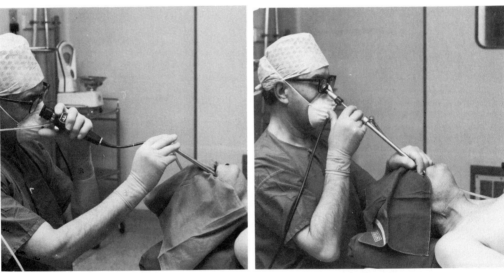

Fig. 27.7   **Fig. 27.8**

Fig. 27.7   The bronchofibrescope in use. The patient is under intravenous general anaesthetic and muscle relaxant. Oxygen venturi ventilation is in operation. The depth of insertion of the fibrescope is being controlled by the operator's right hand; the direction of the tip by his left. Any necessary suction is controlled by the left thumb here seen being applied to the black-grommetted control hole, punched in the side of the suction tube.

Fig. 27.8   Rigid bronchoscope in use. The larynx has been passed and the trachea entered. (Stradling: *Diagnostic Bronchoscopy — An Introduction.*)

inserted through a rigid bronchoscope or endotracheal tube under general anaesthesia (Fig. 27.8).

If local analgesia is to be employed (in addition to premedication) the 4 per cent lignocaine (xylocaine) is sprayed into the nostril and also the throat. The fibrescope is lubricated with 2 per cent lignocaine (xylocaine) gel and the distal lens coated with a little silicone liquid

to prevent misting (Clarke, 1975). The instrument is inserted through the nose and gently maneouvred round the turbinates, into the naso pharynx and thence behind the epiglottis to the larynx.

The larynx is then inspected and 2 ml of 4 per cent lignocaine (xylocaine) instilled directly on to the larynx. This usually causes the patient to cough and splutter a little for a few seconds, but after a pause of about 60 seconds, the bronchoscope can be carefully steered through the larynx and into the trachea. Further doses of 2 per cent lignocaine (xylocaine) are instilled into the trachea and main bronchi as the examination proceeds.

The trachea, carina and both right and left bronchial trees are examined. Biopsies are taken with forceps if any lesions are present, and under direct vision lung areas can be brushed or plugs of mucus aspirated for histology or microbiology.

The bronchofibrescope is removed, and the premedication usually wears off after a few hours.

Mediastinoscopy

Definition

Examination of the mediastinal lymph glands or tumours, with an endoscope similar to a rigid bronchoscope.

Position

Supine.

Instruments

Mediastinoscope (Carlins)
Biopsy forceps
Bronchus sponge holder
Sponge-holding forceps, 5
Towel clips, 5
Scalpel handle No. 3 with 15 blade (Bard Parker)
Dissecting forceps, toothed, small
Dissecting forceps, non-toothed, medium
Scissors, curved on flat 13 cm (5 in) (Mayo)
Small needle holder (Kilner)
Diathermy leads, electrodes and lead anchoring forceps
Syringe, 20 ml with long fine needles
Suction tubing, long fine suction nozzles and tube anchoring forceps
Local anaesthesia requisites (Fig. 11.60)
2 (3/0) Chromic catgut or synthetic absorbable on medium, half circle round bodied needle for subcutaneous sutures
2 (3/0) Synthetic non-absorbable or silk on small curved cutting needle for skin.

Outline of procedure

A short transverse incision is made above the supra sternal notch, and the pre-tracheal fascia is exposed. A plane beneath the pre-tracheal fascia is developed by blunt dissection and the mediastinoscope introduced and advanced toward the mediastinum.

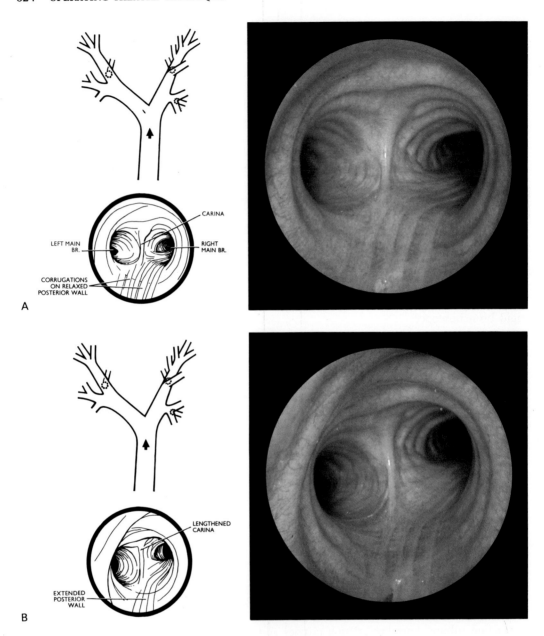

Fig. 27.9 View during bronchoscopy. (A and B) Normal carina. Changes with quiet respiration. The keel-like carinal edge is sharp and prominent as its name implies. The bronchial cartilage outlines are clearly seen beyond the carina, more so in the straighter right main bronchus, which is normally visible to a greater depth than the left. Posterior longitudinal mucosal corrugations are well seen, particularly in the lower trachea and the right main bronchus. The forward protrusion of the posterior walls during the expiratory phase, or during relaxation under general anaesthesia, is slight in normal subjects. It is rapidly abolished by raising the intrabronchial pressure, either by inspiration or ventilation; the lumina become more circular in outline and the transverse muscle bands may be seen more readily, in this case particularly in the left main bronchus.

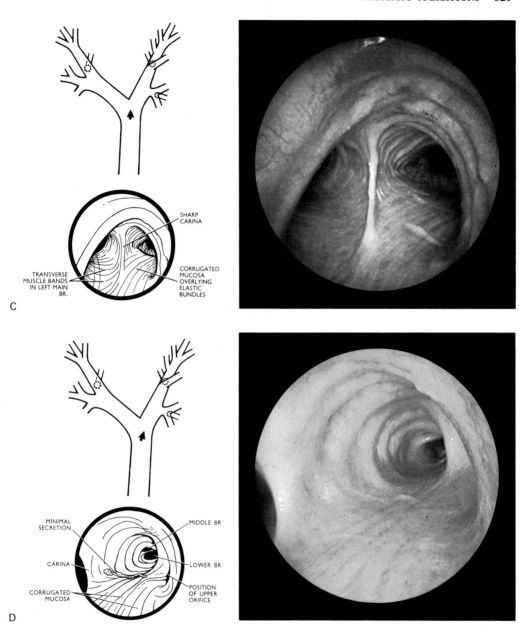

(C) Normal carina. The carinal edge in this case is extremely sharp. The submucosa is thin, showing some senile atrophy, and the mucosa is drawn tightly over the carina and cartilages. The posterior longitudinal mucosal corrugations outlining the elastic bundles, can be seen clearly but are not prominent. The mucosa is a little reddened and there is an increase in secretion due to mild bronchitis. The minor ecchymosis, seen on the anterior tracheal wall in the upper part of the picture, is due to slight pressure from the bronchoscope tube. (D) Normal right main bronchus. The cartilage outlines are well seen through the mucosa as far as the final division into middle and lower bronchi. The inferior lip of the upper bronchial orifice stands out well, making the orifice itself easy to locate. The longitudinal mucosal corrugations on the posterior wall are not unduly prominent and the carina, in the left foreground, is sharp. The minimal secretion, seen on the posterior wall, has been swept into a transverse string by the bronchoscope tube.

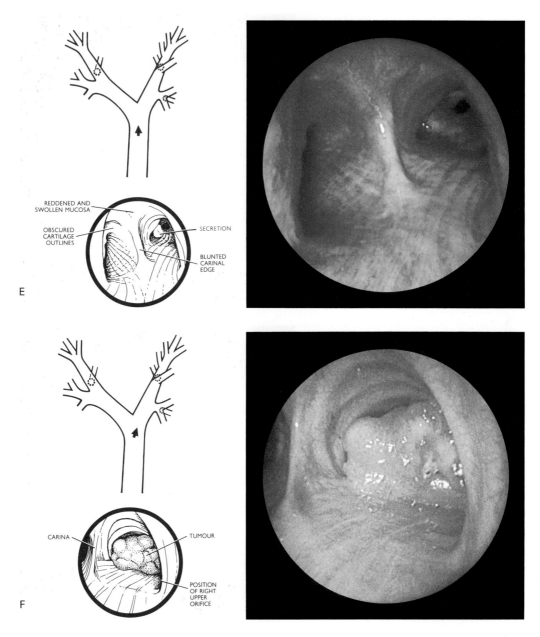

(E) Chronic bronchitis. Main bifurcation. The mucosa is generally reddened and some swelling is evident: cartilage outlines are less well-defined than usual. Some increase in mucoid secretion is present, seen distally in the right main bronchus. Longitudinal mucosal corrugations are clearly visible on the posterior bronchial and tracheal walls. Bronchoscopy was performed for right middle lobe collapse following a recent bronchitic exacerbation. Removal of the obstructing secretions led to rapid recovery. (F) Chondroma. Right main bronchus. Partially occluding the right main bronchus is a large, irregular tumour arising from cartilage in the lateral bronchial wall, just beyond the upper bronchial orifice. The tumour was of hard consistency with healthy, smooth, overlying mucosa and was successfully removed by bronchotomy. Histology: simple chondroma. (Stradling.)

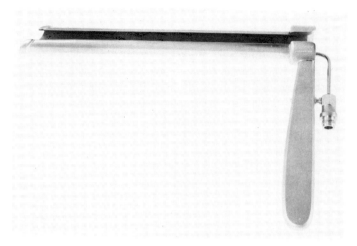

Fig. 27.10   Carlins mediastinoscope. (Genito Urinary Manufacturing Co. Ltd.)

Manipulation of the scope enables visualisation of the trachea bifuration, bronchi, aortic arch and associated lymph nodes. Lymph nodal tissue for biopsy is aspirated to exclude vascular structure, and a piece of tissue excised for histology.

If bleeding occurs, pressure may be applied with a swab on a bronchus swab holder. If necessary diathermy may be used. The incision is closed first by suturing the subcutaneous tissue and then skin.

It is usual to combine this procedure with bronchoscopy (Cook, 1976).

Intercostal tube drainage (for empyema or haemothorax)

Definition

The insertion of a tube for the drainage of a collection of pus or blood in the pleural cavity.

Position

Generally sitting with support.

Instruments

Sponge-holding forceps (Rampley), 5
Towel clips, 5
Scalpel handle No. 3 with No. 11 blade (Bard Parker)
Trocar and cannula
Catheter, self-retaining (De Pezzer or similar, size 24 Charrière gauge)
Catheter introducer
Syringe and wide-bore needles
Underwater seal apparatus or pump
Local anaesthesia requisites (Fig. 11.60)
2 (3/0) Synthetic non-absorbable or silk on medium curved cutting needle *may* be required
    to secure the catheter.

Outline of procedure

Under local anaesthesia, a stab incision is made in the chest wall, and á trocar and cannula introduced between two ribs into the empyema cavity or haemothorax. The trocar is removed and the catheter introduced through the cannula, which is then removed. To prevent collapse of the lung and to allow drainage of pus or blood, the open end of the catheter is connected to an underwater seal apparatus and/or mechanical pump.

One or two skin sutures are inserted, left untied and rolled up in a small piece of gauze. These are tied immediately when the tube is removed, so that a pneumothorax, possibly of 'tension' type, does not occur.

An underwater seal apparatus consists of a sterile glass bottle, generally of 2 litres capacity, half-filled with sterile water and closed with a cap which incorporates two tube connections. One tube connection terminates below the water level in the bottle and the other terminates just inside the cap. The former connection is coupled to the chest tube and the latter remains open to the atmosphere.

The underwater seal apparatus reproduces the negative pressure which should be in the pleural cavity, and prevents air from entering from the atmosphere, but allows pus and air to escape from the expanding lung as the patient breathes out deeply. The pus collects in the bottle and the air bubbles out through the water. Any tendency to back suction will only result in the fluid being drawn slightly up the drainage tube connection.

Alternatively, a suction machine creating a small amount of air displacement may be used, and in this case the drainage tubing is connected to the collection bottle fitted to the apparatus. A disposable pleural drainage unit (Thoraseal) is illustrated in Figure 27.30 (page 843).

Care must be taken that the drainage bottle is not elevated above the level of the patient. If this occurs, fluid may aspirate from the bottle and enter the patient's chest.

Decortication of the lung (for empyema or haemothorax)

Definition

Stripping or peeling off the fibrin layer from the lung following empyema or haemothorax, to allow full pulmonary expansion and obliteration of the empyema cavity.

Position.

Lateral chest (Figs. 5.14).

Instruments

As for thoracotomy.

Outline of procedure

The approach is as for thoracotomy. All free clot is removed from the pleural cavity, and the fibrin layer peeled off the lung to allow full re-expansion. Drainage tubes are introduced at the apex and base of the chest, and are connected to underwater seals or suction apparatus. These drainage tubes are to allow the escape of air and exudate.

Thoracotomy

Definition

Opening the chest cavity as a preliminary to surgery of the thoracic organs.

Position

Lateral chest (Fig. 5.14).

Instruments

General set (Figs. 14.1 to 14.28)
Artery forceps, curved on flat (Kelly Fraser), 50
Artery forceps, straight, 20 cm (8 in) (Spencer Wells), 12
Long-toothed and non-toothed dissecting forceps, 25 cm (10 in)
Long scissors, curved (Nelson)
Small rugine (Faraboeuf)
Large rugine (Mitchell)
Rib raspatory (Doyen), left and right side
Bone-holding forceps (Fergusson) (Lion)
Gouge or bone-nibbling forceps, angled on side
Gouge or bone-nibbling forceps, angled on flat
Rib shears (Exner)
Rib shears (Price Thomas) (A variety of other rib shears may be required according to
    the site of thoracotomy.)
Rib approximator (Morriston)
Sponge-holding forceps (Rampley), 4
Lung artery forceps, right angled (O'Shaughnessy), 6
Lung artery forceps, curved on flat (Roberts or Tudor Edward), 20, lung artery forceps,
    curved on flat (Moynihan) (cholecystectomy) or (Gordon Craig), 6
Lung-holding forceps (Duval), 5
Large aneurysm needle, Nelson right and left, 3 of each
Lung retractors (Deaver or alternatively Allison 'fish slice' type), 2
Bronchus clamp (Thompson)
Lung tourniquet (Roberts-Nelson)
Long needle holder (Halstead)
Deep retractor (Winsbury–White)
Deep retractor (Worrall)
Double rib spreader (Tudor Edwards), complete with one set of blades
    Rib spreader keys
    Two sets of alternative sizes of blades
Suction tubing, nozzles and tube anchoring forceps
Diathermy leads, electrodes and lead anchoring forceps
2, 2.5 and 3 (3/0, 2/0 and 0) Synthetic non-absorbable or silk on a small or medium
    half-circle round-bodied needle for transfixion sutures
4, 5 or 6 (1, 2 or 3) Chromic catgut, synthetic absorbable or silk for ligatures
5 or 6 (2 or 3) Chromic catgut, Synthetic absorbable or non-absorbable, or stainless steel
    wire or large half-circle round-bodied needles for rib closure
3 (0) Synthetic non-absorbable or silk on large curved or straight cutting needles for skin.

Figs. 27.11 to 27.23   Thoracic instruments. (Chas. F. Thackray Ltd.)

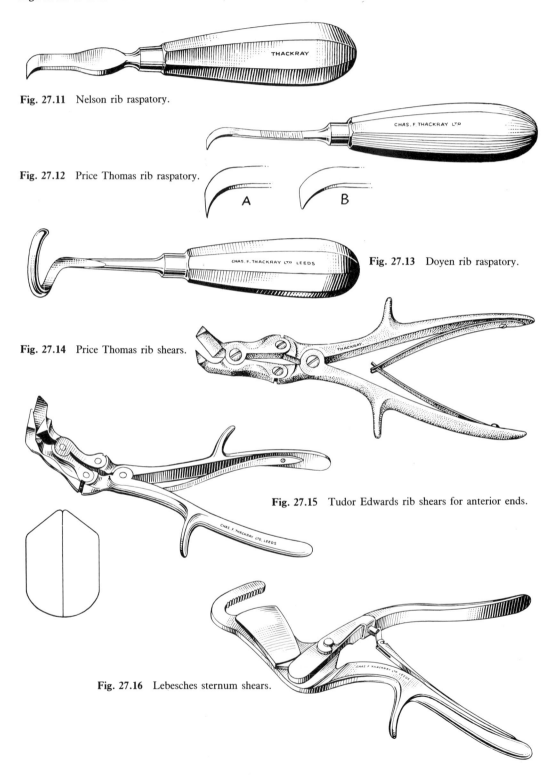

Fig. 27.11   Nelson rib raspatory.

Fig. 27.12   Price Thomas rib raspatory.

Fig. 27.13   Doyen rib raspatory.

Fig. 27.14   Price Thomas rib shears.

Fig. 27.15   Tudor Edwards rib shears for anterior ends.

Fig. 27.16   Lebesches sternum shears.

Fig. 27.17 Morriston Davies rib approximator.

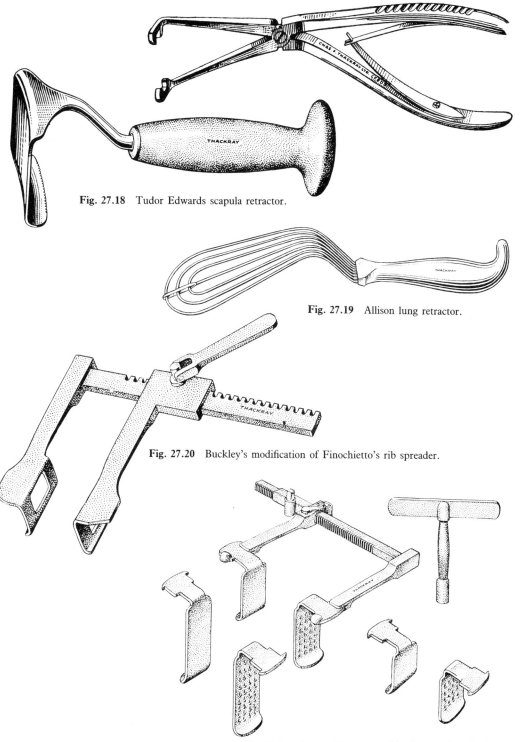

Fig. 27.18 Tudor Edwards scapula retractor.

Fig. 27.19 Allison lung retractor.

Fig. 27.20 Buckley's modification of Finochietto's rib spreader.

Fig. 27.21 Tudor Edwards double rib spreader with key.

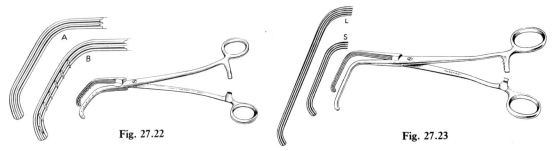

Fig. 27.22

Fig. 27.23

Fig. 27.22 (left) Price Thomas bronchus clamp. (A) Plain jaws. (B) 'Spiked' jaws.

Fig. 27.23 (right) Bickford bronchus clamp. (L) Large jaws. (S) Small jaws.

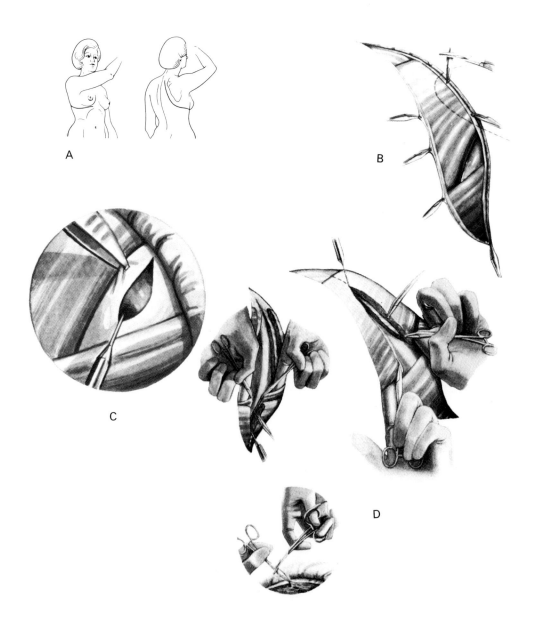

A

B

C

D

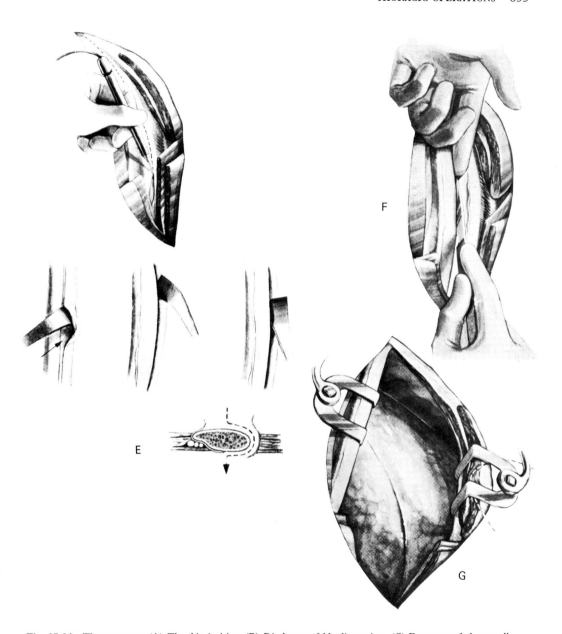

Fig. 27.24 Thoracotomy. (A) *The skin incision*. (B) *Diathermy of bleeding points*. (C) Exposure of chest wall. Entrance to muscle planes, incising through the fascial triangle and the underlying thomboid muscle until the chest wall is reached. (D) *Incision of muscles*. The assistant's and the surgeon's index fingers are used to elevate the muscles, and they are then incised with diathermy parallel to the wound, picking up bleeding points meticulously as they meet. In this way, blood loss is kept to a minimum. (E) *Incision and eversion of periosteum*. The periosteum is incised with diathermy in the mid-rib plane. The periosteum of the upper half of the rib is raised to avoid interference with the intercostal neurovascular bundle below the rib. (F) *Entry into pleural cavity*. Entry into the pleural cavity is made by incising through the rib bed.

An intercostal incision is seldom employed, but some surgeons still prefer to resect the rib subperiosteally. Should subsequently the size of the thoracotomy appear to be restrictive, an increase in access can always be gained by prolonging the incision forwards, if necessary to the sternal border. (G) *Introduction of retractor*. Adhesions in the neighbourhood of the incision between the chest wall and lung are first divided so that a large self-retaining retractor of the Tudor Edwards or Price Thomas type may be introduced, spreading the wound widely without tearing the lung. (Cleland: *Surgery — Thorax*).

Outline of procedure

The site of the incision depends upon which part of the chest contents is to be approached. The incision may be posterolateral, lateral or anterolateral, and may be placed overlying the upper or lower part of the thorax.

The incision is deepened through fascia and muscle down to the intercostal muscles. Haemostasis is secured with diathermy or ligatures, and the chest is entered either between two ribs or through the bed of an excised rib. In the former case an incision is made through the intercostal muscles, and the pleura opened with scissors. In the latter case the periosteum is reflected off the rib anteriorly with a Faraboeuf's, Sembs or Price Thomas rugine, and posteriorly by passing a Doyen's raspatory around and along the rib. The rib is excised, the pleura opened with scissors and a rib spreader inserted.

After the surgical procedure has been completed, an intercostal drain is inserted (see empyema), usually one apical and one basal. The drain is connected to the underwater seal and the wound is closed. Interrupted sutures of chromic catgut, synthetic absorbable or non-absorbable, or stainless-steel wire are inserted through the intercostal muscles above the upper rib of the wound into the chest cavity, and out again through the intercostal muscles below the lower rib. These sutures are left long until all have been inserted for the entire length of the wound. A rib approximator is used to approximate the ribs and the interrupted sutures are tied. Further interrupted sutures may be inserted to reinforce this suture line. If a drainage tube has been used, this is connected to an underwater seal apparatus and the anaesthetist inflates the lung or lungs.

Interrupted or continuous sutures of chromic catgut, synthetic absorbable or non-absorbable, or stainless steel wire are used to close the intercostal muscles and other chest muscles. The skin is sutured with interrupted synthetic non-absorbable or silk.

Lobectomy or pneumonectomy

Definition

Excision of a lobe of the lung or total removal of the lung.

Position

Lateral chest (Fig. 5.14).

Instruments

As thoracotomy (p. 829).

Outline of procedure

The chest is opened as for thoracotomy, with a posterolateral incision usually over the sixth interspace. The sixth rib, or alternatively the fifth or seventh rib, is excised and the chest entered through the bed of the excised rib.

For lobectomy the affected lobe is held with lung forceps and any adhesions are freed with scissors or dissection swabs until the lobe is only attached by its main bronchus and vessels entering the hilum in the mediastium. The pulmonary artery and vein are isolated and clamped, divided and ligated. The bronchus is identified and clamped across with a special bronchus clamp. The rest of the chest is isolated with moist packs to prevent contamination

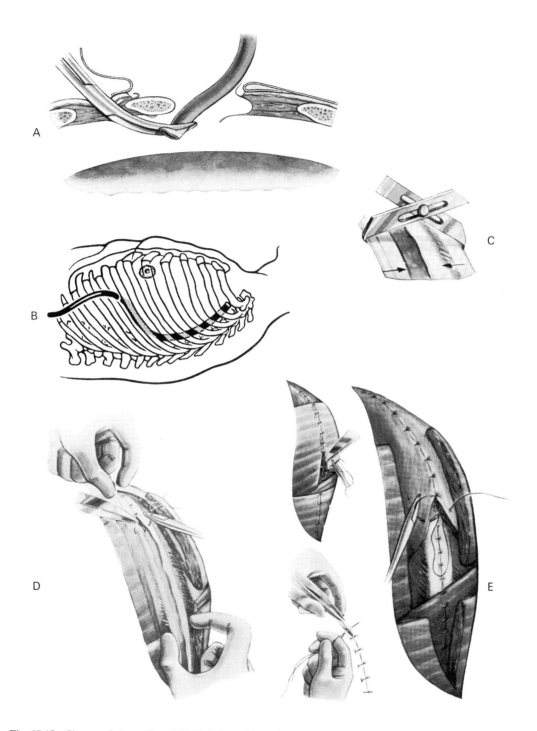

Fig. 27.25 Closure of chest. (A and B) If drainage is required an inter-costal drain is inserted, anterior to the mild axillary line below the incision. (C) Approximation of the ribs with instrument. (D) Periosteum sutured with interrupted thread, catgut or synthetic non-absorbable. (E) Muscle closed in layers with interrupted catgut, synthetic non-absorbable or wire, skin closed with interrupted sutures. (Cleland: *Surgery — Thorax.*)

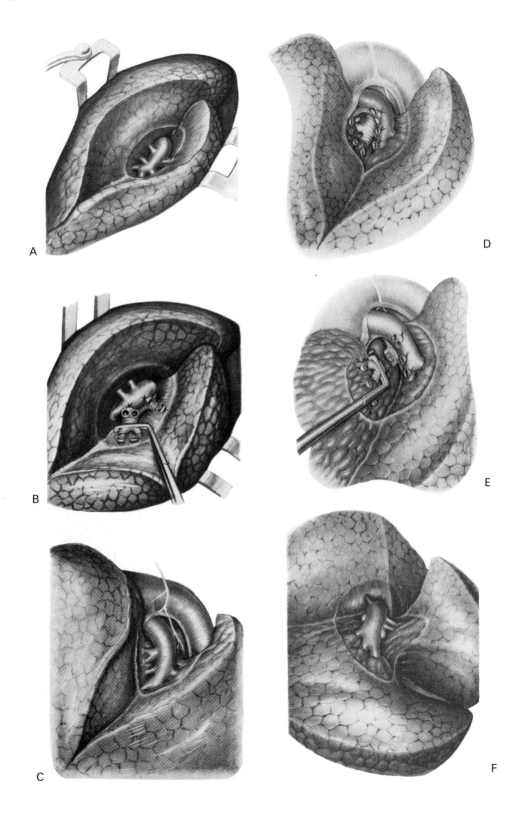

A

B

C

D

E

F

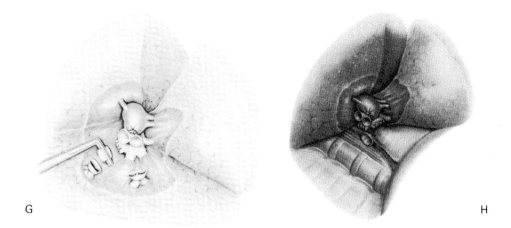

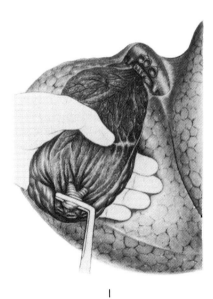

Fig. 27.26 Lobectomy and segmental resection of the lung.

Left lower lobectomy (A) Pulmonary artery and branches exposed. (B) Branches of pulmonary artery leading to lobe divided between ligatures, clamp applied across basal divisions of lower lobe bronchus.

Left upper lobectomy (C) Pulmonary artery and branches to upper lobe exposed. (D) Branches of pulmonary artery leading to upper lobe divided between ligatures. (E) Clamp or clamps are used to close and hold bronchi close to the line of section.

Right lower lobe lobectomy (F) Pulmonary artery and branches to lower lobe exposed. (G) The lower lobe artery has been divided, between ligatures, bronchus to apex of lower lobe divided — sutures on proximal stump shown. (H) The lobe has been removed — bronchial suture lines shown.

Segmental resection (I) After ligation of vessels and clamping of bronchi the segment is 'rolled off'. (Cleland: *Surgery — Thorax.*)

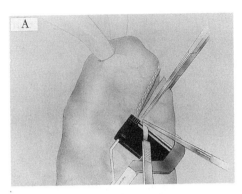
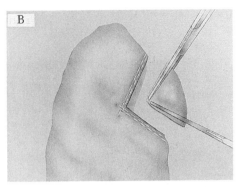

Fig. 27.27 Wedge resection of lung using stapler. (RLGO Stapler, Ethicon Ltd.) A. After identifying the margins of the lesion, the open jaws of the stapler are positioned around the lung tissue and the stapler fired. A clamp is applied on the specimen side and this portion of the wedge cut using the cutting guide on the edge of the stapler anvil. B. Excision of the wedge completed.

as the lung is removed. Either the bronchus is divided by the cut and sew method, whereby sutures are inserted as the bronchus is divided; or a second clamp is applied and the bronchus divided between the two. With the latter method, the bronchus is oversewn before removing the clamp. In both cases a second and sometimes third layer of sutures (chromic catgut, synthetic absorbable or non-absorbable, silk, or stainless steel wire) are inserted to ensure a good closure. Alternatively the bronchus can be closed with a linear stapler (as illustrated in Figure 15.34 — gastrectomy). This technique can be used also for segmental or wedge resection (Fig. 27.27). The stump of the bronchus is pleuralised, using interrupted synthetic non-absorbable, silk or chromic catgut. At this stage the surgeon may instil 500 ml of warm saline solution into the pleural cavity. The anaesthetist then inflates the lungs to ascertain whether the bronchial suture line is secure; the appearance of bubbles indicates a leak.

For pneumonectomy the operative procedure is similar, but the dissection is more extensive, and the total lung is removed. The pericardium is incised and the dissection of the major vessels carried out through this opening in some cases.

If the pericardium has been opened, it is sutured with chromic catgut, synthetic absorbable or silk on a non-traumatic needle after haemostasis has been checked. In most instances, chest drains are not inserted following pneumonectomy. However, a PVC 20 Charierre tube may be left in situ and occluded with a spigot. Any subsequent mediastinal shift detected by radiological examination can be corrected with a Maxwell miniature artificial pneumo-thorax apparatus. The maximum air removed in these circumstances is limited to two litres (at any one time).

The chest is closed as for thoracotomy. Cryotherapy may be applied to intercostal nerves following any thoracotomy. This provides analgesia for a prolonged period and simplifies post-operative chest physiotherapy. The cryoprobe is described in Chapter 3, page 98.

Thoraco-abdominal approach for oesophagogastrectomy

Definition

Removal of part of the oesophagus and stomach for high gastric ulcer or tumour, oesopha-geal varices or oesophageal tumour. The operation is performed through a combined thoracic

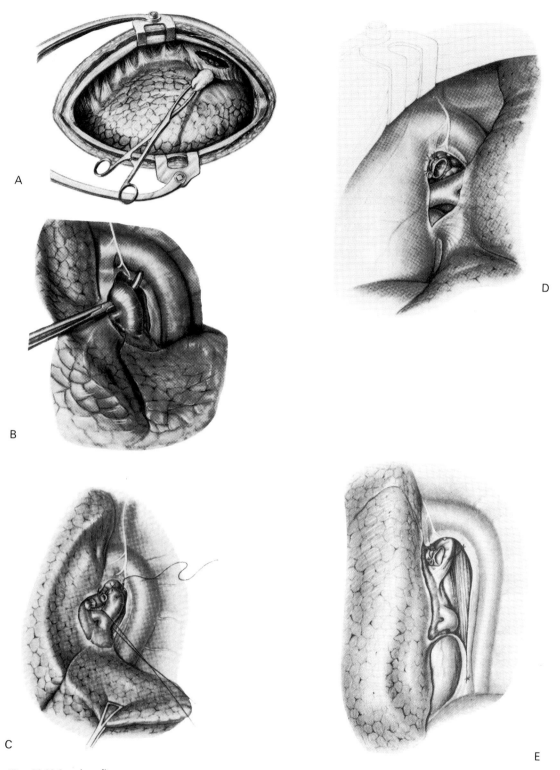

Fig. 27.28 (continued)

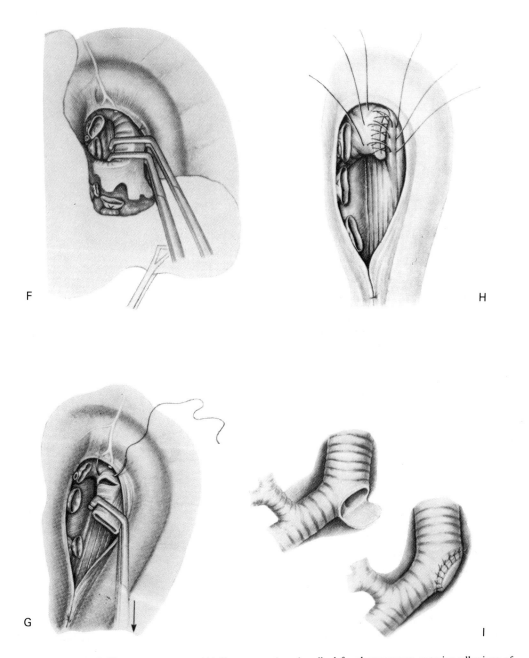

Fig. 27.28 Simple (left) pneumonectomy. (A) Chest opened as described for thoracotomy, anterior adhesions of lung to chest wall being freed by blunt dissection. (B) Pulmonary artery dissection — the vagus nerve has been cut distal to its recurrent laryngeal nerve. (C) Artery ligated by passing a strong thread suture round it. (D) Lung retracted to expose the anterior aspect of the hilum — superior pulmonary vein dissected out and divided between ligatures. (E) Exposure of inferior pulmonary vein, pulmonary ligament divided — pericardium visible behind lung. (F) Bronchus clamped, bronchial artery ligated ready for division. (G) Bronchial incision started close to carina, retraction suture for lifting stump from mediastinum. Continuous suture of thread or wire to close bronchus. (H and I) Alternative method of closure of bronchus. (Cleland: *Surgery — Thorax.*)

and abdominal incision. (Alternatively, laporatomy first to mobilise the stomach and perform a pyloroplasty followed by repositioning of the patient to make a thoracotomy incision to complete the resection.)

Instruments

As for thoracotomy, page 829, plus:
 5 (2) Chromic catgut, synthetic absorbable or silk or wire on a medium half-circle round-bodied needle for diaphragm
 5 (2) Chromic catgut or synthetic absorbable on a large half-circle cutting needle for abdominal muscles.

Outline of procedure

A thoraco-abdominal incision is made, extending transversely across the epigastrium from the umbilicus, along the sixth or seventh intercostal space, to 5 cm (2 in) from the spine, i.e., behind the scapula. The sixth or seventh rib may be resected in the usual manner if insertion of a rib spreader indicates possible fracture of the ribs. The costal cartilage is cut across the diaphragm and peritoneum opened.

The tumour is palpated and resectibility determined. The oesophagus and upper end of the stomach are freed carefully, and vessels ligated with chromic catgut, synthetic absorbable or silk. Nylon tape may be passed around the oesophagus for traction during dissection. Clamps are applied across the cardia of the stomach which is transected (if a tumour is present it would be distal to this point) and the lesser curvature narrowed by resection and closure with 2.5 or 3 (2/0 or 0) chromic catgut or synthetic absorbable on a non-traumatic needle.

Two occlusion clamps are applied across the oesophagus and the lesion is removed by dividing between the two clamps. The stomach is delivered into the chest and an end to end anastomosis made to the oesophagus with 'through and through' interrupted chromic catgut or synthetic absorbable non-traumatic sutures or by using an intra-luminal stapler (Figure 15.42), a similar technique being employed to that adopted for large bowel anasthomosis. The suture line is reinforced anteriorly and posteriorly with a serosa closure of interrupted silk sutures.

If the lesion is extensive, a total gastrectomy may be performed (Chapter 15) with oesophago-jejunostomy.

The diaphragm is closed with interrupted chromic catgut, synthetic absorbable, non-absorbable, or silk sutures, and the peritoneum with a continuous chromic catgut or synthetic absorbable suture. The chest cavity *may* be irrigated and an intercostal drainage tube is inserted through the eighth intercostal space. The chest muscles are sutured with interrupted chromic catgut, synthetic absorbable or wire, followed by interrupted synthetic non-absorbable for the skin.

The intercostal tube from the chest is connected to an underwater seal bottle.

Repair of diaphragmatic hernia (thoracic approach)

Definition

The repair of an abnormal opening in the diaphragm (usually at the oesophageal hiatus), which allows a sliding hernia of stomach into the chest.

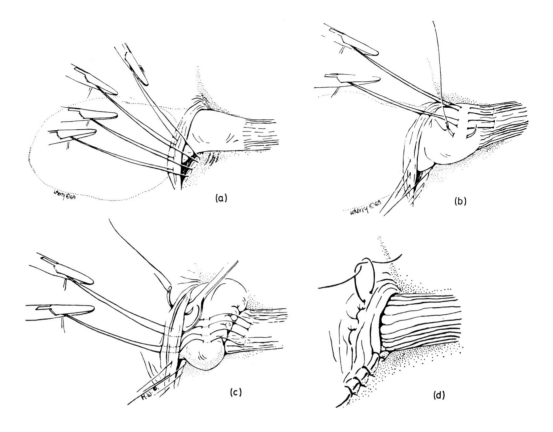

Fig. 27.29 The Belsey 'Mark IV' technique, viewed through left thoracotomy with patient lying on right side: (A) crural approximation sutures; (B) fastening stomach to oesophagus above the cardia; (C) placing second row of mattress sutures with the aid of cocktail spoon; (D) the completed repair. (Irvine: *Modern Trends in Surgery.*)

Position

Lateral chest (Fig. 5.14).

Instruments

As for thoracotomy (p. 829).

    Long tissue forceps (Littlewood or Vulsellum), 4

    Ligatures and sutures as for thoracotomy

    2.5 (2/0) Synthetic absorbable, silk or stainless steel wire on a small half-circle
       round-bodied needle for diaphragm repair

    Nylon tape or fine rubber tubing for oesophageal retraction.

Outline of procedure

A left posterolateral incision is made through the seventh intercostal space, and the chest opened as for thoracotomy. (A rib may, or may not be resected.) Rib spreaders are inserted,

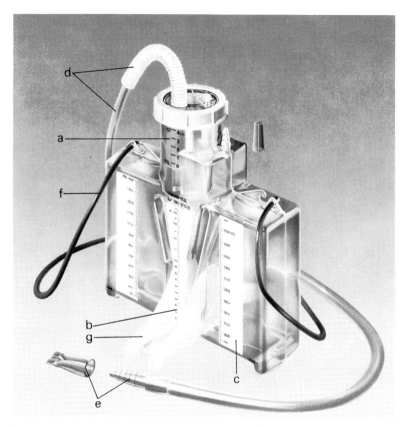

Fig. 27.30 Thora-seal is a sterile plastic disposable pleural drainage unit which incorporates many innovative design features. It is convenient, uncomplicated and economical to use which facilitates clinical assessment and management. Thora-seal features:
A Self-monitoring underwater seal which ensures that there is no progressive resistance to drainage;
B Fine graduations which make the unit suitable for both adult and paediatric drainage;
C Write-on drainage record column;
D Clear milkable drainage tube with an anti-kink collar device;
E Thoracic step connector with protective cap;
F Adaptable strap which can be used as a bed-frame hanger, hand or shoulder strap;
G Sturdy disposable plastic floor stand.
The unit offers a double non-woven fabric drape technique which provides a sterile field during set up and facilitates aseptic transfer.
(Sherwood Medical Industries Ltd.)

the mediastinal pleura opened, and the oesophagus mobilised and retracted with the nylon tape or rubber tubing.

The hernial orifice is identified, an incision made in the left dome of the diaphragm and the herniated organs returned to the abdomen. The edges of the orifice are grasped with tissue or Vulsellum forceps and the opening is repaired with interrupted synthetic non-absorbable, or silk or stainless steel wire sutures which are left long and are tied when all have been inserted. The incision in the left dome of the diaphragm is repaired in a similar manner.

The mediastinal pleura is approximated over the oesophagus and the chest closed in the manner usual for thoracotomy.

Sometimes the operation is performed through an abdominal or thoraco-abdominal incision, as described for oesophagectomy.

REFERENCES AND FURTHER READING

CLELAND, W. P. (1968) *Surgery — Thorax*. London: Butterworths.
COOK, F. (1976) *Nursing Times*, 1718.
CLARKE, S.W. (1975) *Nursing Mirror*, 47, November 27.
IRVINE, W. T. (1971) *Modern Trends in Surgery — 3*. London: Butterworths.
STRADLING, P. (1986) *Diagnostic Bronchoscopy*, 5th edn. Edinburgh: Churchill Livingstone.

28

Cardiovascular operations

This is a highly specialised and relatively new branch of surgery. The equipment and instruments used are extensive in range and often include many items which are of personal use only to a particular surgeon. In the following chapter it is possible only to cover those basic instruments for some cardiovascular procedures.

The reader is referred to Chapter 11 for a description of cardiac stimulant drugs, and Chapter 3 for the use of electric defibrillators and pacemakers which play an important part in heart operations.

A large proportion of heart and major blood vessel operations in the chest are performed under extracorporeal circulation (cardiopulmonary bypass), sometimes combined with cold cardioplegia (Norman, 1981). With extracorporeal circulation, the blood is diverted from the heart and the circulation maintained by means of a mechanical pump or pumps and oxygenator (heart/lung machine, e.g., Bentley membrane oxygenator system). To achieve cold cardioplegia, the patient's body temperature is first lowered to 30°C by physical cooling under anaesthesia; after cardiopulmonary bypass has been established, the temperature can be lowered still further to 23°C or exceptionally 15°C. This is achieved by lowering the temperature in the oxygenator heat exchanger.

During operation the patient lies on, and is covered by special blankets which help to control the hypothermia. These blankets are made up of a series of rubber or plastic tubes through which fluid from a hypothermia machine circulates. The temperature of this fluid is adjusted to individual requirements and rewarming is started as soon as the patient is on the operating table.

Intracardiac procedures

Considerable developments have taken place, and intracardiac surgery is now an expanding specialty. There are many variations of technique for the same type of operation, each giving successful results in the hands of a particular team. Newer and more efficient prosthetic valve replacements are being designed, and in the not too distant future the use of auxiliary ventricles will become commonplace.

Cardiac surgery is complex and requires a specialised team of surgeons, anaesthetists, cardiologists, physiologists, technicians and nurses. Space will not permit more than a brief outline of surgical procedures for it would be easy to devote the entire book to describing these. In order to generalise, the descriptions depart from the format of the book hitherto. Exceptions are the descriptions of coarctation of the aorta and patent ductus arteriosus.

Intracardiac lesions vary considerably in severity, and in some cases the diseases overlap requiring several distinctly separate operative procedures during surgery. These lesions can be described as (A) acquired and (B) congenital. They are listed together with the corrective surgery.

(A) Acquired lesions

Mitral stenosis
1. Closed valvulotomy
2. Open valvulotomy (under direct vision)
3. Valve replacement

Mitral insufficiency
1. Valvuloplasty
2. Valve replacement

Tricuspid stenosis, and/or insufficiency aortic stenosis, and/or insufficiency
1. Open valvulotomy
2. Valvuloplasty
3. Valve replacement

Coronary heart disease
1. Revascularisation of the coronary arteries

Occlusive disease of the aorta
1. Graft replacement
2. Bypass
3. Thromboendarterectomy

Thoracic aortic aneurysm
1. Repair procedure
2. Graft replacement

Chronic heart disease
1. Transplantation

(B) Congenital defects

Pulmonary stenosis
1. Valvulotomy

Atrial septal defect

Ventricular septal defect

Tetralogy of Fallot
1. Repair procedure

Patent ductus arteriosis
1. Ligation and division

Coarctation of the aorta
1. Resection and end to end anastomosis
2. Resection and graft

Cardiopulmonary bypass — an overview

Maintaining a patient's circulation by temporarily bypassing the blood from the heart enables protracted intracardiac operative procedures to be undertaken. Regardless of design the heart-lung machines, as they are known, consist basically of an oxygenator, arterial and venous pumps, heat exchanger, filters, and arterial, venous and cardiotomy blood reservoirs.

The oxygenator takes the place of the patient's lungs by removing excess carbon dioxide from the venous blood and providing oxygenation to arterial blood. This is achieved usually by separating the blood into a thin film or flow which then is exposed to an oxygen rich environment where the interchange of gases takes place.

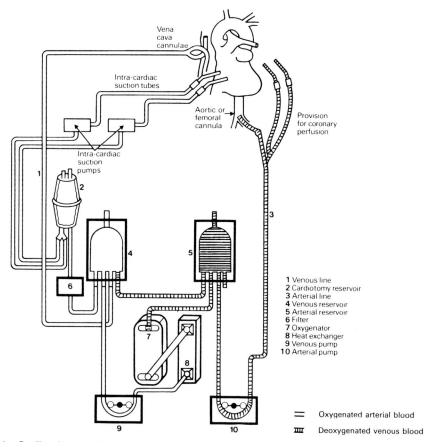

Fig. 28.1 Cardiopulmonary bypass twin pump system.

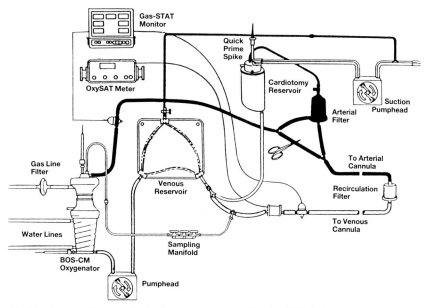

Fig. 28.2 Cardiopulmonary bypass, single pump system using Bentley BOS-CM system. (Bentley Edwards.)

The pumps, usually a set of rollers rhythmically massaging the outside of the arterial and venous tubes, maintain the flow of blood from the patient to the machine, and back after oxygenation. The output of the pump depends on the speed of rotation and therefore the perfusion rate can be varied but should approximate the resting cardiac output.

The heat exchanger is used to lower or raise the temperature of the blood after it has passed though the pump/oxygenator. In conjunction with suitable drugs, the heat exchanger provides a means of rapidly inducing cardioplegia if required.

The filter is interposed between the cardiotomy reservoir and the venous reservoir. If a bubble oxygenator is used, it is necessary to interpose an arterial filter coated with a defoaming agent, between the oxygenator and the arterial line.

The arterial and venous reservoirs are joined by a recirculation tube to form the reservoir set. The venous reservoir is connected to the filter and cardiotomy reservoir, and has connections for venous drainage from the patient and delivering venous blood to the oxygenator. The arterial reservoir is connected to the exit part of the oxygenator and the arterial line back to the patient.

The cardiotomy reservoir collects blood suctioned from the heart or thoracic cavity. Its functions are to deform and remove debris from blood being returned from the operative site, to the extracorporeal circuit.

Oxygenators

Oxygenators can be divided into two main classes — *bubble oxygenators* and *membrane oxygenators*.

Bubble oxygenators are probably still the most generally used; many bypass procedures world wide are undertaken using this technique. The apparatus is efficient, provides minimal blood trauma, is cost effective and convenient to set up and operate, particularly for shorter routine procedures.

The technique consists simply of oxygenation by diffusing oxygen gas bubbles into venous blood (Fig. 28.3). 'Foaming' will occur, therefore the oxygenated blood must then be 'defoamed' and filtered before it can be returned to the patient. The direct gas and blood contact during lengthy bypass procedures can result in protein denaturation, loss of platelet function and haemolysis.

Membrane oxygenators provide oxygenation by the interposition of a thin, highly gas permeable membrane between the gas and flow of venous blood (Fig. 28.4). A pressure gradient is established, whereby oxygen will diffuse across the membrane into the blood when the partial pressure for oxygen in the ventilating gas is higher than the partial pressure for oxygen in the venous blood. Removal of excess carbon dioxide follows the same principle. If the partial pressure of carbon dioxide (Pco_2) of venous blood is higher than the Pco_2 of the ventilating gas, carbon dioxide will diffuse from the blood across the membrane and out into the ventilating gas.

Three types of membrane oxygenators are presently available:

Plate oxygenators consist of a series of folded rectangular membranes; blood flows on one side of each plate while gas flows on the other (Fig. 28.5). Because of the drag on the surface of the membrane, blood closer to the membrane flows at a lower velocity than that in the centre of the blood path and unfortunately creates a barrier to the transfer of oxygen to the mainstream blood. This is called the boundary effect (Fig. 28.6). Oxygenators use various mechanical methods to minimise this problem. These include mixing screens which provide an uneven blood flow path to increase gas transfer; shims which actually compress the blood

Figs. 28.3–28.9 Principles of bubble and membrane oxygenators. (*The Principles and Benefits of Membrane Oxygenation* — Bentley Edwards.)

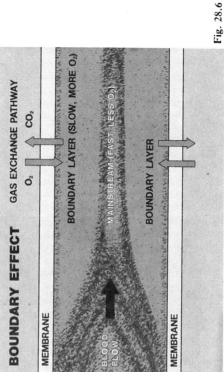

OXYGEN SIDE

PAPER
MESH
MICROPOROUS
POLYPROPYLENE
MEMBRANE

BLOOD SIDE

BLOOD FILM
SPACER

PLATE MEMBRANE

Fig. 28.5

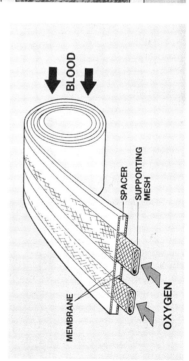

BOUNDARY EFFECT   GAS EXCHANGE PATHWAY

MEMBRANE

O_2 CO_2

BOUNDARY LAYER (SLOW, MORE O_2)

MAINSTREAM (FAST LESS O_2)

BOUNDARY LAYER

BLOOD
FLOW

MEMBRANE

Fig. 28.6

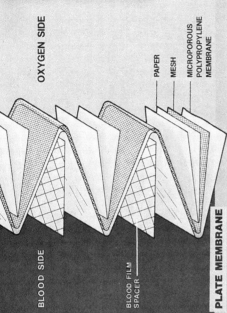

BLOOD
FLOW

OXYGEN

DIFFUSION
PLATE

Fig. 28.3

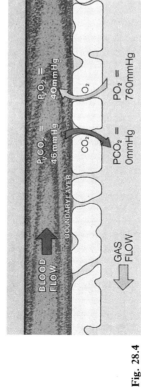

$P_vO_2 =$
40mmHg

O_2

$PO_2 =$
760mmHg

$P_vCO_2 =$
46mmHg

CO_2

$PCO_2 =$
0mmHg

BOUNDARY LAYER

BLOOD
FLOW

GAS
FLOW

Fig. 28.4

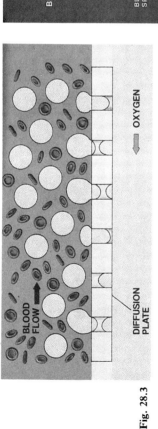

BLOOD

SPACER
SUPPORTING
MESH

MEMBRANE

OXYGEN

Fig. 28.7

Fig. 28.3 Bubble oxygenation which diffuses gas bubbles into venous blood. **Fig. 28.4** Membrane oxygenation where venous blood flows along one side of the membrane and gas on the other side. **Fig. 28.5** Plate oxygenators showing the plate membrane. **Fig. 28.6** The boundary layer effect on gas exchange. **Fig. 28.7** Coil oxygenator.

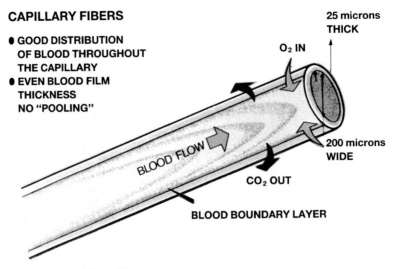

Fig. 28.8   Capillary fibres used in capillary oxygenators.

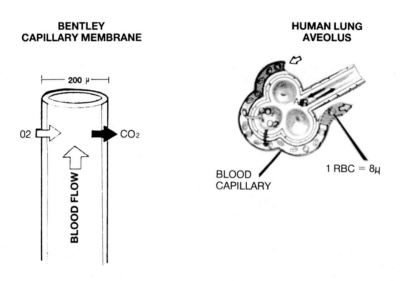

Fig. 28.9   Gas exchange in Bentley capillary oxygenator and human lung.

film into a thinner surface, thus making gas transfer more efficient; and pulsing devices which agitate the blood in the oxygenator.

Coil oxygenators are similar to plate oxygenators except that the ventilating gas flows in a spiral through a series of sheet membranes, while blood flows on a parallel axis to the cylinder (Fig. 28.7).

Capillary oxygenators employ thousands of cylindrically shaped, hollow, microporous fibres through which the blood flows; the ventilating gas surrounds each fibre. A separate blood phase is created inside the fibres and a gas phase outside the fibres. The uniformly thin fibres provide a maximum blood film thickness of 100 microns (distance from the centre of the fibre channel to the surface of the fibre membrane) (Figs. 28.8–28.9).

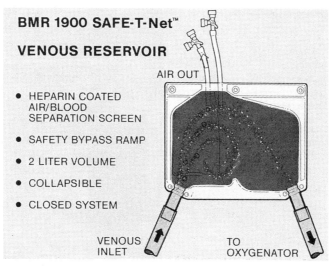

Fig. 28.10 BMR venous blood reservoir. (Bentley Edwards.)

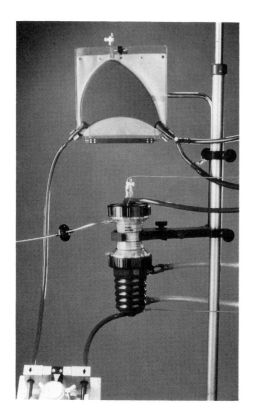

Fig. 28.11 *Top* — venous blood reservoir.
Middle — capillary oxygenator.
Bottom — roller pump.

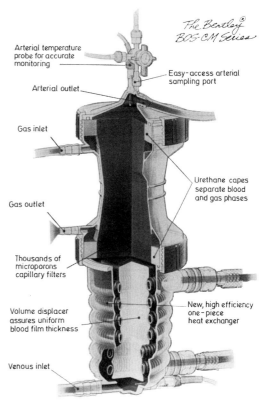

Fig. 28.12 Capillary membrane oxygenator.
(BOS-CM, Bentley Edwards.)

Capillary oxygenators require no mixing screens or other mechanical assist devices. Each fibre acts as an independent oxygenation column so that a loss in a few fibres will not significantly affect performance. In addition, the cylindrical shape of the membrane provides maximum frontal surface area so that excellent gas transfer capabilities may be designed into a relatively compact apparatus. An example of this type of oxygenator is the Bentley BOS-CM System.

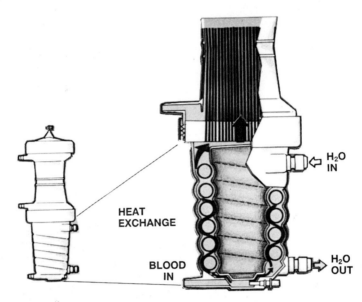

Fig. 28.13 Capillary membrane oxygenator — flow dynamics, heat exchange module. (BOS-CM, Bentley Edwards.)

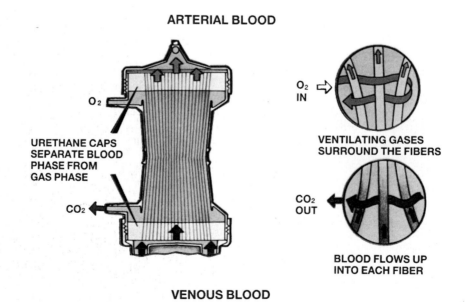

Fig. 28.14 Capillary membrane oxygenator — flow dynamics, oxygenation module. (BOS-CM, Bentley Edwards.)

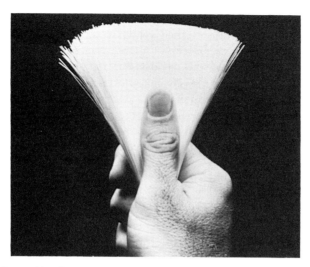

Fig. 28.15 Capillary fibres which form the oxygenation columns. (BOS-CM, Bentley Edwards.)

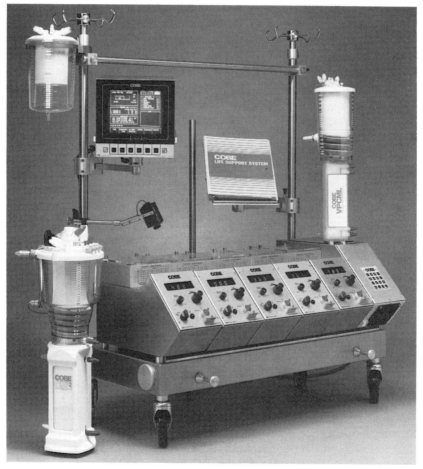

Fig. 28.16 Computerised perfusion control console suitable for use with disposable oxygenators such as the BOS-CM and COBE VPCML and CML2. (COBE Laboratories Inc.)

The BOS-CM system is a single pump system (Fig. 28.2). Venous blood is drained by gravity from the patient into the soft shell venous reservoir (Figs. 28.10 and 28.11). The venous blood is pumped from the reservoir to the oxygenator (Figs. 28.12–28.14), where the blood is temperature regulated and oxygenated, and then delivered to the patient.

Venous reservoir (Fig. 28.10 and Fig. 28.11 top). This provides effective separation of air from blood. Any venous air present enters the reservoir and is directed upwards into the Safe-T-Net separation screen, and continues to the air purge line where it is removed. The 100 micron polyester screen is coated with a thin layer of heparin to inhibit thrombus formation, and to enhance wettability, thereby making the debubbling process more efficient. Should the blood volume level fall, the soft shell of the 1900 ml capacity reservoir collapses, inhibiting the passage of air.

Oxygenator flow dynamics (Figs. 28.13 and 28.14). Venous blood enters the BOS-CM oxygenator at the base. The walls of the oxygenator and hidden volume displacer are moulded to conform to the shape of the heat exchange coil. Blood is then uniformly directed over and around the heat exchanger which provides rapid cooling and thorough rewarming. The corrugated coil is a single piece design which minimises possible water to blood leaks, and is capable of water flow rates of 10 litres per minute at 75 p.s.i. The clear plastic housing permits complete visibility.

The microporous capillary fibres of the BOS-CM capillary membrane permit efficient, controllable gas transfer. There are approximately 50,000 fibres in each oxygenator which function as independent oxygenation columns (Fig. 28.15). The fibres are several inches long and encased at the top and bottom in medical grade urethane (Fig. 28.14). Blood flows through each fibre and the result is a consistent predictable gas transfer.

Figure 28.16 illustrates a computerised perfusion pump control console which is suitable for use either with the BOS-CM perfusion system or other membrane systems such as the COBE, VPCML and CML2.

Cannulation

Cannulation is performed as a prelude to connecting the patient to the heart/lung machine. Venous blood is collected either from the superior and inferior venae cavae or the right atrium. If the venae cavae are cannulated Portex polyvinyl catheters 8 mm ($\frac{5}{16}$ in) are used; cannulation of the right atrium requires a larger size of catheter, 13 mm ($\frac{1}{2}$ in). A further plastic cannula is inserted into the left ventricle and connected to the venous blood reservoir on the heart/lung machine. This collects any blood pooling in the ventricular cavity, and is used to remove air from the heart immediately after bypass is stopped. A further suction line is also used to return aspirated blood into the venous blood reservoir.

Oxygenated arterial blood is returned either to a cannula inserted into the aorta or a cannulated femoral artery. The latter procedure is generally nowadays restricted to cardiopulmonary bypass for the repair of aortic aneurysms, or sometimes in review operations where there may be danger of damaging the heart on re-opening.

During cannulation the polyvinyl catheters are inserted with their obturators in position, an exception being the finer femoral catheters. After insertion, these obturators are removed and the proximal end of the catheter clamped shut. The catheters are then connected to the heart/lung machine with polyvinyl tubing. This is done carefully under a constant flow of sterile saline to ensure air free connections. All tubing is secured to the drapes with sutures or towel clips, to prevent accidental withdrawal of the cannulae. If the myocardium is likely to be deprived of blood while the heart is ischaemic e.g., during aortic valve replacement, coronary cannulae are inserted to perfuse the coronary system. Before going on bypass,

intracardiac pressures are taken with a needle connected to a fluid filled manometer line incorporating a transducer, (this converts pressure to an electrical signal which is then amplified and displayed on a cardiac monitor). Normal values to be expected, are right atrium — 6 mm, right ventricle — 25/0 mm, left atrium — 11 mm, left ventricle — 12/0 mm and aorta — 120/0 mm (Linley, 1976). These values can of course vary considerably in the diseased heart. The measurements are checked again at the end of the procedure.

After total body heparinisation, removal of the clamps on the tubing puts the patients on partial bypass, that is some blood still passes into the heart. Complete bypass is accomplished by passing tourniquets around the venae cavae where they join the heart. These consist of 6 mm ($\frac{1}{4}$ in) wide nylon tape passed around the venae cavae with both ends threaded through a 10 cm (4 in) length of No. 5 rubber tubing. Tightening the rubber tubing down on to the tape constricts the venae cavae and prevents blood entering the heart. The patient is then on total bypass.

Instruments required

Thoracotomy
   General basic
   Sponge holding forceps, (Rampley), 4
   Artery forceps, curved on flat (Kelly Fraser), 50
   Artery forceps, straight, 20 cm (8 in) (Spencer Wells), 10
   Long toothed and non-toothed dissecting forceps, 25 cm (10 in)
   Long dissecting forceps, toothed, fine (Waugh)
   Long dissecting forceps, non-toothed, fine (Waugh)
   Long needle holders, (Potts Smith, Holmes Sellor, etc.) 2
   Long scissors, curved, 25 cm (Nelson)
   Rib approximator (Morriston)
   Sternal saw (splitter), pneumatic
   Lung artery forceps, right angled (O'Shaughnessy), 6
   Lung artery forceps, curved on flat (Roberts or Tudor Edward), 20
   Lung artery forceps, curved on flat (Moynihan, Cholecystectomy) or (Gordon Craig), 6
   Large aneurysm needle (Nelson) right and left, 3 of each
   Deep retactors — various
   Double rib spreader (Tudor Edwards), complete with one set of blades, rib spreader keys, two sets of alternative blades
   Various vascular clamps, Satinsky, Brock, Potts Smith, Craford etc. (pp. 856–857)
   Tissue forceps, Potts, 6
   Suction tubing, nozzles and tube anchoring forceps
   Diathermy leads, electrodes and lead anchoring forceps.
   Graduated jug for saline
   Irrigation syringe and catheter
   Coronary suction tip 2, and tubing
   Assorted stop cocks, connectors and needles, etc.
   Recording catheters and insertion needles
Cannulation and bypass
   Polyvinyl cannulae pressure recording catheters/needles with connections to pressure tubing for cannulation
   Connectors to attach catheters to heart/lung machine tubing
   Nylon tape 6 mm ($\frac{1}{4}$ in) wide, 35 cm (14 in) long with 10 cm (4 in) lengths of No. 5 rubber tubing to act as tourniquets for major vessels

Figs. 28.17 to 28.25   Cardiovascular instruments. (Genito Urinary Manufacturing Co. Ltd.)

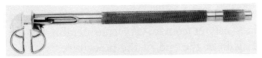

Fig. 28.17   Aorta clamp, Potts-Smith.

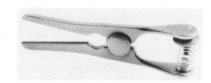

Fig. 28.18   Bulldog clamp, straight, Glover, 6.5 cm (2½ in) long.

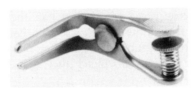

Fig. 28.19   Bulldog clamp, Glover, right angle, 6 cm (2¼ in) long, 27 mm jaw length.

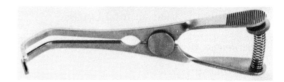

Fig. 28.20   Bulldog clamp, Glover, Satinsky shape jaws, 6.5 cm (2¼ in) long.

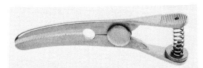

Fig. 28.21   Bulldog clamp, Potts', half-curved, 4 cm blades.

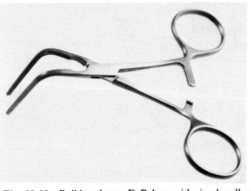

Fig. 28.22   Bulldog clamp, DeBakey, with ring handles, right angle jaws, 10.5 cm (4⅛ in) long.

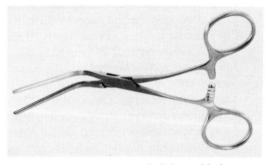

Fig. 28.23   Bulldog clamp, DeBakey, with ring handles, 45° angle jaws, 12.5 cm (5 in) long.

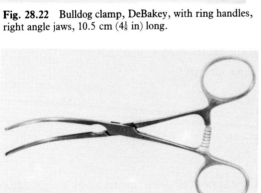

Fig. 28.24   Bulldog clamp, DeBakey, with ring handles, curved on flat, 12.5 cm (5 in) long.

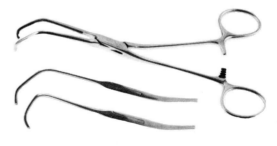

Fig. 28.25   Vessel clamp, Waterston's, delicate model, 16 cm (6½ in) long with 1.5 cm and 2 cm straight portion of jaws.

Figs. 28.26 to 28.31 Cardiovascular instruments (*cont'd.*) (Genito-Urinary Manufacturing Co. Ltd.)

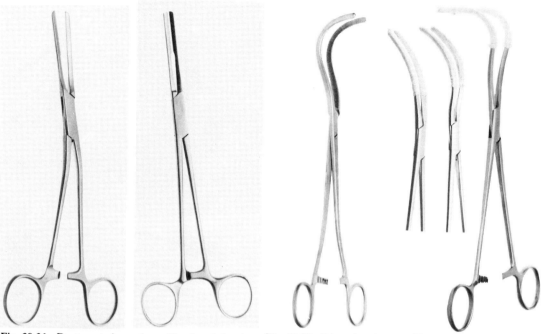

Fig. 28.26 Ductus arteriosus clamp, Potts' angled and straight, 20 cm (8 in) long.

Fig. 28.27 Dissecting clamp, Crafoord's, full curve.

Fig. 28.28 Auricular clamps, Brock's, set of three varying curves.

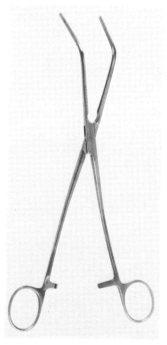

Fig. 28.29 Multi-purpose clamp, DeBakey, obtuse angle 60°, 24 cm (9½ in) long with 4 cm jaws.

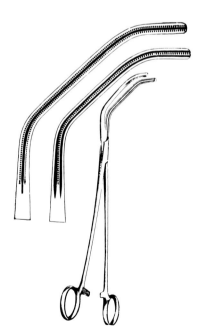

Fig. 28.30 Vascular clamp, Satinsky's, with 4 cm and 5 cm straight portion of jaws.

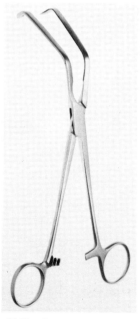

Fig. 28.31 Aorta clamp, Brock's, with Potts' teeth, 4 cm straight portion of jaws.

Figs. 28.32 to 28.39 Cardiovascular instruments. (Genito-Urinary Manufacturing Co. Ltd.)

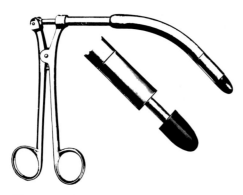

Fig. 28.32 Cardiac punch, Brock's, for infundibular stenosis, 7.5 mm, 10 mm and 12 mm blade.

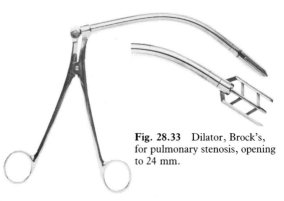

Fig. 28.33 Dilator, Brock's, for pulmonary stenosis, opening to 24 mm.

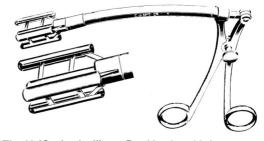

Fig. 28.35 Aortic dilator, Brock's, three blade.

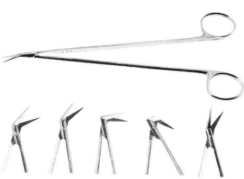

Fig. 28.34 Dissecting scissors, Hedgeman's, delicate, angled on edge 25°, 19 cm (7½ in) long.

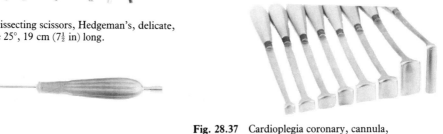

Fig. 28.37 Cardioplegia coronary, cannula, Brainbridge's, 50° and 90° angle, 3.0 mm dia. distal end, with 5 mm olive for ¼ in tubing, stainless steel.

Fig. 28.36 Cardiac retractors, Brainbridge's, 23 cm (9 in) long.

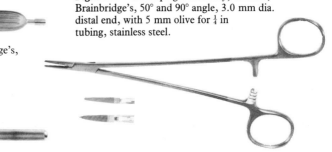

Fig. 28.38 Needle holder, Abrams, modified Sellors', for fine non-traumatic needles, 20 cm (8 in) long.

Fig. 28.39 Needle holder, DeBakey, with extended ring on one side, 19 cm (7¾ in) long.

Closure

3 or 2.5 or 2 (0 or 2/0 or 3/0) Synthetic absorbable, non-absorbable, silk or chromic catgut on medium half-circle round-bodied needle for pericardium retraction and closure sutures

2.5 to 0.7 (2/0 to 6/0) Synthetic non-absorbable or silk, on small curved non-traumatic round-bodied or taper-cut needle for vascular sutures, valve replacements and closure of the atrium. The size varies according to the vessel and surgeon's preference. A size 3(0) may be used for closing ventricular incisions, combined with a Teflon felt reinforcing buttress. This may also be used as a purse-string suture for the cannulation sites, and appendage in closed mitralvalvulotomy.

4, 5 or 6 (1, 2 or 3) Chromic catgut or synthetic non-absorbable or silk for ligatures

4, 5 or 6 (1, 2 or 3) Chromic catgut or stainless steel wire on large half-circle round bodied needles for sternal closure

4 (1) Chromic catgut or synthetic absorbable on medium half circle cutting needles for muscle

2.5 or 3 (2/0 or 0) Chromic catgut or synthetic/absorbable for sub-cutaneous sutures

3 (0) Synthetic non-absorbable or curved or straight cutting needles for skin.

Drainage tubing for pericardium and pleural cavity (if opened).

Special instruments

Valvulotomy

Dilators, valvulotomes (Brock, etc.), various sizes

Scissors, angled (Potts), set of 3

Leaflet retractors

Valve replacement

Prosthetic heart valve, e.g., Starr Edwards, heterograft

Valve holder

Scissors, angled (Potts), set of 3

Suture to secure valve, usually 2.5 (2/0) synthetic non-absorbable on double ended 25 mm taper cut non-traumatic needle

Septal defects

Teflon or similar prosthetic repair material for patch

Suitable sutures are detailed above.

Types of valve replacement. Often by the time the patient presents himself for the treatment of an acquired heart valve malfunction, the valves are so affected by calcification or disorganisation, that valve replacement, not repair is the preferred procedure (Paneth, 1975).

Replacement valves can be considered under two headings:

1. *Mechanical valves* — (a) ball and socket, e.g., Starr-Edwards, De Bakey, Magovera-Cromie., (b) Floating discs, e.g., Bjork-Shiley.

2. *Biological valves* — (a) homograft fresh free or mounted, and preserved free or mounted; (b) heterograft preserved mounted.

The mechanical valves in group 1, although having superior mechanical durability compared with the biological graft, exhibit thrombogenic tendency to a greater or lesser degree. This requires anti-coagulant therapy for an indefinite period.

Conversely although biological valves have a greater mechanical failure rate, they are for all practical purposes free from the danger of formulation of thrombus. Patients do not require anticoagulant therapy to avoid thrombus interfering with valve function or causing systemic embolism.

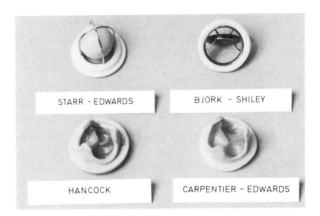

STARR - EDWARDS

BJORK - SHILEY

HANCOCK

CARPENTIER - EDWARDS

Fig. 28.40   Heart valve replacements. (Courtesy E. Lockie and *Nursing Times.*)

Preparation of homograft is difficult and time consuming. They must be removed within 12 hours of death and after antibiotic sterilization, are stored at 4°C for a limited period; usually not more than 14 days.

There has been an increasing use of heterograft valves, in the form of porcine valves, prepared in gluteraldehyde and mounted on a frame (Lockie, 1975; Pagliero, 1975). These pig valves are preserved by a special tanning technique to render the valve leaflets more durable. They are not viable when implanted but this is not disadvantageous compared with initially viable homograft. Examination of implanted valves after predetermined periods has shown that the viable valves quickly lost all living cells. In addition, homografts in many instances became distorted and damaged, probably due to inflammatory rejection, whereas this was avoided by non-viable valve transplant (Lockie, 1976).

Careful consideration is necessary before deciding whether a hetero valve graft or a mechanical valve should be the method of choice. For example, a young woman of child bearing age may be more suitable for a heterograft to avoid continuous anticoagulant therapy. Similarly, a manual labourer may be subjected to frequent minor injuries, especially to his limbs (Gilbert, 1972). In cases of re-operation due to failure of a valve graft, the patient may demand the superior durability of a mechanical valve. In all instances meticulous care, in preparation of grafts, sterilisation and surgical technique are paramount in rate of success.

Procedures

Mitral valvulotomy. The chest is opened through a right posterior lateral incision (Fig. 28.41) or median sternotomy split. The pleura is opened with scissors and a rib spreader inserted. With the posterior lateral approach it may be necessary to resect a rib; the lung is retracted.

For closed valvulotomy. The pericardium is incised and retracted with interrupted silk sutures. The left appendage is identified and an appendage clamp applied. A purse-string suture may be placed in position beneath the clamp. An opening is made in the appendage tip and the clamp loosened to admit the surgeon's finger. (The purse-string suture may be tightened if there is a leak of blood.) If dilatation of the stenosed valve is impossible with the surgeon's finger, he withdraws it and inserts a dilator. After adequate dilatation has been accomplished, the dilator is removed and the appendage clamp applied. The opening in the

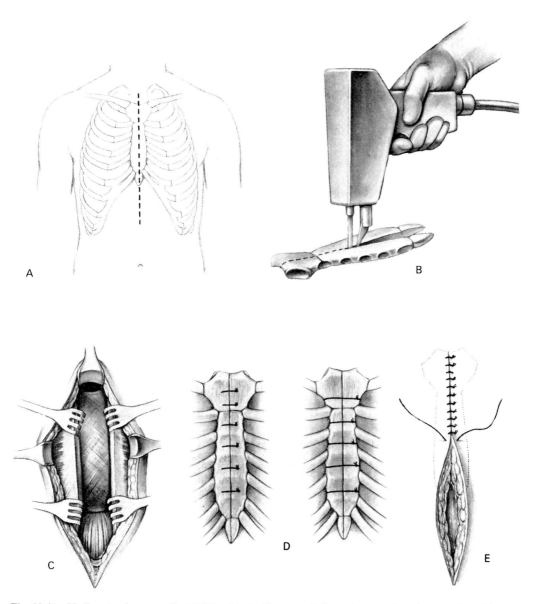

Fig. 28.41 Median sterniotomy split. (A) The skin incision extends from the sternal notch to a point midway between the xyphoid and the umbilicus. (B) A pneumatic saw is utilised to split the sternum. (C) The split sternum is separated to expose the pericardium. (D) Closure of the sternum can be accomplished by sutures passed through holes in the sternum or by encircling sutures. (E) The subcutaneous tissue and skin are closed. (*A Digest of Cardiac and Vascular Procedures*, Ethicon Ltd.)

appendage tip is closed with two rows of 2 (3/0) synthetic non-absorbable or silk on non-traumatic needles.

Alternatively, a dilator may be passed from the ventricle. In this case the instrument is introduced through the ventricle wall, and after dilatation the opening in the myocardium is closed with 2 (3/0) synthetic non-absorbable or silk on non-traumatic needles.

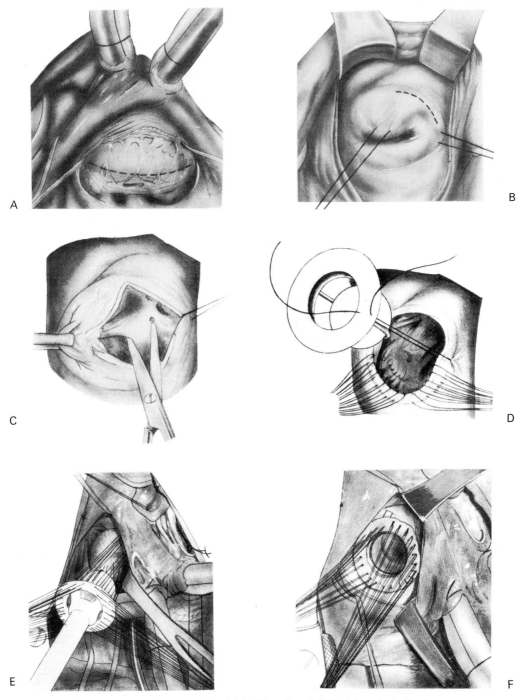

Fig. 28.42 Mitral valve replacement (A) left atrial incision. (B and C) Excision of mitral valve — stay sutures placed in mitral leaflets to facilitate exposure, excision started along attached margin of aortic leaflet, division of posterior papillary complex, followed by division of anterior papillary complex and incision of remaining attached portions of the aortic and mural leaflets. (D) Doubled armed sutures in position through mural leaflet portion of the mitral annulus, sutures being placed through the remainder of annulus, method of attachment to cloth portion of valve prosthesis. (E and F) All sutures in position, prosthesis is passed down into its bed. (Cleland: *Surgery–Thorax.*)

The pericardium is irrigated with warm saline and sutured with interrupted 2 (3/0) silk on round-bodied needle. The chest is closed in the usual manner.

For open valvulotomy the chest is entered through a right posterior lateral incision or mediastinal split, the pericardium is opened and secured to the chest wall with 2 or 2.5 (3/0 or 2/0) synthetic non-absorbable or silk etc.

After the establishment of total bypass, an incision is made into the left atrium. The mitral valve is opened under direct vision and the atrium then closed with 3 (0) synthetic non-absorbable or silk. The patient is put onto partial bypass by releasing the venae cavae tourniquets, clamps are then placed on the tubing leading to the heart/lung machine and the bypass is discontinued. Filling of the heart chambers is started before the final sutures are tied, in order to evacuate the air. After removing the cannulae, the incisions in the atrium are closed with 3 (0) synthetic non-absorbable or silk, and the chest is closed in the routine manner.

Mitral valve replacement. Similar to the above except the valve is excised and a valve prosthesis inserted and secured with 2.5 (2/0) synthetic non-absorbable or silk.

Mitral valvuloplasty. Similar to valvulotomy except the incompetent valve is plicated with sutures of 2 or 2.5 (3/0 or 2/0) synthetic non-absorbable or silk.

Tricuspid valvulotomy, valvuloplasty, or valve replacement. Essentially the same as the mitral procedures described except the right atrium is opened to visualise the valve.

Aortic valvuloplasty or valve replacement. During this procedure, which is performed under bypass, the normal coronary circulation will be compromised. It is essential to incorporate coronary perfusion in the bypass and this can be accomplished in several ways. A tube from the main arterial supply is split into two with a Y connection. The two tubes are then used to perfuse both coronary arteries, one method being via hand-held metal suction ends.

The venous blood is collected from the right atrium via a 13 mm ($\frac{1}{2}$ in) Portex polyvinyl atrium catheter. Total bypass is accomplished by clamping the main pulmonary artery. Frequently the bypass is combined with hypothermia to minimise the hazards associated with interrupting the normal coronary blood supply.

After establishing complete bypass the aorta is clamped, incised and coronary perfusion started. Aortic valvulotomy, reconstructive valvuloplasty or valve replacement is then performed using 2.5 (2/0) synthetic non-absorbable etc. on a 17 taper cut needle. After this has been completed the aorta is closed rapidly, for in order to do so the coronary perfusion has to be stopped. Saline 'slush' is often put into the chest cavity to produce some local hypothermia thereby protecting the myocardium until normal coronary circulation is started. Partial bypass is started by unclamping the pulmonary artery, and when the patient's condition is satisfactory, this is discontinued and the chest closed in the normal manner. The sternum is generally approximated with stainless steel wire size No. 25 SWG.

Pulmonary valvulotomy. This can be performed under hypothermia without cardiopulmonary bypass. The approach is through a sternal splitting incision with the patient supine. Tape tourniquets are placed in position round the major vessels (aorta, venae cavae and pulmonary vessels).

A Potts clamp (which constricts only one third of the vessel lumen) is placed on the pulmonary artery a few centimetres from the valve, and a longitudinal incision of about 2 cm is made in the segment held by the clamp. The heart is emptied of blood by tightening the tourniquets on the venae cavae, and when the chambers are empty the pulmonary artery and aorta are occluded. A careful note is made of the time that the tourniquets are applied. Pulmonary valvulotomy is then performed under direct vision after removing the Potts clamp. This is then reapplied to the pulmonary artery and the circulation started again, usually within 3 minutes or so of its cessation, by releasing the tourniquets. (First the venae

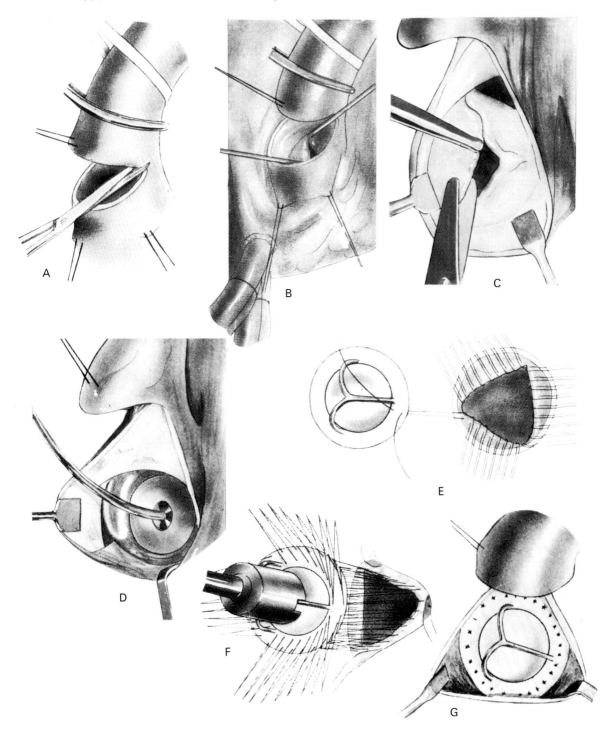

Fig. 28.43 Aortic valve replacement. (A and B) Aortic cross-clamped, opened transversely; aortic valve being palpated. (C) Excision of aortic valve. (D) Measurement of aortic root and annulus to determine type of prosthesis. (E and F) Double armed sutures are used to secure cloth edge of valve prosthesis, these are tied after the valve (G) has been passed down in place. (Cleland: *Surgery–Thorax*.)

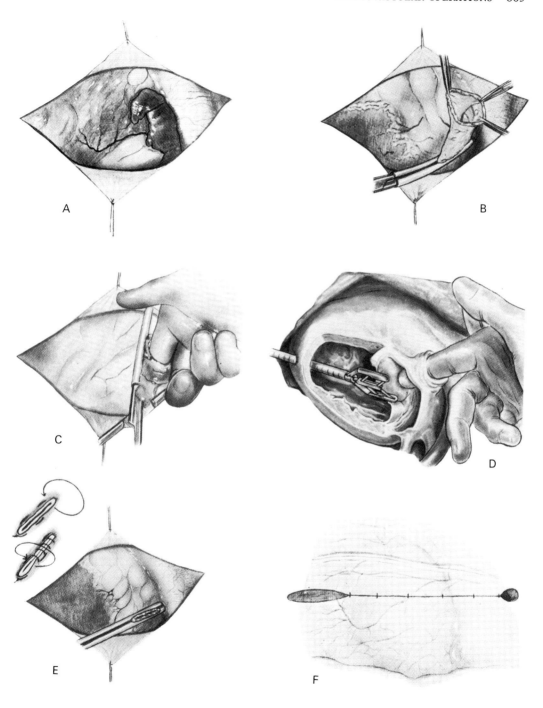

Fig. 28.44 Mitral valvulotomy. (A) Non crushing clamp applied to base of appendage, tip of appendage amputated to provide a lumen sufficient to admit index finger to second interphalangeal joint. (B) Momentary release of clamp to wash out any loose thrombi. (C) Palpation of valve; it may be possible to dilate the valve with the index finger or dilator from this approach. (D) Transventricular dilatation. (E and F) Suture of appendage. Inset in (F) Suture of the pericardium. (Cleland: *Surgery–Thorax.*)

cavae constrictions are released, then the pulmonary artery side clamp is applied, and finally the pulmonary artery and aorta tourniquets released.) The opening in the pulmonary artery is closed with 1 (5/0) synthetic non-absorbable or silk on a non-traumatic needle. If ventricular fibrillation is present, this is dealt with by electrical stimulation.

It should be noted that various arterial clamps may be used to occlude the major vessels as an alternative to tourniquets.

With the indirect Bourie procedure, a Bisch dilator (or Bisch knife) is passed into the right ventricle through the myocardium, pushed through the valve, opened 15 or 20 mm, thereby dilating the valve or cutting in two planes. The opening in the myocardium is closed with 2 (3/0) synthetic non-absorbable or silk etc. on a non-traumatic needle.

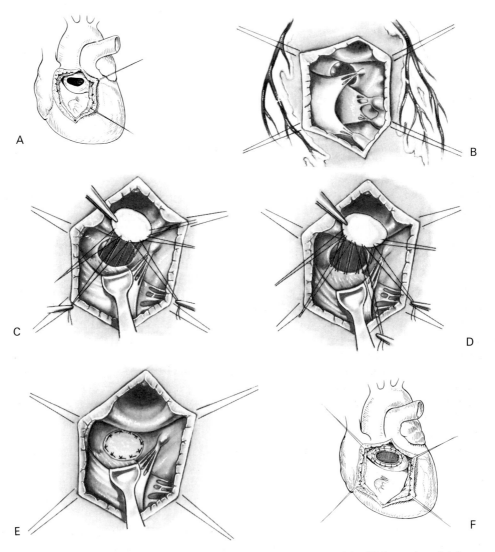

Fig. 28.45 Ventricular septal defect. (A) Seen through incision in right ventricle. (B) Inspection of defect before repair. (C and D) Mattress sutures are first placed in the margins of the defect and through the Teflon patch. (E and F) When all sutures are passed, the patch is lowered down and the sutures tied. Additional reinforcing sutures may be required after testing for completeness of closure. (Cleland: *Surgery–Thorax.*)

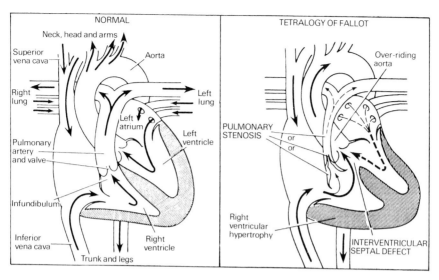

Fig. 28.46 Normal heart and vessels as compared with characteristics of Tetralogy of Fallot. (Courtesy Evans and *Nursing Times*.)

Intraventricular pressures are reassessed, and the pericardium is irrigated and closed as described before.

The chest is closed in the normal way.

Atrial septal defect. One of the most common of the congenital cardiac defects, it causes shunting of blood from the left to the right side of the heart. The gradual pressure build up and volume in the right heart and increased pulmonary resistance eventually causes a reverse of this shunt from right to left with consequent right heart failure. Surgical treatment of this condition consists of repairing the defect under direct vision, with complete bypass.

The approach is normally via a sternal splitting incision and the procedure approximates that for open mitral valvulotomy. A thoracotomy approach may be adopted for young females for cosmetic reasons. The right atrium is opened and the intraseptal defect either sutured, or repaired with a Teflon patch. The atrioventricular valves may also require some reconstructive surgery. The atrium is closed with 3 (0) synthetic non-absorbable or silk, bypass discontinued and the chest closed in the usual manner.

Ventricular septal defect. This again produces a left to right shunt of blood within the heart which may eventually 'balance' due to an increase in the right ventricular and pulmonary pressures. The reconstructive procedure is similar to repair of atrial septal defect except that the right ventricle is incised, and is closed with 3 (0) synthetic non-absorbable or silk combined with Teflon patches.

Tetralogy of Fallot. This is a simultaneous occurrence of pulmonary stenosis, intraventricular septal defect, dextraposition of the aorta and hypertrophy of the right ventricle. This resuts in increased pressure within the right ventricle due to pulmonary stenosis and a right to left shunt of blood via the ventricular septal defect with decreased oxygenation of the systemic blood.

The corrective procedure is similar to aortic valvulotomy under direct vision, and repair of the ventricular septal defect. The patient is placed on complete bypass.

During all open heart surgery it is generally necessary to arrest the heart beat by using a fibrillator which administers a constant D.C. shock. The effect is reversed with a defibrillator.

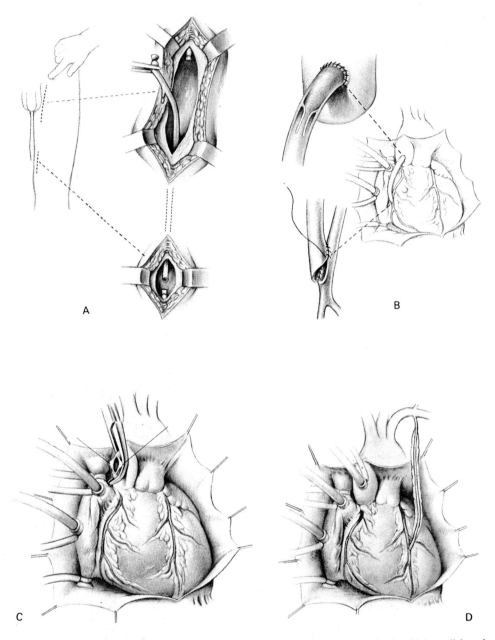

Fig. 28.47 Coronary artery bypass — saphenous vein. (A) Two incisions are made in the thigh medial to the femoral pulse. The saphenous vein is ligated and cut, then withdrawn through the upper incision. (B) A median sternotomy incision is made. The heart is cannulated through right atrial incisions near the superior and inferior vena cavae. Return cannula is placed in the ascending aorta or femoral artery. The proximal aorta is partially clamped to isolate site for creation of ostium. (C) The saphenous vein, reversed flow direction, is sutured to the aortic ostium. Care is taken that the distal end is used so valves do not interfere with blood flow. The bypass is completed by an end-to-side anastomosis to the coronary artery at a point distal to the obstruction. The purse string sutures are tied and the cannula entrances repaired. The internal mammary artery may be used for bypass procedure instead of the saphenous vein. After dissection of the artery from its origin, the vessel is connected end-to-side, to the coronary artery distal to the area of obstruction. (D) The pericardium is not reapproximated; however, the vein graft or the internal mammary artery graft is protected by loosely inherent pericardium or pleura. (*A Digest of Cardiac and Vascular Procedures*, Ethicon Ltd.)

Revascularisation of the coronary arteries. There are several operations carried out in the surgical treatment of coronary heart disease. Varied success has been reported on performing myocardial mammary artery implantation, coronary endarterectomy, and saphenous vein graft between the aorta and coronary artery beyond the blocked segment (Rowe, 1978). Of these, the latter procedure has gained a degree of popularity in the United Kingdom (Waugh, 1975). An appropriate length of long saphenous vein is removed from either leg, and the cut side branches are ligated; it is then placed in heparinised saline solution. Alternatively, if the patient has had an operation for varicose veins, the vein graft may be removed from the arm.

The heart is approached through a sternum-splitting incision; the pericardium is opened and cardio pulmonary bypass established. An 1 cm incision is made longitudinally in the coronary artery beyond the stenosed segment. The end of the vein graft is cut obliquely and anastomosed end-to-side to the slit in the coronary artery, using 0.75 (6/0) synthetic non-absorbable. It is essential to ensure that the vein is anastomosed the correct way round i.e., valves opening towards the coronary anastomosis.

The vein graft is then cut to the required length, and anastomosed end-to-side to the aorta after removing a 7 mm disc of aortic wall. If necessary, further bypass grafts are inserted and the heart is then allowed to take over the circulation, cardio pulmonary bypass being discontinued.

Great care is taken to secure haemostasis. Heparinisation of the patient is reversed and drainage tubes inserted in the pericardial cavity and chest cavity just behind the sternum. The chest is closed in the usual way.

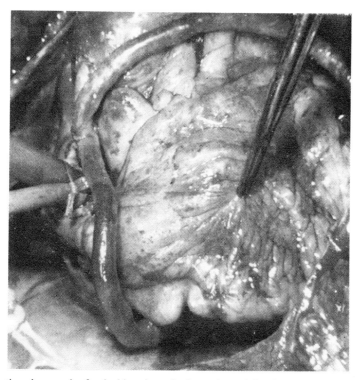

Fig. 28.48 Operative photograph of a double vein graft. One vein graft has been attached to the aorta, whereas the other has been attached to the previously inserted vein graft as an end-to-side anastomosis. It courses transversely across the field to connect to the anterior descending coronary artery. The initial graft was anastomosed distally to the termination of the right coronary artery. (Irvine: *Modern Trends in Surgery.*)

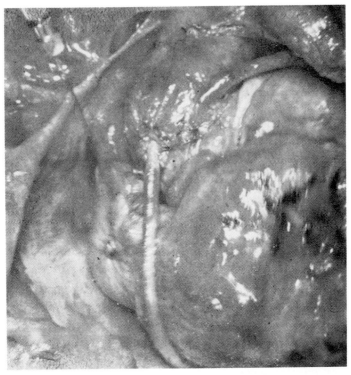

Fig. 28.49   Operative photograph of double vein grafts implanted in the aorta. The vein graft in the centre of the field was anastomosed distally to the anterior descending coronary artery, while the graft in the upper right portion of the field was attached to the circumflex coronary artery. (Irvine: *Modern Trends in Surgery.*)

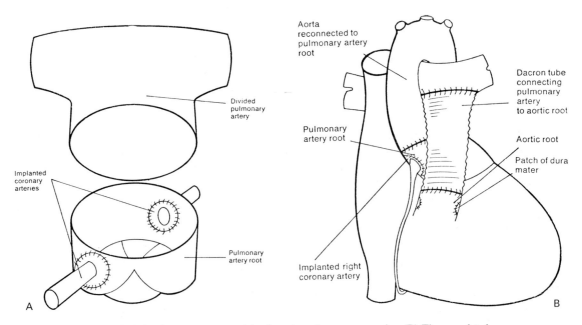

Fig. 28.50   (A) Divided pulmonary artery and implantation of coronary arteries. (B) The completed 'transposition' operation. Aorta connected to left ventricle, pulmonary artery connected to right ventricle. (Foster: *Nursing Times.*)

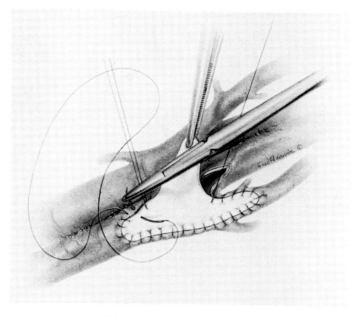

Fig. 28.51   Synthetic vascular patch. (GORETEX, W. L. Gore and Associates (UK) Ltd.)

Transposition of the great arteries. (TGA) One of the commonest forms of cyanotic congenital cardiac defects, TGA generally consists of the aorta arising from the right ventricle and the pulmonary artery from the left ventricle. The result of this is two completely separate circulations, and for a baby to survive at birth a ventricular septal defect, (VSD) atral septal defect (ASD) or patent ductus arteriosus must be present (Foster and Hibbert, 1977).

For many years the only operative surgery possible consisted of a physiological type of correction, where the pulmonary venous blood was redirected to the right ventricle and systemic venous return redirected into the left ventricle (Mustard operation). Now in certain cases, it is possible to transpose the great arteries to their anatomically correct ventricles.

The pulmonary artery is divided transversely above the pulmonary valve. The right ventricle is incised and the ASD or VSD repaired with a Dacron patch. The right and left coronary arteries are excised with a disc of aorta, and anastomosed to the sides of the pulmonary artery root. The holes left in the aorta are repaired either with a patch of Dacron, reinforced expanded polytetra fluoroethylene (Gore-Tex) or Dura mater. The aorta is then divided and anastomosed to the pulmonary artery root.

To achieve continuity between the aortic root and the pulmonary artery, it is usual to interpose a connecting Dacron tube. The cardiopulmonary bypass is discontinued and the chest closed in the usual manner.

Thoracic aortic aneurysm. This is performed through a left posteriolateral thoracotomy.

With the repair procedure, the distal portion of the aneurysm is clamped across both proximally and distally. The aorta is divided and sutured circumferentially back on itself to close the false channel. The aorta is then re-anastomosed.

Replacement with a graft of woven Dacron or aortic homograft is accomplished after excising the aneurysm between two aortic clamps. The graft is sutured with 2.5 (2/0) synthetic non-absorbable.

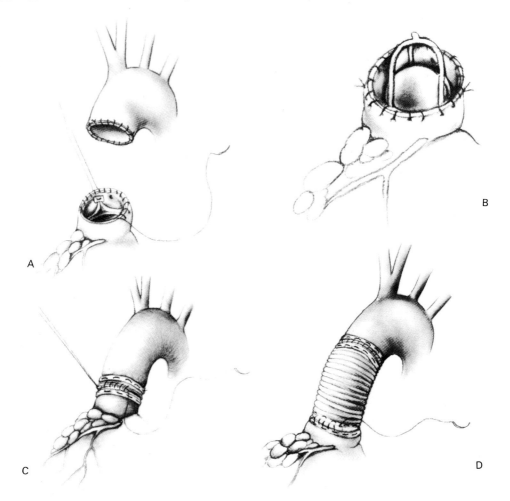

Fig. 28.52   Thoracic aortic aneurysm. (A) The aorta is divided through the intimal tear, and catheters inserted into one or both coronary artery orifices for perfusion with cooled blood from the oxygenator. The separated intima and adventibia are sutured circumferentially. (B) It may be necessary to insert a valve prosthesis if the aortic valve has been deformed. (C) Anastomosis of the aorta. (D) Insertion of a Teflon aortic graft. (Cleland: *Surgery–Thorax.*)

Correction of patent ductus arteriosus

Definition

The ligation or division of a patent ductus which is a remnant of foetal circulation and allows blood to pass from the aorta into the pulmonary artery.

Position

Right lateral chest (Fig. 5.14).

Instruments

As for thoracotomy (p. 829)
   Ductus clamps (Potts) 3

Aortic clamp (Potts)
Large bulldog clamps (Potts), 3
Scissors, angled (Potts Smith), set of 3
Long needle holders (Potts Smith or Holmes Sellor, etc.), 2
Irrigation syringe, rubber catheter and sterile warm saline
Nylon tape or fine rubber tubing prepared for tourniquets
Routine thoracotomy ligatures and sutures
Sterile liquid paraffin
3 (0) synthetic non-absorbable or silk for ligation of ductus
2 (3/0) Synthetic non-absorbable or silk on a small half-circle round-bodied needle for mediastinal pleura
1 (5/0) Synthetic non-absorbable or silk on a small curved non-traumatic needle for ductus suture.

Outline of procedure

A left posterolateral incision is made and the chest entered through the fourth interspace or the bed of a resected fifth rib. A rib spreader is inserted and the lung retracted to expose the region of the ductus and the mediastinal pleura which is incised.

The aortic arch and pulmonary artery are dissected free on both sides of the ductus, using blunt and sharp dissection. In order to allow adequate mobilisation, some small vessels in the ductus region may require ligation. The vagus nerve is identified and retracted with tape or rubber tubing.

The ductus may be ligated with 3(0) synthetic non-absorbable or silk ligatures or ligaclips (page 231) which are placed at the aortic and pulmonary end of the ductus. Alternatively, the ductus may be divided after placing ductus clamps near to the pulmonary artery and aortic junction. With the latter method, the ductus is then divided and the ends closed with a continuous 1 (5/0) synthetic non-absorbable or silk on a non-traumatic needle, followed by an outer layer of interrupted sutures.

The clamps are then removed, haemostasis is secured and the mediastinal pleura sutured over the operation area with 2 (3/0) synthetic non-absorbable or silk. The chest cavity is irrigated with saline and the thorax closed in the usual manner, with underwater drainage.

Correction of coarctation of the aorta

Definition

Resection of a congenital narrowing of the arch or descending part of the aorta, and re-establishment of aortic continuity by end to end anastomosis.

Position

Right lateral chest (Fig. 5.14).

Instruments

As for thoracotomy (p. 829)
    Coarctation clamps, straight and curved (Craoford, Potts, etc.), 2 of each
    Clamps (Blalock), 2

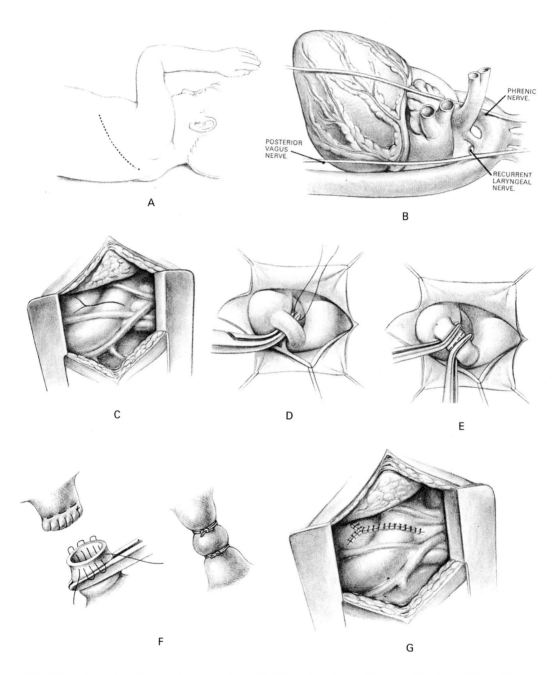

Fig. 28.53 Correction of patent ductus arteriosus. (*A Digest of Cardiac and Vascular Procedures, Ethicon Ltd.*)
(A) The approach is through a left posterior lateral incision. (B) The relationship of the nerves that are
encountered is shown. (C) An incision is made through the mediastinal pleura and the pleura is retracted.
(D) The patent ductus is freed by blunt dissection, and an encircling suture positioned. (E) The ductus is
clamped prior to occlusion if it is to be divided. (F) Two methods of occluding patent ductus arteriosus, namely
division and double ligation. (G) The mediastinal pleura is closed.

Large bulldog clamps (Potts), 6
Various other arterial clamps (Blalock, etc.)
Long dissecting forceps, toothed, fine (Waugh)
Long dissecting forceps, non-toothed, fine (Waugh)
Long fine scissors (tonsil or McIndoe)
Long needle holders (Potts Smith for Holmes Sellor, etc.), 2
Irrigation syringe, rubber catheter and sterile warm saline
Nylon tape or fine rubber tubing prepared for tourniquets
Routine thoracotomy ligatures and sutures
Sterile liquid paraffin
2 (3/0) Synthetic non-absorbable or silk on a small half-circle round-bodied needle for
    mediastinal pleura
1 (5/0) Synthetic non-absorbable or silk on a small curved non-traumatic needle for
    anastomosis
Prepared homograft or fabric prosthesis may be required (Chapter 27).

Outline of procedure

A left posterolateral incision is made and haemostasis of the many collateral vessels is
secured. The chest is entered through the fourth interspace or bed of a resected fifth rib.
A rib spreader is inserted, the lung retracted, and the mediastinal pleura incised to expose
the aortic arch. The aorta is freed by sharp and blunt dissection and tapes or rubber tubing
passed above and below the stenosed area. Alternatively, arterial clamps may be employed.

Vessels which leave the aorta at the point of resection are ligated, and this may include
the left subclavian artery which commonly rises at the stenosis.

The vagus nerve is identified and retracted before applying coarctation clamps or Blalock
clamps above and below the stenosed segment, which is then excised. The gap is closed
either by end to end anastomosis with 1 (5/0) synthetic non-absorbable or silk, or the interposition of a homograft or fabric (Teflon) tube prosthesis. The homograft or fabric prosthesis
is anastomosed to each end of the cut aorta in the usual manner.

Haemostasis secured, the mediastinal pleura is sutured over the operation area, and the
chest cavity irrigated before closing in the usual manner, with underwater drainage.

Heart transplantation

Note: Human orthoptic cardiac transplantation is now (Laguea *et al.*, 1979) a well established procedure (Ballinger *et al.*, 1972; Jamieson *et al.*, 1979; Laguea *et al.*; 1979; Jamieson
and Stinson, 1985; Cory Pearce, 1981). The ethical aspects of donor selection and the problems of immune reaction will remain for some time to come, although great advances have
been made during the past decade.

Position and instruments

As for major intra cardiac surgery (p. 855).

Outline of procedure

Donor operation. Until 1979, it was necessary to undertake a transplant immediately
following removal of the donor heart in an adjacent operating theatre. However, following

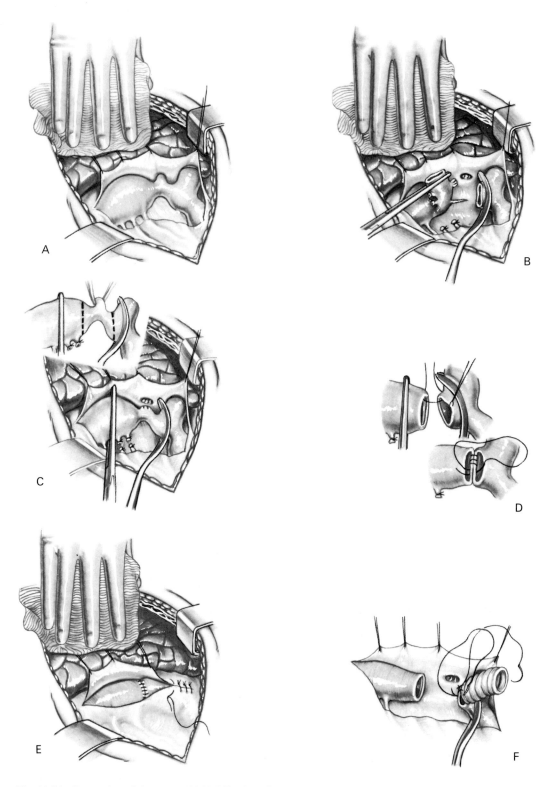

Fig. 28.54 Coarctation of the aorta. (A) Mobilization of the aorta. (B) Control of the right intercostal arteries. (C) Occlusion of the aorta and excision of coarctation. (D) Anastomosis. (E) Removal of clamps — additional sutures may be required to control oozing. (F) Teflon graft replacement for long coarctations. (Cleland: *Surgery–Thorax.*)

the development of a technique at Stanford University Medical Centre, California (Jamieson *et al.*, 1979), it is now quite usual to remove donor hearts in distant centres and transport them within three hours to the recipient. This is provided the myocardial temperature is reduced sufficiently to preserve the donor heart.

In this instance, a cardiac team travels to the hospital concerned to remove the heart. A thorough examination of the donor is undertaken to exclude congenital cardiac defects or cardiac trauma. If the donor is suitable, he is taken to the operating theatre where the heart is exposed and thoroughly examined. After pronouncement of death, heparine is administered, the heart arrested, followed by infusion of cold cardioplegic solution through the coronary arteries. After mobilisation, the venae cavae and pulmonary veins are divided at the atrium. Transection of the pulmonary artery is carried out following division of the atrial septum. The aorta is divided beyond the coronary ostia, the heart filled with cold cardioplegic solution, and placed in cold saline at 4°C. Transferring to several further bowls of cold saline ensures maximum cooling. The heart is finally placed in a sterile plastic bag of cold saline, covered with several more sterile plastic bags and stored in an ice container for rapid transport to the recipient.

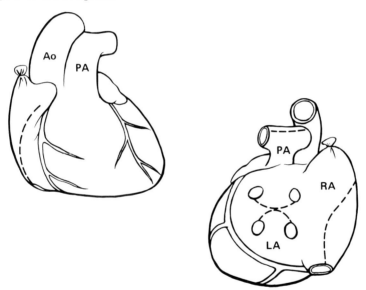

Fig. 28.55 Preparation of the donor heart. The superior vena cava is tied. The right and left pulmonary arteries are opened opposite the main pulmonary artery. The pulmonary veins are joined to open out the left atrium. A curved linear is made in the right atrium for subsequent anastomosis (avoiding the sinu-atrial node). (Russell: *Recent Advances in Surgery.*)

Throughout this procdure, communication is maintained with the recipient hospital so that removal of the donor heart can be coordinated with the start of the recipient operation.

Recipient operation. On arrival, the donor heart is removed from the protective bags, and still kept in cold saline, is dissected and tailored to fit the recipient vessels. This usually consists of trimming fat off the aorta and pulmonary artery, followed by an incision from the inferior vena cava towards the superior vena cava, curving upwards to the right atrial appendage and avoiding the sinuatrial node (Jamieson *et al.*, 1979). This opens up the right atrium. The left atrium is then opened up by incisions connecting the pulmonary veins on the posterior surface of the heart.

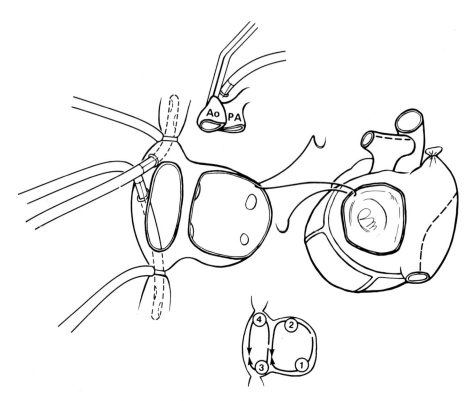

Fig. 28.56 Implantation of the heart. The anastomosis is begun at the level of the upper pulmonary vein (the left atrial appendage in the donor). The sequence of atrial anastomosis is shown. (Russell: *Recent Advances in Surgery.*)

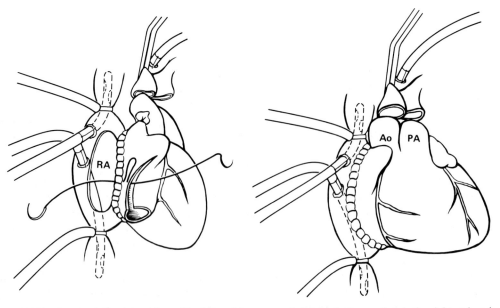

Fig. 28.57 Suture of the right atrium. The left atrial anastomosis having been completed, the right atrium is anastomosed; the septum of the recipient is doubly sewn. (Russell: *Recent Advances in Surgery.*)

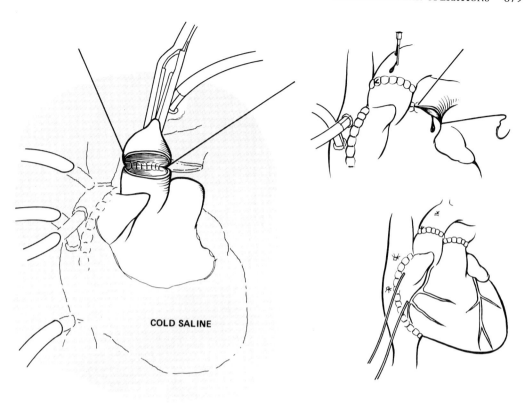

COLD SALINE

Fig. 28.58   The aortic and pulmonary artery anastomoses. The aortic anastomosis is performed first. The heart is preserved by continuous topical irrigation with cold saline. After removal of air from the heart, the aortic clamp is removed. Note the needle in the ascending aorta to vent any remnants of air. Coronary sinus return is to the caval cannulae. The pulmonary artery anastomosis is performed last. (Russell: *Recent Advances in Surgery.*)

After exposure of the heart, the recipient is placed on cardiopulmonary bypass. As there must be complete absence of tubes in the region of the heart, peripheral cannulation of the venae cavae is carried out through the right internal jugular and left saphenous veins.

Occlusion of the intra pericardial venae cavae is achieved with rubber tourniquets. The pulmonary trunk and aorta are mobilised just above their semi lunar valves, and the atria are excised, leaving adequate intact portions of the right and left atrial walls and atrial septum. The redundant heart tissue is then removed.

The donor heart is placed in position, and sutures at each end of the atrial cavity (of the recipient) are united to the extent of the donor heart left atrium. Simple over and over sutures are then used to unite first the left atria, and then the right atria. Preservation of the myocardium is continued by continuous pericardial irrigation with cold saline. On completion of the atrial anastomosis, irrigation of cold saline is continued through a tube inserted through the left atrial appendage. This maintains cooling and helps to expel air from the left atrium and ventricle.

The aortic anastomosis is carried out and just before the suture line is complete, any air remaining in the chambers of the heart is expelled by manipulation of the heart and inflation of the lungs. The aortic clamp is removed to allow perfusion of the coronary vessels by blood returning from the cardiopulmonary bypass machine.

The heart is generally in ventricular fibrillation at this time and the pulmonary artery anastomosis is carried out. The donor pulmonary artery is occluded, the venae cavae tourniquets released and a needle inserted in the apex of the ascending aorta to allow any residual air to be expelled. The heart usually defibrillates spontaneously; if not a small electric shock restores sinus rhythm.

Temporary cardiac pacing wires are positioned on the donor right atrium. These are for direct ECG recording and pacing if necessary. After a 20 minute period of partial bypass, the cardiopulmonary bypass is discontinued, and the chest closed in the usual manner, meticulous care being taken with haemostasis, apposition of tissues and insertion of the two chest drains. It is usual to leave an indwelling catheter inserted suprapubically to minimise the risk of transurethral infection.

REFERENCES AND FURTHER READING

BALLINGER, W. F., TREYBAL, J. C. AND VOSS, A. B. (1972) *Alexander's Care of the Patient in Surgery*. C. V. Mosby Co.

CLELAND, W. P. (1968) *Surgery — Thorax*. London: Butterworths.

CORY-PEARCE, R. (1981) *Heart Transplantation Nursing* 32, 1420–1422, Medical Education International Ltd.

EVANS, J. (1978) *Nursing Times*, 918.

FOSTER, G. A. (1977) *Nursing Times*, 1193.

GILBART, R. (1972) *Nursing Times*, 1439.

ILLINGWORTH, C. (1973) *A short Textbook of Surgery*. Edinburgh: Churchill Livingstone.

IRVINE, W. T. (1971) *Modern Trends in Surgery*. London: Butterworths.

JAMIESON, S., STINSON, E. AND SHUMWAY, N. (1979) *Nursing Mirror*, **24,** June 21st.

JAMIESON, S. W. AND STINSON, E. B. (1985) Cardiac transplantation, In *Recent Advances in Surgery*, pp. 141–151. Edinburgh: Churchill Livingstone.

LAGUEA, J., CROWIE, D., WALKER, C. AND WILLIAMS, J. (1976) *Nursing Mirror*, **19,** November 29th.

LINLEY, G. (1976) *Nursing Mirror*, **52,** June 24th.

LOCKIE, E. (1976) *Nursing Times*, 1190.

NORMAN, A. (1981) Cold cardioplagia, *Nursing Mirror*, **xvii,** September

PAGLIERO, K. M. (1975) *Nursing Times*, 925.

PANETH, M. (1975) *Nursing Mirror*, **58,** August 7th.

ROSS, et al. (1976) *British Medical Journal*, **1,** 1109.

ROWE, G. C. (1978) *Lancet*, **i,** 264.

WRIGHT, J. E. C. (1975) *Nursing Mirror*, **53,** August 7th.

29

Abdominal vascular operations

Excision and graft for aneurysm of the aorta

Definition

Excision of a dilated portion of the abdominal aorta (dissecting aneurysm) and insertion of a synthetic fabric prosthesis, e.g., PTFE, Dacron.

Position

Supine.

Instruments

General set (Figs. 14.1 to 14.28)
Laparotomy set (Figs. 15.1 to 15.7)
Long fine dissecting forceps, toothed, 20 cm (8 in) (Waugh Micro), 2
Lone fine dissecting forceps, non-toothed, 20 cm (8 in) (Waugh Micro), 2
Dissecting forceps, toothed, 25 cm (10 in)
Dissecting forceps, non-toothed, 25 cm (10 in)
Long scissors, curved on flat, 23 cm (9in) (Nelson)
Scissors, curved on flat, 18 cm (7 in) (Mayo)
Scissors, angled (Potts Smith), set of 3
Vena cava occlusion clamps, 2
Aortic clamps (Potts), 2
Large bulldog clamps, 6
Small bulldog clamps, 6
Long needle holders (Potts Smith or Holmes Sellor, etc.), 2
Polythene tubing or nylon tape
20 ml syringe, needles and blunt cannula
Heparin 5,000 units in 2 ml and protamine sulphate 50 mgm (*Note.* 1 mg of heparin is equivalent to 100 units, and for neutralisation the equivalent of 1 mg of protamine sulphate or polybrene is given for each 100 units of heparin.)
Prosthesis, e.g. PTFE (Goretex), Dacron (Vacutek-Triaxial)
Laparotomy ligatures and sutures
2 and 1 (3/0 and 5/0) Synthetic non-absorbable or silk., on small curved arterial needles for anastomosis
Occlusion cuffs (tourniquets) for both thighs.
Cardiopulmonary bypass equipment may be required

Outline of procedure

Cardiopulmonary bypass may be carried out (Chapter 28, page 885) if the lesion extends above the diaphragm (Seifert, 1986).

A midline or left paramedian incision is made from the xyphisternum to the symphysis pubis. The bowel is retracted with moist packs and the posterior peritoneum opened over the aorta. The ureters are identified and retracted, and the inferior mesenteric artery is divided between ligatures.

The aorta is mobilised above the aneurysm and the aorta or the iliac vessels below, and polythene tubing or nylon tape passed round them. Adjoining vessels are retracted in a similar manner, and after systemic heparinisation, the aorta above the aneurysm (but below the renal arteries) is occluded with an occlusion clamp. The common iliac arteries are occluded with bulldog clamps, the aneurysm is mobilised and the anterior wall excised.

The aortic defect is bridged with a bifurcated fabric prosthesis (e.g., thin PTFE (Goretex), Dacron (Vascutek), Fig. 29.2), and the anastomosis carried out with continuous non-absorbable sutures. Synthetic fabric prostheses of Dacron are either of the knitted or woven type. The knitted type have a wider mesh and required 'pre-clotting'. This is done by immersing the graft for at least 20 min in 30 ml of patient's blood taken before heparinisation. However, one type (Vascutek-Triaxial) has a very dense knitted structure with a low porosity

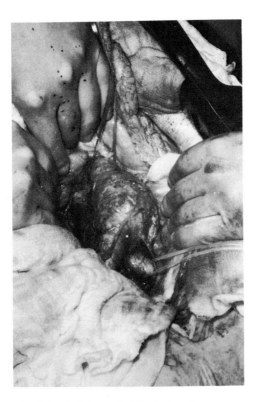
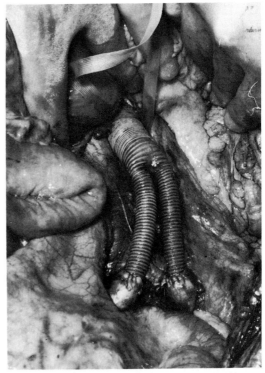

Fig. 29.1 (left) A small abdominal aortic aneurysm exposed at operation, tapes around normal vessels in vicinity of aneurysm. These will be clamped and ligated before the anterior wall of the aneurysm is excised.

Fig. 29.2 (right) Bifurcated Dacron graft replacing the aneurysm seen in Fig. 29.1. (Courtesy Mr A. P. Wyatt, F.R.C.S. and *Nursing Mirror*.)

and velour surfaces. It is claimed that this provides a structure with good resistance to post-operative dilatation, a decrease in thrombogenicy and improved external tissue encasement during subsequent healing. After the anastomoses are completed, the clamps are carefully released one after another to test the integrity of the suture line. If necessary, the anastomoses may be reinforced with further interrupted sutures of non-absorbable material. Thigh occlusion cuffs may be applied and inflated before release of the iliac occlusion clamps, and gradually released subsequently to avoid possible fall of blood-pressure. The action of the heparin is neutralised by the appropriate amounts of protamine sulphate.

Should occlusion of the aorta above the renal arteries be required, hypothermia, a temporary bypass graft, or an extracorporeal circulation may be required.

The posterior peritoneum is closed with absorbable sutures and the abdominal aspirated free of blood before closure of the wound. Tension sutures are usual as paralytic ileus is frequent.

Splenorenal shunt

Definition

Anastomosis between the splenic and renal veins to relieve hypertension in the portal venous system.

Position

Supine or right lateral chest for a left side approach.

Instruments

Abdominal approach. As for laparotomy (p. 411)
Thoraco-abdominal approach. As for thoracotomy (p. 829)
Both routes: additional instruments

Long fine dissecting forceps, toothed, 20 cm (8 in) (Waugh Micro), 2
Long fine dissecting forceps, non-toothed, 20 cm (8 in) (Waugh Micro), 2
Dissecting forceps, toothed, 25 cm (10 in)
Dissecting forceps, non-toothed, 25 cm (10 in)
Long scissors, curved on flat, 23 cm (9 in) (Nelson)
Aorta clamps (Potts and Blalock), 2 of each, optional
Large bulldog clamps (Potts), 6
Small bulldog clamps, 6
Long needle holders (Potts Smith or Holmes Sellor, etc.), 2
Manometer, three-way tap, rubber or plastic tubing and exploration needle
Polythene tubing or nylon tape
20 ml syringe, needles and blunt cannula
Heparin 5,000 units in 2 ml and protamine sulphate 50 mg
Laparotomy or thoracotomy ligatures and sutures
1 and 0.75 (5/0 and 6/0) Synthetic non-absorbable or silk, on small curved non-traumatic arterial needles for anastomosis.

Outline of procedure

For abdominal approach, a long, left paramedian incision with 'T' or 'L' extension as required is made and the peritoneum opened in the usual manner.

For thoraco-abdominal approach, the incision is made through the bed of the ninth rib which is resected, and extends across the epigastrium transversely. The left diaphragm is divided and a rib spreader inserted to obtain exposure.

The pressure in the splenic vein may be measured with a needle and manometer before mobilising the spleen, either directly from the vein or by splenic puncture. The spleen is freed and removed as described for splenectomy in Chapter 15, but leaving a maximum length of the vein by mobilising from the tail of the pancreas. The splenic vein is divided distal to the occlusion clamp applied close to the hilum of the spleen.

The left kidney is exposed and mobilised, and the renal vein is identified and marked with polythene tubing or nylon tape. Occlusion clamps or tubing tourniquets with rubber stops are applied to the renal vein to isolate a suitable segment for the anastomosis. It is wise to have temporary control of the renal artery with occlusion clamps at this stage also. The end of the splenic vein is trimmed before making an end to side anastomosis with 1 or 0.75 (5/0 or 6/0) non-absorbable sutures. Alternatively, a nephrectomy may be carried out to

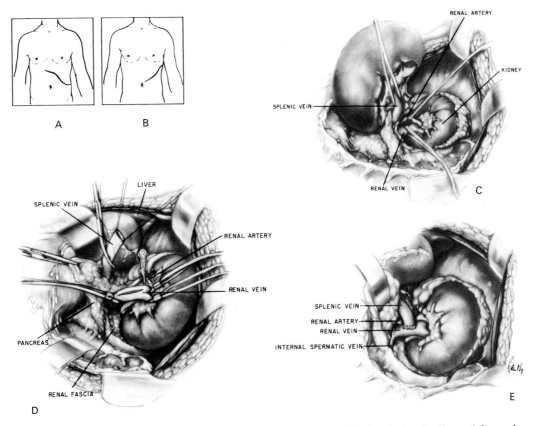

Fig. 29.3 Splenorenal shunt. (A and B) Site of incision. (C) Spleen mobilised, splenic vein dissected free and held with tape. (D) Kidney exposed, spleen removed, splenic vein transected, renal vein occluded with tape-tourniquet, before longitudinal incision made at site of anastomosis. (E) Splenorenal anastomosis completed. (Robb: *Vascular Surgery.*)

permit end to end anastomosis to the renal vein, but this method is avoided if at all possible. Heparin may be injected systematically before the clamps are applied and the anastomosis made, followed by an injection of the appropriate amounts of protamine sulphate after release of the clamps.

The wound is closed in the usual manner for laparotomy or thoracotomy.

Portacaval shunt

Definition

Anastomosis between the portal vein and the inferior vena cava.

Position

Supine or left lateral chest for a right side approach.

Instruments

As for splenorenal shunt except that the operation is on the other side.

Outline of procedure

The exposure is identical to that for splenorenal shunt but on the right side.

The portal vein and inferior vena cava are mobilised in the usual manner and either an end to side anastomosis or side to side anastomosis made. A laterally placed partial occlusion clamp on the inferior vena cava avoids obstruction to the venous drainage of the kidneys and lower part of the body during the formation of the shunt.

REFERENCES AND FURTHER READING

ROBB, C. (1976) *Vascular Surgery*. London: Butterworths.
WYATT, A. R. (1976) *Nursing Mirror*, **52**, August 11–19.
SEIFERT, P. C. (1986) Dissecting Aortic Aneurysms. *AORN J*. **43**, No 2 pp 443–450

30

Peripheral vascular operations

Development of the binocular operating microscope has enabled considerable advances to be made in the field of microsurgery (see Chapter 13). This is particularly so in peripheral vascular operations. Previously, the surgeon was restricted to operations on vessels which were large enough to visualise either by normal eyesight, or by limited magnification afforded by using spectacles or binocular lenses. Using an operating microscope and the ultra-fine suture needles and suture material now available, it is possible to repair blood vessels and nerves with a diameter of only 1 mm or less. This technique has revolutionised the surgery of trauma, enabling reimplantation of digits which previously would have been amputated.

Microvascular surgery requires meticulous, painstaking technique. The principles of vascular anastomosis is described in some of the operations included in this chapter. For more detail, the reader is advised to consult a specialised text book on the subject. However, the basic technique can be appreciated in the following illustrations and Figures 30.5 to 30.11 give some indication of the delicate instrumentation required.

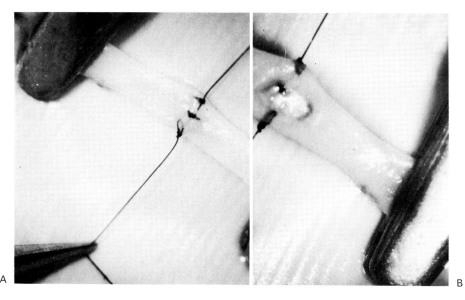

Fig. 30.1 Microvascular repair of a 1 mm vessel. (A) Three sutures have been inserted on the anterior wall. The clear circle of one of the sutures is evident. (B) The clamps have been turned over and the gaping posterior vessel edges are obvious. The posterior repair is completed in a similar fashion after inserting a central suture first. (O'Brien.)

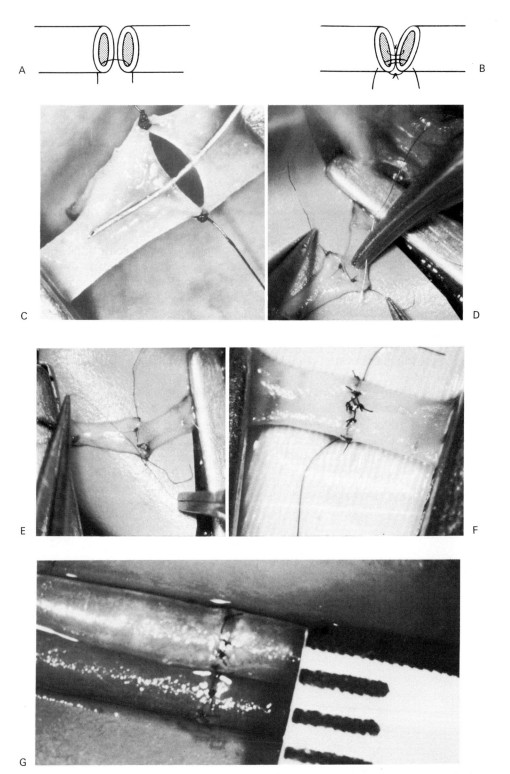

Fig. 30.2 Repair of 1 mm vein. (A to C) Sometimes, in a confined space, it may be necessary to repair the posterior vessel edges first from an anterior approach after placing guide sutures. (D) The posterior repair of the vein is almost complete. The micro needle holder grasps the metallized needle of the nylon microsuture. (E) A final suture is being placed in the posterior wall of the 1 mm vein repair, tying the suture with the needle holder in the right hand and number 5 jeweller's forceps in the left hand. (F) Completed posterior wall repair. (G) Final microvascular repair, the scale is measured in millimetres. (O'Brien: *Microvascular Reconstructive Surgery.*)

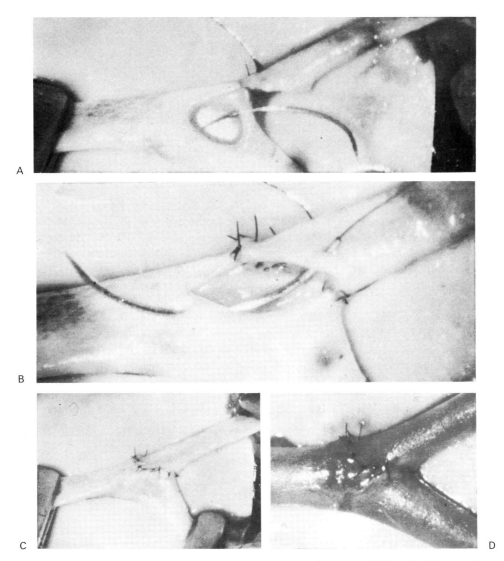

Fig. 30.3 End to side anastomosis of an 0.9 mm artery using 0.2 (10/0) nylon. (A) Second guide suture being inserted. (B) Posterior wall repair completed — central anterior suture being inserted. (C) Anterior wall repair completed. (D) Patent anastomosis on release of clamps. (O'Brien: *Microvascular Reconstructive Surgery.*)

Operations for varicose veins (Trendelenburg's operation and vein stripping)

Definition

Ligation and division of the long saphenous vein at the point where it joins the femoral vein and of the terminal long saphenous vein tributaries. In the stripping operation, a flexible stripper is used to remove a length of the diseased vein from the leg.

Position

Supine, with the legs slightly abducted.

Instruments

General set (Figs. 14.1 to 14.28)
Vein stripper, if stripping operation is to be performed
2.5 and 3 (2/0 and 0) Chromic catgut, synthetic absorbable or non-absorbable, or silk for
    ligatures
3 (0) Chromic catgut or synthetic absorbable on a small half-circle round-bodied needle
    for deep sutures
2.5 (2/0) Synthetic non-absorbable or silk on a medium curved or straight cutting needle
    for skin sutures.

Outline of procedure

For Trendelenburg's operation an incision is made in the upper thigh, parallel to the crease
in the groin over the saphenous opening. Dissection is made through the fat down to the
point where the saphenous vein joins the femoral vein. (Small tributaries are ligated as
the dissection proceeds.) The saphenous vein is isolated, divided, and both ends ligated at
the femoral junction. The wound is closed in layers. The operation may require to be
supplemented by ligation of the deep perforating veins, or stripping.

For the stripping operation, before the groin wound is closed, an incision is made at the
ankle and a stripper threaded up the saphenous vein to the groin. The lower part of the
divided saphenous vein in the ankle is secured to the bulbous end of the stripper by a
ligature, and the whole withdrawn through the groin incision, thereby pulling the saphenous
vein out of the leg. The short saphenous vein is treated by division and ligation at the
sapheno-popliteal junction and stripped between there and an incision on the outer side of
the tendino Achilles. A crêpe bandage is applied after the wounds have been closed. The
patient has the foot of his bed elevated on blocks after operation, but is mobilised as soon
as possible.

Arterial and venous embolectomy

Definition

Removal of a blood clot which has become impacted in an artery or vein and is interfering
with the circulation below that point. The most common sites for an arterial embolism to
occur are at the arterial bifurcations, such as that of the abdominal aorta, the femoral and
popliteal arteries. Similarly, venous emboli are also common at venous bifurcations such as
the junction of the vena cava with the common iliac vessels. This is an emergency operation.

Position

Depends upon the site of the embolus.

Instruments

General set (Figs. 14.1 to 14.28)
Scalpel handle No. 9 with No. 15 blade (Bard Parker)
Fine dissecting forceps, toothed (Gillies), 2
Fine dissecting forceps, non-toothed (McIndoe), 2
Fine dissecting forceps, micro (various sizes and shapes)

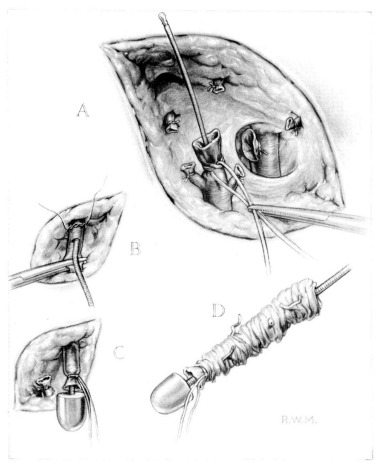

Fig. 30.4 Stripping operation for varicose veins. (A) Trendelenburg operation. Long saphenous vein ligatured and divided at junction with femoral. Tributaries divided between ligatures. (The stripper will not be seen emerging from the cut saphenous vein until a later stage of the operation.) (B) Lower end of long saphenous vein exposed in front of medial malleolus. Stripper inserted, and ligature around vein ready to be tied.
(C) Ligature tied to anchor vein against acorn-head of stripper, and vein divided. (D) The complete vein after avulsion, telescoped against the head of the stripper. (Farquharson and Rintoul: *Textbook of Operative Surgery*.)

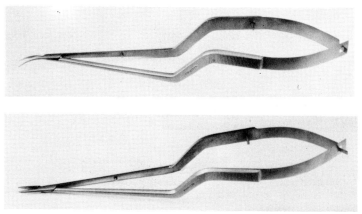

Fig. 30.5 Microscissors. (Genito Urinary Manufacturing Co. Ltd.)

Figs. 30.6 to 30.11   Micro instruments (Chas. F. Thackray Ltd.)

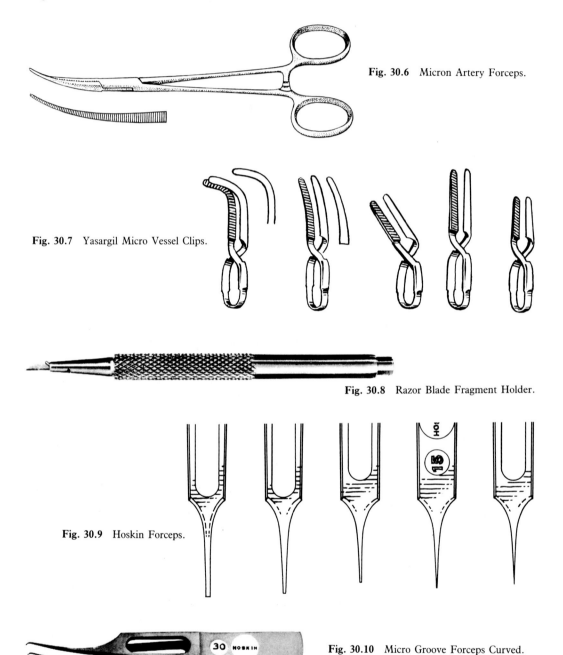

Fig. 30.6   Micron Artery Forceps.

Fig. 30.7   Yasargil Micro Vessel Clips.

Fig. 30.8   Razor Blade Fragment Holder.

Fig. 30.9   Hoskin Forceps.

Fig. 30.10   Micro Groove Forceps Curved.

Fig. 30.11   Micro Groove Forceps Straight.

Fine scissors, curved on flat, 10 cm (4 in) (Kilner or iris)

Fine needle holders, 2

Fine needle holders, micro, 2

Vascular occlusion clamps (Yasargil, Carrel) 6 or more will be needed

Suction tubing, fine nozzles, rubber catheter with connection

Irrigation syringe, rubber catheter and non-pyrogenic saline

20 ml syringe, needles and blunt cannula

Fogarty embolectomy catheters 3FG to 7FG (Balloon inflation according to catheter size, i.e., 0.5 ml to 2.5 ml)

Fogarty irrigating catheters 4FG to 6FG (Balloon inflation according to catheter size, i.e., 0.5 ml to 2.5 ml)

Heparin 5,000 units in 2 ml and protamine sulphate 50 mg

Local anaesthetic requisites may be required (Fig. 11.60)

2.5 and 3 (2/0 and 0) Chromic catgut, synthetic absorbable or non-absorbable, or silk for ligatures

1.5, 1 or 0.7 (4/0, 5/0 or 6/0) synthetic non-absorbable or silk on a small curved non-traumatic arterial needle for vascular suture

Appropriate sutures for that area of the body.

Outline of procedure

Method 1. An incision is made over the point at which the embolus has lodged. Dissection is made down to the vessel and an adequate exposure obtained. Polythene tubing or nylon tape is passed round the vessel and any immediate branches above and below the clot. This tubing or tapes can be threaded through short pieces of rubber or plastic tubing, as shown in Fig. 30.12, which can be slid down to occlude the vessel. Alternatively, bulldog or other vascular occlusion clamps (e.g., Carrel's) are applied to occlude the vessels. Heparin solution may be injected systemically before the application of clamps. An incision is made in the vessel wall and the clot milked or suctioned out. After as much of the clot as can be seen and palpated has been removed, the patency of the vessels below the thrombosed section is checked by momentarily releasing the constrictions and allowing the blood to flow. When the surgeon is satisfied that all the thrombus has been removed, the vessel incision is closed with 1 (5/0) synthetic non-absorbable or silk and if the heparin has been injected, it is neutralised with protamine sulphate, following which the blood circulation is recommenced.

The wound is closed in layers.

Method 2. Using the Fogarty embolectomy balloon catheter for saddle emboli, iliac artery and peripheral artery emboli.

Bilateral incisions are made over the common femoral arteries and the superficial and deep femoral arteries are isolated. After applying suitable arterial clamps, incisions are made at the junction of the superficial and deep femoral arteries. Appropriate sizes of embolectomy catheters are threaded distally as far as they will go, inflated with fluid and withdrawn to remove the distal thrombus. After removal, 20 mg of heparin in 50 ml of saline is injected into the distal arterial tree via irrigation catheters. This procedure is repeated by passing a catheter through the common femoral artery and into the aorta, inflating the balloon with fluid and withdrawing to extract the thrombus.

The incisions in the vessels are then closed with 1 or 0.7 (5/0 or 6/0) synthetic non-absorbable or silk and the groin incision is closed in the usual manner.

Method 3. Vein emboli. Using the Fogarty embolectomy balloon catheter for ileo-femoral emboli. An incision is made over the sapheno-femoral junction on the unaffected side. The

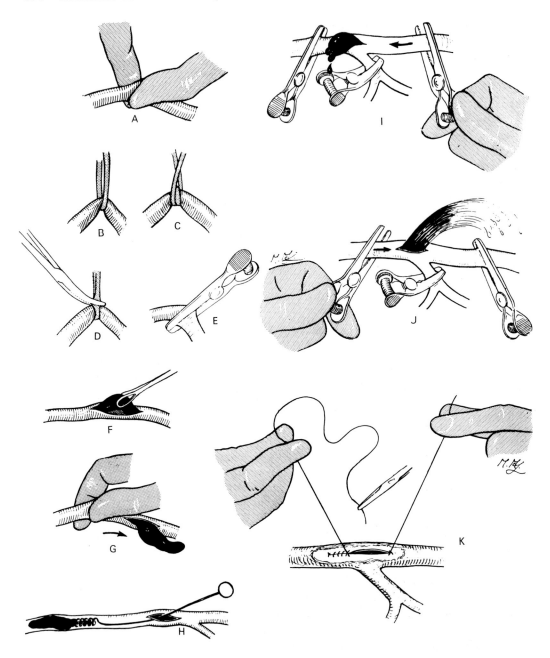

Fig. 30.12 Embolectomy (A to E) methods of temporary control of the artery. (F to H) Clot may be removed by extraction, 'milking' or a 'corkscrew' wire. (I to J) Testing for patency of the artery. (I) Backflow indicates clearance to at least one sizable branch but this is not necessarily sufficient. (J) Full flow from above — this must be an obvious full bore flow to be accepted as evidence of complete clearance above the arteriotomy. A conical and arterial cannula attached to a syringe filled with saline can also be used to test for patency. (K) Resuture of the arteriotomy. (Martin: *Indications and Techniques in Arterial Surgery*.)

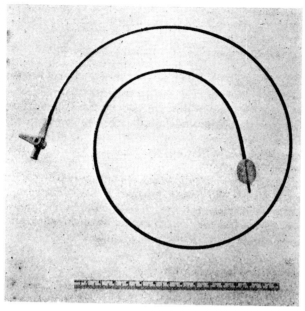

Fig. 30.13   Fogarty embolectomy catheter. (Genito-Urinary Mfg. Co. Ltd.)

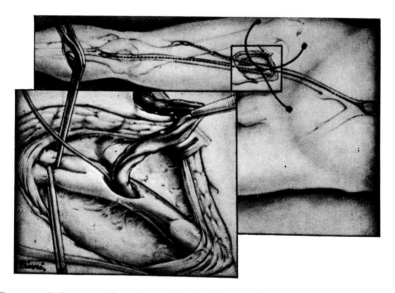

Fig. 30.14   Fogarty embolectomy catheter in use. (Genito-Urinary Mfg. Co. Ltd.)

largest major tributary is isolated, ligatured distally and its stump utilised to introduce an embolectomy catheter. The catheter is passed up the iliac vein to the vena cava where it is left uninflated.

An incision is then made in the femoral triangle on the affected side and the common, superficial and deep femoral vessels identified. If dissection is difficult the balloon catheter already inserted is inflated with fluid to prevent movement of emboli up the vena cava.

Through a venotomy at the junction of the superficial and deep femoral veins on the affected side, a further balloon is introduced until it is obstructed by the previously inflated catheter. It is then inflated and withdrawn until it lies within the proximal iliac vein segment — the first catheter is then deflated.

A second catheter is then inserted proximally into the affected side and when it reaches the inflated balloon, is itself inflated with fluid. Withdrawal of this catheter extracts the thrombus. Further catheters may be inserted distally into the limb to extract distal thrombus after which 20 mg of heparin in 50 ml of saline is injected.

Femoral popliteal bypass graft

Definition

The creation of a channel for arterial blood to bypass an occluded segment of the femoral artery. The patient's long saphenous vein or synthetic tubular graft may be used. (Alternatively thromboendarterectomy may be performed although percutaneous transluminal angioplasty under X-ray control is becoming more common.) This procedure consists of the insertion of a catheter through the ipsilateral common femoral artery and passed retrograde for iliac obstruction and antegrade for superficial femoral obstruction. The catheter splits the thick mature plague forming the site of stenosis, or the final artery closure, along its sides where it joins the normal intima and adventitia. 'The dilatation is then free to stretch up the media and adventitia of the remaining portion of the arterial circumference, to restore a normal lumen, with the loosened plaque still held securely at its upper and lower ends and perhaps along one side as well' (Eastcott, 1984). Alternatively, disobliteration may be undertaken with a laser endoscope, but if unsuitable, thromboendarterectomy may be performed as an alternative procedure.

Position

Supine, with the leg slightly abducted and flexed.

Instruments

> As arterial embolectomy, minus embolectomy catheters
> Graft introducing tube and obturator
> Long crocodile forceps
> Solution for inflating vein graft which is made up at commencement of operation as follows:
>> Normal saline 500 ml
>> Heparin 5,000 units in 1 ml and 50 mg protamine sulphate (or Polybrene)
>> Procaine hydrochloride 2 per cent, 10 ml.
> Or synthetic vascular graft

Outline of procedure

For a vein graft longitudinal incisions, separated by small skin bridges, are made over the course of the long saphenous vein from the groin crease to behind the knee. (This relieves tension from the suture line and preserves skin vitality.) The long saphenous vein is exposed and inspected. If found suitable it is removed at a later stage in the operation.

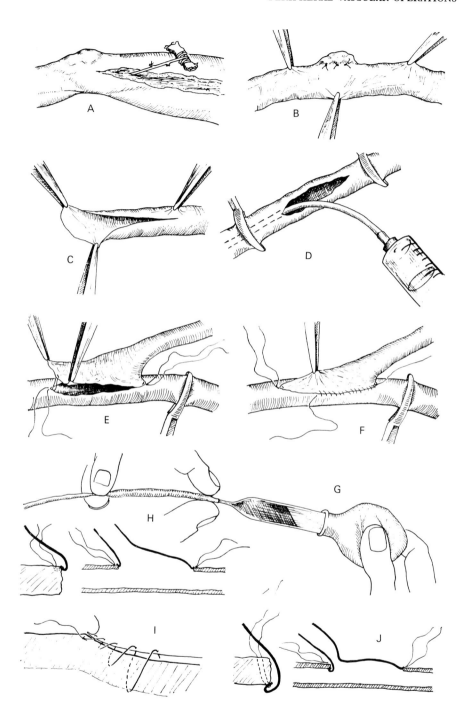

Fig. 30.15 Technique of femoro-popliteal by-pass operation. (A) Removal of vein. (B) Suture of localized varix. (C) Preparation of end of vein. (D) Injection of heparin solution into distal segment of artery. (E) Mattress sutures in place. (F) Completion of suturing. (G) Distension of segment of vein. (H) Mattress suture taking the adventitia of the thickened artery. (I) Progressively deeper bites of artery. (J) Constriction of vein graft if initial bite is too deep. (Martin: *Indications and Techniques in Arterial Surgery*.)

Systemic heparinisation with 5,000 units in 2 ml is now carried out. The common femoral artery and its branches in the femoral triangle are exposed and isolated with tapes of polythene tubing. The popliteal artery is also exposed and mobilised so that it may be brought up into the superficial part of the wound. In order to select a patent length of healthy artery suitable for receiving the distal end of the graft, it may be necessary to divide both the tendon of adductor magnus and the medial head of the gastrocnemius muscle. Small arterial branches are controlled either with small bulldog clamps or double-looped slings of strong silk or polyester.

After ligating its tributaries, the vein is removed and cleaned of adventitia. To test for leaks and size, the proximal end of the vessel is clamped and a suitable arterial cannula tied into the distal end. Using a 20 ml syringe the vein is 'blown up' with a solution of saline/heparin/procaine. Sections of the vein which appear narrow may be due to spasm or constricting adventitia; removal of the latter will allow it to dilate. If a synthetic fabric vein graft is being used, this may require pre-clotting by immersion of the graft for at least 20 minutes, in 30 ml of the patient's blood taken before heparinisation.

The graft introducing tube is inserted, with gentle pressure, from the popliteal fossa, through the adductor canal to emerge in the groin incision. The synthetic fabric graft or reversed vein graft is pulled through the tube with long forceps. The tube is then removed and the proximal end of the vein or synthetic graft anastomosed (only three-quarters of the anastomosis being completed at this stage) end-to-side to the popliteal artery using 1 or 0.7 (5/0 or 6/0) synthetic non-absorbable or silk as a continuous running suture. The proximal anastomosis of the narrow (distal) end of the vein to the common femoral artery, also end-to-side is completed. Distal, then proximal clamps are released to test for distal reverse flow and to wash out any clots from the graft. The clamps are then re-applied, the distal anastomosis completed and the clamps removed for a second time.

Surgicel may be applied locally to control small leaks, but larger ones will require insertion of further sutures. Heparinisation is reversed with appropriate amounts of protamine sulphate.

Wounds are closed with interrupted skin sutures only with closed suction drainage (Redivac, Activac, Portavac).

Disobliteration (Re-bore thromboendarterectomy)

Definition

Removal of a central atheromatous obstructive core of an artery leaving an outer layer which is free from disease, usually performed on the aorta, iliac, femoral, or popliteal arteries, also the vertebral, subclavian and carotid arteries. This may be performed as a non-invasive procedure under X-ray control, using a laser endoscope.

Position and instruments

As femoral popliteal bypass graft
Cannon's endarterectomy ring strippers or similar.

Outline of procedure

A long thromboendarterectomy may be performed if the long saphenous vein is not suitable

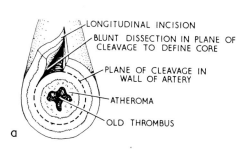

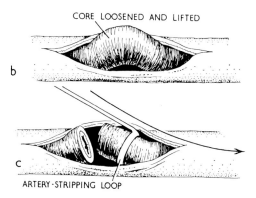

Fig. 30.16 Disobliteration or 'rebore': (A) is the cross-section of the diseased artery. The dotted line shows the plane of cleavage within the wall of the artery around the atheromatous inner layer and the solid centre of old thrombosis. In (B) the core has been lifted out and in (C) the core has been divided and an artery stripping loop threaded over it, preparatory to being thrust up the affected length of artery. (Figures 30.16 and 30.17 by kind permission of Prof. A. Harding Rains and the *Nursing Times*, published May 1964.)

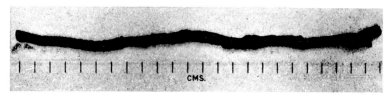

Fig. 30.17 The atheromatous core after it has been stripped out of the femoral artery (the mark indicates 1 cm).

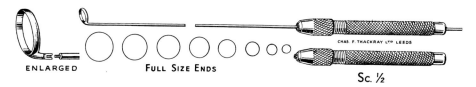

Fig. 30.18 Cannon endarterectomy ring strippers.

as a graft (see previous operation). This may occur if the vein is too narrow, or has been thrombosed, or is varicose, or absent.

The thromboendarterectomy is carried out from patent artery above to patent artery below, through multiple arteriotomies. These are repaired using patches of vein graft or Dacron to prevent narrowing.

Through the arteriotomies, the atheromatous core is divided and the loop of the instrument is threaded over one end of the core. Holding this core with artery forceps, the loop is pushed along the plane of cleavage between the core and the vessel wall thereby effecting separation.

At the most distal arteriotomy, the intima is tacked down to the subjacent media by 3 or 4 0.7 (6/0) synthetic non-absorbable or silk sutures tied on the outside. This prevents flap formation or 'dissection' which results in occlusion.

There are a number of ring strippers and dissectors in use including Cannon's ring strippers and MacDonald's dissector. A method has been developed using high pressure CO_2 gas which acts in a similar manner.

Short occlusions are treated by localised thromboendarterectomy and the arteriotomy is repaired by vein or Dacron patches.

REFERENCES AND FURTHER READING

EASTCOTT, H. H. G. (1984) Peripheral angioplasty. In *Angioplasty*, Edited by R. J. Vecht. London: Pitman
FARQUHARSON, E. L. AND RINTOUL, R. F. (1972) *Textbook of Operative Surgery*. Edinburgh: Churchill Livingstone.
MARTIN, P. (1968) *Indications and Techniques in Arterial Surgery*. Edinburgh: Churchill Livingstone.
O'BRIEN, B. McC. (1977) *Microvascular Reconstructive Surgery*. Edinburgh: Churchill Livingstone.

31

Plaster of Paris technique

For further details of plaster techniques, the reader is referred to *Handbook of Plaster Techniques* by E. Narborough and G. Densley, published by Smith and Nephew Medical Ltd.

Although metal and wooden splints are still used for the immobilisation of some fractures, plaster of Paris has almost entirely superseded these, and offers many advantages. The basic constituent of plaster of Paris is crystalline gypsum or calcium sulphate which is quarried in rock form. The gypsum is ground into a fine powder and heated under controlled conditions to evaporate most of the water content to form plaster of Paris. The powder is mixed with chemical solvents and cellulose. Combined with a heating process, the liquid is impregnated on to an open woven, interlocked fabric which holds the plaster uniformly. The impregnated fabric can then be fashioned into bandages and slabs of various sizes. The addition of resin to the basic process of manufacture helps to minimise plaster loss after moistening the bandage, thereby reducing the number of bandages needed for each cast.

Gypsona, manufactured by Smith & Nephew Medical Ltd., is a brand of plaster of Paris which is used extensively in orthopaedics today. This chapter provides a basic outline of plaster procedure related to the operating theatre and readers are referred to *Handbook of Plaster Techniques* for a more extensive exposition.

Requirements for plaster of Paris application

A deep pail or bowl for soaking the plaster bandages. (This should be three parts filled with tepid water 25 to 35°C.)
Plaster bandages of various widths
Prepared slabs in Gypsona dispenser
Cotton bandages 5 cm and 7.5 cm (2 in and 3 in)
Crepe bandages of various widths
Macintoshes, or disposable paper towels
Plaster wool and orthopaedic felt for padding
Tubular stockinet of various widths
Plaster scissors (usually of the Böhler type)
Heavy angled dressing scissors
Plaster shears
Plaster benders
Plaster knife
Tape measure and marking pencil
A suitable table top or glass sheet for the preparation of slabs

Dusting powder or olive oil may be needed for application to the patient's skin before
plastering is commenced, especially if a tight plaster cast is being applied
An electric plaster saw may be required for the removal of a dry cast.

Application of plaster of Paris

Some surgeons prefer to apply their own plaster casts but this may be left to experienced
plaster staff who specialise in the art.

The person applying plaster usually wears rubber boots and apron. Rubber gloves may
be worn although this is a matter for individual preference.

Plaster slabs

Some operations such as tendon suture of the hand and certain fresh fractures require only
the application of a plaster slab for immobilisation, followed by a gauze or crêpe bandage.
This provides a well-fitting splint which is quick to prepare and easy to remove for dressings,
etc.

There are four methods of preparing plaster slabs:

(a) By unrolling dry plaster bandages,
(b) By unrolling wet plaster bandages,
(c) By using 5 or 6 thickness plies material from a dry plaster dispenser,
(d) The pattern technique.

(a) The slab is prepared from either dry or wet Gypsona plaster bandages folded out on
a smooth surface. The most usual way is to use dry plaster bandages, for the operator may
measure and cut the slab at his own speed without fear of the plaster setting before this has
been completed.

The dry bandage is placed alongside the limb and the length required marked with a
pencil or cut. Alternatively, a tape measure may be used and the length required marked
on a bandage which has been unrolled sufficiently on the table-top. The necessary thickness,
usually four to six layers, is obtained by unwinding the bandage 'to and fro'. Care must be
taken to ensure that all layers extend for the same distance and short ends are discarded.
Ten per cent additional length is allowed for shrinkage.

To apply, the slab is lightly folded from each end to the centre, immersed in water and
immediately removed (Fig. 31.2). After submergence, surplus water may then be removed

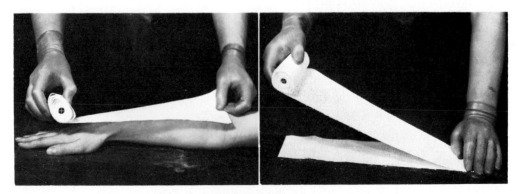

Fig. 31.1 Dry method of preparing plaster slabs.

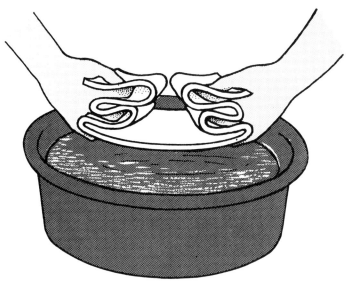

Fig. 31.2 Method of wetting a plaster slab.

by compression, which must be moderately light, for strong squeezing will cause quick setting and vice versa.

After extending the squeezed slab, it is placed on the table-top and carefully smoothed out to remove air bubbles. Failure to do this may cause the finished slab to crack or crumble after application.

Widths of slabs vary according to the individual surgeon's requirements, but the nurse will find generally that a 10 to 15 cm (4 to 6 in) wide slab is suitable for the forearm or a child's leg, but a 15 to 20 cm (6 to 8 in) wide slab will be needed for the lower limb. A larger cast such as a spica may incorporate wider slabs described in the pattern technique.

(b) With this method the bandage is unrolled for about 5 cm (2 in), *held* (not gripped) in the hand and lowered into the water until all bubbling has ceased, usually 5 to 10 seconds. Gripping of the bandage should be avoided because it tends to force plaster out of the fabric. The bandage is then lifted out of the water, and the two edges squeezed towards the centre and each other with the thumb and forefinger of each hand. This will allow excess moisture to run out of the bandage, but will retain the greater part of the plaster.

The slab is made by pressing the end of the bandage on to the table-top and holding it there with the left hand. The bandage is then unrolled with the right hand, 'to and fro', to form the correct length and thickness of slab. The air bubbles are smoothed out and the slab applied immediately. The nurse will find it useful to place a stout rod through the centre core of the bandage before unrolling during the preparation of a slab.

(c) The required length of 6 thickness plies (5 thickness low plaster loss) is withdrawn from a dry plaster dispenser. This is quicker and more reliable than the unrolling method. The slab is applied as described under (a).

(d) Another method is the pattern technique by which standard dry plaster slabs are prepared before they are required, using wide Gypsona material.

The patterns described in this chapter are for hip, shoulder and spinal jacket.

The patterns allow for shrinkage after the slabs have been moistened. If the slabs are cut to individual measurements and not the patterns, 10 per cent should be added to these measurements to compensate for this shrinkage.

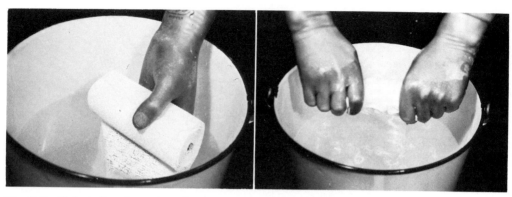

Fig. 31.3 Method of wetting a plaster bandage.

The slabs are moistened by submerging flat in a sink filled to a depth of 8 to 10 cm (3 to 4 in). The surplus water is removed by drawing the slab over the edge of the sink as it is lifted out. Air bubbles are expressed by smoothing the slab on the table-top, after which it is applied immediately, moulded to the part, and held in place by open wove or Gypsona bandages.

Any slab may be reinforced to withstand additional stress by ridging or girdering. Ridging consists of raising the centre of the slab for 10 mm ($\frac{3}{8}$ in) along its length, after which it is applied carefully to the cast. Girdering is accomplished by superimposing a ridged slab which is about 10 cm shorter than the underlying one.

If the cast has dried, the surface should be roughened and moistened before the application of further slabs.

Application of plaster bandages

Plaster bandages may be used either to make a cast or to complete one after slabs have been applied.

Bony prominences are padded with plaster wool or felt after applying tubular stockinet if required. The stockinet should be longer than the completed plaster to allow turning back for 2.5 cm (1 in) or so just before the final bandages are applied.

The bandages of correct size are immersed one at a time in tepid water and held there until bubbling stops. The bandage is removed by holding at the ends, which are gently squeezed towards the centre and then pulled back into shape (Fig. 31.3). They are applied, using even tension circular turns with no reversing and with a rolling action, not as an ordinary bandage. Any threads which work free from the bandage as it is applied should be cut away, otherwise tightening may occur afterwards. Each turn of the bandage should cover approximately two-thirds of the previous turn. Smooth pleats can be made in the upper or lower edges of the bandage, to allow it to 'sit' evenly when following the contour of a limb. A pause is made after each bandage has been applied, to mould the plaster to the part and allow the layers to set. As the finished plaster cast should be an homogenous mass rather than a series of layers, the moulding is very necessary, together with the exclusion of air between each plaster bandage.

The nurse holding the limb should support it with extended palms to avoid indentations from her finger tips which can cause pressure sores at the point of indentation. She should be very careful to maintain the correct position during the whole period of application.

After application, the plaster cast should be supported on macintosh covered pillows until it has dried. Drying may be hastened in the ward with a heat cradle, but care must be taken to protect exposed areas of the patient's skin from burns, especially if he is unconscious.

An unpadded plaster is very rarely applied to fresh fractures due to the subsequent swelling which always occurs. Even with padding, it may be necessary to bi-valve or cut the plaster along its entire length to allow for this swelling. As the swelling subsides and the plaster becomes loose, it may need to be reapplied (with little padding) to ensure immobilisation.

If it is known that a plaster cast may require splitting, a greased rubber or plastic tube should be placed anteriorly along the length of the limb before plastering is commenced. This tube may be pulled out of the completed plaster easily, leaving a channel inside which simplifies cutting afterwards.

Control of setting time

Normally tepid water (25 to 35°C) should be used for moistening plaster bandages; cold water may cause involuntary muscular contractions if the patient is conscious, and hot water will cause the plaster to set too quickly.

Gypsona bandages set in four to six minutes using tepid water. It is possible to retard this setting time by adding borax to the water.

The setting may be retarded for 1 minute by adding two heaped teaspoonfuls of borax to 1 gal (0.5 per cent); for 7 minutes by adding four level dessertspoonfuls of borax to 1 gal (0.75 per cent); and for 15 minutes by adding one heaped tablespoonful of borax to 1 gal.

TYPES OF PLASTER CASTS

ARM

Colles' fracture

After reduction, the hand is maintained in a position of full pronation and ulnar deviation. A simple fracture is then immobilised with an incomplete forearm plaster, and a severe fracture is immobilised with a mid-arm pronation plaster.

For an incomplete plaster, the elbow is flexed to 90 degrees and the arm is covered with stockinet or a thin layer of plaster wool bandage. A dorsal slab is made from 15 cm (6 in) wide 5 or 6 ply plaster bandage, the length of the slab being 15 cm (6 in) more than the measurement from the elbow to the metacarpo-phalangeal joints. The slab is applied and extends 2.5 cm (1 in) from the olecranon process (where it is folded obliquely to avoid pressing into the antecubital fossa when the elbow is flexed) to 13 mm ($\frac{1}{2}$ in) proximal to the metacarpo-phalangeal joints. The slab must be well moulded and extend round the ventral surface of the radius and base of the first metacarpal to prevent radial deviation. The slab is fixed to forearm with a *wet* gauze bandage or a crêpe bandage which is applied from the elbow to the wrist where it is carried across the palm.

For a complete plaster, stockinet is applied and the elbow flexed to 90 degrees with full

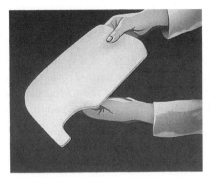

Fig. 31.4 Fabrication of plaster slab.

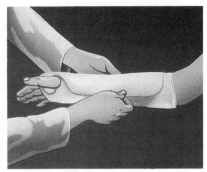

Fig. 31.5 Application of wet plaster slab.

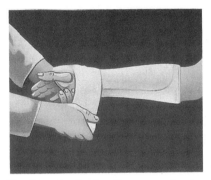

Fig. 31.6 Application of wet gauze bandage.

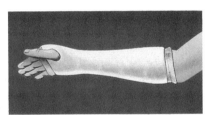

Fig. 31.7 Completed plaster cast.

Figs. 31.4–31.7 Colles' fracture. (*Handbook of Plaster Techniques.*)

pronation of the hand. Plaster wool bandage is used at the elbow and at mid-arm. A short Colles' plaster is applied as previously described, followed by a U-slab made from 10 cm (4 in) wide 5 or 6 ply plaster bandage which is applied to the upper arm. This slab is secured with a wet gauze bandage or crêpe bandage, followed by a 10 cm (4 in) wide by 2.74 m (3 yd) plaster bandage, which extends below for one turn only.

Both these plasters may be completed after swelling has subsided by applying plaster bandages circular fashion round the forearm and upper arm.

Alternatively, a completed plaster cast may be applied over plaster wool bandage and is changed for a skin-tight plaster when swelling has subsided.

Scaphoid fracture

The wrist is maintained in a position of radial deviation and dorsiflexion. A modified short arm Colles' plaster which incorporates the thumb up to the distal joint is applied. The slab is prepared by cutting a notch to accommodate the thumb, and it is then bound to the dorsum of the arm and hand with a *wet* gauze bandage in the usual manner.

When the swelling has subsided, the plaster is completed with circular turns of two 10 cm (4 in) wide by 2.74 m (3 yd) plaster bandages. Alternatively, a completed padded cast may be applied at first and renewed when it becomes loose.

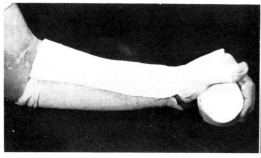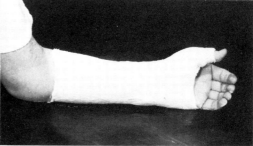

Fig. 31.8 Scaphoid fracture; dorsal slab applied.   **Fig. 31.9** Scaphoid fracture; plaster cast completed.

Fractures of the radius and ulna

There are two types of plasters — full flexed elbow and straight arm. The flexed elbow plaster is most generally used unless contraindicated by the position of the fracture, as straight arm plasters tend to cause a stiff elbow joint, especially in adults.

For a flexed arm plaster, the forearm is generally in a position of mid-pronation, although some fractures may require full pronation or supination. The fracture is reduced with counter-traction applied by means of a sling round the upper arm. Stockinet is applied, followed by plaster wool bandage round the wrist, elbow and upper arm. A U-slab is prepared from 10 cm (4 in) 5 or 6 ply wide 2.74 m (3 yd) plaster bandage and is applied along the dorsal aspect of the forearm, extending from 13 mm ($\frac{1}{2}$ in) behind the knuckles, round the elbow and along the palmar aspect to finish at the wrist crease. This slab is retained with a few turns of a circular plaster bandage and after it has set the counter-traction sling is removed.

A second U-slab is prepared from 10 cm (4 in) 5 or 6 ply wide by 2.74 m (3 yd) plaster bandage sufficiently long to extend from the axilla round the elbow and up the outer aspect of the arm to just below the shoulder. This slab is retained with a few turns of a circular plaster bandage in the usual manner, and the elbow section is strengthened with one 10 cm (4 in) wide by 2.74 m (3 yd) plaster bandage applied obliquely from upper to lower arm round the elbow.

If swelling increases, the gauze bandage is cut and a fresh one applied. As swelling decreases, fresh or additional gauze bandages are applied to take up the 'slack'. When swelling has completely subsided, the cast is completed with circular turns of one or two plaster bandages.

Alternatively, a complete padded plaster may be applied at first, and changed when it becomes loose.

For a straight arm plaster, the elbow is extended and stockinet applied, followed by plaster wool bandages to the wrist, elbow and upper arm. The wrist is placed in a position of pronation and a dorsal slab made from 10 cm (4 in) 5 or 6 ply plaster bandage is applied. This should extend from the axilla to the wrist for olecranon fractures, and from just below the axilla to 13 mm ($\frac{1}{2}$ in) proximal to the metacarpal heads for all forearm fractures. The slab is held in position by a wet gauze bandage, and when swelling has subsided the cast is completed with plaster bandages in the usual way.

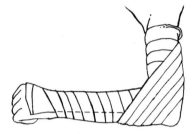

Fig. 31.10 Forearm fractures, flexed elbow plaster. U-slab applied to forearm and secured with circular turns of plaster bandage.

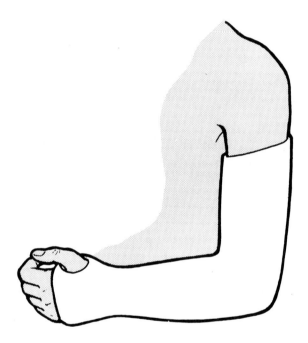

Fig. 31.11 Full arm plaster cast completed.

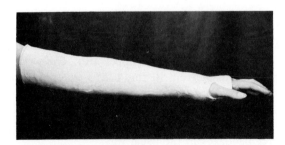

Fig. 31.12 Forearm fractures; straight arm plaster cast completed.

Fractures of the humerus

Middle and upper third. The patient stands or sits with his trunk inclined towards the injured side and his upper arm hanging vertically. The forearm is supported with the elbow flexed to 90 degrees and adhesive felt is applied to pad the outer end of the clavicle and acromium process. A thin layer of plaster wool bandage may be applied from the elbow to the axilla and any tendency to outward angulation of a high shaft fracture is countered with a pad of wool placed to keep the elbow away from the body.

A slab is made from 15 cm (6 in) 5 or 6 ply plaster bandage, and is applied from within 2.5 cm of the axilla, along the inner aspect of the arm, round the elbow, up the outer aspect of the arm and over the shoulder to the acromio-clavicular joint where 15 cm (6 in) excess (allowed in the slab length) is turned back and secured with strapping. The slab is bound to the arm with a *wet* crinx which is covered with a crêpe bandage, and the forearm is supported with a collar and cuff sling.

Lower third. A U-slab is applied in the manner just described, and a strip of wet lint is placed over the forearm and lower part of the U-slab. A short slab about 40 cm (16 in)

Fig. 31.13–31.16   U-slab or hanging slab for upper and middle third fractures of the humerus. (*Handbook of Plaster Techniques.*)

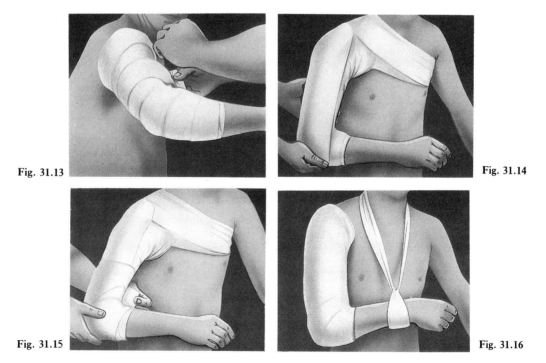

Fig. 31.13

Fig. 31.14

Fig. 31.15

Fig. 31.16

Fig. 31.13   Stockinette and wool padding is used to protect any bony prominences.

Fig. 31.14   Slab applied from the acromio-clavicular joint, down the lateral aspect of the humerus, under the medial aspect of the olecranon, and under the humerus to within 2.5 cm of the axilla.

Fig. 31.15   Slab is held in place with a wet crinx bandage which in turn is covered with a crêpe bandage.

Fig. 31.16   Arm supported with collar and cuff sling.

long is prepared and applied to the dorsal aspect of the forearm. This slab extends from the wrist to just above the elbow, and is secured with a *wet* gauze bandage or crêpe bandage. The wet lint prevents adherence of the two slabs so that the lower slab can be removed after an interval of two weeks or so.

Alternatively, a padded complete plaster may be applied at first and renewed if necessary.

SHOULDER

Shoulder abduction spica

This is used for some humeral or shoulder fractures and post-operative immobilisation for shoulder arthrodesis or recurrent dislocation of the shoulder.

The cast is applied with the patient seated on a backless stool or supported sitting up on the operation table. The arm is abducted about 60 degrees from the side, being carried well forward in front of the coronal plane and with some 15 degrees lateral rotation. The correct position for ankylosis should enable the hand to reach the mouth by flexion of the elbow alone. An assistant supports the elbow and forearm.

A stockinet vest is applied followed by adhesive felt pads over the iliac crests, either side of the spinous process, across the clavicle on the affected side and under the elbow with a small hole to accommodate the medial epicondyle. Plaster wool bandages are then applied to cover the area to be enclosed.

A light layer of plaster bandage is applied over the plaster wool. Plaster slabs, 15 cm (6 in) wide, are applied from the iliac crests under the axilla to the elbow; from the axilla on the sound side across the affected shoulder and upper arm, anteriorly and posteriorly (Fig. 31.17). In addition 15 cm (6 in) wide slabs can be applied from the suprasternal notch to the symphysis pubis and posteriorly from the seventh cervical vertebra to the sacrum. The cast is completed with circular plaster bandages. The arm section is then applied with circular plaster bandages.

If a strut is desired, this may be made from the cores of the bandages, cut to length, covered with plaster material and fixed between the body and arm with a few turns of plaster bandage.

The cast is trimmed as indicated in Figure 31.20 and the edges made neat by turning back and securing the edges of the stockinet lining.

LEG

Fractures of the tarsus, metatarsus, internal and external malleoli, and stable Potts fractures

These fractures are immobilised with below-knee casts. The fracture is reduced (if necessary) and the knee flexed as shown over a padded knee rest with the foot dorsiflexed and the leg supported by an assistant. Stockinet and plaster wool bandage are then applied from just below the knee to the toes.

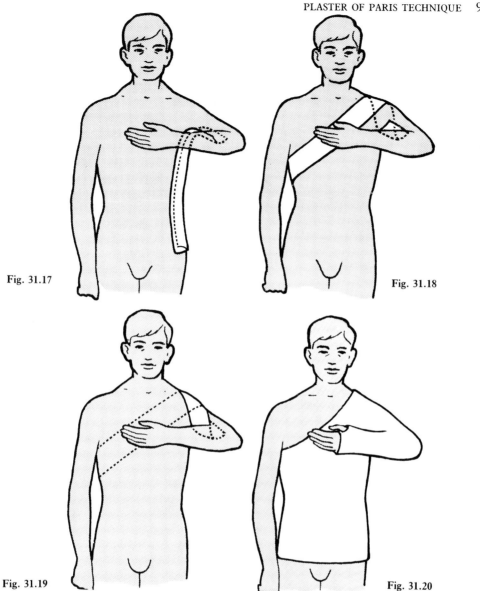

Fig. 31.17

Fig. 31.18

Fig. 31.19

Fig. 31.20

Figs. 31.17–31.20 Method of applying plaster slabs for shoulder abduction plaster; and completed cast.

A plaster stirrup may then be prepared from 10 cm (4 in) plaster bandages and applied commencing just below the knee, continuing down the leg, round the heel, to finish just below the knee on the outer side where any excess is turned back. This stirrup is bound loosely in place with a plaster bandage.

A back slab is prepared from 15 cm (6 in), 5 or 6 ply plaster bandage (10 or 12 ply if the plaster stirrup has not been used) and is applied extending from just below the knee, round the heel (where a cut is made to accommodate the ankle) and along the sole of the foot where excess slab is temporarily dropped over the toes, or in front of the surgeon's knees if the plaster is being applied with the leg flexed over the end of the table

Figs. 31.21–31.22   Below knee plaster, non-weight bearing. (*Handbook of Plaster Techniques.*)

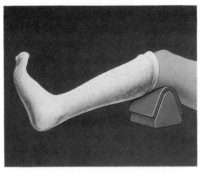 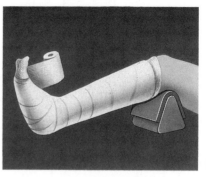

Fig. 31.21   **Fig. 31.22**

Fig. 31.21   Stockinette and padding applied from the base of the toes to within 2.5 cm of the popliteal crease.

Fig. 31.22   Application of plaster bandage, starting spirally from the toes from the outside to the inside of the limb. Usually four bandages are required; sometimes dorsal slabs are used and held in position by two bandages. Excess padding and stockinette is turned back over the cast, and another plaster bandage used to fix the plaster edges and complete the cast.

Figs. 31.23–31.25   Below-knee plaster cast, alternative method.

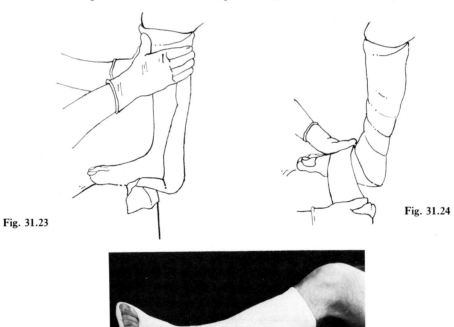

Fig. 31.23

Fig. 31.24

Fig. 31.25

Fig. 31.23   A back slab is applied and excess turned back temporarily in front of the surgeon's knees.

Fig. 31.24   Plaster bandages are applied spirally to secure back slab; note how toe platform is formed.

Fig. 31.25   Below-knee plaster cast completed.

(Figs. 31.23–31.24). The slab is secured with two 15 cm (6 in) wide by 2.74 m (3 yd) plaster bandages from just below the knee to include the ankle. The excess slab is turned back to make a double thickness of plaster which extends just beyond the toes (toe platform). This foot portion of the slab is secured with one or two 10 cm (4 in) wide by 2.74 m (3 yd) plaster bandages and another similar bandage is applied round the ankle to provide reinforcement. The toe platform portion of the slab must not be bent upwards, as contracture of the extensor tendons may occur.

Severe Potts fractures; fractures of the lower third of the tibia; and fractures of the upper tibia when the patient is immobilised in bed.

These fractures are immobilised with mid-thigh casts. If the fracture is comparatively stable, the below-knee portion of the cast is applied first as described previously, but with the stockinet extended to mid-thigh. Plaster wool bandage is then applied round the knee joint and thigh.

Anterior and posterior slabs 76 cm (30 in) long are each prepared from two 15 cm (6 in) wide by 2.74 m (3 yd) plaster bandages. These are applied from a point 20 cm (8 in) below

Figs. 31.26–31.28 Above-knee plaster cast. (*Handbook of Plaster Techniques.*)

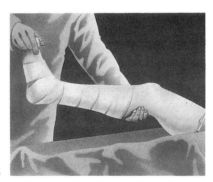

Fig. 31.26

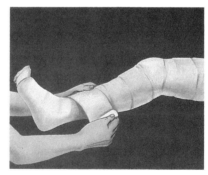

Fig. 31.27

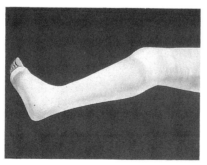

Fig. 31.28

Fig. 31.26 Stockinette padding is applied from the toes to within 2.5 cm of the gluteal fold. The leg is held in a slightly flexed position (10–15°) from the extended position.

Fig. 31.27 The below knee section is applied in a similar fashion to that illustrated in Figures 31.21–31.22. The upper section is then completed with circular turns of plaster bandages, if necessary applying a figure of eight reinforcement around the knee.

Fig. 31.28 Completed above-knee plaster cast.

the knee joint to mid-thigh, where any excess bandage is turned back. The slabs are secured to the limb in the usual manner with two 15 cm (6 in) wide by 2.74 m (3 yd) plaster bandages.

If the fracture is unstable, it is usually easier to apply the upper and lower portions of the cast in one operation. A thin layer of plaster wool is applied to the limb and the fracture is reduced. The limb is supported by two padded wedges, as illustrated, one under the knee joint and one under the fracture, or alternatively, this second wedge is dispensed with and the fracture area supported by an assistant.

Two anterior slabs may be used and are prepared from six layers of wide plaster material, or alternatively, from 15 cm (6 in) wide 2.74 m (3 yd) plaster bandages. These slabs are applied on each side, from mid-thigh along the anterolateral aspect of the limb, and round the sole of the foot. They are moulded carefully and secured with two 15 cm (6 in) wide by 2.74 m (3 yd) plaster bandages, leaving two small gaps where the limb is supported by the wedges or assistant.

When the anterior slabs have set, the lower wedge or support is withdrawn and a back slab may be made from two 15 cm (6 in) wide by 2.74 m (3 yd) plaster bandages is applied from behind the knee to the toes, where it forms the toe platform. The slab is secured with two 15 cm (6 in) wide by 2.74 m (3 yd) plaster bandages applied spirally.

The knee wedge is removed and another back slab prepared from two 15 cm (6 in) wide by 2.74 m (3 yd) plaster bandages. This slab is applied to the back of the thigh, extending down beyond the knee, and is secured with two 15 cm (6 in) wide by 2.74 m (3 yd) plaster bandages.

When the swelling has subsided and the plaster becomes loose, it will be changed to a full length tuber bearing plaster, which is in effect a mid-thigh cast extending to the tuber ischii where it is padded similarly to a walking caliper.

HIP

Hip spica

This is used for immobilisation of infective conditions of the knee, femur and hip; fractures of the femur and hip; osteotomy of the femur; pelvic injuries and arthrodesis of the hip. The double hip spica is the cast most frequently applied in theatre and this will be described.

The patient is placed on extension apparatus as illustrated, and all bony prominences are padded with adhesive felt, i.e., the anterior superior iliac spines, the sacrum, head of the fibula, both malleoli and the tendo achillis. Stockinet is applied to the trunk and legs. Other padding depends upon the type of patient. A thin patient will require a good deal of padding in the form of plaster wool, whereas a stout patient will require very little.

The cast consists of a series of circular bandages and reinforcing slabs, 15 cm (6 in) wide applied as illustrated in Fig. 31.30. The hip section is reinforced by slabs positioned anteriorly and posteriorly from the lower ribs on each side around the hip to the groin and also from the lower ribs down to the lateral side of the knee. The cast is completed by circular bandages; 20 cm (8 in) used in a figure of eight manner around the pelvis and the hip, and 15 cm (6 in) bandages from the hip joint to the knee joint.

Using the pattern technique the main part of the spica consists of slabs which are made from wide plaster material. For a double hip spica five slabs are required: a posterior section

Figs. 31.29–31.32 Hip spica. (*Handbook of Plaster Techniques.*)

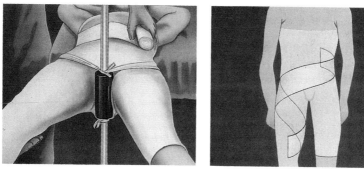
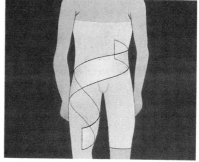

Fig. 31.29

Fig. 31.30

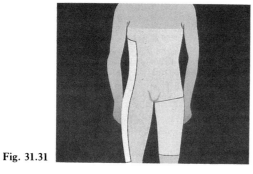
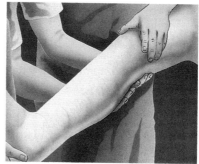

Fig. 31.31

Fig. 31.32

Fig. 31.29 The patient supported on a hip prop or fracture table; stockinette and wool padding applied.

Fig. 31.30 Circular slab wound figure of eight fashion from the front of the cast, around the leg, to the front of the cast.

Fig. 31.31 Longitudinal slab applied to the lateral aspect of the limb and hip.

Fig. 31.32 Cast completed with circular plaster bandages.

of seven or eight layers, two anterior sections of four layers, a complete long leg section of eight layers, and a thigh and pelvic section of eight layers. One heaped tablespoonful of borax may be added to a sink filled with tepid water to a depth of about 8 cm (3 in), and this retards setting of the plaster and allows time for adequate moulding.

The posterior body section is soaked, drained, smoothed and applied. The slab is moulded carefully and secured with a few turns of a 20 cm (8 in) wide by 2.74 m (3 yd) plaster bandage.

The first anterior body section is then soaked, drained, smoothed and applied, followed by the second anterior section which is reversed so that each thigh section can be moulded carefully round the upper part of the leg.

The long leg section is then soaked, drained, smoothed and applied to the lateral aspect of the body, thigh and lower leg, so that the pelvic section stretches roughly from the opposite anterior superior iliac spine to the tuber ischii on the slab side, and the leg section extends down to the foot stirrup. The thigh and leg sections are carefully moulded and the back of the hip is reinforced with the surplus material remaining from the cut slabs.

The short thigh section is soaked, drained, smoothed and applied to the opposite pelvis and thigh. This section is finished just proximal to the knee joint so that full flexion is possible afterwards. The ankle section is completed with 10 cm (4 in) wide by 2.74 m (3 yd) plaster bandages and this may be extended to include the foot if required.

The whole spica is secured firmly with several 15 and 20 cm (6 and 8 in) wide plaster bandages and the stockinet is turned back at the upper and lower limits of the plaster in the usual manner. If the spica is required to incorporate the upper ribs, the depth of body sections must be increased accordingly.

SPINE

Spinal jacket

This is used for immobilisation of a fractured spine. The patient is placed in a position of hyperextension between two tables or standing erect. Cervical traction may be used if standing, to give extension to the spine and to overcome spasm of the erector spinae muscles. Stockinet is applied to the trunk and leg and adhesive felt pads are applied to the manubrium sternum, the symphysis pubis and over the fracture area.

Stockinet is applied followed by felt padding over the iliac crests and down either side of the spinous processes. The whole area is covered with plaster wool compressed with a light covering of plaster bandages. An anterior slab is applied (as illustrated in Fig. 31.35) followed by 15 or 20 cm (6 or 8 in) plaster bandages to complete the cast (Fig. 31.37).

Plaster cast-alternative materials

Plaster of Paris is likely to remain the dominant material used in the foreseeable future for splinting fresh fractures and for immobilisation following operative procedures. Alternatives have been tried, particularly in the field of orthopaedics where lightness, high strength to weight ratio and durability of casts are important for the active patient and the elderly. In the past, attempts have been made to achieve these requirements by using fibreglass bandages which were activated by immersion in acetone. Because of the flammable nature of the acetone and a tendency for adverse skin reactions to occur, these early developments proved unsuitable. Now manufacturers have discovered how to utilise synthetic materials which do not require solvent activation.

An example called Dynacast XR, developed by Smith and Nephew, is an orthopaedic synthetic casting bandage which combines the advantage of fibreglass reinforcement with activation by water. Dynacast XR is a combination of fibreglass substriate and polyurethane resin which stretches lengthways, widthways and on the bias. This makes application easy; it can be moulded around the joints without the need to tuck and fold, thereby eliminating the danger of ridges which can cause pressure points. The material sets quickly and provides a smooth, rigid, light weight cast that will withstand wear and tear.

Dynacast XR has a high moisture vapour permeability which helps to prevent skin maceration and other problems associated with long term casts. Bivalving and the insertion of windows in orthopaedic casts for patient comfort is easily achieved. *Dynocast is not suitable*

Figs. 31.33–31.35   Plaster jacket. (*Handbook of Plaster Techniques.*)

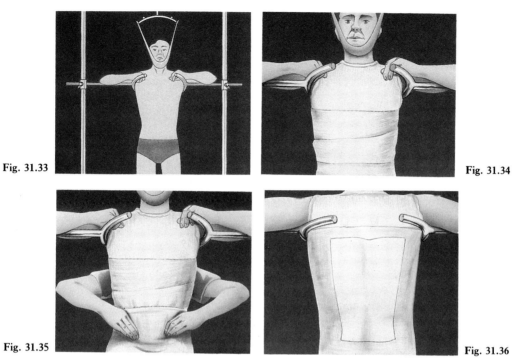

Fig. 31.33

Fig. 31.34

Fig. 31.35

Fig. 31.36

Fig. 31.33   Position of patient, standing, supported.

Fig. 31.34   Stockinette and wool padding applied around the body and orthopaedic felt to the spinous processes and iliac crests.

Fig. 31.35   The jacket is fabricated using an anterior slab held in place with circular plaster bandages.

Fig. 31.36   Wet slab applied over ventral spine.

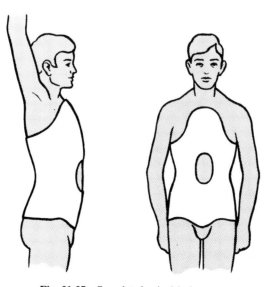

Fig. 31.37   Completed spinal jacket.

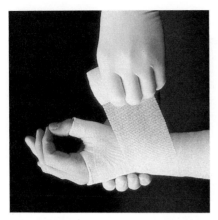

Fig. 31.38   The application of Dynacast XR bandage to forearm.

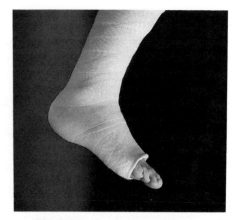

Fig. 31.39   Completed Dynacast.

for fresh fractures unless there is no danger of swelling. The following procedure is recommended by the manufacturer:

1. Apply stockinette and undercast padding.
2. Use warm water.
3. Wear gloves to prevent resin adhering to the skin.
4. Open only one bandage at a time.
5. Immerse the bandage for 2–5 seconds. Squeezing the bandage two to four times during immersion will speed up the setting time.
6. Overlap the bandage by one half of its width.
7. Moulding time is 3–5 minutes, dependent upon the immersion techniques.
8. Weight-bearing is possible in 30 minutes.

32

Radioactive materials in the theatre

There is a variety of radio-isotopes used during diagnostic and treatment procedures. Many of these are utilised in the radiodiagnostic or nuclear medicine departments and are unlikely to form part of operating department procedures. The following gives an outline of those isotopes which may be used in the operating theatre, together with basic guidelines for the protection of staff.

RADIUM

Radium is an element emitting powerful rays which are used for the destruction of malignant or other abnormal tissue.

These rays are energy liberated as a result of constant disintegration of the element, and consist of three forms: alpha, beta and gamma radiation. It is gamma rays which are utilised for therapeutic purposes, the alpha and beta rays generally being excluded by using metal screens made of platinum 0.5 to 1.0 mm thick, although beta rays are sometimes used therapeutically.

Radium is generally used in the form of radium sulphate and is virtually indestructible, for its 'half-life' is about 1,700 years.

Over-exposure to the radiation from radium or radioactive products is dangerous, and care must be taken to ensure that this does not occur, either to the patient or staff.

Radium needles and tubes

Practically all the radium used medically today is prepared as needles or tubes. The needles, made from platinum, are hollowed to contain the radium salt and have a trocar point and an eye to which thread may be attached. Radium for use in gynaecology is in tubes, having no trocar and sometimes an eye. There are varying sizes of needles and tubes containing from 0.5 to 50 mg of radium salt.

If needles are used individually, they are threaded with strong silk, tying the thread near but not on the eye, and leaving it about 15 cm (6 in) long. The silk threads may be of different colours, according to the strength of radium packed in the needle, and may help in the sorting and handling of various types, although the needles are engraved accordingly and vary in length. The knot should not be tied actually on the eye for it may break during or after insertion into the tissues.

Larger amounts of radium may be prepared by packing various sizes of needles or tubes into a silver or plastic box or tubes, making applicators which are covered with plastic or rubber before disinfection and insertion.

The needles and applicators are disinfected by pasteurization in a suitable container, care being taken to avoid tangling of the threads. These should be clipped individually with artery forceps or arranged in slots incorporated in the container.

OTHER RADIOACTIVE PRODUCTS FOR THERAPEUTIC USE

Radium is being superseded by isotopes prepared by treating elements in the atomic reactor.

Radioactive cobalt, Co 60, 'half-life' of 5.3 years, and *radioactive caesium 137*, 'half-life' 30 years, has replaced radium to some degree. The cobalt/caesium element is placed in the atomic reactor and after radioactivation is prepared as needles and tubes in a similar manner to radium. Large amounts of radioactive cobalt Co 60 or caesium 137 are also incorporated in the beam unit for teletherapy.

Radioactive tantalum wire and radioactive gold-198 seeds 'half-life' 2.7 days are often used therapeutically, the radioactive gold seeds having superseded radon. As the emanation is for a limited time, these seeds may be left buried in the tissues, but are sometimes removed owing to the value of the containers.

All these radioactive isotopes require very careful handling as the radiation may be equally lethal to that of a similar amount of radium or radon.

Methods of radium application

1. *Surface application* is made by embedding the needles or applications in a mould made from plaster of Paris, Stent composition, Acrylic, or sorbo rubber, etc. These moulds are placed in position over the area being treated for the requisite period.

2. *Teletherapy* is a form of treatment with a large amount of radioactive cobalt Co 60 or caesium 137 which is enclosed in a thick lead-walled chamber having an aperture through which the rays may be directed on to the area being treated. This is often called the radium or cobalt beam unit, but alternately deep X-rays are used, generated by machines using several million volts of electricity.

3. *Interstitial irradiation* is applied by inserting radium needles, radioactive tantalum wire or radioactive gold seeds into the tissues.

4. *Cavitary irradiation* is applied by inserting applicators into the natural cavities of the body, e.g., vagina or cervical canal.

Of the four methods of radium or radioactive isotopes application, only the last two are generally performed in the theatre. Surface application and teletherapy are performed on patients in the radiotherapy department either as inpatients or outpatients.

A technique called 'after loading' may be used with cobalt-60 or caesium 137, whereby the empty containers are positioned in the patient before the radioactive tubes are inserted within them (Mould, 1978). This reduces the radiation dose to those personnel involved in the operation.

Safety precautions during the handling of radioactive products — guidelines

1. Health District Policies based on national guidance issued by the Radiology and Nuclear Medicine Department must be observed (NATN, 1983; DHSS, 1972; DHSS, 1965)

2. Radiation Safety officers should be appointed to be responsible for implementation of these policies.

3. An official warning notice should be displayed on the door to the theatre in which radio-isotopes are present.

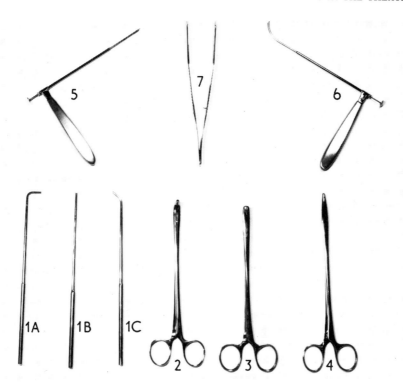

Fig. 32.1 Radium insertion instruments.
1. A, B, C, Radium needle probes.
2., 3., 4. Radium needle insertion forceps (Finzi).

5., 6. Radon seed introducers (Christie Cancer Hospital).
7. Radium needle-holding forceps (Chester Williams).

4. An official warning notice should accompany patients who are being treated with radio-isotopes and all staff should be instructed regarding the safest side of the bed or trolley by which to stand during post-operative transfer to recovery and the ward.

5. Pregnant or possibly pregnant staff should in no circumstances remain in the theatre when radio-isotope procedures are being carried out.

6. All radioactive needles, applicators, wires, seeds are manipulated with long-handled forceps, the jaws of which are covered with rubber or plastic. *On no account should they be picked up by hand.*

7. All radioactive products must be carried in a special lead-lined container during transport between radium safe and the theatre. This container should be carried by the long handle or strap provided.

8. Any preparation of needles, wires or applicators must be performed behind special lead screens, using the long manipulation forceps. All staff involved must wear lead aprons and use lead-lined tables for this preparation.

9. Proximity to radioactive products should be minimal. All persons coming into regular contact with these are issued with personal monitoring films from which the physicist can determine the radiation dose received by the person concerned. Blood tests may be made regularly to ensure that the white cell-count remains within normal limits, especially if a suspected high dose has been recorded on the monitoring film. There must be a planned rotation programme for staff dealing with radio-isotopes, to safeguard against over-exposure to radiation.

10. The theatre sister or nurse is responsible for checking the radium, etc., when it arrives at the theatre and after disinfection.

Used needles and applicators are entered on the record sheet, and unused ones checked and placed in the transport container for immediate return to the radium custodian. If it is necessary to keep radioactive materials in the theatre for any length of time, a special lead-lined safe must be provided and the key retained by the person accepting responsibility for the materials.

11. The success of the treatment is dependent upon a carefully calculated dosage. The time at which the radium treatment is due to start and terminate must be carefully noted and strictly adhered to, for the time of contact with the tissues is one factor which affects dosage.

It is usual to use special record charts for the guidance of ward staff and others responsible during the course of treatment. In theatre on this card or chart are entered all relevant details, including the number, strength and position of needles, applicators, wires or seeds. The time inserted and time due for removal is also entered on this record chart. This record is sent to the ward when the patient returns. There may also be a duplication which is returned to the radium custodian after the radioactive products have been inserted.

Radium, cobalt and other products are very valuable as well as very dangerous. Careful checking at each stage of handling is important to avoid accidental loss. Radium containers left lying about the wards or departments, or radium needles, etc., which may have slipped out of their proper place and are lying in contact with healthy tissues are in the first case a danger to the staff, and in the second case a danger to the patient.

Misplacement or loss of any radioactive element must be reported immediately either to the radiotherapist or to the physicist. Strict observance of the instructions regarding handling of the radioactive materials makes this work completely safe nowadays.

REFERENCES

DEPARTMENT OF HEALTH AND SOCIAL SECURITY (1965) *The Safe use of Ionising Radiation — A Handbook for Nurses*, Radioactive substances Advisory Committee. London: HMSO
DEPARTMENT OF HEALTH AND SOCIAL SECURITY (1972) *Codes of Practice for the Protection of Persons against Ionizing Radiation arising from Medical and Dental Use*. London: HMSO
MOULD, R. F. (1978) *Nursing Mirror*, **15**, August 31, September 23.
NATIONAL ASSOCIATION OF THEATRE NURSES (1983) Guidelines — protection of staff during radiological procedure including radio-isotopes, *Codes of Practice — Guidelines to the Total Patient Care and Safe Practice in Operating Theatres*, Harrogate; NATN

Appendix

Table I Showing the pressure/temperature relationship of phase boundary steam and the actual temperatures achieved in an sterilizer chamber with partial air discharge

lb p.s.i.	Pure steam and complete air discharge		Two-thirds air discharge 20 in vacuum		One-half air discharge 15 in vacuum		One-third air discharge 10 in vacuum	
	Degrees C	Degrees F	Degrees C	Degrees F	Degrees C	Degrees F	Degrees C	Degrees F
15	121	250	115	240	112	234	109	228
20	126	259	121	250	118	245	115	240
25	130	267	126	259	124	254	121	250
30	135	275	130	267	128	263	126	259

This chart indicates the importance of temperature, as pressure which is a mixture of air and steam has a much lower temperature than that of pure steam. Partial air discharge means a much longer sterilization period than if complete air discharge had been achieved from the chamber.

Table II Medical gas cylinder capacities and pressures

Gas	Pressure of a full cylinder (lb p.s.i.)	(kPa approx)	Capacities of cylinders in common use	
			Boyle's machine	Transportable circle circuit machines
Oxygen, O_2	1,500/2,000	10350/13800	24 cubic feet	36 or 72 gallons
Nitrous oxide, N_2O	600/700	4140/4830	200 gallons	100 or 200 gallons
Carbon dioxide, CO_2	1,000		2 pounds weight	2 pounds weight
Cyclopropane, C_3H_6	90		40 or 80 gallons	40 or 80 gallons

Table III Calibrations of rotameters on anaesthesia machines

Gas	Calibration	Maximum measurable flow per minute
Oxygen, O_2	In 100 ml divisions	2,000 ml or 2 litres
Carbon dioxide, CO_2	. . .	. . .
Nitrous oxide, N_2O	In 1,000 ml or 1 litre divisions	10 litres
Cyclopropane, C_3H_6	In 50 ml divisions	750 ml

Note: A bypass is usually incorporated adjacent to the flowmeter bank whereby an increased flow of oxygen can be obtained. This increased flow is not measurable without additional instruments, but in the case of oxygen is probably in the region of about 6 to 8 litres per minute.

Table IV Recommended sizes of twist drills to be used for various screws or bolts

Screw or bolt, outside diameter	*Drills, outside diameter*
Finger screws, 1.6 mm ($\frac{1}{16}$ in)	No. 55, 1.2 mm ($\frac{3}{64}$ in)
Wood screws, 2.8 mm ($\frac{7}{64}$ in)	2.3 mm ($\frac{3}{32}$ in)
Wood screws, 3.6 mm ($\frac{7}{64}$ in)	2.8 mm ($\frac{7}{64}$ in)
Sherman, Phillips, or cruciform screws — 3.6 mm $\frac{9}{64}$ in	No. 31 (3.0 mm)
4.0 mm ($\frac{5}{32}$ in)	3.6 mm ($\frac{9}{64}$ in), or 3.2 mm ($\frac{1}{8}$ in)
Transfixion screws, 4.4 mm ($\frac{11}{64}$ in)	3.6 mm ($\frac{9}{64}$ in), cancellous bone; 4.0 mm ($\frac{5}{32}$ in), cortical bone
Wilson bolts, 3.6 mm ($\frac{9}{64}$ in)	3.6 mm ($\frac{9}{64}$ in)
Barr bolts, 4.3 mm ($\frac{11}{64}$ in)	4.0 mm ($\frac{5}{32}$ in)
Johannson lag screws, 4.0 mm ($\frac{5}{32}$ in) (shaft diameter)	4.8 mm ($\frac{3}{16}$ in) for 3.2 mm ($\frac{1}{8}$ in) depth, followed by 4.0 mm ($\frac{5}{32}$ in) for total depth of screw
Venable hip screws, 6.4 mm ($\frac{1}{4}$ in)	No. 4 (5.3 mm)
Venable hip screws, 5.5 mm ($\frac{7}{32}$ in)	4.8 mm ($\frac{3}{16}$ in)
AO system, 4.5 mm cortex screws and 6.5 mm cancellous bone screws	3.2 mm for thread hole; 4.5 mm for gliding hole

Method of reproofing Ventile or Scotchguard in the laundry*
(Based on a 250-lb load)

After washing and rinsing the material three times, the machine is filled with cold water to a 30 cm (12 in) dip.

Add $3\frac{1}{4}$ pints of 50 per cent acetic acid previously diluted with an equal amount of cold water and rotate the machine for 3 minutes.

Add 25 lb of Mystolene M. K. 7 † previously diluted with its own weight of cold water and raise the temperature slowly to 49°C to 54.5°C, when the milky liquor should have cleared. Turn off the heat and continue running the machine for a further 2 to 3 minutes.

Run the liquor to waste and add cold water until the materials are cool enough to handle when they can be removed, hydro-extracted and finished in the usual way.

This method produces a reproofed dense fabric which possesses more advantages than most disposable products yet available. It is a method which can easily be absorbed into the normal hospital laundry service and has the advantage that larger pieces than one square yard can be used. (The average size of a disposable drape.) The latter are useful as water-repellent layers in theatre packs or perhaps as drapes for lotion bowl stands.

There is no reason why the material should not be used as ordinary drapes, and it is particularly suited to making up abdominal 'slit' sheets. Used over the incision area in conjunction with Vi-Drape or similar plastic, the water-repellent sheet is ideal, particularly where excessive soiling is likely to occur, as in Caesarean section.

Test circuit for extra low voltage equipment/lamps.

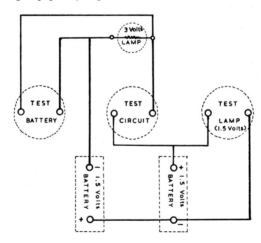

* Nursing Times, 11th December 1964
† Mystolene M. K. 7 obtainable from Catomance Ltd, 96 Bridge Road, Welwyn Garden City, Herts.

Glossary of technical terms and words commonly used in the theatre

Some of the technical terms used in the theatre often appear very complicated, and may be rather difficult to understand at first.

Definitions of some of the more common suffixes and roots may help in understanding descriptions of various operations and instruments sets.

SUFFIXES

— desis: a fusion operation, e.g., arthrodesis or fusion of a joint.
— ectomy: describes the removal or excision of a structure, e.g., gastrectomy, or excision of the stomach.
— graphy: representing, recording or describing, e.g., ventriculography.
— otomy: refers to incising or dividing a structure, e.g., laparotomy, making an opening into the abdomen; or tenotomy, dividing a tendon.
— ostomy: making an artificial opening between one organ and another, or one organ and the surface of the body, e.g., gastroenterostomy, an opening between the stomach and small intestine; gastrostomy, an opening between the stomach and the surface of the abdomen, usually for the purpose of feeding.
— orrhaphy: a repair operation, e.g., herniorrhaphy, repair of a hernia; perineorrhaphy, repair of the perineum.
— oscopy: inspection of the interior of a duct, cavity or organ by means of an endoscopic instrument. These instruments usually incorporate their own illumination in the form of a minute electric lamp (or bundle of optic fibres which transmit light to the area being examined) and often having magnifying viewing attachments, e.g., the cystoscope, for examining the bladder; the sigmoidoscope, for examining the sigmoid flexure of the colon.
— pexy: suturing or fixing in place, e.g., nephropexy, suturing a 'wandering' kidney to the posterior abdominal wall.
— plasty: is used to describe a plastic operation for the repair of tissues or organs which have been damaged by injury or disease, e.g., rhinoplasty, the rotation of a skin flap from the forehead and scalp, to cover a defect of the nose; arthroplasty, an operation on a joint to increase mobility.

ROOTS

Adeno:	gland, e.g., Adenoma
Angio:	vessel, e.g., Angiography
Arthro:	joint, e.g., Arthroplasty
Broncho:	bronchus, e.g., Bronchoscopy
Cardio:	heart, e.g., Cardiotomy
Cholecyst:	gall bladder, e.g., Cholecystectomy
Col:	colon, e.g., Colectomy
Colpo:	vagina, e.g., Colporrhaphy
Cranio:	skull, e.g., Cranioplasty
Cysto:	sac containing fluid, e.g., Cystectomy
Gastro:	stomach, e.g., Gastrectomy
Herni:	abnormal aperture, e.g., Herniorrhaphy
Hyster:	uterus, e.g., Hysterectomy
Laryn:	larynx, e.g., Laryngoscopy
Mast:	breast, e.g., Mastectomy
Nephr:	kidney, e.g., Nephrectomy
Oöphor:	ovary, e.g., Oöphorectomy
Orchid:	testis, e.g., Orchidectomy
Osteo:	bone, e.g., Osteotomy
Pharyng:	throat, e.g., Pharyngotomy
Pneum:	lung, e.g., Pneumonectomy
Prostate:	prostate, e.g., Prostatectomy
Pyel:	kidney or pelvis, e.g., Pyelolithotomy
Rhino:	nose, e.g., Rhinoplasty
Thoraco:	chest, e.g., Thoracotomy
Ureter:	ureter, e.g., Ureterolithotomy
Vulv:	vulva, e.g., Vulvectomy

Adenoidectomy: Removal of adenoid tissue from the naso-pharynx.

Adrenalectomy: Excision of an adrenal gland for tumour, treatment of hypertension or relief of pain in malignant conditions, e.g. carcinoma of breast.

Advancement: An operation to correct squint, also known as strabismus operation.

Albee's operation: *Hip* — arthrodesis effected by removing the upper surface of the femur and corresponding edge of acetabulum; *spine* — arthrodesis effected by splitting spinous processes and inserting a bone graft obtained from the tibia.

Anastomosis: The establishment of an intercommunication between two hollow organs, blood vessels or nerves.

Antisepsis: The use of a disinfectant compatible with living tissue.

Antiseptic: A chemical agent used in antisepsis.

Angiography: Serial X-ray examination of the cerebral vascular tree following injection of radio-opaque medium into a neck artery.

Antrostomy: Making an opening into the maxillary antrum to provide external drainage. The Caldwell Luc operation is an extensive form of antrostomy.

Appendectomy: Removal of the appendix.

Arteriectomy: Excision of an artery or part of an artery.

Arteriorrhaphy: Suturing an artery.

Arteriotomy: Incision of an artery.

Arthrectomy: Excision of a joint.

Arthrodesis: An operation to permanently stiffen a joint and performed to prevent movement by obliterating the joint.

Arthrography: X-ray examination of a joint, often after the injection of a radio-opaque substance.

Arthroplasty: An operation to effect increased movement of a joint. The operation usually consists of replacing the joint surface or surfaces with a metallic or plastic prosthesis.

Arthroscopy: Examination of the interior of a joint by means of an arthroscope.

Arthrotomy: Incising a joint for the purpose of examination or subsequent drainage.

Bactericide: A chemical agent which under defined conditions is capable of killing bacteria but not necessarily bacterial spores.

Bacteriostasis: A state of bacterial population in which multiplication is inhibited.

Bacteriostat: A chemical agent which under defined conditions induces bacteriostasis.

Bankhart's operation: For recurrent dislocation of the shoulder — repair of the glenoid rim defect supplemented by plication of the joint capsule and subscapularis muscle.

Bilroth's operation: A partial gastrectomy with either (1) anastomosis of the remaining section of the stomach to the duodenum or (2) closure of the lines of section followed by gastrojejunostomy.

Biopsy: Excision of small piece of tissue for examination.

Biocide: A loose term which embraces the more specific terms bactericide, fungicide, virucide, sporicide and algicide but not pesticide.

Blalock's operation: Performed usually for Fallot's tetralogy — anastomosis of the pulmonary artery (distal to a pulmonary stenosis) to a branch of the aorta.

Bronchoscopy: Examination of the interior of the bronchial tree by means of a bronchoscope. Certain operative manipulations are possible through the instrument, including removal of a foreign body or section of a growth for pathological investigation.

Caesarean section: Removal of a fetus at or near term through an abdominal incision.

Capsulectomy: Excision of a capsule — generally a joint, lens or kidney.

Capsulotomy: Incision of a capsule, e.g. that surrounding the lens of the eye.

Caudal block: *See* Epidural.

Cervicectomy: Amputation of the uterine cervix.

Cholecystectomy: Excision of the gall-bladder.

Cholecystenterostomy: Constructing an opening between the gall-bladder and the small intestine for the drainage of bile. This is performed when there is an obstruction of the common bile duct as may occur by pressure due to a growth, e.g. carcinoma of the head of pancreas.

Cholecystotomy: Making an opening into the gall-bladder, generally for the removal of gall-stones.

Choledochotomy: Making an opening into the common bile duct generally for the removal of stones.

Chordotomy: The division of nerve tracts within the spinal cord.

Circumcision: Excision of the prepuce or foreskin.

Coccygectomy: Excision of the coccyx.

Colpotomy: Incision of the vaginal wall, usually performed to drain an abscess in the pouch of Douglas through the vagina.

Colectomy: Excision of a portion or whole of the colon.

Colostomy and Caecostomy: These are terms used when making a fistula or an opening between the colon or caecum and the surface of the abdomen, to act as a temporary or permanent anus for the discharge of faeces. The most common sites for colostomy are at the level of the transverse or pelvic colon.

Colporrhaphy: A repair operation of the vaginal wall in the treatment of pelvic prolapse. Prolapse of the uterus and stretching of the anterior vaginal wall may cause the bladder and urethra to bulge into the vaginal canal, creating the condition known as cystocele. Similarly, a posterior prolapse, with stretching of the posterior vaginal wall, allows prolapse of the rectum, forming a rectocele. A cystocele is treated by the operation of anterior colporrhaphy, and a rectocele by posterior colporrhapy. Both these operations are often combined with perineorrhapy.

Commissurotomy: Splitting a stenosed valve, e.g. mitral or aortic.

Corneoplasty: Excision of opaque corneal tissue and replacement with a healthy, transparent, human donor cornea (Keratoplasty).

Craniectomy: Denotes removal of bone from skull vault, e.g. osteoplastic flap.

Cranioplasty: A plastic operation on the skull.

Craniotomy: This is a term used when opening the cavity of the skull, e.g. in the treatment of cranial injuries such as depressed fracture; for the removal of an intracranial tumour; for the drainage of an abscess.

Cryosurgery: Using the effect of freezing on tissue in surgery.

Culdoscopy: Examining the uterus by passing a culdoscope through the posterior vaginal fornex behind the uterus to enter the peritoneal cavity.

Curettage: The removal of tissue by means of a curette, or spoon, using a scraping action. The most frequent curettage is that of the interior of the uterus and the removal of overgrown lymphatic tissue in the nasopharynx (adenoids).

Cyclotomy: An incision through the ciliary body as a drainage operation for the relief of glaucoma.

Cystectomy: Excision of the urinary bladder, most commonly for a malignant tumour.

Cystodiathermy: The application of a diathermy current to the walls of the urinary bladder via a cystoscope or by open operation.

Cystoscopy: Inspection of the interior of the bladder by means of an examining cystoscope. An operating cystoscope may be used for catheterising the ureters, cauterising papillomata, and obtaining a biopsy of bladder or tumour tissue. A resectoscope is used for resecting part of the prostate via the urethra.

Cystostomy: Temporary or permanent suprapubic drainage of the bladder.

Dacryocystectomy: Excision of part of all of the lacrymal sac.

Dacryocystorhinostomy: Performed for obstruction of the nasolacrymal duct to establish drainage from the lacrymal sac to the nose.

Debridement: Thorough cleasing of a wound, removal of foreign matter, and damaged or infected tissue.

Decortication: Excision of the cortex or outer layer of an organ, e.g. visceral pleura of the lung.

Diathermy: A high-frequency electric current in the form of electromagnetic waves. These waves are concentrated at the point of the surgeon's electrode, producing great heat which is utilised to coagulate the tissues (e.g. sealing blood-vessels). When the frequency of the current is increased, the diathermy electrode may be used like a knife to divide the tissues, giving minimal coagulation.

Diathermy snare: Snare, which may be passed through the operating channel of an

endoscope, designed for the removal of polyps and larger biopsy specimens by electrosurgical techniques.

Disinfection: The reduction of contamination by micro-organisms to a level acceptable for a defined purpose.

Disinfectant: A chemical agent used for disinfection.

Disobliteration: Endarterectomy — removal of intimal plaques which are blocking an artery — rebore.

Dissect: To cut or separate tissues.

Duodenoscopy: Endoscopic examination of the duodenum; by implication, of the upper or proximal duodenum, to the exclusion of the lower or distal portion.

Ectopic gestation: The implantation and development of a fertilised ovum outside the uterus, most frequently in a Fallopian tube. Rupture of the ectopic gestation causes severe bleeding and shock, requiring urgent surgical intervention.

Embolectomy: An operation for the removal of an embolus, usually a blood-clot, from an artery.

Encephalography: X-ray examination of the ventricular system and subarachnoid spaces surrounding the brain by fractional replacement of cerebrospinal fluid with a water-soluble radio-opaque contrast medium. *See also* Ventriculography

Endarterectomy: *See* Disobliteration.

Endoscopic retrograde cholangiography (ERC): Technique for radiological visualisation of the biliary tree by retrograde injection of a water soluble radio-opaque contrast medium, following endoscopic intubation of the papilla of Vater with a suitable catheter.

Endoscopic retrograde cholangio-pancreatography (ERCP): Technique whereby ERC and ERP are performed at the same examination.

Endoscopic retrograde choledochography: *See* Endoscopic retrograde cholangiography.

Endoscopic retrograde pancreatography (ERP): Technique for radiological visualisation of the pancreatic duct system by retrograde injection of contrast medium, following endoscopic intubation of the papilla of Vater with a suitable catheter.

Endoscope: An instrument, whether flexible or rigid, for the performance of endoscopic examinations.

Endoscopy: Internal examination of cavities or hollow organs (e.g. pleural cavity, rectum, oesophagus, bladder, bronchial tree) by means of specially designed instruments, not necessarily incorporating a fibre-optic viewing bundle or utilising fibre-optic illumination.

Enteroscopy: Endoscopic examination of part or all of the small bowel; by implication of part or all of the small bowel, to the exclusion of the upper or proximal duodenum.

ERC: *See* Endoscopic retrograde cholangiography and Endoscopic retrograde choledochography.

ERCP: *See* Endoscopic retrograde cholangio-pancreatography and Endoscopic retrograde choledocho-pancreatography.

ERP: *See* Endoscopic retrograde pancreatography.

Enterostomy: The establishment of an intestinal fistula.

Enucleation: Removal of the eye is described under this heading. The term means also the removal of a tumour as a whole, compared to its removal in sections (eviscerate or gut).

Epididymectomy: Excision of the epididymis, which is a series of tubules lying behind the testis, and continuous with the vas deferens.

Epidural block: Injection of local anaesthetic, usually into the lumbar or caudal region before surgery or for prolonged analgesia.

Episiotomy: Involves the incision of the perineum during labour, to prevent excessive laceration.

Excision: Cutting away or taking out.

Fasciotomy: Incision of fascia.

Fenestration: Establishment of a fenestra or window in the horizontal semicircular canal to re-establish sound conduction to the inner ear of a patient suffering from otosclerosis.

Fibre-optic endoscope: An instrument for fibre-optic endoscopic examinations; one or more fibre-optic bundles must form an integral part of such an instrument, which may be rigid, semi-rigid or flexible.

Fibre-optic endoscopy: Internal examination of cavities or hollow organs (e.g. peritoneal cavity, gut, bladder, bronchial tree) by means of fibre-optic instruments, i.e. fibre-optic endoscopes.

Fibre-optic illumination: System employing a proximal light source, a fibre-optic light cable, and sometimes a light carrier.

Fibre-optic light cable: Fibres carrying light to a fibre-optic endoscope or to the connecting post of a rigid endoscope.

Fibre-optic light Exit: Distal end of fibre-optic illumination bundle or bundles opening onto distal tip of endoscope.

Fothergill's operation: Colpoperinorrhaphy including amputation of the cervix — i.e. repair of a cystocele and rectocele. *See also* Manchester repair.

Fulguration: Destruction of tissue by diathermy.

Fungicide: A chemical agent which under defined conditions is capable of killing fungi.

Fungistasis: A state of fungal population, the development of which is inhibited.

Fungistat: A chemical agent which under defined conditions induces fungistasis.

Gallie's operation: Radical repair of a hernia using fascia latal strips taken from the lateral aspect of the thigh.

Ganglionectomy: Excision of a ganglion.

Gastrectomy: Excision of the stomach. The most usual operation is partial gastrectomy in the surgical treatment of gastric or duodenal ulcers. Total gastrectomy, although a relatively infrequent operation, is generally reserved for malignant conditions.

Gastroenterostomy: Making an opening between the stomach and small intestine, usually the jejunum, for the purpose of short-circuiting the stomach contents, which normally pass through the pylorus into the duodenum.

Gastroscopy: Inspection of the stomach cavity via the oesophagus, or via a gastrostomy, using a gastroscope.

Gastrostomy: Making an artificial opening between the stomach and the abdominal surface for the purpose of feeding. This is generally done for the patient having an oesophageal stricture which cannot be relieved by dilation with bougies.

Gastrotomy: Opening the stomach for the purpose of exploration, or the removal of a foreign body.

Gilliam's operation: Shortening of the round ligament to correct retroversion of the uterus. *See also* Hysteropexy, Ventrosuspension.

Girdlestones operation: The original procedure is described as removal of part of the acetabulum and the femoral head and neck with a muscle mass stitched between the bone ends. Nowadays, removal of part of the femoral head and neck only is often called Girdlestones.

Glossectomy: Excision of the tongue.

Haemorrhoidectomy: The ligation and excision of internal piles.

Harris' operation: A transvesical, suprapubic prostatectomy.

Hemicolectomy: Excision of approximately half of the colon.

Hepatectomy: Excision of part of the liver.

Herniorrhaphy: The repair of an abnormal aperture in the walls of a cavity which has allowed the protrusion of a viscus. An example of this is the direct inguinal herniorrhaphy in which a sac containing viscera protruding from the abdomen through Hesselbach's triangle is obliterated.

Herniotomy: A simple operation for hernia, with return of hernia contents to their normal position and ligation of the sac.

Hymenectomy: Excision or trimming of an imperforate or rigid hymen.

Hypophysectomy: Excision of the pituitary gland.

Hysterectomy: Removal of the uterus via the abdomen or vagina. A subtotal hysterectomy means the removal of the body of the uterus, but leaving the cervix: total hysterectomy implies excision of the entire uterus: pan-hysterectomy generally means the excision of the uterus, Fallopian tubes and ovaries also: radical hysterectomy describes removal of the uterus, appendages, upper part of the vaginal and adjacent connective tissue. This latter operation is known also as Wertheim's operation.

Hysteropexy: A plastic operation on the uterus performed in the treatment of a retroverted uterus. *See also* Ventrosuspension.

Hysterotomy: Opening into the uterus usually for the removal of a fetus a good period before term.

Iridectomy: Removal of a section of the iris of the eye, thus forming an artificial pupil. This is performed as a preliminary to cataract extraction and in the relief of tension in glaucoma.

Ileocolostomy: A fistula or opening made between the ileum and colon to by-pass an obstruction or inflammation.

Ileocystoplasty: A plastic operation, utilising a section of isolated ileum to increase the urinary bladder.

Ileostomy: A fistula or opening made between the ileum and the surface of the abdomen.

Ileoureterostomy: Transplantation of the lower ends of the ureters into an artificial bladder formed from an isolated loop of ileum which is made to open on to the surface of the abdomen.

Jejunostomy: Making an opening into the jejunum.

Keller's operation: For hallux valgus or rigidus — excision of the proximal half of the proximal phalanx, also exostosis of the metatarsal head.

Keratectomy: Excision of a portion of the cornea.

Keratoplasty: *See* Corneoplasty.

Laminectomy: Cutting through the removal of the spinal laminae as a preliminary approach to the spinal cord or intervertebral discs.

Laparotomy: Opening the abdominal cavity for the purpose of inspection of, or operation upon the organs within. An emergency laparotomy is performed for many conditions which come under the heading 'acute abdomen'. When an accurate diagnosis is uncertain this may reveal acute appendicitis, perforated ulcers of the stomach or bowel, intestinal obstruction, e.g. malignant growth, strangulated hernia etc.

Laryngectomy: Excision of the larynx.

Laryngofissure: Splitting the thyroid cartilage of the larynx to expose the vocal cords.

Laryngoscopy: Inspection of the interior of the larynx, either by means of an illuminated laryngoscope (direct laryngoscopy), or by a mirror and reflected light (indirect laryngoscopy). The anaesthetist uses a laryngoscope to inspect the entrance to the larynx and to assist in the insertion of an endotracheal tube into the trachea by direct vision.

Laryngotomy: Opening the larynx to introduce a tube for the purpose of aiding respiration. This operation should more correctly be termed laryngostomy, meaning a temporary

or permanent opening into the larynx. Like tracheostomy, this operation is often performed in cases of extreme urgency when the glottis is blocked.

Leucotomy: An operation in the frontal area of the brain for division of some white nerve fibres. Performed for relief of certain mental conditions associated with extreme anxiety or emotional stress.

Light carrier: Fibres used in rigid endoscopes to transmit light from the light source to the distal tip.

Lithotomy: Incision for removal of a stone or calculus.

Lithotrity or **Litholapaxy:** The crushing and removal of a calculus or stone lying in the bladder by using a lithotrite passed per urethra.

Lobectomy: Excision of one lobe of the lung.

Lymphadenectomy: Excision of a lymph node or nodes.

Manchester repair: Colpoperinorrhaphy including amputation and reconstruction of the cervix. *See also* Fothergill's operation.

Mastectomy: Removal of the breast. This operation is performed for carcinoma of the breast and is generally combined with some form of radiotherapy. A more extensive operation called radical mastectomy involves excision of the breast, together with the underlying pectoral muscles and adjacent lymph glands.

Mastoidectomy: The removal of diseased mastoid air cells as a result of mastoiditis.

Meniscectomy: Removal of a torn semilunar cartilage, usually from the knee joint.

Micro-organism: A loose term embracing algae, fungi, bacteria, protozoa and viruses.

Myomectomy: Removal of a fibroid from the uterus.

Myringotomy: Incision of the tympanic membrane of the ear to allow drainage of the middle ear.

Nephrectomy: Removal of a kidney.

Nephropexy: A plastic operation to secure a 'wandering kidney' to the posterior abdominal wall.

Nehprostomy: Making an opening between the pelvis of the kidney and the abdominal surface for the purpose of drainage. It is usual to employ a self-retaining catheter, such as the De Pezzer type, which may be connected to a suitable receptable.

Nephrotomy: Incising the kidney, usually for the removal of a renal calculus. The operation is then called nephrolithotomy.

Neurectomy: Excision of a part of a nerve.

Neuroplasty: Surgical repair of nerves.

Neurorrhaphy: Anastomosis of the two ends of a divided nerve.

Neurotomy: Incision into a nerve.

Non-coherent bundle: A bundle of coated (clad) light transmitting fibres in which the fibres do not bear the same relationship to each other at each end of the bundle, thus making it impossible for an image to be transmitted.

Oesophagectomy: Excision of the oesophagus, generally for a malignant condition.

Oesophagoscopy: Inspection of the interior of the oesophagus by means of an illuminated oesophagoscope. Biopsy of a tumour or the removal of an impacted foreign body may also be carried out.

Oophorectomy: Excision of one or both ovaries.

Oophorosalpingectomy: Excision of an ovary and its associated Fallopian tube.

Operating channel: Channel in the endoscope through which instruments such as forceps, brushes, catheters and polypectomy snares, may be inserted into the organs or cavity under inspection.

Orchidectomy: Removal of the testis.

Osteoplasty: Any plastic operation on a bone.

Osteotomy: Division of a bone. Normally an osteotome is used for this purpose and the instrument has two bevelled edges as opposed to a chisel which has only one bevelled edge, the other being straight. The operation is generally performed to correct bone deformity, or as a part of an arthroplastic procedure.

Pallidotomy: Division of nerve fibres from the cerebral cortex to the corpus striatum to relieve Parkinson tremor.

Pancreatectomy: Radical excision of the pancreatic head: Excision of the head of pancreas, duodenum, part of the jejunum, stomach, lower half of the common bile duct and part of the pancreatic duct.

Paul-Mikulicz operation: After excising a section of the colon, the two cut ends of the bowel are kept exposed outside the peritoneal cavity on the abdominal surface. After a period these cut ends are anastomosed without the peritoneal cavity being opened.

Pericardectomy: Excision of a thickened pericardium of the heart.

Parathyroidectomy: Excision of one or more parathyroid glands.

Parotidectomy: Excision of the parotid salivary gland.

Patellectomy: Excision of the patella.

Perineorrhaphy: This is the repair carried out when the pelvic floor has become weakened, allowing the uterus to prolapse.

Pharyngolaryngectomy: Excision of the pharynx and larynx.

Pharyngotomy: Opening the pharynx as a preliminary to removing a malignant growth of the upper part of the oesophagus.

Phlebectomy: Excision of a vein or part of.

Phlebotomy: Incision into a vein.

Phrenic avulsion: In order to produce paralysis of one dome of the diaphragm and collapse of the lower part of the lung of that side, the fibres of the phrenic nerve are torn from their attachment. Another operation is crushing of the phrenic nerve to produce a temporary effect.

Pneumonectomy: Excision of one lung in the treatment of malignant conditions and tuberculosis, etc.

Pneumothorax (Artificial): Air in the pleural space. The air is introduced into the pleura via a hollow needle and using the pneumothorax apparatus.

Proctoscopy: Examination of the rectum and anal canal, using a proctoscope.

Prostatectomy: Removal of the prostate gland either suprapubically, transurethrally or by the perineal route.

Pyelography (retrograde): The injection of a water soluble radio-opaque medium into the pelvis of the kidney via the ureteric catheter. Subsequent radiological examination reveals the outline of the renal pelvis on the X-ray plate.

Pyelolithotomy: Removal of a stone from the kidney pelvis.

Pyloro-myotomy: In the treatment of congenital pyloric stenosis in infants, the muscular coat of the pyloric section of the stomach is incised down to the level of the mucosa to provide relief. This is known as Ramstedt's operation.

Pyloroplasty: A plastic operation of the pylorus to widen the orifice.

Radium or radiotherapy:

Atomic or nuclear reactor: A machine for producing radioactive isotopes, such as radioactive iodine and cobalt.

Cobalt: A radioactive isotope, which has a half-life of 5.3 years and decays eventually into nickel.

Disintegration or decay: This is a spontaneous process in which the radioactive material emits an alpha, beta or gamma ray.

Half-life: Radioactive material is made up of a large number of radioactive nuclei. As these disintegrate during the decay of the material and give off alpha, beta or gamma rays, the total number of nuclei in the material diminishes, and consequently the activity of the isotope gradually becomes weaker. The half-life is defined as 'the amount of time which is required for one half of a large number of identical nuclei (making up the isotope) to disintegrate'. For example in the case of radium which has a half-life of roughly, 1,700 years; in 1,700 years the radium will contain half as many radioactive nuclei as when it was formed, and in 3,400 years this figure will be approximately one quarter of the original number of nuclei.

Radiation: The diffusion of rays from a point (in this case gamma rays which cause biological damage of the tissues). Malignant tumours are often more susceptible to radiation than normal tissue but over-exposure to these rays may cause normal tissue to become damaged and produce diseases such as leukaemia (where the white cells of the body are over-produced).

Radium: A radioactive isotope, with a half-life of about 1,700 years.

X-ray: A penetrating electromagnetic radiation which is generated by bombarding a metal target (in the X-ray tube) with energetic electrons. X-rays and gamma rays for practical purposes may really be regarded as the same thing.

Ramstedt's operation: *See* Pyloro-myotomy.

Rectosigmoidectomy: Excision of the rectum and sigmoid colon.

Rhinoplasty: A plastic operation on the nose for reformation due to injury or cosmetic reasons.

Salpingectomy: Excision of a Fallopian tube.

Salpingo-oophorectomy: Excision of a Fallopian tube and ovary.

Shelf operation: Open reduction of congenital dislocation of hip.

Sigmoidoscopy: Inspection of the rectum or sigmoid flexure of the colon, using an illuminated endoscope passed per anum.

Skeletal traction: The insertion of a pin or wire through a bone for the purpose of traction. A Steinmann pin, Kirschner wire, and AO system are the most commonly used, and these may be inserted into the fractured bone itself, or a bone below the fracture forming part of an appendage to it. The most usual sites are the tibial tubercle for fractures of the femoral shaft and the lower tibia for fracture of the tibial shaft.

Splenectomy: Removal of the spleen. The most common condition requiring its removal is traumatic rupture, although certain diseases involving enlargement of the organ may require surgery also.

Stapedectomy: Excision of stapes for otosclerosis and insertion of Teflon piston, vein graft or plug of fat.

Stereotactic surgery: Deep ablative surgery of the white matter, basal ganglia or brain stem projection fibres by electro-coagulation or cryo-probe.

Sporicide: A chemical agent which under defined conditions is capable of killing bacterial spores.

Sterile: Free from all viable organisms.

Sterilization: A process which renders an item sterile.

Sympathectomy: Partial excision of sympathetic nerve.

Synovectomy: Excision of a joint synovial membrane often in rheumatoid conditions.

Tarrsorrhaphy: Suturing the eyelids together as a temporary measure in certain conditions, e.g. fifth cranial nerve damage.

Telescope (laparoscopy): A rigid optical system for examination of internal organs.

Tenoplasty: A plastic operation on a tendon.

Tenorrhaphy: Anastomosis of the two ends of a cut tendon.

Tenotomy: Division of a tendon.

Thoracoplasty: Removal of several ribs on one side to produce collapse of the underlying lung.

Thoracotomy: Opening the chest cavity, e.g. as a preliminary to heart surgery.

Thoracoscopy: Inspection of the pleural space, using a thoracoscope passed through a small incision in the chest wall.

Thromboendarterectomy: Removal of a thrombus from an artery followed by reboring.

Thymectomy: Excision of the thymus.

Thyroidectomy: Removal of approximately seven-eighths of each lobe of the thyroid gland leaving the parathyroid gland intact.

Tip deflection control: Control on the proximal assembly of the endoscope adjusting the amount of deflection of the distal tip. There may be a separate control of tip deflection in each plane, or a combined control of the 'joy-stick' type.

Tonsillectomy: Excision of the tonsils.

Trachelorrhaphy: Repair of a lacerated uterine cervix.

Tracheostomy: Often incorrectly termed tracheotomy, is an operation for the insertion of a tube into the trachea as an aid to respiration. Generally, the trachea is opened at the level of the thyroid isthmus, but in emergency the opening may be made through the upper rings of the trachea. This latter operation is called a 'high tracheostomy', and may be performed rapidly as the tracheal rings are close to the skin.

Trendelenburg's operation: Usually refers to ligation of internal saphenous vein in varicosed leg veins, also an operation describing pulmonary embolectomy.

Trephine operation: This term is applied to the removal of a disc of tissue. Trephining of the skull, in the true sense of the word, involves the removal of a disc of bone, although today craniotomies are usually performed by drilling a hole with suitable perforators and burrs. The resultant pulverised bone may be returned to the hole after operation.

Removal of a small disc of the sclerotic coat of the eye in the treatment of chronic glaucoma is also called trephining.

Trocar (laparoscopy): A puncturing instrument incorporating a sharp obturator or stylet designed to penetrate the peritoneum, and through which the laparoscope is passed.

Trocar valve (laparoscopy): A gas-tight valve incorporated in the trocar, to prevent loss of gas from the peritoneum.

Turbinectomy: Removal of the turbinate bones.

Ureterectomy: Excision of a ureter.

Ureterocolostomy: Transplanatation of the ureters into the colon.

Ureteroileostomy: See ileoureterostomy.

Ureterolithotomy: This describes the operation for opening the ureter to remove a calculus.

Urethrotomy: A rather uncommon operation now for incising the urethra in the treatment of strictures. Internal urethrotomy is performed with a guarded knife passed into the urethra. External urethrotomy involves opening the urethra through an incision made in the perineum.

Vagotomy: Division of the vagus nerves often in conjunction with gastro-enterostomy in the treatment of peptic ulcer or pyloroplasty.

Valvotomy: Incision of a valve generally in the heart of major blood vessels.

Vasectomy: Excision of a section of the vas deferens.

Ventriculo-atrial or **ventriculo-peritoneal shunt:** The establishment of artificial CSF drainage to heart or peritoneal cavity in cases or primary or secondary hydrocephalus (Pudenz or Spitzholter valve).

Ventriculo-cysternostomy: The establishment of artificial drainage between the ventricles and cysterna magna (Torkildsen operation).

Ventriculography: This is radiography of the cerebral ventricles accomplished by removing cerebrospinal fluid and replacing it with a small quantity of water soluble radio-opaque medium, using hollow ventricular needles. Trephine holes are made in the skull and the ventricular needles passed into the ventricles. (*See also* Encephalography.)

Ventro-suspension: A plastic operation on the uterus for shortening the round ligaments which run forward to the inguinal canal, thereby suspending the uterus in the anteverted position. This operation is known also as hysteropexy.

Vulvectomy: Excision of the vulva.

Wertheim's hysterectomy: For carcinoma of the cervix — extensive excision involving the uterus, upper vagina, Fallopian tubes, ovaries and regional lymph glands.

Index